Samaranayake's
Essential Microbiology for Dentistry

Samaranayake's Essential Microbiology for Dentistry

SIXTH EDITION

Lakshman Samaranayake

DSc(*hc*), FRCPath, DDS(*Glas*), FDSRCS (*Ed*), FDS RCPS (*Glas*), FRACDS, FHKCPath, FCDSHK

Professor Emeritus & Immediate-Past Dean of Dentistry, University of Hong Kong, Hong Kong, *King James IV Professor*, Royal College of Surgeons of Edinburgh, UK

Current/Past/ Honorary/Adjunct/Advisory Professor at: University College, London, UK; University of Queensland, Australia; Chulalongkorn University, Thailand; Thammasat University, Thailand; Walalaik University, Thailand; University of Sharjah, UAE; Jiao Tong University School of Medicine, Shanghai, China; University of Indonesia, Indonesia; University of Peradeniya, Sri Lanka; University of Sri Jayewardenepura, Sri Lanka

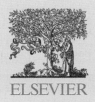

ELSEVIER

Elsevier

First edition 1996
Second edition 2002
Third edition 2006
Fourth edition 2012
Fifth edition 2018
Sixth edition 2025

Notices

ISBN: 9780443117213

Content Strategist: Alexandra Mortimer
Content Project Manager: Ayan Dhar
Design: Matthew Limbert
Marketing Manager: Deborah Watkins

Printed in India by Thomson Press (Ltd)

Last digit is the print number: 9 8 7 6 5 4 3 2 1

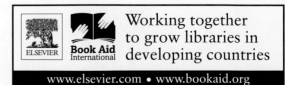

Contents

v

Contents

Welcome to the sixth edition of Smaranayake`s *Essential Microbiology for Dentistry*!

It is now 27 years since the first edition of this tome was published in 1996, and since then the science of microbiomics and infectious diseases has advanced in leaps and bounds. The epochal event that touched the lives of virtually each and every one of us, between the last edition published in 2018 and the current one, was the advent of the severe acute respiratory syndrome—coronavirus 2 (SARS-CoV-2), the agent of the pandemic of Coronavirus Disease 19 (COVID-19). This disease that has now joined forces with other endemic viral infections, such as seasonal influenza, transformed the landscape of infectious diseases and profoundly impacted the practice of dentistry. There are literally thousands of medical and dental publications on the subject, and a distillation of these, relevant to dentistry, is now included in this edition.

The other major reasons for the recent transformational changes in microbiology include the exploding new technologies, such as the so-called second-generation sequencing that has elucidated the hitherto undiscovered dark corners of the world of unculturable oral microbiota. These novel findings have led to a radical rethink on the quantity and quality of the flora that reside in our body, including in the oral cavity. In this sixth edition of this book I have attempted to incorporate the new data as much as possible while maintaining its popular concise, yet comprehensive, outlook.

The fact that you are now reading the sixth edition of this book is testimony to its popularity, with more than 50,000 copies sold on five continents, including Chinese, Polish and Korean translations as well as Middle East editions (Al-Farabi version). However, the e-print version of this book appears to be outstripping the hardbound book sales. For this I am deeply grateful to the microbiology teachers in dental schools/colleges, as well as the undergraduates and the postgraduates who are avid fans worldwide.

In compiling this completely revised sixth edition I have retained the popular features of the last few editions. Other major features of this edition, apart from COVID-19, include expanded sections on the archaeome and its role in oral disease, periodontal microbiota, infection control and novel vaccines, implant-related infections, oral systemic axis, antimicrobial stewardship and the 'one health' concept and dentistry. There is also a companion digital resource of 300 multiple-choice questions that should prove useful for review of learning.

Of course, a tome of this nature cannot be produced without the help of many friends and colleagues. I wish to gratefully acknowledge the legacy authors of several sections of the book who initially contributed to the immunology, oral microbiology and infection control sections of the book, respectively: Dr Brian Jones and Professor Liwei Lu, the University of Hong Kong; Professor Glen C Ulett, Griffith University, Australia; and Dr Caroline Pankhurst, University of London, UK. Their contributions have added immeasurable value to the book. To them, my extreme gratitude.

Once again, I am indebted to the following colleagues worldwide, who graciously permitted the reproduction of their work: Professor H Jenkinson, University of Bristol, United Kingdom (Fig. 3.9); Dr Bernard Low, Malaysia (Fig. 5.1); Professor Willie van Heerden, University of Pretoria, South Africa (Figs. 18.4 and 19.1); Dr Maribasappa Karched of Kuwait University (Fig. 31.2); Dr Leanor Haley, Centers for Disease Control and Prevention, Atlanta, United States (Fig. 22.5); Dr Annette Motte, Free University of Berlin, Germany (Fig. 31.8); and Professor Saso Ivanowski, Griffith University, Australia (Fig. 33.8). Figs. 38.1 and 38.5 are reproduced from UK Health Technical Memorandum No. 01-05, 2009, with permission from Crown Copyright.

As always, the publishing team at Elsevier led by Alexandra Mortimer, Ayan Dhar and Charu Bali from Aptara unceasingly pushed me to beat the deadlines despite my myriad duties. Their professionalism and patience have my admiration and gratitude. Last but not least, Hemamali, Dilani and Asanka have lost some quality family time due to this tome, and I am eternally grateful to them for their tolerance and understanding.

Above all, YOU, the reader, are my most important friend and critic! The many features of this edition are due to your feedback over a quarter century, and I truly hope that the current edition is the finest product thus far. Nevertheless, no book is perfect—so please keep sending your comments, either good or bad, to me at *lakshman@hku.hk* or *uqlsamar@gmail.com*.

Lakshman Samaranayake
Hong Kong
November 2023

Online Study for Students

The latest edition of Samaranayake's *Essential Microbiology for Dentistry* comes with over 300 online multiple-choice questions that aim to reinforce the student's knowledge as well as to provide exam practice for both undergraduate training and the postgraduate exams set by the UK Royal Colleges and other similar international bodies.

Reflecting and mirroring the structure of the main textbook, each online learning module presents a mini-series of multiple-choice questions covering a range of topics that vary from microbial structure and taxonomy to physiology and genetics. Different classes of microbes are sequentially explored, as well as the host immune response and the role of effective chemotherapy. Downstream modules related to the importance of systemic disease, principles of infection control and infection control procedures complete the picture. The number of questions in each module serve to reflect the importance of the topic to dentistry, either in terms of common, and direct, relevance or the potential seriousness of its impact on any individual patient.

Designed to perfectly complement the sixth edition of Samaranayake's *Essential Microbiology for Dentistry*, readers are encouraged to work through each module at their own pace to achieve an overall percentage score at the end of each exercise. This way they can see their grades at a glance across the range of topics to show instantly their areas of strength and those that require additional learning. When ready, readers can reset the program and repeat the process with the aim of reworking each module to raise their overall score.

Prepared by Professor Lakshman Samaranayake, the questions are designed to provide review and exam practice in a relaxed, unpressured environment with the overall aim of improving real exam grades.

To access this helpful online self-assessment tool, please log in to eBooks+.

1 *Why Study Microbiology?*

Microbiology (Greek: *mīkros* small; *bios* life), so called because it primarily deals with organisms too small for the naked eye to see, encompasses the study of organisms that cause disease, the host response to infection and ways in which such infection may be prevented. For our purposes, the subject can be broadly classified into **general**, **medical** and **oral microbiology**.

Dental students need both a basic understanding of general and medical microbiology and a detailed knowledge of clinical oral microbiology in order to diagnose oral microbial infections, which are intimately related to the overall treatment plan for their patients. Moreover, the two major oral disorders—**caries** and **periodontal disease**—that the dental practitioner is frequently called upon to treat are due to changes in the oral bacterial ecosystem including the constituent oral microbiome. A grasp of these disease processes and their sequelae is essential for their appropriate management.

The impact of these infections on the health and welfare of the community is simply astonishing. For instance, periodontal disease has gained the dubious distinction of being the most prevalent disease affecting humankind, as approximately 10% of the human population is considered to be affected by severe periodontitis. Similarly, caries in permanent teeth is considered the most common disease in humans globally with over 2.5 billion people affected, and the disease is ranked first among 328 diseases. It is not surprising, therefore, that caries and periodontal disease are the most costly and chronic diseases that the majority of the population has to contend with during their lifetime. In economic terms, the number of working hours lost due to these infections and the related cost of dental treatment worldwide amount to billions of dollars per annum (e.g., the global economic impact of dental diseases has been estimated to be US $442 billion in 2010). Some fast facts on oral infections and their impact on society are given in Box 1.1.

Another major reason why a good comprehension of microbial infections and their epidemiology is essential for the dental profession is the chronic recurrence of various emerging infections that has revolutionized the **infection control regimens of dentistry** over the last few decades. A stark example is the coronavirus disease 2019 (COVID-19) pandemic due to severe acute respiratory syndrome coronavirus 2 (SARS-CoV-2). The global endemicity of this disease led to the review of infection control regimentation of dentistry with new modified guidelines. Such epidemics that impacted dentistry in the recent past include the hepatitis B

Box 1.1　A Few Fast Facts on Oral Infections and Their Impact on Society

- Oral health is essential to general health and well-being.
- Oral infections may lead to problems with eating, speaking and learning as well as social interaction and employment potential.
- The three oral infectious diseases that most affect overall health and quality of life are caries, severe periodontal disease and associated severe tooth loss.
- In general, by age 8, more than half of children (52%) have had caries in their primary dentition.
- Children from low-income families are twice as likely to have caries as those from higher-income families.
- One in four adults in the United States aged 20–64 years currently has cavities.
- Drinking fluoridated water and getting dental sealants (in childhood) prevent caries and save money by avoiding expensive dental care.
- Tobacco use and diabetes are two major risk factors for periodontal diseases.
- Medical–dental integration between oral health and chronic noncommunicable disease (NCD) prevention programs benefits patients and saves money.

---

epidemic in the 1970s and the advent of the human immunodeficiency virus (HIV) infection in the early 1980s. Additionally, many patients are acutely concerned about possible infection transmission in clinical settings because of the intense, and sometimes unwarranted, publicity given to these matters by the media. The dental practitioner should therefore be conversant with all aspects of infection control in the clinical environment, not only to implement infection control measures but also to advise the dental team (dental surgery assistants, dental hygienists and other ancillary personnel) and to allay patients' unfounded fears. For all these and many other reasons, which the student will discover in this text, the discipline of microbiology is intimately woven into the fabric of dentistry and composes a crucial component of the dental curriculum.

Finally, the advent of COVID-19 is a wakeup call for the dental profession regarding the importance of being eternally vigilant about new microbial diseases that emerge incessantly. The text you are now reading is a primer for understanding and managing such future eventualities, especially in the context of infection control.

A Note on Emerging and Re-emerging Infections

Infectious agents have been adversaries of humans for millennia. Diseases such as plague wiped out civilizations in ancient times, whereas humans have won the battle against microbes in more recent times (e.g., eradication of smallpox). New diseases are given the terms **emerging infections** or **re-emerging infections** (Fig. 1.1), and they are broadly categorized as follows:

- **New infections:** caused by agents such as new influenza virus strains emerging periodically to cause epidemics, as well as the mosquito-borne Zika virus infection.
- **'Old' infections:** known disease entities whose aetiological agents have been recently identified through advances in technology (e.g., *Helicobacter pylori* causing gastric ulcer disease).
- **Re-emerging infections:** diseases that have returned with a vengeance due to genetic and structural transformations and attendant increased virulence of the organism (e.g., drug-resistant *Mycobacterium tuberculosis* with its 'new bag of tricks').

The reasons for their emergence are manifold and include the following:

- **Societal events:** economic impoverishment (especially in the developing world), war and civil conflicts, as well as mass population migration

- **Health care:** new medical devices, organ/tissue transplantation, immunosuppression, antibiotic abuse and contaminated blood and blood products
- **Human behaviour:** increasing number of sexual partners, injectable drug abuse
- **Environmental changes:** deforestation, drought, floods and global warming
- **Microbial adaptation:** emergence of new species from the wild (e.g., HIV), changes in virulence and toxin production and development of drug resistance.

About This Book

This text is divided into six parts in order to highlight the different features of microbiology related to dentistry, but it should be noted that such division is artificial and is merely an attempt to simplify the learning process.

The first few chapters in **Part 1** essentially describe general microbiological features of bacteria and viruses and how they cause human infections (i.e., **pathogenesis**). **Diagnostic microbiology**, by which clinical microbiologists ascertain the nature of agents causing various infections, is described in Chapter 6. The laboratory aspect of this fascinating subject is analogous to the work of a crime detection bureau! When a specimen (e.g., pus, urine) from a patient with an infectious disease is sent to the laboratory for identification of the offending agent, the clinical

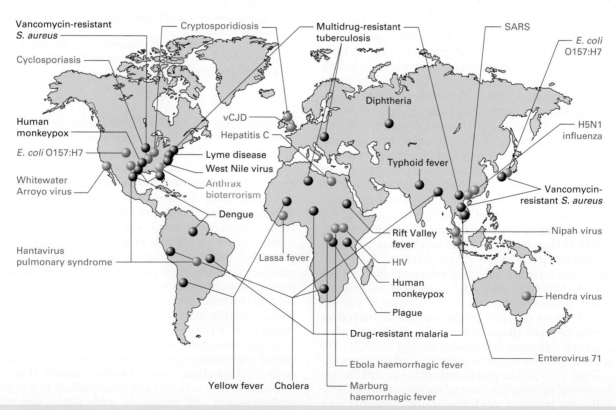

Fig. 1.1   Global prevalence of some emerging and re-emerging diseases. *E. coli, Escherichia coli*; HIV, human immunodeficiency virus; SARS, severe acute respiratory syndrome; *S. aureus, Staphylococcus aureus*; vCJD, variant Creutzfeldt–Jakob disease.

microbiologist utilizes many methods and techniques, as well as a fair amount of thought and contemplation, to identify the pathogen(s) lurking in the clinical sample. In many situations the pathogen may be dead, in which case other, indirect clues via molecular techniques need to be pursued to incriminate the suspect pathogen. Once an offending pathogen is identified, antimicrobial chemotherapy is the mainstay of treatment; a description of chemotherapeutic agents and how they are chosen in the laboratory is given in Chapter 7.

The host responds to infection by mounting an immune response. A highly abbreviated account of **basic immunology** is given in **Part 2**; supplemental reading is essential to augment this material, and the reader is referred to recommended texts for this purpose. Immunological nomenclature is complex and often difficult: a glossary of terms and abbreviations is therefore provided as an appendix.

Although there are thousands of offending pathogens, only some are of direct relevance to dental practice and to the comprehension of the **mechanisms of disease**; these are described in **Part 3**. Arguably this section may appear to be the most daunting part of the book because of the complex nomenclature of microbes; hence only the salient bacterial genera—some of which are more closely related to dental practice (e.g., streptococci) than others (e.g., legionellae)—are outlined. Similarly, the chapters on viruses and fungi are relatively brief, with thumbnail sketches of only the most relevant organisms.

The major **infections of each organ system** are discussed in **Part 4**, with emphasis on those that are most relevant to dentistry. The student is strongly advised to cross-refer to organisms and their characteristics (described in Part 3) when studying this section, as the microbial attributes and the diseases they cause form a single continuum.

Part 5 specifically outlines the **microbial interactions in the craniofacial region**, in both health and disease. This section should be particularly useful for the later years of the dental curriculum, to reinforce the studies in conservative dentistry, periodontics, oral and maxillofacial surgery and oral medicine.

Last but not least, the subject of **cross-infection and its control** in dentistry is encapsulated in **Part 6**, which provides a comprehensive summary of the routine infection control regimens that must be implemented in every dental practice. This new sixth edition also provides the basics of infection control in readily assimilable boxes and describes in detail the transmission-based infection controls that

were the norm during the COVID-19 pandemic period in all dental surgeries. Fortunately, the pandemic requirements for such stringent infection control practices are abating in many regions of the world; however, the reader must be proficient and aware of these additional recommendations in the unfortunate event of a new or recrudescent highly transmissible infection emerging in the future as predicted by a number of authorities. Hence, the relevance of this information in routine dental practice cannot be overemphasized, and a thorough understanding of this material should pay rich dividends in years to come.

As the student will discover, the comprehensive nature of this text has made almost all the materials significant. Thus the reader will be intellectually challenged to learn a new concept or terminology in almost every sentence or phrase. In addition, an attempt has been made to summarize the information as key facts to serve as an *aide-mémoire* at the end of each chapter. It is important, however, that the subject matter is augmented with additional reading, and it is to this end that the list of further readings is given. The self-assessment review questions at the end of each chapter, which may not cover all aspects of the preceding narrative, should help the student to assess knowledge assimilation in key areas.

Finally, in most chapters the text is arranged under the following important features of microbiology, which the student must understand in order to deal with infectious diseases:

- **Epidemiology**: spread, distribution and prevalence of infection in the community
- **Pathogenesis**: the means by which microbes cause disease in humans, an understanding of which is critical for the successful diagnosis and management of infections
- **Diagnosis**: detection of an infection; dependent on the collection of the correct specimen in the most appropriate manner along with subsequent interpretation of laboratory results
- **Treatment**: antibacterial, antifungal or antiviral therapy combined with supportive therapy leading to resolution of most infections
- **Prevention** (prophylaxis): immunization is the most useful mode of preventing diseases such as tetanus and hepatitis B; however, increasing public awareness of diseases and their modes of spread significantly helps to curb the spread of infections in the community (e.g., HIV infection).

Further Reading

Beikler, T., & Flemming, T. F. (2011). Oral biofilm-associated diseases: Trends and implications for quality of life, systemic health and expenditures. *Periodontology, 2000* (55), 87–103.

Bonita, R., Beaglehole, R., & Kjellström, T. (2006). Communicable diseases: Epidemiology surveillance and response. In *Basic epidemiology* (2nd ed., pp. 117–132). World Health Organization.

Jamal, M., Shah, M., Almarzooqi, S. H., et al. (2021). Overview of transnational recommendations for COVID-19 transmission control in dental care settings. *Oral Diseases, 27,* 655–664.

Kassebaum, N. J., Bernabé, E., Dahiya, M., Bhandari, B., Murray, C. J., & Marcenes, W. (2015). Global burden of untreated caries: A systematic review and metaregression. *Journal of Dental Research, 94*(5), 650–658. doi:10.1177/0022034515573272.

Listl, S., Galloway, J., Mossey, P. A., & Marcenes, W. (2015). Global economic impact of dental diseases. *Journal of Dental Research, 94*(10), 1355–1361. doi:10.1177/0022034515602879.

Morse, S. S. (1995). Factors in the emergence of infectious diseases. *Emerging Infectious Diseases, 1,* 7–15.

Qin, X., Zi, H., & Zeng, X. (2022). Changes in the global burden of untreated dental caries from 1990–2019: A systematic analysis for the Global Burden of Disease study. *Heliyon, 8*(9), e10714. doi:10.1016/j.heliyon.2022.e10714.

Samaranayake, L., & Fakhruddin, K. S. (2021). Pandemics past, present, and future: Their impact on oral health care. *Journal of the American Dental Association, 152,* 972–980. doi:10.1016/j.adaj.2021.09.008.

PART 1

GENERAL MICROBIOLOGY

The aim of this section is to present the structural features of microbes and how they cause disease, and a perspective of diagnostic laboratory methods to explain the relationship between the scientific basis of microbiology and its practical application in patient care. Finally, a comprehensive overview of antimicrobial chemotherapy in dentistry is provided, which should be supplemented with additional reading due to its critical relevance to dental care.

- Bacterial structure and taxonomy
- Bacterial physiology and genetics
- Viruses and prions
- Pathogenesis of microbial disease
- Diagnostic microbiology and laboratory methods
- Antimicrobial chemotherapy

2 Bacterial Structure and Taxonomy

Classification of all living beings including microbes has been attempted by many over centuries (Table 2.1). Traditionally, though all were classified into two kingdoms—plants and animals—the classification was arbitrary and based on morphological and growth characteristics. With the development of novel techniques, the latter classification was expanded to include five kingdoms: Monera, Protista, Plantae, Fungi and Animalia. However, the current understanding based on their genetic relatedness is that all forms of life fall into three domains: **archaea**, **bacteria** and **eucarya**. The main differences among archaea, bacteria and eucarya are listed in Table 2.2. Note that archaea and bacteria, taken together, are also known as **prokaryotes** (see later text).

Viruses are not included in this classification as they are unique, acellular, metabolically inert organisms and therefore replicate only within living cells. Other differences between viruses and cellular organisms include the following:

- **Structure**. Cells possess a nucleus or, in the case of bacteria, a nucleoid with DNA. This is surrounded by the cytoplasm where energy is generated and proteins are synthesized. In viruses, the inner core of genetic material is either DNA or RNA, but viruses have no cytoplasm and hence depend on the host for their energy and proteins (i.e., they are metabolically inert).
- **Reproduction**. Bacteria reproduce by **binary fission** (a parent cell divides into two similar cells), but viruses disassemble, produce copies of their nucleic acid and proteins, and then reassemble to produce another generation of viruses. As viruses are **metabolically inert**, they must replicate within host cells. Bacteria, however, can replicate extracellularly (except rickettsiae and chlamydiae, which are bacteria that also require living cells for growth).

Eukaryotes and Prokaryotes

As mentioned, another modification of classifying cellular organisms is to divide them into **prokaryotes (i.e., archaea and bacteria)** and **eukaryotes** (Greek *karyon*: nucleus). Fungi, protozoa and humans, for instance, are eukaryotic, whereas bacteria are prokaryotic. In prokaryotes, the bacterial **genome**, or chromosome, is a single, circular molecule of double-stranded DNA, lacking a nuclear membrane (smaller, single or multiple circular DNA molecules called plasmids may also be present in bacteria), whereas the eukaryotic cell has a true nucleus with multiple chromosomes surrounded by a nuclear membrane.

Bacteria comprise the vast majority of human pathogens, whereas archaea appear rarely to cause human disease and live in extreme environments (e.g., high temperature or salt concentrations). Archaea received little attention traditionally as they cannot be easily cultured in the laboratory. Interestingly, recent studies using novel techniques such as **pyrosequencing** have uncovered their presence in the oral cavity. Some studies have even shown that certain species of archaea are more frequently found in subgingival plaque in periodontal disease.

Morphology

SHAPE AND SIZE

The shape of a bacterium is determined by its rigid cell wall. Bacteria are classified by shape into three basic groups (Fig. 2.1):

1. cocci (spherical)
2. bacilli (rod shaped)
3. spirochaetes (helical).

Some bacteria with variable shapes, appearing as both coccal and bacillary forms, are called **pleomorphic** (*pleo*: many; *morphic*: shaped) in appearance.

The size of bacteria ranges from about 0.2 μm to 5 μm. The smallest bacteria approximate the size of the largest viruses (poxviruses), whereas the longest bacilli attain the same length as some yeasts and human red blood cells (7 μm).

Table 2.1   Differential Characteristics of Major Groups of Organisms

	Bacteria	Mycoplasmas	Rickettsiae	Chlamydiae	Viruses[a]	Fungi
Visible with light microscope	+	+	+	+	−	+
Capable of free growth	+	+	−	−	−	+
Both DNA and RNA present	+	+	+	+	−	+
Muramic acid in cell wall	+	+	+	+	−	+
Rigid cell wall	+	−	+	Variable	−	+
Susceptible to penicillin	Variable	−	−	−	−	−
Susceptible to tetracycline	Variable	+	+	+	−	−
Reproduce essentially by binary fission	+	+	+	+	−	−

[a]Prions (agents responsible for Creutzfeldt–Jakob disease) are not included as their status is unclear.

Table 2.2   Major Differences Among the Three Domains of Life

Bacteria	Archaea	Eucarya
Organization of the Genetic Material and Replication		
DNA free in the cytoplasm	DNA free in the cytoplasm	DNA is contained with a membrane-bound nucleus. A nucleolus is also present
Only one chromosome	Only one chromosome	More than one chromosome. Two copies of each chromosome may be present (diploid)
DNA associated with histone-like proteins	DNA associated with histone-like proteins	DNA complexed with histone proteins
May contain extrachromosomal elements called plasmids	Plasmids may be found	Plasmids only found in yeast
Introns not found in mRNA	Introns not found in most genes	Introns found in all genes
Cell division by binary fission: asexual replication only	Reproduce asexually and spores are not found	Cells divide by mitosis
Transfer of genetic information occurs by conjugation, transduction and transformation (see Chapter 3)	Processes similar to bacterial conjugation enable exchange of genetic material	Exchange of genetic information occurs during sexual reproduction. Meiosis leads to the production of haploid cells (gametes), which can fuse
Cellular Organization		
Cytoplasmic membrane contains hopanoids	Membranes contain isoprenes	Cytoplasmic membrane contains sterols
Lipopolysaccharides and teichoic acids found	No lipopolysaccharides or teichoic acids found	
Energy metabolism associated with the cytoplasmic membrane		Mitochondria present in most cases
Photosynthesis associated with membrane systems and vesicles in cytoplasm		Chloroplasts present in algal and plant cells
		Internal membranes, endoplasmic reticulum and Golgi apparatus present and associated with protein synthesis and targeting
		Membrane vesicles such as lysosomes and peroxisomes present
		Cytoskeleton of microtubules present
Flagella consist of one protein, flagellin	Contains flagella that derive energy from proton pumps	Flagella have a complex structure with 9 + 2 microtubular arrangement
Ribosomes: 70S	Ribosomes behave more like Eucarya when exposed to inhibitors	Ribosomes: 80S (mitochondrial and chloroplast ribosomes are 70S)
Peptidoglycan cell walls	Cell walls lack peptidoglycan	Polysaccharide cell walls, where present, are generally either cellulose or chitin

ARRANGEMENT

Bacteria, whichever shape they may be, arrange themselves (usually according to the plane of successive cell division) as pairs (diplococci), chains (streptococci), grape-like clusters (staphylococci) or as angled pairs or palisades (corynebacteria).

GRAM-STAINING CHARACTERISTICS

In clinical microbiology, bacteria can be classified into two major subgroups according to the staining characteristics of their cell walls. The stain used, called the **Gram stain** (first developed by a Danish physician, Christian Gram), divides the bacteria into **Gram-positive** (purple) and

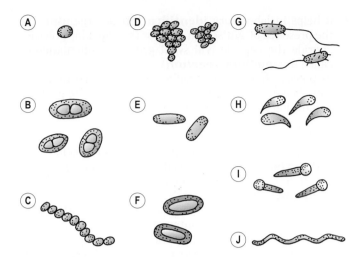

Fig. 2.1   Common bacterial forms. (A) Coccus; (B) capsulated diplococci; (C, D) cocci in chains (e.g., streptococcus) and clusters (e.g., staphylococcus); (E) bacillus; (F, G) capsulated and flagellated bacillus (e.g., *Escherichia coli*); (H) curved bacilli (e.g., *Vibrio* spp.); (I) spore-bearing bacilli (e.g., *Clostridium tetani*); (J) spirochaete.

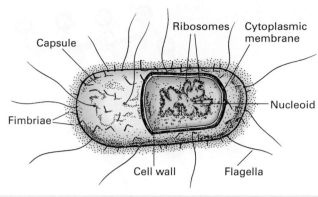

Fig. 2.2   A bacterial cell.

Gram-negative (pink) groups. The Gram-staining property of bacteria is useful both for their identification and in the therapy of bacterial infections because, in general, Gram-positive bacteria are more susceptible to penicillins than Gram-negative bacteria.

STRUCTURE

The structure of a typical bacterium is shown in Fig. 2.2. Bacteria have a rigid cell wall protecting a fluid **protoplast** comprising a **cytoplasmic membrane** and a variety of other components (described later).

Structures External to the Cell Wall

Flagella. Flagella are whip-like filaments that act as propellers and guide bacteria towards nutritional and other sources (Fig. 2.3). The filaments are composed of many subunits of a single protein, **flagellin**. Flagella may be located at one end (**monotrichous,** a single flagellum; **lophotrichous,** many flagella) or all over the outer surface (**peritrichous**). Many bacilli (rods) have flagella, but most cocci do not and are therefore nonmotile. Spirochaetes move by using a flagellum-like structure called the **axial filament**, which wraps around the cell to produce an undulating motion.

Fimbriae and Pili. Fimbriae and pili are fine, hair-like filaments, **shorter than flagella,** that extend from the cell surface. Pili, found mainly on Gram-negative organisms, are composed of subunits of a protein, **pilin**, and mediate the adhesion of bacteria to receptors on the human cell surface, a necessary first step in the initiation of infection. A specialized type of pilus, the **sex pilus**, forms the attachment between the male (donor) and the female (recipient) bacteria during conjugation, when genes are transferred from one bacterium to another.

Glycocalyx (Slime Layer). The glycocalyx is a **polysaccharide coating** that covers the outer surfaces of

many bacteria and allows the bacteria to adhere firmly to various structures—for example, oral mucosa, teeth, heart valves and catheters—and contributes to the formation of **biofilms**. This is especially true in the case of *mutans* streptococci, a major group of cariogenic organisms, which have the ability to produce vast quantities of extracellular polysaccharide in the presence of dietary sugars such as sucrose.

Capsule. An amorphous, gelatinous layer (usually more substantial than the glycocalyx) surrounds the entire bacterium; it is composed of **polysaccharide** and, sometimes, protein (e.g., anthrax bacillus). The sugar components of the polysaccharide vary in different bacterial species and frequently determine the **serological type** within a species (e.g., 84 different serological types of *Streptococcus pneumoniae* can be distinguished by the antigenic differences among the sugars in the polysaccharide capsule). The capsule is important because:

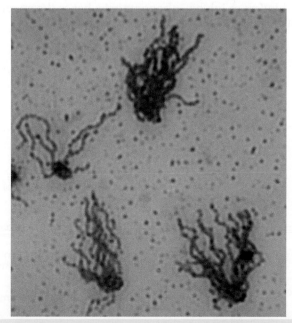

Fig. 2.3 Photomicrograph of a bacterium showing peritrichous flagella. Note the relative length of the flagella compared with the size of the organism.

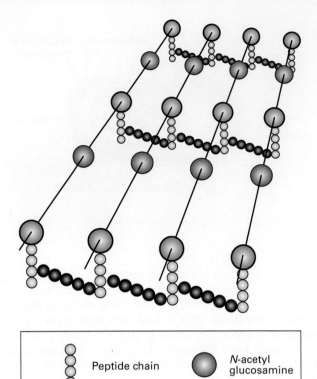

Fig. 2.4 Chemical structure of cross-linking peptidoglycan component of cell wall, common to both Gram-positive and Gram-negative bacteria. (After Sharon, N. (1969). The bacterial cell wall. *Scientific American, 220*, 92.)

- it mediates the **adhesion** of bacteria to human tissues or prosthesis such as dentures or implants, a prerequisite for colonization and infection
- it hinders or inhibits **phagocytosis**; hence the presence of a capsule correlates with virulence

- it helps in laboratory **identification** of organisms (in the presence of antiserum against the capsular polysaccharide the capsule will swell greatly, a phenomenon called the **quellung reaction**)
- its polysaccharides are used as antigens in certain vaccines because they elicit protective antibodies (e.g., polysaccharide vaccine of *S. pneumoniae*).

Cell Wall

The cell wall confers rigidity upon the bacterial cell. It is a **multilayered structure** outside the cytoplasmic membrane. It is porous and permeable to substances of low molecular weight.

The inner layer of the cell wall is made of **peptidoglycan** and is covered by an outer membrane that varies in thickness and chemical composition, depending upon the Gram-staining property of the bacteria (Fig. 2.4). The term 'peptidoglycan' is derived from the peptides and the sugars (glycan) that make up the molecule. (Synonyms for peptidoglycan are **murein** and **mucopeptide**.)

The cell walls of Gram-positive and Gram-negative bacteria have important structural and chemical differences (Fig. 2.5):

- The **peptidoglycan** layer is **common to both Gram-positive and Gram-negative bacteria** but is much thicker in the Gram-positive bacteria.
- By contrast, the Gram-negative organisms have a complex outer membrane composed of **lipopolysaccharide (LPS), lipoprotein and phospholipid**. These form **porins**, through which hydrophilic molecules are transported in and out of the organism. The O antigen of the LPS and the lipid A component are also embedded in the outer membrane. Lying between the outer membrane and the cytoplasmic membrane of Gram-negative bacteria is the **periplasmic space**. It is in this space that some bacterial species produce enzymes that destroy drugs such as penicillins (e.g., β-lactamases). A notable feature is that **LPS is exclusively found in Gram-negative bacteria.**

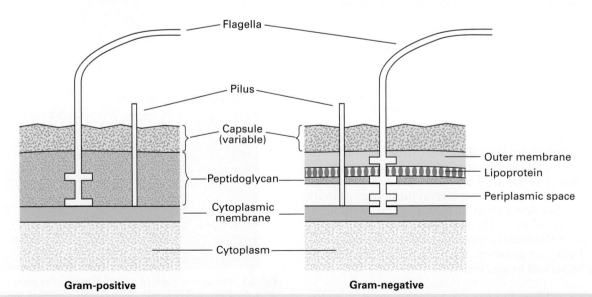

Fig. 2.5 Structural features of Gram-positive and Gram-negative cell walls. (Note the short pilus relative to the much longer flagellum).

- The LPS of Gram-negative bacteria, which is extremely toxic, has been called the **endotoxin**. (Hence, by definition, endotoxins cannot be produced by Gram-positive bacteria, as they do not have LPS in their cell walls.) LPS is bound to the cell surface and is only released when it is lysed. It is responsible for many of the features of disease, such as fever and shock (see Chapter 5).
- The cell walls of some bacteria (e.g., *Mycobacterium tuberculosis*) contain lipids called **mycolic acids**, which cannot be Gram stained, and hence are called **acid-fast organisms** (i.e., they resist decolourization with acid alcohol after being stained with carbolfuchsin).

Bacteria With Defective Cell Walls. Some bacteria can survive with defective cell walls. These include mycoplasmas, L-forms, spheroplasts and protoplasts.

Mycoplasmas do not possess a cell wall and do not need hypertonic media for their survival. They occur in nature and may cause human disease (e.g., pneumonia).

L-forms are usually produced in the laboratory and may totally or partially lack cell walls. They may be produced in patients treated with penicillin and, like mycoplasmas, can replicate on ordinary media.

Both **spheroplasts** (derived from Gram-negative bacteria) and **protoplasts** (derived from Gram-positive bacteria) lack cell walls, cannot replicate on laboratory media and are unstable and osmotically fragile. They require hypertonic conditions for maintenance and are produced in the laboratory by the action of enzymes or antibiotics.

Cytoplasmic Membrane

The cytoplasmic membrane lies just inside the peptidoglycan layer of the cell wall and is **a unit membrane** composed of a **phospholipid bilayer** similar in appearance to that of eukaryotic cells. However, eukaryotic membranes contain sterols, whereas prokaryotes generally do not (the only exception being mycoplasmas). The membrane has the following major functions:

- active transport and selective diffusion of molecules and solutes in and out of the cell
- electron transport and oxidative phosphorylation, in aerobic species
- synthesis of cell wall precursors
- secretion of enzymes and toxins
- supporting the receptors and other proteins of the chemotactic and sensory transduction systems.

Mesosome. This is a convoluted invagination of the cytoplasmic membrane that functions as the origin of the transverse septum that divides the cell in half during cell division. It is also the binding site of the DNA that will become the genetic material of each daughter cell.

Cytoplasm

The cytoplasm comprises an inner, nucleoid region (composed of DNA), which is surrounded by an amorphous matrix that contains ribosomes, nutrient granules, metabolites and various ions.

Nuclear Material or Nucleoid. Bacterial DNA comprises a **single, supercoiled, circular chromosome** that contains about 2000 genes, approximately 1 mm long in the unfolded state. (It is analogous to a single, haploid chromosome.) During cell division, it undergoes semiconservative replication bidirectionally from a fixed point.

Ribosomes. Ribosomes are the sites of **protein synthesis**. Bacterial ribosomes differ from those of eukaryotic cells in both size and chemical composition. They are organized in units of 70S, compared with eukaryotic ribosomes of 80S. These differences are the basis of the selective action of some antibiotics that inhibit bacterial, but not human, protein β-synthesis.

Cytoplasmic Inclusions. The cytoplasm contains different types of inclusions, which serve as sources of stored energy; examples include polymetaphosphate, polysaccharide and β-hydroxybutyrate.

BACTERIAL SPORES

Spores are formed in response to adverse conditions by the medically important bacteria that belong to the genus *Bacillus* (which includes the agent of anthrax) and the genus *Clostridium* (which includes the agents of tetanus and botulism). These bacteria **sporulate** (form spores) when nutrients, such as sources of carbon and nitrogen, are scarce (Fig. 2.6). The spore develops at the expense of the vegetative cell and contains bacterial DNA, a small amount of cytoplasm, cell membrane, peptidoglycan, very little water and, most importantly, a **thick, keratin-like coat**. This coat, which contains a high concentration of calcium dipicolinate, is remarkably resistant to heat, dehydration, radiation and chemicals. Once formed, the spore is metabolically inert and can remain dormant for many years. Spores are called either **terminal** or **subterminal**, depending on their position in relation to the cell wall of the bacillus from which they developed.

When appropriate conditions supervene (i.e., water, nutrients), there is enzymatic degradation of the coat, and the spore transforms itself into a metabolizing, reproducing bacterial cell once again (Fig. 2.6).

Clinical Significance of Bacterial Spores

The clinical importance of spores lies in their extraordinary resistance to heat and chemicals. Hence they can survive in a dormant state for many years in adverse habitats, such as soil, and cause infections once they are implanted into an unsuspecting host through, say, a penetrative injury. Trauma from road traffic accidents and even an innocuous garden fork injury may lead to such infections when sporulation ensues with exotoxin production (e.g., tetanus caused by *Clostridium tetani*; Chapter 13).

The extraordinary ability of bacterial spores to withstand high temperatures is also exploited for evaluating the **sterilization efficacy of autoclaves**. In this case, the spores of *Bacillus stearothermophilus* and related species are used as *biological monitors* to check the efficacy of the autoclaving process (Chapter 38).

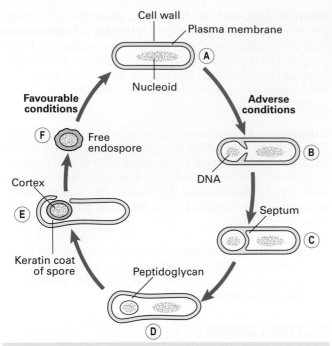

Fig. 2.6 The cycle of sporulation. (A) Vegetative cell; (B) ingrowth of cytoplasmic membrane; (C) developing forespore; (D) forespore completely cut off from the cell cytoplasm; (E) development of cortex and keratin spore coat; (F) liberation of spore and conversion to vegetative state under favourable conditions.

Taxonomy

The systematic classification and categorization of organisms into ordered groups are called **taxonomy**. A working knowledge of taxonomy is useful for **diagnostic microbiology** and for studies in epidemiology and pathogenicity.

As mentioned at the beginning of this chapter, organisms encountered in medical microbiology fall into the domains of bacteria, archaea and eucarya. Although this system of classification is based on the evolutionary relatedness or the genetic homogeneity of the species represented in each domain, a more pragmatic means of classification is employed in the clinical microbiology laboratory. Such bacterial classification is somewhat artificial in that they are categorized according to **phenotypic** (as opposed to **genotypic**) features, which facilitate their laboratory identification. These comprise:

- **morphology** (cocci, bacilli, spirochaetes)
- **staining properties** (Gram-positive, Gram-negative)
- **cultural requirements** (aerobic, facultative anaerobic, anaerobic)
- **biochemical reactions** (saccharolytic and asaccharolytic, according to sugar fermentation reactions)
- antigenic structure (serotypes).

Most of the medically and dentally important bacteria are classified according to their morphology, Gram-staining characteristics and atmospheric requirements. A simple classification of medically important bacteria is given in Figs. 2.7 and 2.8.

GENOTYPIC TAXONOMY

In contrast to the classical phenotypic classification methods previously outlined, **genotypic** classification and speciation of organisms are becoming increasingly important and useful. Genotypic taxonomy exploits the genetic characteristics, which are more stable than the sometimes transient phenotypic features of organisms. These methods essentially evaluate the degree of **DNA homology of organisms** in order to **speciate** them—for example, by assessing molecular guanine and cytosine (GC) content, ribotyping, random amplification of polymorphic DNA (RAPD) analysis and pulsed-field gel electrophoresis (PFGE). Novel bacterial typing methods based on the nucleotide sequences of ribosomal RNA (rRNA) genes have become a robust way of assessing bacterial identity. Further details of these methods are given in Chapter 3.

Additionally, recent research indicates that endogenous bacterial habitats in humans, including the oral

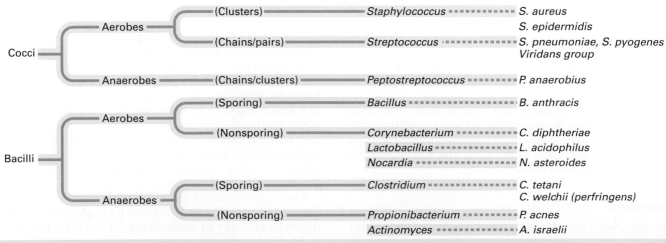

Fig. 2.7 A simple classification of Gram-positive bacteria.

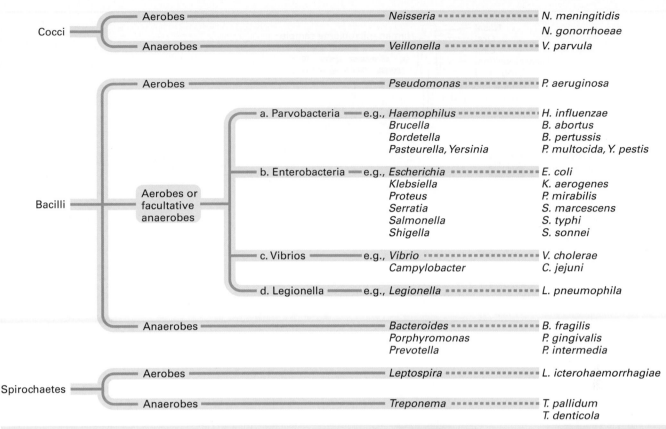

Fig. 2.8   A simple classification of Gram-negative bacteria.

cavity, harbour a flora that cannot be cultured using routine laboratory techniques. These so-called **uncul-turable species** comprise both bacteria and archaea, previously mentioned, and can only be detected by molecular techniques or **metagenomics** (e.g., by direct amplification of 16S RNA). The role of these totally new **phylotypes** of bacteria in either disease or health awaits clarification.

Both the culturable and unculturable organisms (i.e., the total microbial community) including biomolecules within a defined habitat, such as the human body, are given the term **core microbiome**. The total collection of resident microbes within the core microbiome is termed the **microbiota**. The analysis of this microbiome has been greatly facilitated by novel techniques such as **pyrosequencing** (a method of DNA sequencing) and **next-generation sequencing (NGS).** The data from such studies have revealed that the oral cavity in health may contain more than 1000 different phylotypes (Fig. 2.9; also see Chapter 31).

HOW DO ORGANISMS GET THEIR NAMES?

Organisms are named according to a hierarchical system, beginning with the taxonomic rank **domain**, followed by **kingdom, phylum, class, order, family, genus** and **species** (Table 2.3). The scientific name of an organism is classically a binomial of the last two ranks—that is, a com-bination of the generic name followed by the species name, such as *Streptococcus salivarius* and *Homo sapiens* (note that the species name does not begin with a capital letter). The name is usually written in italics with the generic name abbreviated (e.g., *S. salivarius*). When bacterial names are used adjectivally or collectively, the names are not italicized and do not begin with a capital letter (e.g., staphylococcal enzymes, lactobacilli).

Table 2.3   Hierarchical Ranks in Classification of Organisms (e.g., *Lactobacillus acidophilus*)[a]

Taxonomic Rank	Example
Domain	Bacteria
Kingdom	Bacteria
Phylum	Firmicutes
Class	Bacilli
Order	Lactobacillales
Family	Lactobacillaceae
Genus	*Lactobacillus*
Species	*Lactobacillus acidophilus*

[a]*Note:* This is the basic classification, although more modern and detailed classifications are also available with further subcategorization of the taxonomic ranks.

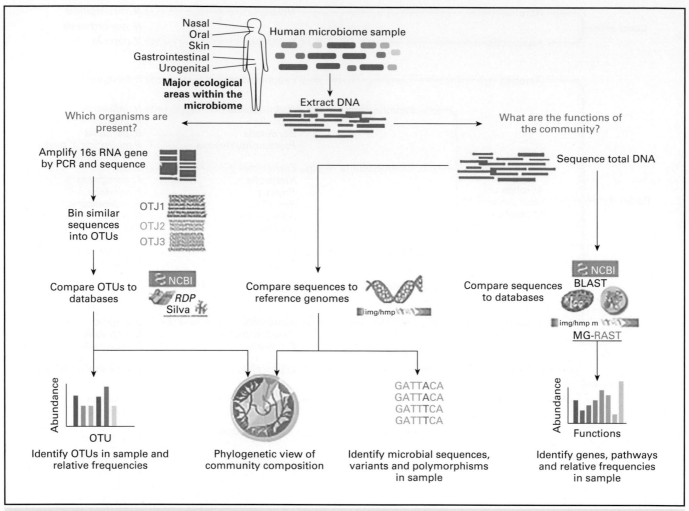

Fig. 2.9 A schematic overview of the uses of bioinformatics for functional metagenome analysis. Microbial community contains numerous bacterial and other species. Once the total DNA has been extracted, the composition of the community is determined by amplifying and sequencing the 16S ribosomal RNA (rRNA) gene. Highly similar sequences are then grouped as operational taxonomic units (OTUs), which are then recognized by comparisons with databases of already recognized organisms. OTUs are then analysed to determine the biomolecular and metabolic functions of the community. (Adapted from Morgan, X. C., Segata N., & Huttenhower C. (2013). Biodiversity and functional genomics in the human microbiome. *Trends in Genetics, 29*[1], 51–58.)

Key Facts

Note: Clinically relevant facts and practice points are *italicized*; key words are in **bold**.

- The word *microorganism* (microbe) is used to describe an organism that cannot be seen without the use of a microscope.
- The main groups of microbes are **algae**, **protozoa**, **fungi**, **bacteria** and **viruses**, with progressively decreasing size.
- All living cells are either **prokaryotic** (archaea and bacteria) or **eukaryotic**.
- Prokaryotes such as bacteria are simple cells with no internal membranes or organelles.
- **Eukaryotes have a nucleus**, **organelles** such as mitochondria and complex **internal membranes** (e.g., fungi, human cells).
- Bacteria are divided into two major classes according to staining characteristics: **Gram-positive** (purple) and **Gram-negative** (pink).
- **Structures external** to the cell wall of bacteria are the **flagella** (whip-like filaments), **fimbriae** or pili (fine, short, hair-like filaments), **glycocalyx** (slime layer) and **capsule**.

- Flagella are used for movement, the fimbriae and pili for adhesion and the glycocalyx for adhesion, protection and biofilm formation.
- Cell wall **peptidoglycan is common to both Gram-positive and Gram-negative bacteria** but thicker in the former; it gives rigidity and shape to the organism.
- Peptidoglycan comprises long chains of N-acetylmuramic acid and N-acetylglucosamine cross-linked by peptide side chains and cross-bridges.
- **Lipopolysaccharides (LPS)** are integral components of the outer membranes of Gram-negative (but not Gram-positive) bacteria; LPS is the endotoxin, and therefore Gram-positive bacteria cannot produce endotoxin.
- Cell walls of some bacteria such as the **mycobacteria** contain lipids (mycolic acids) that are resistant to Gram staining; these bacteria are called **acid-fast organisms**.
- Bacterial cytoplasm contains chromosomal nuclear material: nucleoid, ribosomes, inclusions/storage granules.

- Spore formation or **sporulation** is a **response to adverse conditions** in *Bacillus* spp. and *Clostridium* spp.
- **Taxonomy** (**systematic classification of organisms** into groups) can be performed according to morphology, staining reactions, cultural requirements, biochemical reactions, antigenic structure and DNA composition.

- The total microbial community including biomolecules within a defined habitat, such as the human body, is called the **core microbiome**.
- The total collection of resident microbes within the core microbiome is termed the **microbiota**.

Review Questions (Answers on p. 388)

Please indicate which answers are true and which are false.

2.1. Prokaryotes are different from eukaryotes in that prokaryotes:
   a. have ribosomes
   b. possess Golgi apparatus
   c. have their genetic material organized in the cytoplasm
   d. reproduce by binary fission only
   e. do not have introns in their mRNA

2.2. Bacterial capsule:
   a. mediates adhesion to surfaces
   b. hinders the action of phagocytes
   c. helps in identification
   d. is antigenic
   e. in all species is made up of polysaccharides

2.3. From the following list of bacterial structural components (A–G) match the best fit/association to the descriptors (1–8) given below:
   a. cytoplasmic membrane
   b. ribosomes
   c. cytoplasmic inclusions
   d. spores
   e. nucleoid
   f. fimbriae
   g. flagella
      1. associated with oxidative phosphorylation
      2. mediates cell motility
      3. a source of stored energy
      4. protein synthesis
      5. enables survival under harsh environmental conditions
      6. mediates host attachment
      7. enables selective transfer of molecule in and out of the cell
      8. resembles a single chromosome

Further Reading

Dewhirst, F. E., Chen, T., Izard, I., et al. (2010). The human oral microbiome. *Journal of Bacteriology, 192,* 5002–5017.
Human Microbiome Project Consortium. (2012). Structure, function and diversity of the healthy human microbiome. *Nature, 486,* 2017–2214.

Parahitiyawa, N., Scully, C., Leung, W., et al. (2010). Exploring the oral bacterial flora: Current status and future directions. *Oral Diseases, 16,* 136–145.
Wade, W. G. (2004). Non-culturable bacteria in complex commensal populations. *Advances in Applied Microbiology, 54,* 93–106.

3 Bacterial Physiology and Genetics

Bacterial Physiology

GROWTH

Bacteria, like all living organisms, require nutrients for metabolic purposes and for cell division and grow best in an environment that satisfies these requirements. Chemically, bacteria are made up of polysaccharide, protein, lipid, nucleic acid and peptidoglycan, all of which must be manufactured for successful growth.

Nutritional Requirements

Oxygen and Hydrogen. Both oxygen and hydrogen are obtained from water; hence, water is essential for bacterial growth. In addition the correct oxygen tension is necessary for balanced growth. While the growth of aerobic bacteria is limited by availability of oxygen, anaerobic bacteria may be inhibited by low oxygen tension.

Carbon. Carbon is obtained by bacteria in two main ways:

1. **Autotrophs**, which are free-living, nonparasitic bacteria, use carbon dioxide as the carbon source.

2. **Heterotrophs**, which are parasitic bacteria, utilize complex organic substances such as sugars as their source of carbon dioxide and energy.

Inorganic Ions. Nitrogen, sulphur, phosphate, magnesium, potassium and a number of trace elements are required for bacterial growth.

Organic Nutrients. Organic nutrients are essential in different amounts, depending on the bacterial species:

- Carbohydrates are used as an energy source and as an initial substrate for biosynthesis of many substances.
- Amino acids are crucial for growth of some bacteria.
- Vitamins, purines, and pyrimidines in trace amounts are needed for growth.

REPRODUCTION

Bacteria reproduce by a process called **binary fission**, in which a parent cell divides to form a **progeny** of two cells. This results in a **logarithmic growth rate**—one bacterium will produce 16 bacteria after four generations. The **doubling** or **mean generation time** of bacteria may vary (e.g., 20 min for *Escherichia coli*, 24 h for *Mycobacterium tuberculosis*); the shorter the doubling time, the faster the multiplication rate. Other factors that affect the doubling time include the amount of nutrients, the temperature and the pH of the environment.

BACTERIAL GROWTH CYCLE

The growth cycle of a bacterium has four main phases (Fig. 3.1):

1. **Lag phase**: may last for a few minutes or for many hours, as bacteria do not divide immediately but undergo a period of adaptation with vigorous metabolic activity
2. **Log** (logarithmic, exponential) **phase**: rapid cell division occurs, determined by the environmental conditions
3. **Stationary phase**: reached when nutrient depletion or toxic products cause growth to slow until the number of new cells produced balances the number of cells that die; the bacteria have now achieved their **maximal cell density** or **yield**
4. **Decline** or **death phase**: marked by a decline in the number of live bacteria.

GROWTH REGULATION

Bacterial growth is essentially regulated by the nutritional environment. However, both intracellular and extracellular regulatory events can modify the growth rate. Intracellular factors include:

- **end-product inhibition**: the first enzyme in a metabolic pathway is inhibited by the end product of that pathway
- **catabolite repression**: enzyme synthesis is inhibited by catabolites.

Extracellular factors that modify bacterial growth are:

- **temperature**: the optimum is required for efficient activity of many bacterial enzymes, although bacteria can grow in a wide range of temperatures. Accordingly, bacteria can be classified as:
  - **mesophiles**, which grow well between 25°C and 40°C, comprising most medically important bacteria (that grow best at body temperature)
  - **thermophiles**, which grow between 55°C and 80°C (e.g., *Thermus aquaticus* grows in hot springs, and its enzymes such as *Taq* polymerase are therefore heat resistant, a fact exploited by molecular biologists in the polymerase chain reaction PCR)
    - **psychrophiles**, which grow at temperatures below 20°C
- **pH**: the hydrogen **ion** concentration of the environment should be around pH 7.2–7.4 (i.e., physiological pH) for optimal bacterial growth. However, some bacteria (e.g., lactobacilli) have evolved to exploit ecological niches, such as carious cavities where the pH may be as low as 5.0.

AEROBIC AND ANAEROBIC GROWTH

A good supply of oxygen enhances the metabolism and growth of most bacteria. The oxygen acts as the hydrogen acceptor in the final steps of energy production and generates two molecules: hydrogen peroxide (H_2O_2) and the free radical superoxide (O_2). Both of these are toxic and need to be destroyed. Two enzymes are used by bacteria to dispose of them: the first is **superoxide dismutase**, which catalyses the reaction:

$$2O_2 + 2H^+ \rightarrow H_2O_2 + O_2$$

and the second is **catalase**, which converts hydrogen peroxide to water and oxygen:

$$2H_2O_2 \rightarrow 2H_2O + O_2$$

Bacteria can therefore be classified according to their ability to live in an oxygen-replete or an oxygen-free environment (Fig. 3.2, Table 3.1). This has important practical implications, as clinical specimens must be incubated in the laboratory under appropriate gaseous conditions for the pathogenic bacteria to grow. Thus bacteria can be classified as follows:

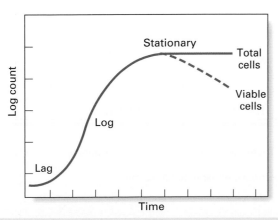

Fig. 3.1 Bacterial growth curve. Lag, lag phase of growth; Log, logarithmic phase of growth.

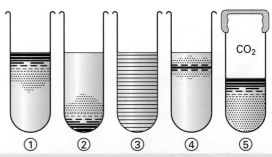

Fig. 3.2 Atmospheric requirements of bacteria, as demonstrated in agar shake cultures. (1) obligate aerobe; (2) obligate anaerobe; (3) facultative anaerobe; (4) microaerophile; (5) capnophilic organism (growing in carbon dioxide-enriched atmosphere). (See also Table 3.1.)

Table 3.1 Effect of Oxygen on the Growth of Bacteria

Degree of Oxygenation	Term	Example
Oxygen essential for growth	Obligate aerobe	*Pseudomonas aeruginosa*
Grows well under low oxygen concentration (5%)	Microaerophile	*Campylobacter fetus*
Grows in the presence or absence of oxygen	Facultative anaerobe[a]	*Streptococcus milleri*
Only grows in the absence of oxygen	Obligate anaerobe	*Porphyromonas gingivalis*

[a]Facultative anaerobes may be subgrouped as capnophiles or capnophilic organisms if they grow well in the presence of 8–10% carbon dioxide (e.g., *Legionella pneumophila*).

- **obligate (strict) aerobes**, which require oxygen to grow because their adenosine triphosphate (ATP)-generating system is dependent on oxygen as the hydrogen acceptor (e.g., *M. tuberculosis*)
- **facultative anaerobes**, which use oxygen to generate energy by respiration if it is present but can use the fermentation pathway to synthesize ATP in the absence of sufficient oxygen (e.g., oral bacteria such as *mutans* streptococci, *E. coli*)
- **obligate (strict) anaerobes**, which cannot grow in the presence of oxygen because they lack either superoxide dismutase or catalase, or both (e.g., *Porphyromonas gingivalis*)

- **microaerophiles**, which grow best at a low oxygen concentration (e.g., *Campylobacter fetus*).

Bacterial Genetics

Genetics is the study of inheritance and variation. All inherited characteristics are encoded in DNA, except in RNA viruses.

THE BACTERIAL CHROMOSOME

The bacterial chromosome contains the genetic information that defines all the characteristics of the organism. It is a single, continuous strand of DNA (Fig. 3.3) with a closed, circular structure attached to the cell membrane of the organism. The average bacterial chromosome has a molecular weight of 2×10^9.

Replication

Chromosome replication is an accurate process that ensures that the progeny cells receive identical copies from the mother cell. The replication process is initiated at a specific site on the chromosome (*oriC* site) where the two DNA strands are locally denatured. A complex of proteins binds to this site, opens up the helix and initiates replication. Each strand then serves as a template for a complete round of DNA synthesis, which occurs in both directions (bidirectional) and on both strands, creating a **replication bubble** (Fig. 3.4). The two sites at which

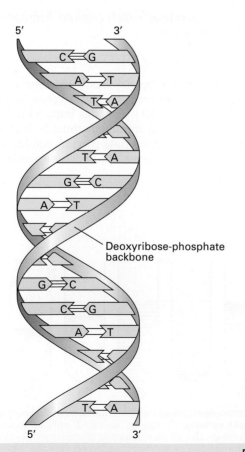

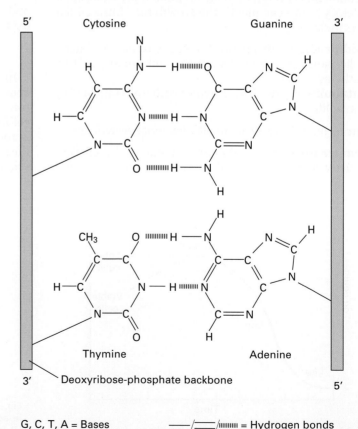

Fig. 3.3 The structure of DNA.

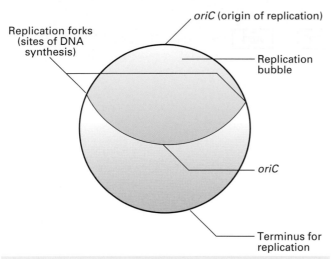

Fig. 3.4   **Bidirectional replication of a circular bacterial chromosome.**

the replication occurs are called the **replication forks**. As replication proceeds, the replication forks move around the molecule in opposite directions opening up the DNA strands, synthesizing two new complementary strands until the two replication forks meet at a termination site. Of the four DNA strands now available, each daughter cell receives a parental strand and a newly synthesized strand. This process is called **semiconservative replication**. Such chromosomal replication is synchronous with cell division, so that each cell receives a full complement of DNA from the mother cell.

The main enzyme that mediates DNA replication is **DNA-dependent DNA polymerase**, although a number of others take part in this process. When errors occur during DNA replication, repair mechanisms excise incorrect nucleotide sequences with nucleases, replace them with the correct nucleotides and relegate the sequence.

Bacteria have evolved mechanisms to delete foreign nucleotides from their genomes. **Restriction enzymes** are mainly used for this purpose, and they cleave double-stranded DNA at specific sequences. The DNA fragments produced by restriction enzymes vary in their molecular weight and can be demonstrated in the laboratory by gel electrophoresis. Hence, these restriction enzymes are used in many clinical analytical techniques to cleave DNA and to characterize both bacteria and viruses.

Genes

The genetic code of bacteria is contained in a series of units called **genes**. As the normal bacterial chromosome has only one copy of each gene, bacteria are called **haploid** organisms (as opposed to higher organisms, which contain two copies of the gene and hence are **diploid**).

A gene is a chain of **purine** and **pyrimidine** nucleotides. The genetic information is coded in triple nucleotide groups or **codons**. Each codon or triplet nucleotide codes for a specific amino acid or a regulatory sequence (e.g., start and stop codons). In this way, the structural genes determine the sequence of amino acids that form the protein, which is the gene product.

The genetic material of a typical bacterium (e.g., *E. coli*) comprises a single circular DNA with a molecular weight of about 2×10^9 and composed of approximately 5×10^6 base pairs, which in turn can code for about 2000 proteins.

GENETIC VARIATION IN BACTERIA

Genetic variation can occur as a result of mutation or gene transfer.

Mutation

A mutation is a change in the base sequence of DNA, as a consequence of which different amino acids are incorporated into a protein, resulting in an altered phenotype. Mutations result from three types of molecular change, as follows.

Base Substitution. This occurs during DNA replication when one base is inserted in place of another. When the base substitution results in a codon that instructs a different amino acid to be inserted, the mutation is called a *missense mutation*; when the base substitution generates a termination codon that stops protein synthesis prematurely, the mutation is called a *nonsense mutation*. The latter always destroys protein function.

Frame Shift Mutation. A frame shift mutation occurs when one or more base pairs are added or deleted, which shifts the reading frame on the ribosome and results in the incorporation of the wrong amino acids 'downstream' from the mutation and in the production of an inactive protein.

Insertion. The insertion of additional pieces of DNA (e.g., transposons) or an additional base can cause profound changes in the reading frames of the DNA and in adjacent genes (Fig. 3.5).

Mutations can be induced by chemicals, radiation or viruses.

Gene Transfer

The transfer of genetic information can occur by:

- conjugation
- transduction
- transformation
- transposition.

Clinically, the most important consequence of DNA transfer is that antibiotic-resistant genes are spread from one bacterium to another.

Conjugation. This is the mating of two bacteria, during which DNA is transferred from the donor to the recipient cell (Fig. 3.6A). The mating process is controlled by an **F (fertility) plasmid**, which carries the genes for the proteins required for mating, including the protein pilin, which forms the sex pilus (conjugation tube). During mating, the pilus of the donor (male) bacterium carrying the F factor (F+) attaches to a receptor on the surface of the recipient (female) bacterium. The latter is devoid of an F plasmid (F−). The cells are then brought into direct contact with each other by 'reeling in' of the sex pilus. Then the F factor DNA is cleaved enzymatically, and one strand is transferred across the bridge into the female cell. The process

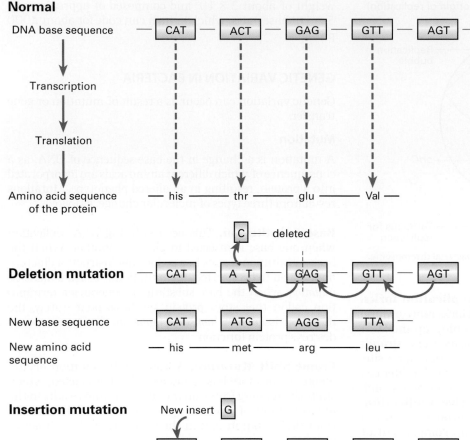

Normal

DNA base sequence — CAT — ACT — GAG — GTT — AGT —

Transcription

Translation

Amino acid sequence of the protein — his — thr — glu — Val —

C — deleted

Deletion mutation — CAT — A T — GAG — GTT — AGT —

New base sequence — CAT — ATG — AGG — TTA —

New amino acid sequence — his — met — arg — leu —

Insertion mutation   New insert G

CAT — ACT — GAG — GTT — AGT

New base sequence — CAG — TAC — TGA — GGT — TAG —

New amino acid sequence — glu — tyr — cys — gly —

Fig. 3.5 Events that entail mutation: the effect of the deletion and insertion of a single base on the amino acid sequence (and the quality of the protein thus produced) is shown.

is completed by synthesis of the complementary strand to form a double-stranded F plasmid in both the donor and recipient cells. The recipient now becomes an F+ male cell that has the ability to transmit the plasmid further. The new DNA can integrate into the recipient's DNA and become a stable component of its genetic material. Complete transfer of the bacterial DNA takes about 100 min.

Transduction. Transduction is a process of DNA transfer by means of a bacterial virus: a **bacteriophage (phage)**. During the replication of the phage, a piece of bacterial DNA is incorporated, accidentally, into the phage particle and is carried into the recipient cell at the time of infection (Fig. 3.6B). There are two types of transduction:

1. Generalized transduction occurs when the phage carries a segment from any part of the bacterial chromosome. This may occur when the bacterial DNA is fragmented after phage infection and pieces of bacterial DNA the same size as the phage DNA are incorporated into the latter.
2. Specialized transduction occurs when the phage DNA that has been already integrated into the bacterial DNA

is excised and carries with it an adjacent part of the bacterial DNA. Phage genes can cause changes in the phenotype of the host bacterium—for example, toxin production in *Corynebacterium diphtheriae* is controlled by a phage gene. This property is lost as soon as the phage DNA is lost in succeeding reproductive cycles.

Plasmid DNA can also be transferred to another bacterium by transduction. However, the donated plasmid can function independently without recombining with bacterial DNA. The ability to produce an enzyme that destroys penicillin (β-lactamase) is mediated by plasmids that are transferred between staphylococci by transduction.

Transformation. Transformation is the transfer of exogenous bacterial DNA from one cell to another. It occurs in nature when dying bacteria release their DNA, which is then taken up by recipient cells and recombined with the recipient cell DNA. This process appears to play an insignificant role in disease (Fig. 3.6C).

Transposition. Transposition occurs when transposable elements (transposons) move from one DNA site to

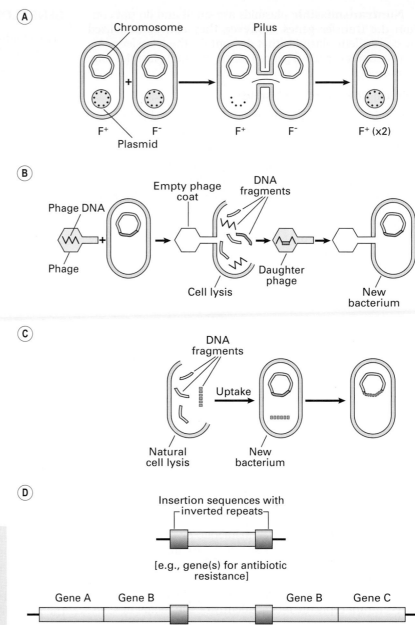

Fig. 3.6 Gene transfer. (A) Conjugation: transfer of a plasmid gene by conjugation (see text); (B) transduction: phage-mediated gene transfer from one bacterium to another; (C) transformation: gene transfer by uptake of exogenous bacterial DNA by another bacterium in the vicinity (not mediated by plasmid or phage); (D) transposition: transposons (jumping genes) can move from one DNA site to another, thereby inactivating the recipient gene and conferring new traits such as drug resistance.

another within the genome of the same organism (e.g., *E. coli*). The simplest transposable elements, called *insertion sequences*, are less than 2 kilobases in length and encode enzymes (transposase) required for 'jumping' from one site to another (Fig. 3.6D).

Recombination

When the DNA is transferred from the donor to the recipient cell by one of the above mechanisms, it is integrated into the host genome by a process called *recombination*. There are two types of recombination:

1. **Homologous recombination**, in which two pieces of DNA that have extensive homologous regions pair up and exchange pieces by the processes of breakage and reunion
2. **Nonhomologous recombination**, in which little homology is necessary for recombination to occur.

A number of different enzymes (e.g., endonucleases, ligases) are involved in the recombination process.

PLASMIDS

Plasmids are extrachromosomal, double-stranded circular DNA molecules within the size range 1–200 MDa. They are capable of replicating independently of the bacterial chromosome (i.e., they are replicons). Plasmids occur in both gram-positive and gram-negative bacteria, and several different plasmids can often coexist in one cell.

Transmissible plasmids can be transferred from cell to cell by conjugation. They contain about 10–12 genes responsible for synthesis of the sex pilus and for the enzymes required for transfer; because of their large size, they are usually present in a few (one to three) copies per cell.

Nontransmissible plasmids are small and do not contain the transfer genes. However, they can be mobilized by co-resident plasmids that do contain the transfer gene. Many copies (up to 60 per cell) of these small plasmids may be present.

Clinical Relevance of Plasmids

A number of medically important functions of bacteria are attributable to plasmids (i.e., are plasmid coded). The plasmid-coded bacterial attributes include:

- antibiotic resistance (carried by R plasmids)
- the production of colicins (toxins that are produced by many species of enterobacteria and are lethal for other bacteria)
- resistance to heavy metals such as mercury (the active component of some antiseptics) and silver—mediated by a reductase enzyme
- pili (fimbriae), which mediate the adherence of bacteria to epithelial cells
- exotoxins, including several enterotoxins.

TRANSPOSONS

Transposons, also called **jumping genes**, are pieces of DNA that move readily from one site to another, either within or between the DNAs of bacteria, plasmids and bacteriophages. In this manner, plasmid genes can become part of the chromosomal complement of genes. Interestingly, when transposons transfer to a new site, it is usually a copy of the transposon that moves, while the original remains in situ (like photocopying). For their insertion, transposons do not require extensive homology between the terminal repeat sequences of the transposon (which mediate integration) and the site of insertion in the recipient DNA.

Transposons can code for metabolic or drug resistance enzymes and toxins. They also may cause mutations in the gene into which they insert or may alter the expression of nearby genes.

In contrast to plasmids or bacterial viruses, transposons cannot replicate independently of the recipient DNA. More than one transposon can be located in the DNA—for example, a plasmid can contain several transposons carrying drug-resistance genes. Thus transposons can jump from:

- the host genomic DNA to a plasmid
- one plasmid to another
- a plasmid to genomic DNA.

Recombinant DNA Technology in Microbiology

By definition, every classified species must have somewhere on its genome a unique DNA or RNA sequence that distinguishes it from another species. In diagnostic microbiology, this attribute is used to identify microbes where the DNA sequence of the offending pathogen can be identified by means of a number of clever techniques, using clinical samples from the patient.

GENE CLONING

Gene cloning is the artificial incorporation of one or more genes into the genome of a new host cell by various genetic recombination techniques.

The candidate DNA is first extracted from the source, purified and cut or cleaved into small fragments by restriction enzymes, leaving 'sticky ends'. These are then inserted into a vector DNA, first by cutting the vector DNA with the same enzyme so as to produce complementary sticky ends. The sticky ends of the vector and the candidate DNA are then tied or ligated together using enzymes called **DNA ligases** to produce a recombinant DNA molecule. This process can also be used for cloning RNA, when complementary copies of DNA are produced by **reverse transcription** using reverse transcriptase enzymes. The vector used for gene transfer is usually a plasmid or a virus.

The vector with the integrated DNA has to be inserted into a cell in order to obtain multiple copies of the organism that express the selected gene. This can be done by:

- **transformation** (see above)—very popular owing to its simplicity, but competent cells need to be found
- **electroporation**—an electric current induces pores on the cell membrane for vector entry
- **gene gun**—tungsten or gold particles are coated with the vector and propelled into cells by a helium burst
- **microinjection**—direct manual injection of the vector into a cell by a glass micropipette.

The insertion of the vector containing the recombinant DNA does not necessarily mean that all the progeny bacteria will contain the inserted element, because the vector integration process is somewhat random. In order to select the clone of bacteria that expresses the recombinant gene, other devious manoeuvres have to be adopted. For instance, one can choose a plasmid vector that carries resistance to antibiotics A and B. If the foreign DNA is inserted in the middle of gene *A* that confers resistance to antibiotic A, then this gene will be inactivated as a consequence. In this manner, bacteria with the cloned foreign DNA can be selected and are called the **gene library**.

GENE PROBES

DNA Probes

Used extensively in diagnostic microbiology, gene probes are pieces of DNA that are labelled radioactively or with a chemiluminescent marker. The probes carry a single strand of DNA analogous to the pathogen that is sought in the clinical sample. There are different types of DNA probes:

- **Whole DNA probes** are derived from chromosomal DNA and are used to seek organisms where the genome is not well characterized. Owing to their relatively large size, nonspecific reactions are common and the method is not very reliable.
- **Cloned DNA** probes are similar to whole DNA probes but are smaller, and the reaction is more specific. These are generally targeted at genes unique to the organism sought.

Oligonucleotide Probes

Oligonucleotide probes are based on the variable region of the 16S ribosomal RNA (rRNA) genes. The nucleotide sequences of the latter gene of a number of microbes have been well characterized, and they are known to be well preserved across species except for several small variable regions. This property is helpful in the construction of specific oligonucleotide probes of about 18–30 bases, which are much more specific than the DNA probes described above.

RNA Probes

Cellular protein synthesis is dependent on rRNA, and any mutation of the rRNA leads to cell death. Further, rRNA is highly species specific, and this property is exploited to produce RNA probes that are useful for both diagnostic microbiology and taxonomic studies. The most commonly used are the 5S, 16S and 23S probes.

DNA/RNA Probes and Oral Microbiology

Cultivation of the complex mixture of bacteria residing in the oral cavity is fraught with problems, and it is now recognized that a number of bacterial genera are difficult or almost impossible to culture. The introduction of DNA and RNA probes has helped us to obtain a more complete picture of the oral flora. For example, commercially available probes can now be used in diagnostic laboratories not only to identify but also to quantify **periodontopathic flora** in subgingival plaque samples obtained from a periodontal pocket (Fig. 3.7). Further, the samples, say in paper points, could be simply sent by post to distant laboratories for identification without the fear of death of organisms and the associated cumbersome culture procedures.

POLYMERASE CHAIN REACTION

Gene-cloning techniques revolutionized molecular biological advances in the 1970s. The analogous event that took place in the late 1980s was the invention of the **polymerase chain reaction (PCR)**. It is a simple technique in which a short region of a DNA molecule—a single gene, for instance—is copied repetitiously by a DNA polymerase enzyme (Fig. 3.8). This technique, in combination with a number of others described below, is used to identify unculturable bacteria from the oral cavity and other body sites (Fig. 3.9).

Materials

The following materials are required:

- the region of the DNA molecule to be amplified
- *Taq* polymerase (a heat-stable enzyme from *T. aquaticus* (hence *Taq*), a bacterium that lives in hot springs)
- deoxyribonucleoside 5′-triphosphate (dNTP): adenine, guanine, cytosine, thymine
- primers (with a known DNA sequence).

Method

1. Choose a region of the DNA molecule where the nucleotide sequences of the borders are known. (The border sequence must be known because two short oligonucleotides must hybridize—one to each strand of the double helix of the DNA molecule—for the PCR to begin.)
2. The double strand of the DNA molecule is first split into single strands by heating at 94°C (**denaturation** step).
3. The oligonucleotides now act as primers for the DNA synthesis and stick (or hybridize) to the region adjacent

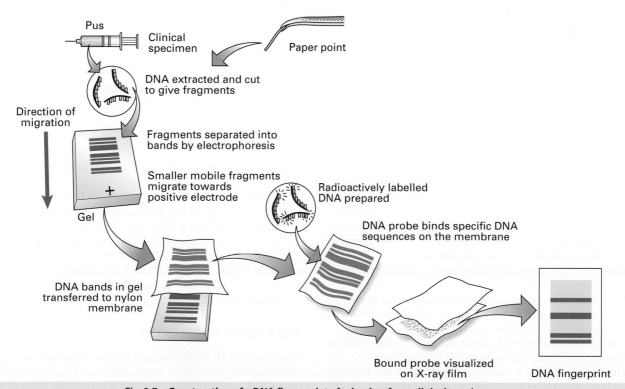

Fig. 3.7   Construction of a DNA fingerprint of microbes from clinical specimens.

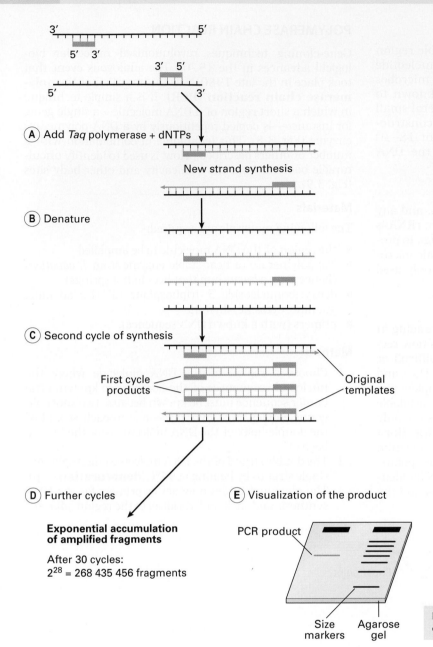

(A) Add *Taq* polymerase + dNTPs

New strand synthesis

(B) Denature

(C) Second cycle of synthesis

First cycle products

Original templates

(D) Further cycles

(E) Visualization of the product

Exponential accumulation of amplified fragments

After 30 cycles:
$2^{28} = 268\ 435\ 456$ fragments

PCR product

Size markers

Agarose gel

Fig. 3.8 The polymerase chain reaction (PCR). dNTP, deoxyribonucleoside 5′-triphosphate.

to the target DNA sequence, thus delimiting the region that is copied and amplified (hybridization step; around 55°C).

4. The DNA polymerase enzyme (*Taq* polymerase) and the nucleotides are added to the primed template DNA and incubated at 72°C for synthesis of new complementary strands or **amplicons** (**synthesis** step).

5. The mixture is again heated to 94°C to detach the newly synthesized strands (amplicons) from the template.

6. The solution is cooled, enabling more primers to hybridize at their respective positions, including positions on the newly synthesized strands.

7. A second round of DNA synthesis occurs (this time on four strands) with the help of the *Taq* polymerase.

8. This three-step PCR cycle of **denaturation–hybridization–synthesis** can be repeated, usually 25–30 times (in a thermocycler), resulting in exponential

accumulation of several million copies of the amplified fragment (amplicons).

9. Finally, a sample of the reaction mixture is run through an agarose gel electrophoresis system in order to visualize the product, which manifests as a discrete band after staining with ethidium bromide (Fig. 3.8).

10. The latter step is obviated in newer variations of PCR such as real-time PCR where the amplicon can be identified using labelled probes and labelled fluorophores.

PCR AND ITS VARIATIONS

The basic PCR methodology is now modified to provide sophisticated analytical tools. The main features of three commonly used variations of PCR—namely nested, mutiplex and real-time PCR—are given below.

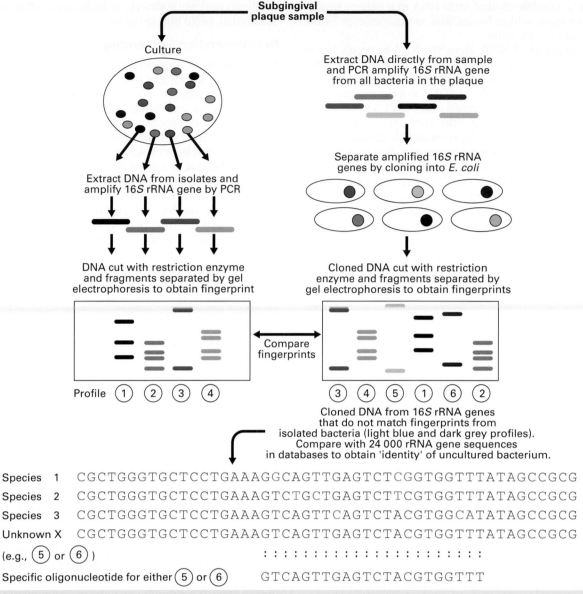

Subgingival plaque sample

Culture

Extract DNA directly from sample and PCR amplify 16S rRNA gene from all bacteria in the plaque

Extract DNA from isolates and amplify 16S rRNA gene by PCR

Separate amplified 16S rRNA genes by cloning into *E. coli*

DNA cut with restriction enzyme and fragments separated by gel electrophoresis to obtain fingerprint

Cloned DNA cut with restriction enzyme and fragments separated by gel electrophoresis to obtain fingerprints

Compare fingerprints

Profile ① ② ③ ④

③ ④ ⑤ ① ⑥ ②

Cloned DNA from 16S rRNA genes that do not match fingerprints from isolated bacteria (light blue and dark grey profiles). Compare with 24 000 rRNA gene sequences in databases to obtain 'identity' of uncultured bacterium.

Species 1   CGCTGGGTGCTCCTGAAAGGCAGTTGAGTCTCGGTGGTTTATAGCCGCG

Species 2   CGCTGGGTGCTCCTGAAAGTCTGCTGAGTCTTCGTGGTTTATAGCCGCG

Species 3   CGCTGGGTGCTCCTGAAAGTCAGTTCAGTCTACGTGGCATATAGCCGCG

Unknown X   CGCTGGGTGCTCCTGAAAGTCAGTTGAGTCTACGTGGTTTATAGCCGCG

(e.g., ⑤ or ⑥)   :

Specific oligonucleotide for either ⑤ or ⑥   GTCAGTTGAGTCTACGTGGTTT

Fig. 3.9 Use of polymerase chain reaction (PCR) technology to identify unculturable bacteria obtained from a subgingival plaque sample. (Modified from Jenkinson, H and Dymock, D. (1999). Dental Update 26: 191–197, by permission of George Warman Publications (UK) Ltd.)

Nested PCR

Here, two sets of primers are used: the first set is used for the primary amplification round. The second primer set, specifically chosen to anneal with an internal sequence of the amplicon, reamplifies the latter 'specific' sequence; nested PCR has increased sensitivity compared to conventional PCR.

Multiplex PCR

In this method, more than one locus of the nucleotide is simultaneously amplified using multiple sets of primers, thus saving time and resources; mutiplex PCR has increased specificity and can identify organisms more accurately.

Real-Time PCR

Conventional PCR requires gel electrophoresis for analysis of the amplicons. In real-time PCR, this step is automatically performed in real time, and the target sequence is identified within a closed system, using either labelled fluorophores or other similarly labelled probes. Further advantages are the versatility of the system, enabling (1) analysis of multiple amplicons at specific time sequences during a reaction period, (2) semiquantitative estimation of the yield, and (3) multiplex evaluation of the products (see above). The disadvantage is the relatively expensive technology.

Why Is PCR so Widely Used?

Some reasons why the use of PCR is so widespread:

- **To study minuscule quantities of DNA**. As a single DNA molecule is adequate for an amplification reaction (hence its use in forensic studies, archaeology and palaeontology).
- **Use in rapid clinical diagnostic procedures**. The sensitivity of the PCR has resulted in its use in rapid diagnosis of viral, bacterial, fungal and other diseases. For

instance, amplification of viral DNA in a patient sample could be made within hours, and sometimes even before the onset of symptoms.

- **Amplification of RNA**. Here, the RNA molecule has to be first converted to single-strand complementary DNA (cDNA) with an enzyme called *reverse transcriptase* (as it transcribes the RNA code into DNA in a reverse manner). Once this initial step is carried out, the PCR primers and *Taq* polymerase are added; afterwards, the experimental procedure is identical to the standard technique.
- **Comparison of different genomes**. Random amplification with short lengths of primers can be used in **phylogenetics**, the study of evolutionary history and lines of descent of species or groups of organisms. This technique is called **random amplification of polymorphic DNA (RAPD)**.

OTHER TECHNIQUES FOR GENETIC TYPING OF MICROORGANISMS

Restriction Enzyme Analysis

A genetic 'fingerprint' of the organism is obtained by extracting its DNA and cutting or cleaving the DNA at specific points by **restriction endonucleases**. The DNA fragments so generated are run on an agarose electrophoresis gel and viewed under ultraviolet illumination after staining with ethidium bromide. The profiles of the bands produced on the gel (the 'fingerprints') can be compared or contrasted with those from other strains. This was the original molecular method used for genotyping organisms, but it has been supplanted by newer methods that are more discriminatory.

Restriction Fragment Length Polymorphism

In restriction fragment length polymorphism (RFLP), the DNA is first cleaved using restriction endonucleases and separated on the agarose gel. Afterwards, the separated fragments are transferred by blotting onto a nitrocellulose or nylon membrane by a method called **Southern blotting**, and DNA probes constructed from genes of known organisms (species or strains) are then hybridized to the membrane; these will bind to complementary sequences in the DNA fragments on the membrane, revealing the species or strain identity.

Pulsed-Field Gel Electrophoresis

Pulsed-field gel electrophoresis (PFGE) is similar to RFLP. Here, the chromosomal DNA of an organism is cut into relatively large pieces by restriction enzymes and the resultant fragments are separated in an agarose gel with the help of a pulsed electric field, in which the polarity is regularly reversed. Large pieces of chromosomes usually do not separate in conventional agarose gels, hence the necessity of the pulsed/reversed electric field.

Pyrosequencing

Pyrosequencing is one of the most novel and reliable techniques of DNA sequencing. It is based on the *sequencing by synthesis* principle, so-called as it relies on the detection of pyrophosphate release on nucleotide incorporation, rather than chain termination with dideoxynucleotides used in PCR techniques. It uses chemiluminescence enzyme reactions and photodetection techniques that are highly automated, rapid and sensitive.

Next-Generation Sequencing

Next-generation sequencing (NGS), also known as *high-throughput sequencing* or *massively parallel sequencing*, is the catch-all term used to describe a number of different modern sequencing technologies (e.g., Illumina, Ion Torrent). NGS permits sequencing numerous samples of DNA and RNA much more quickly and cheaply than the previous technology and has revolutionized microbiology.

The technique is rather complex and requires sophisticated and expensive equipment, and hence only specialist centres can perform NGS analyses. This said, with the wide use of NGS technology the cost of the machinery is rapidly declining and the methodology should be widely available for clinical use in the not-too-distant future.

A discussion of NGS technology is beyond the remit of this book, but the major steps are shown in Fig. 3.10.

NGS techniques are now widely used in the analysis of the oral microbiome. An example of a so-called 'heat tree' of microbial genera forming an endodontic infection is shown in Fig. 3.11. This figure shows the hierarchical pattern of the prevalence of both the cultivable and uncultivable flora in an endodontic infection, beginning with the more common taxa in the central root of the tree and progressing into the less common taxa at the tips of the branching tree at the periphery.

The Era of '-omics'

With the advent of the new millennium, there has been an explosion of digital and computer technology, the use of which has led to a parallel advancement of the knowledge of our biosphere. This in turn has led to focal developments of subdisciplines such as genomics, proteomics and metabolomics—the so-called '-omics' era. These new technologies have had a significant impact on the identification of microbes, particularly those that could not be cultured in the laboratory (unculturable bacteria), and on the elucidation of their pathogenic mechanisms such as resistance to antibiotics. Indeed, a new term **oralome** has been recently coined for the 'biosphere' of the oral cavity as described in detail in Part 5 of this book. A brief introduction to the various -omics domains are given in the following sections.

GENOMICS

Genomics refers to the study of the identity of all genes within the chromosome of a cell. The human animal and microbial genome sequencing projects have thus far provided a rich genetic resource to better understand human diseases including oral diseases. As mentioned in Chapter 2, the development of technologies such as microarray analysis have helped microbiologists to explore patterns of gene expression in various infectious diseases, and their pathogenic mechanisms—for example, in periodontal disease. The subcategory of functional genomics deals with the organization of the genes and their expression patterns under defined conditions.

The development of computer models for high-throughput analyses of genomic data has simplified the exploration of gene expression profiles in both eukaryotes and prokaryotes.

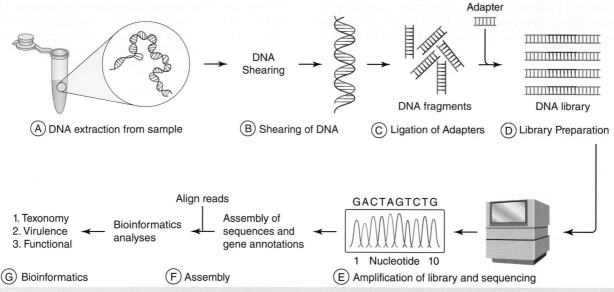

Fig. 3.10   Workflow of next-generation sequencing (NGS) technology (diagrammatic).

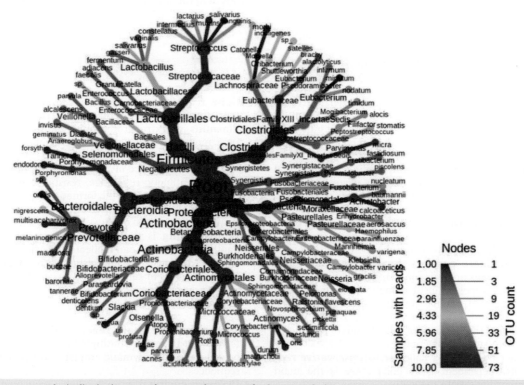

Fig. 3.11   A heat-tree analysis displaying prominent taxa in a case of primary endodontic (root canal) infection. This figure shows the hierarchical pattern of the prevalence of both the cultivable and nonculturable flora in an endodontic (root canal) infection, beginning with the more common taxa in the central root of the tree (dark red) and progressing into the less common taxa at the tips of the branching tree at the periphery (blue). OTU, Operational taxonomic unit.

Furthermore, **DNA microarray technologies** help investigators to evaluate gene expression on a genome-wide basis, providing a 'global' perspective of how an organism responds to a specific stress, drug or toxin.

PROTEOMICS

Proteomics is defined as the study of the myriad of proteins expressed by the genome of an organism, cell or tissue type. Proteomics builds on and complements the knowledge gained from genomics by revealing the levels, activities, regulation and interactions of every protein in an organism or a cell. Study of the proteome is more complex than that of the genome, as the number of proteins in an organism/cell is considered many orders of magnitude greater than that of the number of genes.

Such complexity is further confounded by the dynamic changes in the proteome in response to the environment and also the multiple possible interactive combinations among proteins. **Protein chips** that can simultaneously identify large numbers of proteins are helpful in unravelling such complexity.

TRANSCRIPTOMICS

Transcriptomics is a related branch of molecular biology that deals with the study of messenger RNA molecules produced in an individual or population of a particular cell type.

METABOLOMICS

Metabolomics is defined as the scientific study of chemical processes involving metabolites of a cell or an organism. While proteomic analyses do not tell the whole story of what might be happening in a cell, metabolic profiling can give an instantaneous snapshot of the physiology of that organism. This has led to the development of a further domain known as **interactomics**. The latter is defined as a discipline involving the intersection of bioinformatics and biology that deals with studying both the interactions and the consequences of those interactions between and among

proteins, and other molecules within an organism. The network of all such interactions is called the *interactome*. In essence, interactomics aims to compare networks of interactions (i.e., interactomes) between and within species in order to elucidate how the traits of such networks are either preserved or varied.

One of the current challenges of science is to integrate proteomic, transcriptomic, metabolic and interactomic data to provide a more complete picture of living organisms.

BIOINFORMATICS

Bioinformatics is an essential component of the -omics era. The avalanche of information spewed out by, for instance, NGS and similar techniques cannot be sorted using traditional methods. Hence new computational methods and their application to the solution of biological problems, often via the **mining** of information databases, have been developed over the last decade or so. This rapidly developing field is called **bioinformatics** and forms a crucial pivotal point for -omics technology. As bioinformatics occupies a central role in a broad spectrum of biological research, its analytical toolkits are equally diverse and complex.

Key Facts

- Bacteria, like all living organisms, require oxygen, hydrogen, carbon, inorganic ions and organic nutrients for survival.
- Other factors that modify growth are end-product inhibition and catabolite repression, as well as the temperature and pH of the medium.
- Bacteria reproduce by **binary fission**, leading to logarithmic growth of cell numbers; the doubling or mean generation time of bacteria can vary from minutes to hours or days.
- Bacterial growth in laboratory media can be divided into a **lag phase**, **log phase**, **stationary phase** and **decline phase**.
- Depending on their oxygen requirements, bacteria can be divided into **obligate aerobes, facultative anaerobes, obligate anaerobes** and **microaerophiles**.
- Bacterial chromosomes comprise a single, continuous strand of DNA with a closed, circular structure attached to the cell membrane.
- DNA replication is the synthesis of new strands of DNA using the original DNA strands as templates.
- DNA replicates by a process called *semiconservative replication;* DNA-dependent DNA polymerase is the main enzyme that mediates DNA replication.
- Restriction enzymes of bacteria delete foreign nucleotides from their genomes. These enzymes are therefore extremely useful in molecular biological techniques.
- Genetic variations in bacteria can occur by either mutation or gene transfer.
- **Mutation**, a change in the base sequence of the DNA, can be due to either base substitution frame shifts or insertion of additional pieces of DNA.

- **Gene transfer** in bacteria may occur by **conjugation, transduction, transformation or transposition**.
- **Plasmids** are extrachromosomal, double-stranded circular DNA molecules capable of independent replication within the bacterial host.
- The clinical relevance of plasmids lies in the fact that they code for antibiotic resistance, resistance to heavy metals, exotoxin production and pili formation.
- **Transposons** are 'jumping genes' that move from one site to another either within or between the DNA molecules.
- **Gene cloning** is the introduction of foreign DNA into another cell where it can replicate and express itself.
- **Gene probes** used in diagnostic microbiology are labelled (with chemicals or radioactively) pieces of DNA that can be used to detect specific sequences of DNA of the pathogen (in the clinical sample) by pairing with the complementary bases.
- The **polymerase chain reaction (PCR)** is a widely used technique that enables multiple copies of a DNA molecule to be generated by enzymatic amplification of the target DNA sequence.
- **Pyrosequencing** is a rapid, reliable sequencing method of relatively short DNA templates based on real-time (quantitative) pyrophosphate release and is a valuable tool for identification of bacteria (particularly unculturable).
- **Next-generation sequencing (NGS)** is a general term used to describe a number of different modern sequencing technologies

Review Questions (answers on p. 388)

Please indicate which answers are true and which are false.

3.1   With regard to bacterial growth, which of the following statements are true?
    a. autotrophic bacteria can use carbon dioxide as the sole source of carbon
    b. the growth of facultative anaerobes is arrested in the presence of oxygen
    c. a new progeny of cells are formed as a result of sporulation
    d. the logarithmic growth phase of bacteria precedes the lag phase
    e. some bacteria can grow at 80°C

3.2   Plasmid-coded bacterial attributes include:
    a. antibiotic resistance
    b. production of exotoxins
    c. resistance to disinfectants
    d. transfer of genetic material
    e. production of endotoxins

3.3   With regard to transposons, which of the following are true?
    a. they are also called jumping genes
    b. they can replicate independently of the chromosome or the plasmid
    c. they can cause mutations
    d. they mediate antimicrobial resistance
    e. a bacterial chromosome can have only one transposon

Further Reading

Alberts, B., Johnson, A., Lewis, J., Raff, M., Roberts, K., & Walter, P. (2007). *The molecular biology of the cell* (5th ed.). Garland.

Beebee, T., & Burke, J. (1992). *Gene structure and transcription* (2nd ed.). IRL Press/Oxford University Press.

Moat, A. G., Foster, J. W., & Spector, M. P. (2002). *Microbial physiology*. Wiley-Liss.

Mukherjee, S. (2016). *The gene: An intimate history*. Scribner.

4 Viruses and Prions

Viruses are one of the smallest forms of microorganism and infect most other forms of life: animals, plants and bacteria. They can also cause severe acute oral and orofacial disease, produce oral signs of systemic infection and be transmitted to patients and dental staff. The main features that characterize viruses are:

- **small size** (10–100 nm), averaging about one-tenth the size of a bacterium
- **genome** consisting of either DNA or RNA but never both; single- (ss) or double-stranded (ds); linear or circular (the encoding of the whole of the genetic information as RNA in RNA viruses is a situation unique in biology)
- **metabolic inactivity** outside the cells of susceptible hosts; viruses lack ribosomes: the protein-synthesizing apparatus (the corollary of this is that viruses can only multiply inside living cells—that is, they are **obligate intracellular parasites**).

Structure

Viruses consist of a nucleic acid core containing the viral genome, surrounded by a protein shell called a **capsid** (Figs. 4.1 and 4.2). The entire structure is referred to as the **nucleocapsid**. This may be 'naked', or it may be 'enveloped' within a lipoprotein sheath derived from the host cell membrane. In many viruses (e.g., orthomyxoviruses,

paramyxoviruses), the ensheathment begins by a budding process at the plasma membrane of the host cell, whereas others, such as herpesviruses, ensheath at the membrane of the nucleus or endoplasmic reticulum.

The protein shell or capsid consists of repeating units of one or more protein molecules; these protein units may go on to form structural units, which may be visualized by electron microscopy as morphological units called **capsomeres** (Fig. 4.1). Genetic economy dictates that the variety of viral proteins be kept to a minimum as viral genomes lack sufficient genetic information to code for a large array of different proteins. In enveloped viruses, the protein units, which comprise the envelopes and are visualized electron microscopically, are called 'peplomers' (loosely referred to as 'spikes').

VIRAL NUCLEIC ACID

Viral nucleic acid may be either DNA or RNA—never both. The RNA, in turn, may be single stranded (ss) or double stranded (ds), and the genome may consist of one or several molecules of nucleic acid. If the genome consists of a single molecule, which may be linear or have a circular configuration. The DNA viruses all have genomes composed of a single molecule of nucleic acid, whereas the genomes of many RNA viruses consist of several different molecules or segments, which are probably loosely linked together in the virion.

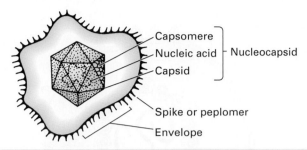

Fig. 4.1   **Viral structure (schematic).**

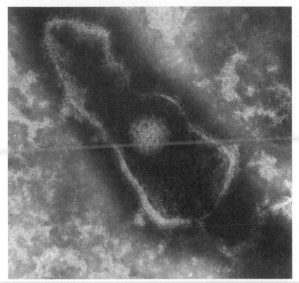

Fig. 4.2   **Scanning electron micrograph of a herpesvirus.** Note the extensive outer lipid envelope and the icosahedral nucleocapsid.

VIRAL PROTEIN

In terms of volume, the major bulk of the virion is protein, which offers a protective sheath for the nucleic acid. The viral protein is made up of two or three different polypeptide chains, although in some only one kind of polypeptide chain may be present. Virion surface proteins may have a special affinity for receptors on the surface of susceptible cells and may bear antigenic determinants.

Although most viral proteins have a structural function, some have enzymatic activity. For instance, many viruses, such as the human immunodeficiency virus (HIV), contain a reverse transcriptase, whereas several enzymes (e.g., neuraminidase, lysozyme) are found in larger, more complex viruses.

VIRAL LIPIDS AND CARBOHYDRATES

In general, lipids and carbohydrates of viruses are only found in their envelopes and are mostly derived from the host cells. About 50–60% of the lipids are phospholipids; most of the remainder is cholesterol.

VIRUS SYMMETRY

The nucleocapsids of viruses are arranged in a highly symmetrical fashion (symmetry refers to the way in which the protein units are arranged). Three kinds of symmetry are recognized (Fig. 4.3):

- **Icosahedral symmetry**. The protein molecules are symmetrically arranged in the shape of an icosahedron (i.e., a 20-sided solid, each face being an equilateral triangle). Herpesviruses are an example (Figs. 4.1 and 4.2).
- **Helical symmetry**. The capsomeres surround the viral nucleic acid in the form of a helix or spiral to form a tubular nucleocapsid. Most mammalian RNA viruses have this symmetry, where the nucleocapsid is arranged in the form of a coil and enclosed within a lipoprotein envelope.
- **Complex symmetry**. This is exhibited by a few families of viruses—notably the retroviruses and poxviruses.

Taxonomy

Vertebrate viruses are classified into families, genera and species. The attributes used in classification are their symmetry, the presence or absence of an envelope, nucleic acid composition (DNA or RNA), the number of nucleic acid strands and their polarity. Classification of some of the recognized families of RNA and DNA viruses is given in Table 4.1. (*Note*: to memorize which viruses contain DNA, remember the acronym PHAD: P is for papova and pox, H for herpes and AD for adenoviruses. Most of the remainder are RNA viruses, including the self-evident picornaviruses.)

The following is a concise description of the families of mammalian viruses.

DNA VIRUSES

Papovaviruses

Papovaviruses are small, icosahedral DNA viruses with a capacity to produce tumours in vivo and to transform cultured cell lines. The name *papova* is an acronym derived from the papillomavirus, polyomavirus and vacuolating agent simian virus 40 (SV40), which make up this family.

Papillomavirus. This genus contains human serotypes that cause benign skin tumours or warts and both oral and skin papillomas (e.g., hand and plantar warts). Although they were regarded as a cosmetic nuisance rather than a specific disease, it is now known that the papillomaviruses may be involved in genital and oral cancers.

Polyomavirus. This genus contains the polyomavirus of mice and SV40 of monkeys, which are used in experimental carcinogenesis in these animals.

Adenoviruses

Adenoviruses are icosahedral DNA viruses, commonly associated with respiratory and eye infections in humans. These viruses were so named because they were first isolated from cultured adenoid tissue eliciting cytopathic effects. Syndromes associated with adenoviruses include:

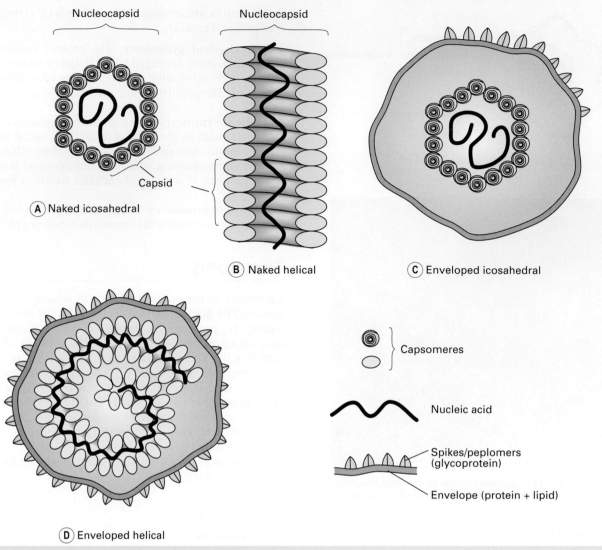

Fig. 4.3   Structural components and symmetry of different viruses. (A) Naked icosahedral; (B) naked helical; (C) enveloped icosahedral; (D) enveloped helical.

- acute febrile pharyngitis (primarily in infants and children), often indistinguishable from pharyngitis due to β-haemolytic streptococci
- acute adult respiratory disease, ranging from pharyngitis to pneumonia
- ocular infections.

Herpesviruses

Herpesviruses are the predominant viral cause of oral infections in humans; often the infections are latent and recurrent.

Structure. These enveloped, icosahedral viruses are 180–200 nm in diameter and contain a linear dsDNA molecule. The Herpesviridae family has over 100 members that spread widely among vertebrates and invertebrates, and new species are continuously being added. Owing to the disruption of the outer lipid envelope, herpesviruses are unstable at room temperature and are rapidly inactivated by lipid solvents such as alcohol and other common disinfectants.

During reproduction, maturation of the progeny begins in the nucleus of the host cell, which buds through the nuclear membrane and acquires the viral envelope. Typical and highly pathognomonic **intranuclear inclusions** are therefore found in cells that have undergone active virus replication. As many herpesviruses can fuse with the cells they infect, **polykaryocytes** or **giant cells** readily appear in tissue lesions. Such cells (e.g., Tzanck cells or nuclear inclusions (Lipschutz bodies)) are hallmarks of herpetic infections.

Different herpesviruses cause a variety of infectious diseases, some localized and some generalized, often with a vesicular rash. Herpesviruses establish latent infection, which can be readily reactivated by immunosuppression (Table 4.2).

The nomenclature of herpesviruses is contentious; there is thus a historical or a traditional (trivial) nomenclature and an official name for each virus (Table 4.3). The herpesviruses that commonly infect humans can be distinguished by their antigenic and genomic profiles, although they cannot be differentiated by electron microscopy owing

Table 4.1 Classification of Some of the Viruses Causing Human Disease

Morphology	Virus
DNA	
Enveloped, double-stranded nucleic acid	Herpesviruses
	Herpes simplex virus
	Varicella-zoster virus
	Epstein–Barr virus
	Cytomegalovirus
	Human herpesvirus 6
	Poxviruses
	Vaccinia
	Orf
Enveloped, single-stranded	Parvoviruses
Nonenveloped, double-stranded	Adenoviruses
	Papovaviruses
	Polyomaviruses
	Papillomaviruses
	Hepadnaviruses
	Hepatitis B virus
RNA	
Enveloped, single-stranded	Orthomyxoviruses
	Influenzavirus
	Paramyxoviruses
	Parainfluenza
	Respiratory syncytial
	Mumps
	Measles
	Togaviruses
	Rubella
	Retroviruses
	Human immunodeficiency viruses HTLV-I, HTLV-II
	Rhabdoviruses
	Rabies
Nonenveloped, double-stranded	Reoviruses
	Rotavirus
Nonenveloped, single-stranded	Picornaviruses
	Rhinovirus
	Enterovirus
	Coxsackievirus
	Echovirus
	Poliovirus

HTLV-I, Human T cell leukaemia virus type I.

Table 4.2 Latent Viruses Relevant to Dentistry

Virus	Site of Latency
Herpes simplex virus	Trigeminal ganglion
Varicella-zoster virus	Sensory ganglia
Epstein–Barr virus	Epithelial cells
	B lymphocytes
Cytomegalovirus	Salivary gland cells
Papillomaviruses	Epithelial cells
Human immunodeficiency viruses	Lymphocytes and other CD4+ cells (see Chapter 30)

to identical capsid morphology. They also have a universal ability to establish latent infection in the host in which they reside, and they manifest a number of common epidemiological features. Herpes simplex virus, herpes zoster virus, Epstein–Barr virus, human cytomegalovirus and herpesviruses 6 and 8 can all cause infections in oral and perioral tissues (Fig. 4.4); see Chapter 35 for details.

Poxviruses

The poxviruses are the largest viruses to infect humans or animals. Molluscum contagiosum in humans is caused by a poxvirus, as is smallpox, which is now a disease of only historical interest. Humans occasionally acquire infection by animal poxviruses (e.g., cowpox).

Parvoviruses

Parvoviruses are icosahedral viruses with ssDNA. Three serologically distinct types of autonomous parvoviruses are recognized in human disease. The first group is found in stool specimens, the second (the B19 virus) in the serum of asymptomatic blood donors, and the third has been recovered from synovial tissues of rheumatoid arthritis patients. The B19 virus is responsible for a febrile illness, particularly in children, manifesting as a maculopapular rash.

The exanthem is characterized by a fiery-red rash on the cheeks—the 'slapped-cheek' syndrome (also termed *fifth disease*).

Hepadnaviruses

Hepadnaviruses are small, spherical DNA viruses causing hepatitis, chronic liver infections and possibly liver cancer. They are of particular interest in dentistry because of their mode of transmission via blood and saliva (see Chapter 29).

Table 4.3 Official and Trivial Nomenclature of Human Herpesviruses (Family Herpesviridae)

Subfamily Species	Official Name	Trivial Name	Acronym
Alphaherpesvirinae	Human herpesvirus 1	Herpes simplex virus 1	HSV-1
	Human herpesvirus 2	Herpes simplex virus 2	HSV-2
	Human herpesvirus 3	Varicella-zoster virus	VZV
Betaherpesvirinae	Human herpesvirus 5	Cytomegalovirus	HCMV
	Human herpesvirus 6	—	HHV-6
Gammaherpesvirinae	Human herpesvirus 4	Epstein–Barr virus	EBV
	Human herpesvirus 7	—	HHV-7
	Human herpesvirus 8	Kaposi's sarcoma herpesvirus	HHV-8

HCMV, Human cytomegalovirus.

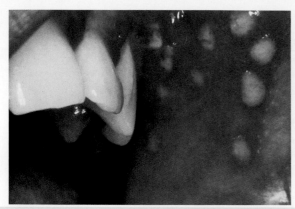

Fig. 4.4   Primary herpes simplex infection of the oral mucosa.

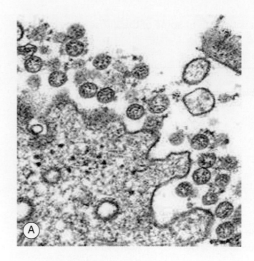

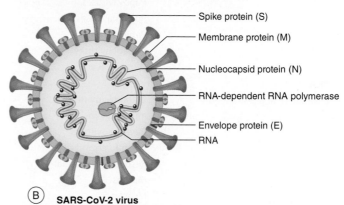

Spike protein (S)

Membrane protein (M)

Nucleocapsid protein (N)

RNA-dependent RNA polymerase

Envelope protein (E)

RNA

(B)   **SARS-CoV-2 virus**

Fig. 4.5   (A) Morphology of SARS-CoV-2. Transmission electron microscope image of SARS-CoV-2 spherical viral particles emerging from an infected epithelial cell. (B) Structural components of SARS-CoV-2. (Modified from the US Centers for Disease Control Image Library.)

RNA VIRUSES

Picornaviruses

Picornaviruses are the smallest family of RNA viruses but incorporate a very large group of viruses, including the genus *Enterovirus*. Human enteroviruses have been further subdivided into three major subgroups:

- polioviruses
- echoviruses (acronym for 'enteric cytopathogenic, human, orphan')
- coxsackieviruses (Coxsackie, a town in the United States) types A and B.

The enteroviruses reside and multiply asymptomatically in the gut but may cause a spectrum of disease ranging from mild undifferentiated rashes, respiratory infections and pharyngitis (coxsackie A) to more serious diseases, including carditis (coxsackie B), which may be lethal in the newborn (see Chapters 21 and 35).

Orthomyxoviruses

Orthomyxoviruses are RNA viruses with a tubular nucleocapsid and a lipoprotein envelope. Influenza A viruses of birds, mammals and humans are in this category. Some of these viruses—for example, Asian influenza viruses—may cause severe and often fatal generalized infections. The nomenclature of these viruses is based on the first letter H and N of the spike glycoproteins **haemagglutinin** and **neuraminidase**, respectively. Thus the earliest recognized virus was termed H1N1, followed by H2N2 and so on. The current 'bird-flu virus' that recently caused sporadic human infections in Asia is termed H5N1. As the latter outbreaks indicate that H5N1 virus has crossed the species barrier from birds to humans, there is great concern that human-to-human transmission of this rather virulent virus may create a worldwide pandemic of avian flu. There have been more than 100 human fatalities associated with avian flu transmitted directly from avian sources to humans, but cases of human-to-human transmission of this virus appear to be extremely rare (Chapter 23).

Paramyxoviruses

Paramyxoviruses are large, pleomorphic enveloped RNA viruses. The family contains four common and important human pathogens: **measles**, **mumps**, **parainfluenza** and **respiratory syncytial viruses**. Paramyxoviruses are a common cause of croup (laryngotracheobronchitis), whereas respiratory syncytial viruses cause regular winter epidemics of bronchiolitis/pneumonitis in infants.

Coronaviruses

Coronaviruses are enveloped RNA viruses with a helical nucleocapsid. The viruses are so called because their surface spike proteins (S proteins) resemble a crown (or *corona*, *Latin* for 'crown') when visualised through microscopy (Fig. 4.5).

Coronaviruses infect both animals and humans. Most human infections lead to mild upper respiratory tract infections including the common cold syndrome. Human coronaviruses infect the respiratory tract by the airborne route (i.e., by inhalation or aerosols generated by coughs and sneezes of infected individuals). Additionally, inanimate reservoirs (i.e., fomites) are a secondary factor in transmission. Rhinoviruses together with coronaviruses are the major agents of the common cold. A coronavirus that crossed the 'species barrier' from civet cats in China to humans is the agent of **severe acute respiratory syndrome (SARS)**. The latter infection—considered the first emerging infection of the new millennium—spread worldwide in 2003, causing many deaths, particularly among health care workers

(Chapter 23). Human coronaviruses are also implicated in gastroenteritis in infants.

Another well-known coronavirus infection led to the pandemic of **coronavirus diseases 2019 (COVID-19)**. This was caused by the **severe acute respiratory syndrome coronavirus 2 (SARS-CoV-2)** that originated in Wuhan, China, in 2019. Globally, as of September 2023, over 7 million have succumbed to COVID-19 with over 770 million confirmed cases detected. The disease is now considered an endemic infection in many geographic regions (see Chapter 30).

Retroviruses

Retroviruses are large, spherical enveloped RNA tumour viruses characterized by a unique genome, a unique enzyme and a unique mode of replication. The viral genome RNA is first transcribed into DNA by a virus-specific enzyme: reverse transcriptase. This DNA can then serve as a template for messenger RNA (mRNA) synthesis. The RNA viruses infecting humans comprise a single taxonomic group with three subfamilies:

- **lentiviruses** cause slowly progressive disease and include HIV types 1 and 2 (see Chapter 30)
- **oneoviruses** include those that cause tumours: human T cell leukaemia virus type I (HTLV-I), the agent of adult T cell leukaemia–lymphoma (ATLL), and HTLV-II, associated with hairy cell leukaemia
- **spumaviruses** are not recognized human pathogens.

Other RNA Viruses

Other RNA viruses that are important but are not known to cause oral disease or to be directly relevant to dentistry include togaviruses, arenaviruses, rhabdoviruses and filoviruses.

VIROIDS

As a result of advances in molecular biology, two new classes of infectious agents, **prions** and **viroids**, have been discovered. These are the smallest known agents of disease. Viroids cause diseases in plants and comprise naked, covalently linked, closed circles of ssRNA, less than 300–400 nucleotides in length. Despite their minute size, they replicate using host cell enzymes. Viroids are not associated with human disease, thus far. (Prions are discussed at the end of this chapter.)

Viral Replication

Viral replication (Fig. 4.6) is a highly complex process, and only a brief summary is given here. There are a number of general steps in the replication cycle of all viruses: **adsorption, penetration, uncoating and eclipse, transcription, synthesis of viral components, assembly** and **release of virions**. In some viruses, however, these steps may not be clearly defined and may overlap (e.g., penetration

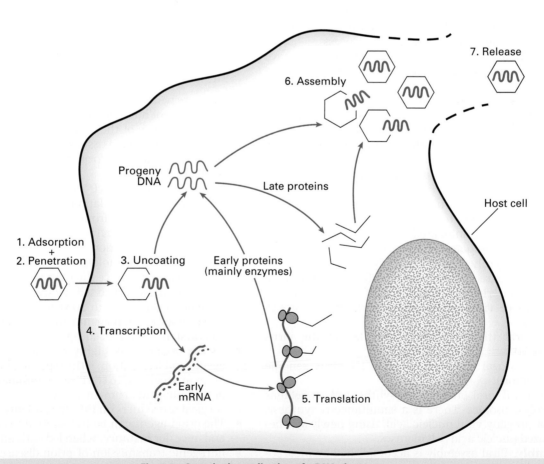

Fig. 4.6   Steps in the replication of a DNA virus.

and uncoating). It is noteworthy that in some families (e.g., Herpesviridae) many of the critical events occur in the cell nucleus, whereas others (e.g., Picornaviridae) multiply exclusively within the cytoplasm. The period between infection and the production of the new virion (**eclipse** or **latent period**) could be as short as 3 h (e.g., Orthomyxoviridae) or as long as several months or years (e.g., HIV).

Fig. 4.6 depicts the steps in the replication of a DNA virus. However, this picture has to be somewhat modified when RNA viruses are considered, as the basic unit of information is now RNA instead of DNA. The strategies of viral replication become more complex when ds rather than ss viruses, and those with RNA of positive polarity and negative polarity, are considered. The basic steps in replication are:

1. **Adsorption** or **attachment** of the virus particle to the specific receptors of the host cell plasma membrane. Firm attachment requires the presence of receptors for the virus on the plasma membrane (e.g., orthomyxoviruses and paramyxoviruses bind via an envelope protein, known as haemagglutinin, to certain glycoproteins or glycolipids on the host cell).

2. **Penetration** or **uptake**. The process by which the virus or its genome enters the host cell cytoplasm. Penetration can be achieved by three separate mechanisms:
   - **endocytosis**: most of the virions taken up by endocytosis appear to be degraded by lysosomal enzymes and therefore fail to initiate infection, but this is the normal route to successful infection by many viruses
   - **fusion**: direct fusion of the viral envelope with the plasma membrane of cells allows the nucleocapsid of some viruses to be released directly into the cytoplasm without an intervening phagocytic process
   - **translocation**: some nonenveloped viruses have the capacity to pass directly through the plasma membrane.

3. **Uncoating** and **eclipse**. After penetration, there is a period during which no intact infectious virus can be detected. This *eclipse phase* begins with uncoating of the lipid membrane and protein capsid surrounding the nucleic acid viral core. As uncoating proceeds, the viral nucleic acid becomes free to act as a template for the synthesis of virus mRNA.

4. **Transcription**. The virus mRNA codes for the synthesis of enzymes necessary to complete the process of uncoating itself and also to initiate early steps in viral replication. When the virus initiates the reproductive cycle within the host cell, the synthesis of host cell RNA is halted, and host ribosomes are free to receive viral mRNA and provide a focus for transcription and synthesis of viral proteins.

5. **Synthesis of viral components**. Viral proteins are of two types:
   - structural (the proteins that make up the virus particle)
   - nonstructural (enzymes required for virus genome replication).
     Structural viral proteins are synthesized on cellular polyribosomes. There is a simultaneous synthesis of progeny viral nucleic acid, using newly synthesized nucleic acid polymerases.

6. **Assembly**. Viral assembly is accomplished by incorporation of viral nucleic acid into putative capsomeres—**procapsids**. Assembly may occur in the cell nucleus, cytoplasm or (with enveloped viruses) at the plasma membrane.

7. **Release** may occur either through gradual budding, in the case of enveloped viruses, or by sudden rupture.

The foregoing is a brief, composite picture of processes involved in viral multiplication. It should be noted that the replication cycle of each family of viruses has unique characteristics that differ from other viruses.

Pathogenesis of Viral Infections

See Chapter 5.

Cellular Antiviral Response

The antiviral response is mostly mediated immunologically and is described in Part 2.

Prions and Prion Diseases

Prions (proteinaceous infectious particles) are unique elements in nature, and they are the agents of a group of chronic diseases called *prion diseases* or **transmissible spongiform encephalopathies**. Essentially, they infect the nerve tissues of animals and humans and manifest with long incubation periods lasting up to decades. The relevance of this chronic disease to dentistry relates to (1) the realization that the infectious agent is extremely difficult to destroy and (2) the probability of infection transmission (variant Creutzfeldt–Jakob disease (vCJD)) in clinical settings.

The following are the major features of prions:

- They are neither viruses nor viroids.
- Prions do not have either DNA or RNA.
- The native form of the prion protein, a normal constituent of healthy neural tissues, is designated PrP^c, whereas the disease-related isoform derived from the latter is designated PrP^{Sc}.
- The abnormal form, PrP^{Sc}, is derived from the native precursor by a posttranslational process leading to a conformational change from an α-helical structure to an insoluble β-sheet structure.
- PrP^{Sc} resists destruction and accumulates in the neural tissues, causing vacuolation of cells, leading to a sponge-like appearance (hence the term *spongiform*).
- They have the ability to self-replicate but with a very long incubation period (up to 20 years in humans).
- The prototype prion agent caused scrapie, a central nervous system disease in sheep.
- As the organism is highly resistant to heat, chemical agents and irradiation, either special autoclaving procedures are required to sterilize contaminated instruments or disposable instruments/materials have to be used for surgical procedures on infected patients.
- The prion agent can be transmitted to cows, mink, cats and mice, for instance, when fed with infected material.
- Iatrogenic transmission of prion disease by neurosurgical instruments has been reported.

MAJOR PRION-INDUCED DISEASES OR TRANSMISSIBLE SPONGIFORM ENCEPHALOPATHIES

Kuru

Kuru is the fatal neurological disease first described in societies in Papua New Guinea who consumed human brain. It is no longer prevalent owing to the cessation of this practice.

Creutzfeldt–Jakob Disease

Creutzfeldt–Jakob disease (CJD) is a globally prevalent, rare, chronic encephalopathy; 10% of cases are **familial** and carry the mutated prion gene; the remainder are either **acquired** or **sporadic**. Onset is in middle to late life (age 40–60 years); the clinical course lasts for about 7–18 months.

Variant Creutzfeldt–Jakob disease

A variant form (vCJD) is localized to Europe, especially the United Kingdom; it almost always affects teenagers or young adults. The disease is spread by consumption of prion-infected animal tissues.

PATHOGENESIS

Prions appear to replicate incessantly, first in lymphoid tissue, then in brain cells where they produce intracellular vacuoles and deposition of altered host prion protein (PrP^{Sc}). These vacuoles give rise to the spongelike appearance of the brain on microscopic examination. The disease is uniformly fatal.

TRANSMISSION

Kuru is transmitted in infected human brain by cannibalism. Other modes of CJD transmission are mostly unknown. There are a few reports of possible iatrogenic transmission by medical and surgical procedures; hereditary acquisition occurs in familial cases; contaminated food (beef from cattle with 'mad cow' disease or bovine spongiform encephalopathy) is thought to cause acquired disease.

PREVENTION AND DENTAL IMPLICATIONS

- There is no treatment for or vaccine against prion-induced disease.
- Hence, the only preventive measure is to not consume suspect food (especially any food containing neural tissues).
- The level of infectivity in oral and dental tissues is uncertain, although in one in vitro study of the dental pulp of eight patients, no prion particles could be detected.
- A few retrospective studies indicate no evidence of dental procedures increasing transmission risk, and published iatrogenic transmission studies show no evidence of associated dental procedures.

Due to the inconclusive data on prion transmission, there was a transatlantic divide between the infection control practices in dentistry a few years ago. However, there is now a consensus among the American, British, Australian and European guidelines.

The current guidelines promulgated by the US Centers for Disease Control and Prevention, on this subject state that the general infection control practices, such as standard infection control procedures (see Chapter 37) recommended by national dental associations, are sufficient when treating patients with transmissible spongiform encephalopathy (TSE) during procedures *not* involving neurovascular tissue. Although there is insufficient data indicating transmission of TSEs through major dental procedures, when treating such patients the following extra precautions should be taken:

- Use single-use items and equipment (e.g., needles, burrs, root canal broaches and anaesthetic cartridges).
- Reusable dental broaches and burrs that may have become contaminated with neurovascular tissue should be destroyed after use (by incineration).
- Procedures involving neurovascular tissue should be scheduled for end of day to permit more extensive cleaning and decontamination.

Key Facts

- Viruses are **obligate intracellular parasites**, which are metabolically inert and can only replicate within living cells.
- The virus genome has either DNA or RNA but never both.
- The genome is protected by an outer protein coat (capsid) composed of capsomeres; *nucleocapsid* is the term given to the protein and the viral genome complex.
- The nucleocapsid of viruses is arranged in one of three spatial configurations: **icosahedral, helical** or **complex symmetry**.
- When a lipoprotein surrounds the virus, it is called an *envelope*. Nonenveloped viruses are called *naked viruses*.
- **Peplomers** (spikes) are glycoprotein extensions from the envelope and play a role in the attachment of the virus to the target host cells.
- Viruses are classified into families, genera and species. The attributes used in classification are their symmetry, the

presence or absence of envelope, nucleic acid composition (DNA or RNA), the number of nucleic acid strands and their polarity. In practice, 'common names' are routinely used when describing viruses.

- The stages of viral replication are adsorption, penetration, uncoating, transcription and translation of the genome, assembly of the virus particles and release.
- **Prions** are unique as they are devoid of nucleic acids and are made of self-replicating, low-molecular-weight proteins (PrP); their mode of replication is unclear as yet.
- The human transmissible spongiform encephalopathies (e.g., kuru, CJD) are caused by prions.
- Special precautions for patients with any form of CJD are not required for routine dental procedures, but strict adherence to standard precautions is essential.

Review Questions (answers on p. 388)

Please indicate which answers are true and which are false.

4.1 Viruses:
a. are in general 300–500 nm in size
b. contain either RNA or DNA as the genetic material
c. are termed *naked* if the envelope does not contain spikes
d. exhibit mainly icosahedral or helical symmetry
e. are able to replicate on serum-containing media

4.2 Viruses may cause human diseases by:
a. direct invasion
b. immune mechanisms
c. production of toxins
d. immunosuppression
e. inducing malignant transformation

4.3 Which of the following statements on human viral infections are true?
a. herpesvirus infections are often present with a vesicular rash
b. herpesviruses have the ability to establish latent infections
c. Kaposi's sarcoma is caused by a herpesvirus
d. during viral replication, the transcription phase is followed by the uncoating and eclipse phase
e. measles and mumps are caused by paramyxovirus

4.4 A 30-year-old British man is diagnosed with neurological symptoms compatible with new variant Creutzfeldt–Jakob disease (vCJD). Which of the following statements are true of this infectious agent/infection?
a. the agent is a low-molecular-weight protein devoid of nucleic acids
b. standard precautions are adequate when a dentist attends to this patient
c. the disease has an acute course with eventual resolution
d. a sterilization cycle of 18 min at 134°C is required to destroy the infectious agent
e. dental procedures have been implicated in the transmission of vCJD

4.5 Which of the following statements on viruses are true?
a. bird flu is caused by a coronavirus
b. herpesviruses can stay latent in neural tissue
c. hepadnaviruses are DNA viruses
d. oncoviruses cause leukaemia
e. viruses are metabolically inert

Further Reading

Centers of Disease Control and Prevention. (2021). *Creutzfeldt-Jakob disease, classic CJD: Infection control, iatrogenic transmission of CJD*. https://www.cdc.gov/prions/cjd/infection-control.html.

Evans, A. S., & Kaslow, R. A. (Eds.). (2014). Epidemiologic concepts and methods. In *Viral infections of humans: Epidemiology and control* (5th ed., Ch. 1). Plenum.

Field, D. N., Knipe, D. M., & Howlley, P. M. (Eds.). (2007). *Fields virology* (6th ed.). Lippincott-Raven.

Porter, S. R. (2003). Prion disease: Possible implications for oral health care. *Journal of the American Dental Association, 134*, 1486–1491.

Samaranayake, L. P., Peiris, J. S. M., & Scully, C. (1996). Ebola virus infection: An overview. *British Dental Journal, 180*, 264–266.

Scully, C., & Samaranayake, L. P. (1992). *Clinical virology in oral medicine and dentistry* (Chs. 1 and 2). Cambridge University Press.

5 Pathogenesis of Microbial Disease

If a microorganism is capable of causing disease, it is called a **pathogen**. Fortunately, only a minority of the vast multitude of microorganisms in nature are pathogenic. Whereas some organisms are highly virulent and cause disease in healthy individuals, even with a small inoculum, others cause disease only in compromised individuals when their defences are weak. The latter are called **opportunistic** organisms, as they take the opportunity offered by reduced host defences to cause disease. These opportunists are frequently members of the body's normal flora.

General Aspects of Infection

VIRULENCE

Virulence is a quantitative measure of pathogenicity and is related to an organism's **toxigenic potential** and **invasiveness**. Virulence can be measured by the number of organisms required to cause disease and is designated as LD_{50} or ID_{50}: the LD_{50} is the number of organisms needed to kill half the hosts, and ID_{50} is the number needed to cause infection in half the hosts. These values are determined by inoculation of laboratory animals.

COMMUNICABLE DISEASES

Infections are called *communicable diseases* if they are spread from host to host. Many, but not all, infections are communicable—for example, tuberculosis is communicable, as it

is spread by airborne droplets produced by coughing, but staphylococcal food poisoning is not, as the exotoxin produced by the organism and present in the contaminated food affects only those eating that food. If a disease is highly communicable, it is called a *contagious disease* (e.g., chickenpox).

Depending on the degree of incidence and prevalence of an infectious disease in a community, it may be called an endemic, an epidemic or a pandemic infection:

- An **endemic** infection is constantly present at a low level in a specific population (e.g., endemic malaria in some African countries).

- An infection is an **epidemic** if it occurs much more frequently than usual (e.g., an epidemic of seasonal influenza in the winter).

- An infection is a **pandemic** if it has a worldwide distribution (e.g., COVID-19, and human immunodeficiency virus [HIV] infection).

NATURAL HISTORY OF INFECTIOUS DISEASE

An acute infection generally progresses through four stages:

1. The **incubation period**: This period is the time between the acquisition of the organism or the toxin and the commencement of symptoms (this may vary from hours to days to weeks).
2. The **prodromal period**: Nonspecific symptoms such as fever, malaise and loss of appetite appear during this period.

3. The **acute specific illness**: The characteristic signs and symptoms of the disease are evident during this period.
4. The **recovery period**: The illness subsides and the patient returns to health during this final phase.

A number of organisms may elicit an **inapparent** or **subclinical** infection, without overt symptoms, where the individual remains **asymptomatic** although infected with the organism. On the other hand, once infected, the body may not completely eliminate the pathogen after recovery and some individuals may become **chronic carriers** of the organism (e.g., *Salmonella typhi*, hepatitis B virus); they may shed the organism while remaining healthy. Some infections result in a latent state, after which reactivation of the growth of the organism and recurrence of symptoms may occur at a later stage (e.g., after primary herpes infection, the virus may reside in a latent state in the trigeminal ganglion, causing recurrent herpes labialis from time to time). All of the groups mentioned above including the asymptomatic carriers, and chronic carriers may unknowingly shed pathogenic organisms and spread disease, just as patients with acute symptomatic disease.

Pathogenesis of Bacterial Disease

DETERMINANTS OF BACTERIAL PATHOGENICITY

Bacterial pathogenicity is a vast subject. The following is a brief outline of the ways and means by which bacteria cause disease. The major steps are transmission, adherence to host surfaces, invasiveness, and toxigenicity.

Transmission

Most infections are acquired by **transmission** from external sources—that is, they are **exogenous** in origin. Others are caused by members of the normal flora behaving as opportunist pathogens—that is, they are **endogenous** in origin. Transmission can be by:

- **inhalation:** the airborne route
- **ingestion:** faecal contamination of food and water
- **inoculation:** sexual contact, contaminated needles, skin contact, blood transfusions or biting insects.

There are four important portals (or gates) of entry of pathogens (Table 5.1):

1. skin
2. respiratory tract
3. gastrointestinal tract
4. genitourinary tract.

Adherence to Host Surfaces

Adherence is the first step in infection. Organisms must have the **ability** to stick or **adhere to host surfaces** to be able to cause infection. Some bacteria and fungi have specialized structures or produce substances that facilitate their attachment to the surface of human cells or prostheses (e.g., dentures, artificial heart valves), thereby enhancing their ability to colonize and cause disease. These adherence mechanisms are critical for organisms that attach to mucous membranes; mutants that lack these mechanisms are often nonpathogenic (e.g., the hair-like pili of *Neisseria gonorrhoeae* and *Escherichia coli* mediate their attachment to the urinary tract epithelium; the extracellular polysaccharides of *Streptococcus mutans* help it adhere to enamel surfaces).

Biofilm Formation

Once the organisms adhere to a host surface, they usually tend to aggregate and form intelligent communities of cells called *biofilms*. A **biofilm** is defined as a complex, intelligent and functional community of one or more species of microbes, encased in an **extracellular polysaccharide**

Table 5.1 Portals of Entry of Some Common Pathogens

Portal of Entry	Pathogen	Disease
Skin	*Clostridium tetani*	Tetanus
	Hepatitis B virus	Hepatitis B
Respiratory Tract	*Streptococcus pneumoniae*	Pneumonia
	Neisseria meningitidis	Meningitis
	Haemophilus influenzae	Meningitis
	Mycobacterium tuberculosis	Tuberculosis
	Influenza virus	Influenza
	Rhinovirus	Common cold
	Severe acute respiratory syndrome coronavirus-2 (SARS-CoV-2)	Coronavirus disease-2019 (COVID-19)
	Epstein–Barr virus	Infectious mononucleosis
Gastrointestinal Tract	*Shigella dysenteriae*	Dysentery
	Salmonella typhi	Typhoid fever
	Vibrio cholerae	Cholera
	Hepatitis A virus	Infectious hepatitis
	Poliovirus	Poliomyelitis
Genital Tract	*Neisseria gonorrhoeae*	Gonorrhoea
	Treponema pallidum	Syphilis
	Human immunodeficiency virus (HIV)	Acquired immunodeficiency syndrome (AIDS)
	Candida albicans (fungus)	Vaginitis

matrix and attached to one another or to a solid surface (such as a denture prosthesis or an intravenous catheter). Up to 65% of human infections are thought to be associated with microbial biofilms. **Dental plaque** on enamel surfaces is a classic example of a biofilm. As biofilms are ubiquitous in nature and form on hulls of ships, warm water pipes, dental unit water systems (see Chapter 38) and so on, their study has rapidly evolved during the past few decades, leading to many discoveries on communal behaviour of microbes.

As mentioned, biofilms are intelligent, functional communities. Structurally, they are not flat, amorphous, and compressed but comprise a complex architecture with towers and mushroom- or dome-shaped structures traversed by so called *water channels* that permit transport of metabolites and nutrients (Figs. 5.1–5.3). Bacteria in biofilms maintain the population composition by constantly secreting low levels of chemicals called **quorum-sensing molecules** (e.g., homoserine lactone), which tend either to repel the invading, extraneous 'enemy' organisms or activate the communal bacteria to seek new abodes, and leave the parent brood. Further, specific gene activation may lead to production of virulence factors or reduction in metabolic activity (especially those living deep within the matrix).

It is now known that infections associated with biofilms are difficult to eradicate, as **sessile or biofilm phase organisms** exhibit higher resistance to antimicrobials than their free-living or **planktonic phase** counterparts. The reasons for this appear to be (Fig. 5.4):

- protection offered by the extracellular polysaccharide matrix from the host immune mechanisms (e.g., immunoglobulins, lactoferrin)
- poor penetration of any antimicrobials (prescribed for the specific disease) into the deeper layers of the biofilm
- degradation of these antimicrobials as they slowly penetrate the biofilm
- difference in pH, and redox potential (E_h) gradients not conducive for the optimal activity of any antimicrobials
- gene expression leading to more virulent or resistant organisms.

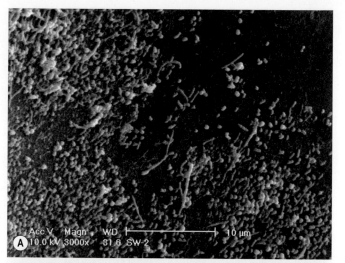

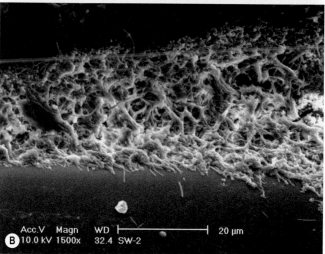

Fig. 5.1 The ultrastructure of (A) an early biofilm on a dental appliance showing the deposition of coccal and bacillary forms; (B) a mature dental plaque biofilm on a dental appliance showing the advancing edge and the complex architecture.
(Courtesy Dr Bernard Low.)

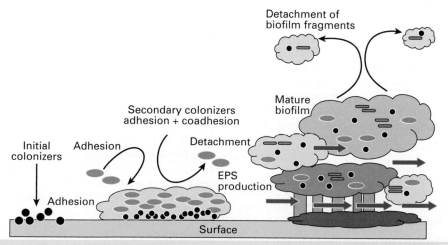

Fig. 5.2 A schematic diagram depicting the various developmental stages of a biofilm from the initial adherent phase *(left)* of the organisms to gradual maturation and subsequent fully developed polymicrobial biofilm (*extreme right*). *EPS,* Extracellular polysaccharide.

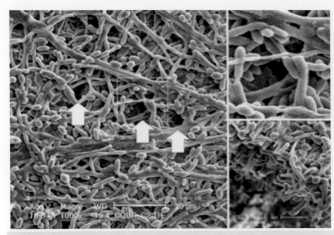

Fig. 5.3 A mature *Candida albicans* biofilm showing water channels (*arrows*) that mediate metabolite and nutrition transfer to and from the biofilm (*inset:* magnified channel architecture).

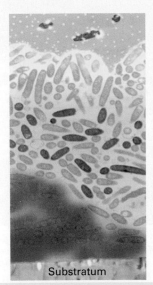

Slow penetration

Antibiotic (yellow) may fail to penetrate beyond the surface layers of the biofilm.

Resistant phenotype

Some of the bacteria may differentiate into a protected phenotypic state (green).

Altered microenvironment

In zones of nutrient depletion or waste product accumulation (red), antibiotic action may be antagonized.

Substratum

Fig. 5.4 Postulated mechanisms of antibiotic resistance in biofilms: The attachment surface is shown at the bottom and the aqueous phase containing the antibiotic at the top. (Modified from Stewart, P.S., & Costerton, J.W. (2001). Antibiotic resistance of bacteria in biofilms. *Lancet, 358,* 135–138.)

Some examples of important recalcitrant human infections mediated by biofilms, which are difficult to manage by antimicrobials alone, include *Pseudomonas aeruginosa* infections of the respiratory tract in cystic fibrosis patients, *Staphylococcus aureus* infections in patients with central venous catheters, chronic candidal infections of HIV-infected individuals, and chronic periodontal infections due to dental plaque biofilms.

Invasiveness

Invasiveness of bacteria plays a critical role in pathogenesis; this property is dependent upon secreted bacterial enzymes. Examples include the following:

- **Collagenase** and **hyaluronidase** degrade the intercellular matrix, permitting easy spread of bacteria through tissues. This is especially important in skin

infections, as these chemicals can break the tough epithelia barrier (e.g., *Streptococcus pyogenes* skin infections).

- **Coagulase**, produced by *Staphylococcus aureus*, accelerates the formation of a fibrin clot (from fibrinogen). It helps protect organisms from phagocytosis by walling off the infected area and by coating the organisms with a fibrin layer.
- **Immunoglobulin A (IgA) protease** degrades protective IgA on mucosal surfaces, allowing organisms such as *N. gonorrhoeae*, *Haemophilus influenzae* and *Streptococcus pneumoniae* to adhere to mucous membranes.
- **Leukocidins** can destroy both neutrophilic leukocytes and macrophages; the periodontopathic organism *Aggregatibacter actinomycetemcomitans* possesses this enzyme. The mutants that do not secrete the enzyme are less virulent.

Other factors also contribute to invasiveness by interfering with the host defence mechanisms, especially phagocytosis:

- The polysaccharide **capsule** of several common pathogens, such as *Streptococcus pneumoniae* and *Neisseria meningitidis*, prevents the phagocyte from adhering to the bacteria. (This can be verified by the introduction of anticapsular antibodies, which allow more effective phagocytosis or opsonization to occur. Thus the vaccines against *Streptococcus pneumoniae* and *N. meningitidis* contain capsular polysaccharides that induce protective **anticapsular antibodies**.)
- The **cell wall proteins** of the Gram-positive cocci, such as the M protein of the group A streptococci and protein A of the staphylococci, are also antiphagocytic (Table 5.2).

Bacterial infection may lead to two categories of inflammation: **pyogenic** (pus producing) and **granulomatous** (granuloma forming).

Pyogenic Inflammation. The neutrophils are the predominant cells in pyogenic inflammation. *Streptococcus pyogenes*, *Staphylococcus aureus* and *Streptococcus pneumoniae* are the common pyogenic bacteria.

Granulomatous Inflammation. Macrophages and T cells predominate in granulomatous inflammation. The most notable organism in this category is *Mycobacterium tuberculosis*, which causes tuberculosis. Here, the bacterial antigens stimulate the cell-mediated immune system, resulting in sensitized T-lymphocyte and macrophage activity. Although the phagocytic activity of macrophages kills most of the tubercle bacilli, some survive and grow within these cells, leading to **granuloma formation**. The organisms reside within **phagosomes**, which are unable to fuse with lysosomes, resulting in protection from degradative enzymes therein. Many fungal diseases are also characterized by granulomatous lesions.

Toxigenicity

Toxin production or toxigenicity is another major mediator of bacterial disease. **Toxins** are of two categories:

Table 5.2   Examples of Surface Virulence Factors That Interfere With Host Defences

Organism	Virulence Factor	Used in Vaccine
Bacteria		
Streptococcus pneumoniae	Polysaccharide capsule	Yes
Streptococcus pyogenes	M protein	No
Staphylococcus aureus	Protein A	No
Neisseria meningitidis	Polysaccharide capsule	Yes
Haemophilus influenzae	Polysaccharide capsule	Yes
Klebsiella pneumoniae	Polysaccharide capsule	No
Escherichia coli	Protein pili	No
Salmonella typhi	Polysaccharide capsule	No
Mycobacterium tuberculosis	Mycolic acid cell wall	No
Fungi		
Cryptococcus neoformans	Capsule	No

Table 5.3   Comparison of the Main Features of Exotoxins and Endotoxins

Property	Exotoxin	Endotoxin
Source	Some species of some Gram-positive and Gram-negative bacteria	Cell walls of Gram-negative bacteria
Origin	Secreted from cell	Cell wall constituent
Chemistry	Polypeptide	Lipopolysaccharide
Toxicity	High (fatal dose of the order of 1 µg)	Low (fatal dose in the order of hundreds of micrograms)
Clinical Effects	Variable	Fever, shock
Antigenicity	Induces high-titre antibodies called antitoxins	Poorly antigenic
Vaccines	Toxoids used as vaccines	No toxoids formed and no vaccine available
Heat Stability	Most are thermolabile (destroyed rapidly at 60°C)	Thermostable at 100°C for 1 h
Typical Diseases	Cholera, tetanus, diphtheria	Sepsis by Gram-negative rods, endotoxic shock

endotoxins and exotoxins. Their main features are shown in Table 5.3.

TOXIN PRODUCTION

Endotoxins

Endotoxins are the cell wall **lipopolysaccharides (LPS)** of Gram-negative bacteria (both cocci and bacilli) and are not actively released from the cell. (*Note:* Thus, by definition, Gram-positive organisms do not possess endotoxins.) Endotoxins cause fever, shock and other generalized symptoms causing endotoxic shock.

A number of biological effects of endotoxins are described in the following text. These are mainly due to the production of host factors such as **interleukin-1 (IL-1)** and **tumour necrosis factor (TNF)** from macrophages:

1. **Fever** is due to the release of endogenous pyrogens (IL-1) by macrophages; these act on the hypothalamic temperature regulatory centre and reset the body *thermostat* at a higher temperature.
2. **Hypotension**, shock and reduced perfusion of major organs due to vasodilatation are brought about by bradykinin release, increased vascular permeability and decreased peripheral resistance.

3. Activation of the **alternative pathway of the complement cascade** results in inflammation and tissue damage.
4. Generalized **activation of the coagulation system** (via factor XII) leads to disseminated intravascular coagulation (DIC), thrombosis and tissue ischaemia.
5. **Increased phagocytic activity** of macrophages and polyclonal B cell activation (but not T lymphocytes).
6. Increased antibody production.

Endotoxin-like effects may also occur in Gram-positive bacteraemic infections. However, as endotoxin is absent in Gram-positive bacteria, other cell wall components, such as teichoic acid or peptidoglycan, are thought to trigger the release of TNF and IL-1 from macrophages.

Exotoxins

Both Gram-positive and Gram-negative bacteria secrete exotoxins (Table 5.4), whereas endotoxin is an integral component of the cell wall of Gram-negative organisms. Hence, by definition, **Gram-positive bacteria do not produce endotoxins**.

Exotoxins, in particular, can cause disease in distant parts of the body as a result of diffusion or carriage of the toxin

Table 5.4   Some Important Bacterial Exotoxins and Their Mode of Action

Organism	Disease	Mode of Action	Toxoid Vaccine
Gram-Positive			
Corynebacterium diphtheriae	Diphtheria	Elongation factor inactivated by ADP-ribosylation	Yes
Clostridium tetani	Tetanus	Tetanospasmin blocks release of the inhibitory neurotransmitter glycine at motor nerve ends	Yes
Clostridium welchii (perfringens)	Gas gangrene	Alpha-toxin: a lecithinase destroys eukaryotic cell membranes	No
Staphylococcus aureus	Toxic shock	Binds to class II MHC protein; induces IL-1 and IL-2	No
Gram-Negative			
Escherichia coli	Diarrhoea	Labile toxin stimulates adenylate cyclase by ADP-ribosylation; stable toxin stimulates guanylate cyclase	No
Vibrio cholerae	Cholera	Stimulates adenylate cyclase by ADP-ribosylation	No
Bordetella pertussis	Whooping cough	Stimulates adenylate cyclase by ADP-ribosylation	No

ADP, Adenosine diphosphate; *IL*, interleukin; *MHC*, major histocompatibility complex.

via systemic routes (e.g., tetanus bacillus infecting a lesion in the foot produces an exotoxin, which causes 'lockjaw,' or spasm of masseter muscles on the face).

Exotoxins are polypeptides whose genes are frequently located on plasmids or lysogenic bacterial viruses. Essentially, these polypeptides consist of two domains or subunits: one for binding to the cell membrane and entry into the cell, and the other possessing the toxic activity.

Exotoxins are highly toxic (e.g., the fatal dose of tetanus toxin for a human can be less than 1 μg). Fortunately, exotoxin polypeptides are good antigens and induce the synthesis of protective antibodies called **antitoxins**, which are useful in the prevention or treatment of diseases such as tetanus. The toxicity of the polypeptides can be neutralized when treated with formaldehyde (or acid or heat), and these **toxoids** are used in protective vaccines because they retain their antigenicity.

Bacterial exotoxins can be broadly categorized as:

- neurotoxins
- enterotoxins
- miscellaneous exotoxins.

Neurotoxins. Tetanus toxin, diphtheria toxin and botulinum toxin are all neurotoxins and their action is mediated via neuronal pathways.

Tetanus toxin, produced by *Clostridium tetani*, is a neurotoxin that prevents the release of the inhibitory neurotransmitter glycine, thus causing muscle spasms (see Fig. 13.4). Tetanus toxin (tetanospasmin) comprises two polypeptide subunits: a heavy chain and a light chain. The former binds to the gangliosides in the membrane of the neuron, whereas the latter is the toxic component. The toxin is liberated at the peripheral wound site but is transmitted to the neurons of the spinal cord either by retrograde axonal transport or in the blood stream. There it blocks the release of the inhibitory transmitter, which leads to sustained and convulsive contractions of the voluntary muscles (e.g., *risus sardonicus*, contraction of the facial muscles; *lockjaw*, contraction of the masseter muscles; see Chapter 13).

Diphtheria toxin, produced by *Corynebacterium diphtheriae*, is synthesized as a single polypeptide with two functional domains. Once secreted, one domain mediates the binding of the toxin to cell membrane receptors; the other domain possesses enzymatic activity and inhibits protein synthesis in all eukaryotic cells. The enzyme activity is highly potent: a single molecule can kill a cell within a few hours. *E. coli*, *Vibrio cholerae* and *Bordetella pertussis* also possess exotoxins that act in a similar manner.

Botulinum toxin, produced by *Clostridium botulinum*, is one of the most toxic compounds known (1 μg will kill a human). The toxin blocks the release of acetylcholine at the synapse, producing paralysis of both voluntary and involuntary muscles. The toxin, encoded by the genes of a bacteriophage, comprises two polypeptide subunits.

Enterotoxins. Enterotoxins act on the gut mucosa and cause gastrointestinal disturbances.

E. coli enterotoxin is of two types: heat labile and heat stable. The heat-labile toxin (inactivated at 65°C in 30 min) is composed of two domains: one binds to a ganglioside in the cell membrane, whereas the other is the active component and mediates synthesis of cyclic adenosine monophosphate (cAMP) in the mucosal cells of the small intestine. This leads to an increase in the concentration of cAMP, which promotes cellular chloride ion excretion and inhibition of sodium ion absorption. The net result is fluid and electrolyte loss into the lumen of the gut (diarrhoea).

The heat-stable toxin of *E. coli* (not inactivated by boiling for 30 min) stimulates guanylate cyclase and thus increases the concentration of cyclic guanosine monophosphate (cGMP), which inhibits the reabsorption of sodium ions and causes diarrhoea (compare with heat-labile toxin). The genes for both toxins are carried on a plasmid.

The enterotoxins produced by the diarrhoea-causing organisms *V. cholerae* and *Bacillus cereus* act in a manner similar to that of the heat-labile toxin of *E. coli*.

Miscellaneous Exotoxins. An array of exotoxins is produced by *Clostridium welchii* and other species of clostridia that cause gas gangrene. These include the α-toxin (a phospholipase that hydrolyses lecithin, present in all eukaryotic cell membranes), collagenase, protease, hyaluronidase and deoxyribonuclease (DNAase). As the names imply, they destroy the cells and the connective tissue by a multiplicity of actions. In addition, a heterogeneous group of toxins with haemolytic and necrotizing activity has been identified in clostridia.

Pathogenesis of Viral Disease

Viral pathogenesis can be defined as the methods by which viruses produce disease in the host. The vast majority of viral infections are **subclinical** (symptomless or asymptomatic) and go almost unrecognized. One individual may succumb to disease with an infection by a virus, whereas another may be entirely asymptomatic when infected by the identical strain of virus. The genetic factors, immunity, nutrition and other host factors influence the outcome of viral infection. The study of viral pathogenesis can be considered at two levels: first, at the level of the virus (parasite) and, second, at the level of the host.

METHODS OF VIRAL ENTRY

As in bacterial infections, viruses gain entry into the host by:

- inoculation (via the skin and mucosa)
- inhalation (via the respiratory tract)
- ingestion (via the gastrointestinal tract).

See Fig. 5.5. (*Note:* Although in this section viruses are considered separately, very similar host defence mechanisms operate to prevent the entry of all other pathogens through these portals.)

Skin and Mucosa

The skin is an effective barrier against viral infection, as the dead cells of the stratum corneum cannot support viral replication. Breach of skin integrity occurs:

- during accidental abrasions or needle-stick injuries that may accidentally occur in dental practice (during vaccination, an avirulent, attenuated virus may be deliberately inoculated into the skin)
- via the bites of arthropod vectors—for example, mosquitoes and ticks (these infect the host either because their saliva is infected as a result of viral multiplication within the arthropod); yellow fever virus in mosquitoes; or because vector mouthparts are contaminated with the virus)
- as a result of deep inoculation into the subcutaneous tissue and muscle, which can follow hypodermic needle injections, tattooing, acupuncture, ear-piercing or animal bites. Once a virus has reached the dermis, it has access to blood and lymphatic vessels as well as to macrophages, so the infection may spread readily (Fig. 5.6).

Oropharynx and Intestinal Tract

Natural defence mechanisms of the mouth and the gastrointestinal tract that prevent viral entry are:

- continuous desquamation of the epithelium or the oral mucosa
- presence of saliva, the mucous layer of the intestine, gastric acid, bile and proteolytic enzymes, all of which nonspecifically inhibit viral entry

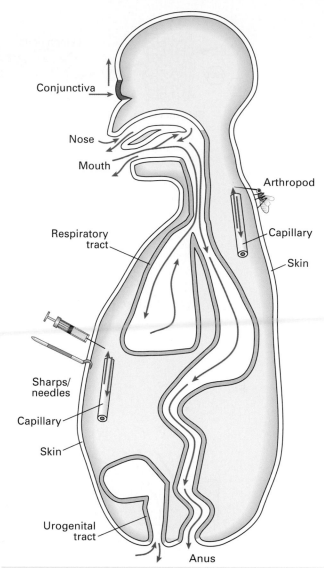

Fig. 5.5   Sites of the body where viral infections may ensue and subsequent shedding may occur.

- mechanical movements of the tongue, cheek, peristalsis and so on
- immune mechanisms (see Chapter 8).

Respiratory Tract

A number of defence mechanisms operate to prevent viral entry through the respiratory tract. These include:

- secretion of mucus by goblet cells; this, propelled by the action of ciliated epithelial cells, clears inhaled foreign material (the mucociliary escalator)
- IgA present in respiratory secretions
- alveolar phagocytic cells.

To gain access to the respiratory tract, viruses need to be primarily in the form of aerosol particles or droplets. Other factors that affect viral respiratory infection include humidity and air temperature (e.g., influenza is more common in the winter) and the physical and chemical properties and structure of the virus particle.

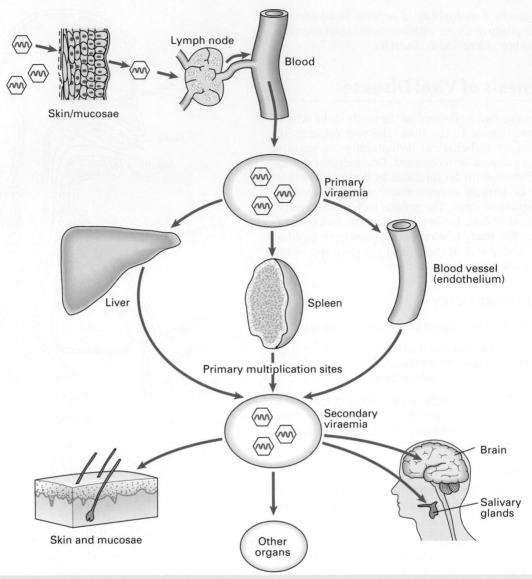

Fig. 5.6   The spread of viral infection in the body. (Note that viruses differ in their replicating sites and target organs.)

Genitourinary Tract

The vagina and urethra can be portals for entry of viral infection. The host factors that can influence viral entry via these routes include:

- natural mucosal desquamation
- vaginal secretions and cervical mucus, which contain both specific and nonspecific defence factors
- intermittent flushing action of urine.

Sexual activity may cause tears or abrasions of the vaginal epithelium or trauma to the urethra, allowing viral ingress. Sexually transmitted viruses in humans include HIV, herpesviruses, human papillomaviruses and most hepatitis viruses.

MECHANISMS OF VIRAL SPREAD IN THE BODY

Viruses, unlike some bacteria, are completely devoid of organelles of transport, and they spread throughout the body by a number of routes. These include:

- direct local spread on epithelial and subepithelial surfaces
- lymphatic spread
- blood stream spread (viraemia)
- central nervous system and peripheral nerve spread.

Local Spread on Body Surfaces

A number of viruses cause disease on epithelial surfaces without systemic spread. Such infections are characterized by:

- their localized nature
- direct viral shedding into the exterior or lumen (e.g., respiratory tract and alimentary tract infections with rhinoviruses and rotaviruses, respectively).

Once an invading virus overcomes the epithelial barrier, it is exposed to the second line of body defences in the form of **phagocytic cells**, predominantly histiocytes of the macrophage series. When the virus is **phagocytosed**, it will be destroyed not only by the low pH conditions in the phagocytic vesicle but also by enzymes in the **phagolysosome**. Some viruses have developed mechanisms to evade this type of defence and, indeed, replicate within the macrophages.

Lymphatic Spread

The phagocytosed and free viral particles lurking beneath the epithelium rapidly enter the subepithelial/mucosal network of lymphatic capillaries and are carried to regional lymph nodes (Fig. 5.6). Lymph nodes serve two main functions:

1. They act as filters of extraneous microbes that gain access to the lymphatic system.
2. They are the sites where immune responses are generated.

Soon after entering the lymph node, viruses are exposed to the macrophages lining the marginal sinus. If the virus is phagocytosed, antigens are presented to the underlying lymphoid cells to evoke an immune response, upon which the outcome of the infection depends. If the virus is inactivated, the infection resolves. However the organism may infect macrophages and lymphocytes if the immune response at this stage is inadequate (e.g., herpesviruses, measles). The virus particles that escape the **nodal filter** can then enter the blood stream via the efferent lymphatics and the thoracic duct (Fig. 5.6).

There is a constant bidirectional movement of macrophages and lymphocytes from the blood into lymph nodes and *vice versa*. Thus, if a virus infects cells in lymph nodes without damaging them, these cells can act as vehicles of virus dissemination. Sometimes, the virus infects and multiplies in lymphatic endothelium, further increasing the virus load reaching the node and hence the lymphatic system. Viruses do not appear to enter the local blood vessels directly, except perhaps when these are damaged mechanically by trauma (e.g., needle-stick injuries, bites). These events are closely followed by a local inflammatory response that alters the eventual outcome of the viral infection, as described in the following section.

Viraemia and Spread to Organs

The entry of virus into the blood and its subsequent spread is called **viraemia**. Once a virus reaches the blood stream, it is effectively disseminated within minutes. The first episode of viral entry into the blood is called a **primary viraemia** (Fig. 5.6). The virus may then be seeded in various distant organs, after which there is further replication at these sites and a second wave of viral entry into the blood stream, a **secondary viraemia**. This is usually larger than the primary viraemia, and the virus is more easily detected in blood samples. The secondary viraemia often leads to infection of other organs.

Viruses may be free in the plasma, in blood cells or in both (Fig. 5.7). Those in the plasma can be cleared relatively easily, but viruses in leukocytes are not easily destroyed. If the infected leukocyte remains healthy, it may disseminate infection to distant body sites. Once a virus reaches an organ, its localization depends on its ability to attach to and grow in vascular endothelial cells, and on phagocytosis by reticuloendothelial cells.

Central Nervous System and Peripheral Nerve Spread

During a viraemia, circulating viruses invade the central nervous system by localizing in the blood vessels of:

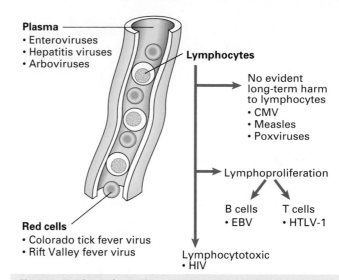

Fig. 5.7   Carriage of some important viruses in different compartments of blood. *CMV*, Cytomegalovirus; *EBV*, Epstein–Barr virus; *HIV*, human immunodeficiency virus; *HTLV-I*, human T-cell leukaemia virus type I.

- the meninges and choroid plexus, with subsequent passage via cerebrospinal fluid into the neural tissues (e.g., mumps virus)
- the spinal cord or brain, with subsequent direct infection (e.g., poliovirus).

The process of localization is enhanced when there is an associated inflammatory focus. Peripheral nerves act as an effective path of transmission for some viruses, such as herpes simplex virus. Viral passage can be either **centripetal** (from body surface inwards), as in rabies, or **centrifugal**, as in reactivation of herpes simplex (herpes labialis) or varicella-zoster virus. This mode of transport is a slow process (mm/h) compared with viraemic spread. Four possible routes of viral transmission in peripheral nerves are known:

1. axon
2. endoneural cell (e.g., Schwann cell)
3. connective tissue space between nerves
4. perineural lymphatics.

VIRUS AND HOST CELL INTERACTIONS

Once the virus enters the host cell, it can interact with the host cell in two main ways:

1. **permissive infection**, in which there is synthesis of viral components, their assembly and release
2. **nonpermissive infection**, in which the infection can result in cell transformation, often with the integration of viral DNA into the host genome.

Permissive Infection

The infection of a cell by a virus may have one or more sequelae (Fig. 5.8). The most common sequela is for the virus to replicate in a lytic or **cytocidal infection**, causing the cells to die and producing an acute illness. A virus-infected cell may die as a result of:

- 'shut-down' of host cell protein and nucleic acid synthesis

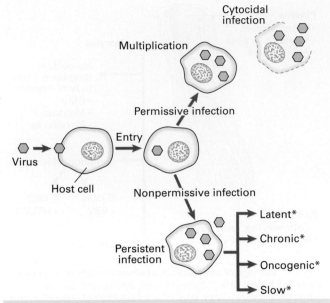

Fig. 5.8   **The possible effects of viruses on host cells.** (*See Fig. 5.9.)

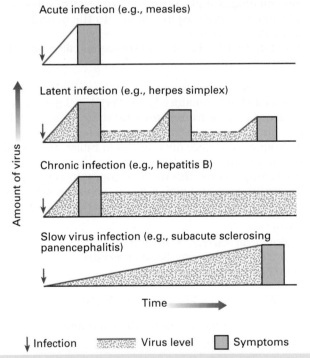

Fig. 5.9   Modes of viral infection, as a function of time (oncogenic infection not shown).

- cell lysis, by the release of progeny virions
- intracellular release of lysosomal enzymes
- damage to cell membranes.

The adverse cellular consequence of viral infection, particularly that observed in virus-infected cells in tissue culture, is termed the **cytopathic effect** (see Chapter 6). During the early phase of infection, before cell death, characteristic alterations in the infected cell membrane may occur. Haemadsorption and giant cell formation are two examples.

Haemadsorption. In viruses that leave the cell by budding through the plasma membrane, viral glycoproteins (destined for the envelope) are first inserted into the membrane. A common envelope protein is haemagglutinin; this protein enables an infected cell to attract red cells at its surface, a phenomenon called *haemadsorption*. Haemadsorption can be used in the laboratory to detect cells infected with certain viruses (e.g., orthoreoviruses and paramyxoviruses).

Giant Cell Formation. Some viruses, such as herpes simplex and HIV, promote cell fusion in which membranes of adjacent cells coalesce to produce multinucleated giant cells (polykaryons, syncytia). Other markers of viral infection include intranuclear or cytoplasmic inclusion bodies.

Nonpermissive Infection

Cell death is not an inevitable accompaniment of viral replication. Sometimes a **persistent infection** may ensue in which there may be viral replication within the cell but the cell remains alive. Many viruses can produce persistent infections. Some relevant examples are hepatitis B virus, papillomaviruses, herpesviruses and retroviruses. Factors that favour persistence include:

- low pathogenicity of the virus
- ineffective or no antibody-mediated or cell-mediated host immune responses
- defective or no interferon production
- infection of lymphocytes and macrophages by the virus.

There are four categories of persistent infection: latent, chronic, oncogenic and slow (Fig. 5.9).

Latent Viral Infections. Latent viral infections occur when viral nucleic acids persist in the cell, usually integrated into the host DNA as a **provirus** (e.g., HIV, herpes simplex virus, varicella-zoster virus). Because herpes simplex infection can be considered as the classic example of latent infection, the mechanism of its persistence is described. After an acute infection, the herpes simplex virus travels along sensory nerve fibres (intra-axonal transport) to the appropriate dorsal root ganglion (e.g., in oral herpes, the virus travels to the trigeminal ganglion). During latency, infectious virus is undetectable, but the virus may be recovered by growing ganglion fragments in tissue culture. The reemergence of virus is prevented, possibly due to host cell–mediated immunity, but when this wanes, there may be recrudescence and shedding of the virus in secretions from the area. Similarly, varicella-zoster virus remains latent for many years and may spontaneously recur as zoster (shingles) on dermatomes supplied by the specific sensory ganglion in which the virus is latent. Latent viral infections are reactivated particularly in immunocompromised patients, who subsequently suffer from infection and excrete the virus (see Chapter 21).

Chronic Infections. Chronic infections occur when viruses persist in quantity in the body over a prolonged period, with or without a history of disease. Chronically infected individuals, who are often asymptomatic, are called **carriers** and are an important potential source of infection for others. Carriers make up a significant but unknown proportion of patients treated by dental health care workers (see Chapter 36). The main difference between chronic and latent infections is that the virus is **continuously detectable** in the former but not in the latter.

Oncogenic Infections. Oncogenic infections are persistent infections in which genetic and developmental factors are important in determining whether a particular virus is oncogenic in a given host (e.g., Epstein–Barr virus causing nasopharyngeal carcinoma and Burkitt lymphoma).

Slow Virus Infections. Slow virus infections are rare, with incubations lasting months or years, leading to severe disability and eventual death (e.g., prion diseases or subacute sclerosing panencephalitis, a late consequence of measles).

TRANSMISSION OF VIRAL INFECTIONS AND INFECTION CONTROL

See Chapters 21 and 36.

HOST DETERMINANTS OF VIRAL INFECTION

The outcome of viral infection in a host depends not only on the type and virulence of the virus but also on host factors, including:

- **immune status** (see Chapter 10)
- **genetic constitution**. Genetic factors are now known to influence susceptibility to infection by herpesviruses, myxoviruses and poxviruses. Susceptibility may also be associated with the presence of the appropriate host cell receptors on target cells.
- **age**. Some viruses (such as mumps, polio, Epstein–Barr virus or hepatitis) tend to produce less severe infection in infants, whereas others (such as respiratory syncytial virus and rotavirus) are more severe in children. The basis for this type of age dependence of viral infection is not clear.
- **miscellaneous factors**. Hormonal and nutritional status may influence the outcome of viral infections, as shown by the fact that a number of viral infections (e.g., polio, hepatitis A and B) are often more severe during pregnancy, and protein malnutrition dramatically exacerbates the severity of measles infection. Personal habits (e.g., cigarette smoking) may influence the outcome of viral infections such as influenza, possibly due to impaired mucociliary clearance in the respiratory tract. Further, it is known that preceding vigorous exercise may accentuate the severity of a subsequent bout of poliomyelitis.

Pathogenesis of Fungal Disease

See Chapter 22.

Koch's Postulates

A wide spectrum of microbes inhabit the human body. Some are permanent residents living as commensals, others are transient organisms and still others are commensals that behave as pathogens under suitable conditions (opportunistic pathogens). Hence, when infection supervenes, it is important to differentiate a commensal from a pathogen in order to identify and eliminate the latter. This problem was encountered in 1877 by Robert Koch, a German general practitioner, when he tried to determine the cause of an anthrax infection in cattle and tuberculosis in humans. Koch defined the criteria for attributing an organism as the cause of specific disease. These criteria, called **Koch's postulates**, are as follows:

1. The organism must be isolated from every patient with the disease, and its distribution in the body must correspond to that of the lesions observed.
2. The organism must be isolated and then cultured outside the body (in vitro) in pure culture.
3. The pure organism must cause the disease in healthy, susceptible animals.
4. The organism must then be recoverable from the inoculated animal.

Currently, these four postulates are complemented by another:

5. The antibody to the organism should be detected in the patient's serum.

Clearly, these are ideal criteria and are not always attainable in practice (e.g., *Mycobacterium leprae*, the leprosy bacillus, cannot be cultured in vitro), but they provide a framework for establishing an aetiological role of organisms in infectious diseases. Furthermore, Koch's postulates are becoming less applicable, with the advent of nucleic acid–based methods of microbial identification. These methods have revealed a great deal about microbes that are associated with pathology, and proving causation has become even more difficult, leading to revision of Koch's postulates (see Further Reading).

Key Facts

- The **virulence** of an organism can be measured by its **toxigenic potential** and **invasiveness**.
- Infections are either **endogenous** or **exogenous**, depending on whether the pathogen is derived from the patient's own flora or from an external source.
- **Transmission** of a pathogen to an infective focus can occur via **inhalation**, **ingestion**, or **inoculation**.
- The **ability** of an organism to **adhere to host surfaces** is a **prerequisite** for initiating infection.
- A **biofilm** is defined as an aggregate of interactive bacteria attached to a solid surface or to each other, encased in an extracellular polysaccharide matrix.
- **Sessile organisms** or attached bacteria within biofilms are more resistant to antimicrobials than their free-living, suspended, **planktonic** counterparts.
- Bacterial infection leads to pyogenic and granulomatous inflammation.
- **Toxins** of bacteria are classified as *endotoxins* or *exotoxins*.
- **Endotoxins** are the **lipopolysaccharide (LPS)** components of cell walls of Gram-negative bacteria, and hence, by definition, Gram-positive bacteria do not produce endotoxins.
- **Exotoxins** can be produced by both **Gram-positive bacteria** and **Gram-negative bacteria**; they are polypeptides whose genes are frequently located on plasmids or lysogenic bacterial viruses.
- **Biological effects of endotoxins** include fever, hypotension, activation of complement cascade, disseminated intravascular coagulation (DIC) and increased phagocytic activity of macrophages.
- **Attenuated exotoxins** of bacteria are called **toxoids**; they are not toxic but are antigenic and hence used in protective vaccines.
- Viruses, once they gain entry, spread throughout the body by direct local spread, lymphatics, blood (viraemia) and the central and peripheral nervous systems.
- Virus entry into a host cell may result in abortive, cytocidal, latent, chronic, oncogenic (transforming) or slow infection.

Review Questions (Answers on p. 388)

Please indicate which answers are true and which are false.

5.1. The effects of endotoxins on the body include:
   a. fever
   b. complement activation
   c. hypertension
   d. disseminated intravascular coagulation
   e. multiple organ dysfunction

5.2. Which of the following statements on bacterial toxins are true?
   a. All Gram-negative bacteria possess endotoxins.
   b. The lethal dose of endotoxin is much higher than exotoxin.
   c. Exotoxins are polypeptides, and endotoxins are lipopolysaccharides.
   d. Endotoxins are poorly antigenic.
   e. The heat-labile enterotoxin of *Escherichia coli* produces the same clinical effects as the cholera toxin.

5.3. Which of the following statements on microbial biofilms are true?
   a. Dental plaque is a highly complex polymicrobial biofilm.
   b. Planktonic bacteria in biofilms aggregate to form mushroomlike structures.
   c. In general, biofilm bacteria are resistant to antimicrobials.
   d. Biofilms in dental unit water lines may pose an infectious threat.
   e. Quorum-sensing molecular signals help maintain the optimal communal size of the biofilm.

5.4. Which of the following statements on viral infections are true?
   a. Most human tumours are caused by oncogenic viruses.
   b. Viral load in the blood is higher during primary viraemia than during secondary viraemia.
   c. Some infections can be diagnosed by isolating the virus in faeces.
   d. A rising antibody titre is helpful in the diagnosis of viral infections.
   e. Giant cell formation is an example of viral cytopathic effect.

Further Reading

Costerton, J. W., Stewart, P. S., & Greenberg, E. P. (1999). Bacterial biofilms: A common cause of persistent infections. *Science, 284*, 1318–1322.

Filoche, S., Wong, L., & Sissons, C. H. (2010). Oral biofilms: Emerging concepts in microbial ecology. *Journal of Dental Research, 89*, 8–18.

Fredericks, D. N., & Relman, D. A. (1996). Sequence-based identification of microbial pathogens: A reconsideration of Koch's postulates. *Clinical Microbiology Reviews, 9*, 18–33.

Inglewski, B. H., & Clark, L. V. (Eds.). (1990). *The bacteria: Molecular basis of bacterial pathogenesis*, (Vol. 11). Academic Press.

Mims, C., Dimmock, N., Nash, A., et al. (1995). *Mims' pathogenesis of infectious disease* (4th ed.). Academic Press.

Seneviratne, C., Jin, L., & Samaranayake, L. (2008). Biofilm lifestyle of *Candida*: A mini review. *Oral Diseases, 14*, 582–590.

Stewart, P. S., & Costerton, J. W. (2001). Antibiotic resistance of bacterial biofilms. *Lancet, 358*, 135–138.

6 Diagnostic Microbiology and Laboratory Methods

Diagnostic Microbiology

Diagnostic microbiology involves the study of specimens taken from patients suspected of having infections. The end result is a report that should assist the clinician in reaching a **definitive diagnosis** and a **decision on antimicrobial therapy**. Hence, clinicians should be acquainted with the techniques of taking specimens and

understand the essential principles and techniques behind laboratory analysis.

The diagnosis of an infectious disease entails a number of decisions and actions by many people. The diagnostic cycle begins when the clinician takes a microbiological sample, and it ends when the clinician receives the laboratory report and uses the information to manage the condition (Fig. 6.1). The steps in the diagnostic cycle are:

1. clinical request and provision of clinical information
2. collection and transport of appropriate specimen(s)
3. laboratory analysis
4. interpretation of the microbiology report and use of the information.

CLINICAL REQUEST

The first stage in the diagnostic cycle comprises the specimen and the accompanying request form. The following, which influence the quality of the specimen, should be noted:

- The clinical condition of the patient: if the patient is not suffering from a microbial infection, then sampling for pathogens would be futile (e.g., tumours, trauma).
- Antibiotic therapy will alter the quality and quantity of the organisms. Hence specimens should be collected before antibiotic therapy, if possible; exceptions are made when the patient is seriously ill, immunologically compromised or not responding to a specific antibiotic, in which case the necessity of obtaining an interim report as a guide to further management justifies such action.

Provision of Clinical Information

The appropriate tests for each specimen have to be selected by the microbiologist according to clinical information given in the accompanying request form. Hence information such as age, main clinical condition, date of onset of illness, recent/current antibiotic therapy, antibiotic allergies and history of previous specimens are all important for the rationalization of investigations and should be supplied with the specimen.

COLLECTION AND TRANSPORT OF SPECIMENS

Always collect appropriate specimens. Specimens should be as fresh as possible: many organisms (e.g., anaerobes, most viruses) do not survive for long in specimens at room temperature. Others, such as coliforms and staphylococci, may multiply at room temperature, and subsequent analysis of such specimens will give misleading results.

Transport specimens in an appropriate medium (see the following section), otherwise dehydration and/or exposure of organisms to aerobic conditions occurs, with the resultant death and reduction in their numbers. The transport medium should be compatible with the organisms that are believed to be present in the clinical sample (e.g., virus specimens should be transported in viral transport medium, which is not suitable for bacteriological samples). Transport specimens in safe, robust containers to avoid contamination.

LABORATORY ANALYSIS

A wide array of specimens is received and analysed by a number of methods in diagnostic microbiology laboratories. The analytical process of a pus specimen from a dental abscess is given as an illustration (Fig. 6.2):

1. Make a **smear** of the specimen, Gram **stain** and examine by microscopy. (A smear is made by spreading a

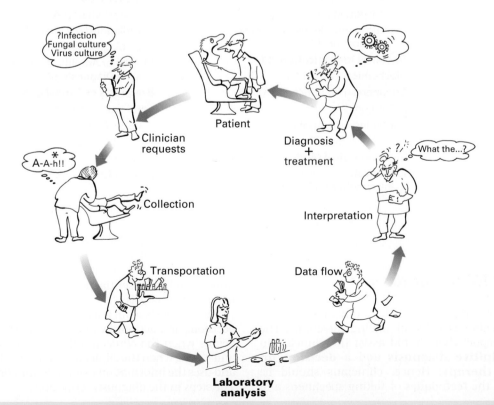

Fig. 6.1 **The cycle of important events in diagnostic microbiology, depicting the interaction between the clinician and the microbiology laboratory.**

small quantity of pus on a clean glass slide and heat fixing.)

2. **Inoculate** the specimen on two blood agar plates for **culture** under aerobic and anaerobic conditions (these plates are referred to as the primary plates).

3. Incubate the blood agar plates for 2–3 days at 37°C (because most oral pathogens are slow-growing anaerobes; for isolating aerobes, an 18-h incubation period is adequate).

4. **Inspect** plates for growth. Note the shapes and size of different colony types for subculture. Infections can be due to one organism (monomicrobial) or more than one organism (polymicrobial), as in the case of the majority of dentoalveolar infections, where samples usually yield a mixture of two or three organisms.

5. **Isolate** the putative pathogen(s) by **subculturing** onto fresh blood agar plate(s) (single organism cultures) and incubating at 37°C for 24–48 h.

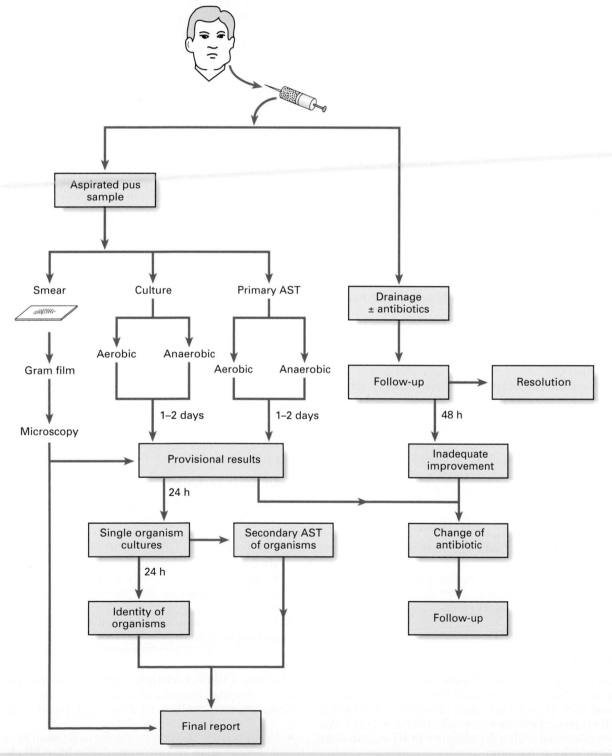

Fig. 6.2   **Laboratory analysis of a pus specimen illustrating the interactions between the laboratory and the clinician.** *AST,* Antibiotic sensitivity test.

6. **Harvest a pure culture** of the pathogen and identify using biochemical reactions, selective media, specific antibody reactions and/or newer polymerase chain reaction (PCR)–based or sequencing techniques (see the following section).

7. **Antibiotic sensitivity tests** can be performed on the mixed growth obtained from pus (primary antibiotic tests) or on the pure organism(s) obtained in step 6 (secondary antibiotic tests; see the following section).

Finally, it should be noted that the microbiologist can issue a provisional report after 2 days but the final report may take longer (Fig. 6.2).

INTERPRETATION OF THE MICROBIOLOGY REPORT AND USE OF INFORMATION

While interpretation of most microbiology reports may be straightforward, there are situations in which the clinician should contact the microbiologist, for example, for guidance in relation to antibiotic therapy and the necessity for further sampling. Good collaboration between the clinician and the microbiologist is essential to achieve optimal therapy.

Laboratory Methods

A number of methods and techniques are used in the laboratory diagnosis of infection; they can be broadly categorized into:

- **noncultural methods**. These are many and varied, and include:
  - *microscopic methods* (light microscopy, electron microscopy)
  - *Molecular Microbiological Methods:* A wide array of molecular microbiological techniques based on PCR is now widely used in diagnostic laboratories (see Chapter 3). These tests are gradually replacing the other traditional methods described below, due to their sensitivity, specificity and rapidity.
- **cultural methods**. Classic methods of diagnosis, in which:
  - solid or liquid media are used for bacterial and fungal growth
  - cultured cells derived from animals and humans are used for viral growth.
- **immunological methods**. These are used to:
  - identify organisms
  - detect antibodies in a patient's body fluids (e.g., serum, saliva), especially when the organism cannot be cultured in laboratory media.

MICROSCOPIC METHODS

Light Microscopy

Bright-Field or Standard Microscopy. Routinely used in diagnostic microbiology, stained smears from lesions are examined with the oil immersion objective (×100) using the ×10 eyepiece, yielding a magnification of × 1000. Wet films are examined with a dry objective (×40; e.g., to demonstrate motility of bacteria).

Dark-Ground Microscopy. The specimen is illuminated obliquely by a special condenser so that the light rays do not enter the objective directly. Instead, the organisms appear bright, as the light rays hit them, against the dark background.

Phase-Contrast Microscopy. Although rarely employed in diagnostic microbiology, this technique may be used to define the detailed structure of unstained microbes.

Fluorescence Microscopy. Fluorescence techniques are widely used, especially in immunology. This method employs the principle of emission of a different wavelength of light when light of one wavelength strikes a fluorescent object. Ultraviolet light is normally used, and the bacteria or cells are stained with fluorescent dyes such as auramine; for example, to detect microbial antigens in a specimen, cells are 'stained' with specific antibodies tagged with fluorescent dyes (immunofluorescence; see below).

Electron Microscopy

In electron microscopy, light waves are replaced by a beam of electrons, which allows resolution of extremely small organisms such as virions (e.g., 0.001 μm). Electron microscopy can be used in diagnostic virology, for instance, for direct examination of specimens (e.g., rotavirus, hepatitis A virus). Approximately 1 million virus particles are needed for such visualization. Clumps of such viral particles can be obtained by reacting the sample with antiviral antibody: immunoelectron microscopy.

LIGHT MICROSCOPY AND STAINS

In light microscopy, bacterial stains are used:

- to visualize bacteria clearly
- to categorize them according to staining properties.

The most commonly used stain in diagnostic microbiology is the Gram stain.

Gram-Stain Technique

1. After heat fixing the dry film (by gently passing through a flame), flood with crystal violet for 15 s. Then wash the excess.
2. Flood with Lugol iodine for 30 s (to fix the stain); wash the excess.
3. **Critical step**. Decolourize with acetone or alcohol for about 5 s. When no blue colour comes off the smear, wash immediately with water.
4. Counterstain with dilute carbolfuchsin for 30 s (or neutral red for 2 min).
5. Wash with water and blot dry.

Staining Characteristics. According to the results of Gram staining, bacteria may be either Gram-positive or Gram-negative (see Figs. 13.2 and 18.1, respectively):

- Gram-positive bacteria retain the violet stain by resisting decolourization and are stained deep **blue-black**.

- Gram-negative bacteria lose the violet stain during decolourization and are therefore counterstained with **pink**, the colour of carbolfuchsin.

Ziehl–Neelsen Technique

Some bacteria, such as tubercle bacilli, are difficult to stain by the Gram method because they possess a thick, waxy outer cell wall. Instead, the Ziehl–Neelsen technique is used. The organisms are exposed to hot, concentrated carbolfuchsin for about 5 min, decolourized with acid and alcohol (hence the term acid- and alcohol-fast bacilli) and finally counterstained with methylene blue or malachite green. The bacilli will stain **red against a blue background**.

Other Stains

A number of other stains are used in microbiology to demonstrate flagella, capsules and granules, and for staining bacteria in tissue sections.

MOLECULAR MICROBIOLOGICAL METHODS

Polymerase Chain Reaction

Very small bacterial numbers (10–100) in patient specimens can be detected using the standard PCR techniques (Chapter 3), whereas more sophisticated techniques can detect one human immunodeficiency virus (HIV) proviral DNA sequence in 10^6 cells. The main advantage of this method is its rapidity (a few hours compared with many days for conventional cultural techniques). However, PCRs may yield nonspecific data; hence judicial selection of primers and careful conduct of the assays (to prevent contaminants giving rise to false-positive results) are important. With the advent of new developments such as microarray technology, PCR-based technology is rapidly replacing traditional techniques in the diagnostic laboratory.

Nucleic Acid Probes

In this technique, a labelled, single-stranded nucleic acid molecule is used to detect a complementary sequence of DNA of the pathogen in the patient sample by hybridizing to it. The probes are obtained in the first instance from naturally occurring DNA by cloning DNA fragments into appropriate plasmid vectors and then isolating the cloned DNA. However, if the sequence of the target gene (in the pathogen) is known, oligonucleotide probes can be synthesized and labelled with a radioactive isotope or with compounds that give colour reactions under appropriate conditions.

This technique is not sensitive for detecting small numbers of organisms (i.e., few copy numbers of the gene) in clinical samples. However, a combination of the PCR technique (to produce high copy numbers) and hybridization with an oligonucleotide probe is likely to be the method of choice in identifying organisms that are slow or difficult to grow in the laboratory.

CULTURAL METHODS

Bacteria grow well on artificial media, unlike viruses that require live cells for growth. **Blood agar** is the most widely used bacterial culture medium. It is an example of a **nonselective** medium, as many organisms can grow on it. However, when chemicals are incorporated into media to prevent the growth of certain bacterial species and to promote the growth of others, **selective media** can be developed (e.g., the addition of bile salts helps the isolation of enterobacteria from a stool sample by suppressing the growth of most gut commensals). Some examples of selective media and their use are given in Table 6.1.

Bacteriological Media

The main constituents of bacteriological media are:

- water
- agar: a carbohydrate obtained from seaweed (as agar melts at 90°C and solidifies at 40°C, heat-sensitive nutrients can be added to the agar base before the medium solidifies)
- growth-enriching constituents: for example, yeast extract, meat extract (these contain carbohydrates, proteins, inorganic salts, vitamins and growth factors for bacterial growth)
- blood: defibrinated horse blood or sheep blood.

Preparation of Solid Media and Inoculation Procedure

When all the necessary ingredients have been added to the molten agar, it is dispensed, while still warm, into plastic or glass **Petri dishes**. The agar will gradually cool and set at room temperature, yielding a plate ready for inoculation of the specimen.

The objective of inoculating the specimen or a culture of bacteria onto a solid medium is to obtain discrete colonies of organisms after appropriate incubation. Hence, a standard technique (Fig. 6.3) should be used. Solid media are more useful than liquid media as they facilitate:

- discrete colony formation, allowing single, pure colonies to be picked from the primary plate for subculture on a secondary plate. The pure growth from the secondary culture can then be used for identification of the organism using biochemical tests, etc.
- observation of colonial characteristics helpful in identification of organisms
- quantification of organisms as **colony-forming units (CFUs)**. This is valuable both in research and in diagnostic microbiology (e.g., if a urine specimen yields more than 10^5 CFU/ml, the patient is deemed to have a urinary tract infection; a mixed saliva sample with more than 10^6 CFU/ml of *Streptococcus mutans* indicates high cariogenic activity).

Liquid Media

Liquid media are used in microbiology to:

- promote growth of small numbers of bacteria present in specimens contaminated with antibiotics; the antibiotic is diluted in the fluid medium, thereby promoting growth of the organism
- promote preferentially the growth of a specific bacterium while suppressing other bacterial commensals present in the sample; these are called **enrichment media** (e.g., selenite F broth used for stool cultures)
- test the biochemical activities of bacteria for identification purposes.

Table 6.1   Some Selective Media Used in Routine Microbiology

Medium	Selective Agents	Differential Substrate (Indicator)	COLONIAL TYPES Selected Organisms I	COLONIAL TYPES Selected Organisms II	Major Organisms Inhibited
MacConkey	Bile salts	Lactose (neutral red)	FERMENTER/RED *Escherichia coli* *Klebsiella*	NONFERMENTER *Salmonella* *Pseudomonas*	Most cocci
Mitis salivarius	Tellurite, crystal violet	Sucrose (trypan blue)	BIG > 2 mm *Streptococcus salivarius*	SMALL < 1 mm *Streptococcus mitis* Other streptococci	Staphylococci, enteric bacilli
Mannitol salt	7.5% NaCl	Mannitol (phenol red)	BIG/YELLOW *Staphylococcus aureus*	SMALL/PINK *Staphylococcus epidermidis*	Streptococci, enteric bacilli
Löwenstein–Jensen	Malachite green	–	ROUGH *Mycobacterium tuberculosis*	SMOOTH/PIGMENTED Atypical mycobacteria	Cocci
TCBS	Thiosulphate, citrate, bile salts, high pH (8.4)	Sucrose (bromothymol blue)	FERMENTER (YELLOW) *Vibrio cholerae* *Aeromonas*	NONFERMENTER *Vibrio parahaemolyticus*	Cocci, enteric bacilli
Thayer–Martin	Antibiotics	–		GREY COLONIES *Neisseria gonorrhoeae* *Neisseria meningitidis*	Gram-positive cocci
Charcoal yeast extract	Cysteine, ferric sulphate	–		CUTGLASS COLONIES *Legionella* spp.	Gram-positive cocci
Sabouraud	Low pH (5.6) ± antibiotics	–		CREAM COLONIES Fungi	Most bacteria

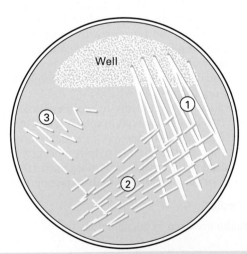

Fig. 6.3   Method of inoculating an agar plate to obtain discrete colonies of bacteria (numbers indicate inoculation steps).

Some examples of solid and liquid media are given in Table 6.2.

Media for Blood Culture

When the infectious agent is circulating in blood (e.g., in septicaemia, endocarditis, pneumonia), the latter has to be aseptically withdrawn by venepuncture and cultured. Blood culture has to be performed on special liquid media, under both aerobic and anaerobic conditions. The blood is aseptically transferred to a rich growth medium (e.g., brain–heart infusion broth) containing anticoagulants (Fig. 6.4). Cultures are checked for turbidity and gas production daily, up to a week (in many laboratories, this process is now automated and machines are used to detect bacterial growth). Positive cultures are sampled, and the organisms are isolated and identified.

Transport Media

Specimens are transported from the clinic to the laboratory in a transport medium, which helps to maintain the viability of the organisms in transit.

Bacteriological Transport Media. A semisolid, nonnutrient agar such as the Stuart transport medium is widely used. It also contains thioglycolic acid as a reducing agent, and electrolytes.

Viral Transport Medium. 'Viral transport medium' is a general term describing a solution containing proteins and balanced salts, which stabilizes the virus during transport. Antimicrobial agents are also added to kill any bacteria present in the sample.

Table 6.2 Constituents and Uses of Some Commonly Used Solid and Liquid Media

Medium	Major Ingredients	Use
Solid Media		
Nutrient agar	Nutrient broth, agar	General purpose
Blood agar	Nutrient agar, 5–10% horse or sheep blood	Very popular, general use
Chocolate agar	Heated blood agar	Isolation of *Haemophilus* and *Neisseria* spp.
CLED agar	Peptone, L-cystine, lactose, etc.	Culture of coliforms
Antibiotic sensitivity	Peptone and a semisynthetic medium	Antibiotic sensitivity tests
Liquid Media		
Peptone	Peptone, sodium chloride, water	General use; base for sugar fermentation tests
Nutrient broth	Peptone water, meat extract	General culture
Robertson's meat medium	Nutrient broth, minced meat	Mainly to culture anaerobes
Selenite F broth	Peptone, water, sodium selenite	Enrichment medium for *Salmonella* and *Shigella* spp.

CLED, Cystine–lactose–electrolyte deficient.

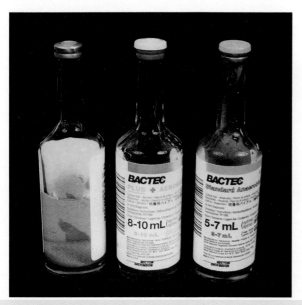

Fig. 6.4   Blood culture bottles: the bottle on the left contains the uninoculated medium.

Atmospheric Requirements and Incubation

Once inoculated, the agar plates may be incubated:

- **aerobically**: but addition of 10% carbon dioxide enhances the growth of most human pathogens
- **anaerobically**: most bacteria, especially the oral pathogens, are strict anaerobes and only grow in the absence of oxygen. Anaerobic conditions can be produced in a sealed jar or in large anaerobic incubators. In either case, the environmental oxygen is replaced by nitrogen, hydrogen and carbon dioxide
- **at body temperature**: 37°C (a few bacteria grow well at a higher or a lower temperature; fungi usually grow at ambient temperature).

Bacterial Identification

When the putative pathogen from the clinical specimen is isolated as a **pure culture**, it is important to identify the organism(s). Bacterial identification (Fig. 6.5) initially entails:

1. inspection of the **colonial characteristics**: size, shape, elevation (flat, convex, umbonate), margin (entire, undulate, filamentous), colour, smell and texture; effect on blood (α-, β- or nonhaemolytic)
2. examination of **microscopic morphology** and **staining characteristics**: a stained film of the colony helps identification
3. identification of **growth conditions**: aerobic, anaerobic, capnophilic (i.e., grows well in carbon dioxide excess); growth on selective and enrichment media.

The foregoing will indicate the major group to which the organism belongs (e.g., streptococci, enterobacteria, clostridia). However, definitive identification to species level requires biochemical tests.

BIOCHEMICAL TESTS

Each bacterial species has a characteristic biochemical profile valuable for its identification. These include:

- **Sugar fermentation and assimilation profile**—the pure culture is incubated with specific sugars and checked for the production of acid or gas or both
- **Enzyme profile**—the organism is incubated with an appropriate enzyme substrate. If the enzyme is secreted by the organism, this will react with the substrate and cause a colour change. In addition, some bacteria can be identified primarily by production of a characteristic enzyme. Thus coagulase produced by *Staphylococcus aureus* clots (or coagulates) plasma and is a specific enzyme for this organism. Another example is lecithinase produced by *Clostridium welchii* (see Chapter 13).

COMMERCIAL IDENTIFICATION KITS

Definitive identification of an organism requires testing for a spectrum of enzymes as well as its ability to ferment (anaerobic breakdown) or assimilate (aerobic breakdown) a number of carbohydrates. This is facilitated by commercially available kits, such as the (analytical profile index [API] and Microgen systems, which incorporate a wide range of the foregoing tests (usually 20) in a single kit system (Fig. 6.6).

Method

A pure culture of the test organism is inoculated into each small well (cupule) containing the appropriate carbohydrate or the chemical and incubated overnight. The resultant

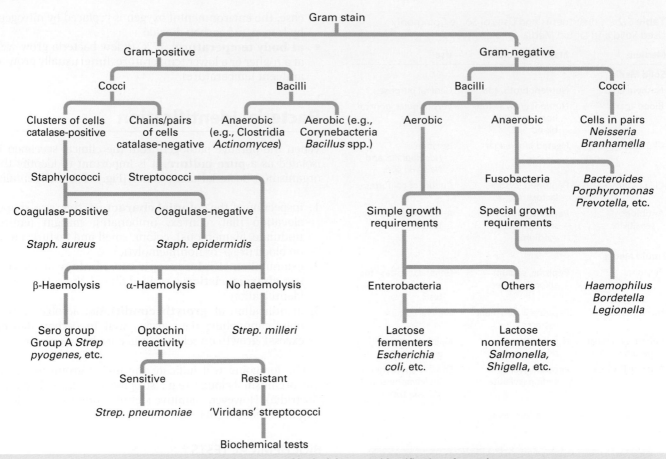

Fig. 6.5   A decision tree used in the laboratory identification of organisms.

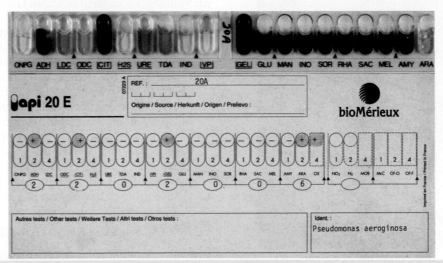

Fig. 6.6   A commercial identification kit of 20 biochemical tests used to speciate (identify to the species level) enterobacteria. Similar kits are used to speciate other genera of bacteria.

colour or turbidity change for each test is then compared with a standard colour chart (provided by the manufacturers) and scored. The numerical profile thus obtained for the organism is compared with a profile compiled from type cultures, and the degree of concordance between the profiles of the two organisms enables identification of the test bacterium.

Sometimes the process of identifying an organism has to be extended further than **speciation** (i.e., identifying the

bacteria beyond the species level) described earlier; this is called **bacterial subtyping**.

SUBTYPING ORGANISMS

It is important to realize that organisms belonging to the same species may have different characteristics (just as individual members of the species *Homo sapiens* vary in characteristics such as skin colour, stature). This is especially important when tracing the epidemic spread of an organism either in the community or in a hospital ward (like tracing a criminal in a vast population). Tracing such an organism can be performed by strain differentiation using the following typing procedures:

- **serotyping**: differentiates bacteria according to antigenic structure
- **biotyping**: differentiates bacteria according to the biochemical reactivity
- **phage typing**: differentiates bacteria on the basis of susceptibility to a panel of known bacteriophages (viruses that kill bacteria)
- **bacteriocin typing**: bacteriocins are potent proteins of bacteria that inhibit the growth of other members of the same class species; a panel of bacteriocins can be used to test the susceptibility of a test organism, and the profile thus obtained used for typing.

GENETIC TYPING

A number of novel genetic typing methods such as those described in Chapter 3 are now available, and these produce very accurate 'fingerprints' of bacteria. These methods are gradually supplanting the foregoing traditional subtyping methods and are likely to replace them in a few years' time. As genetic typing methods are highly discriminatory compared with the foregoing, they are used in both diagnostic and research laboratories to detect **clonality** of organisms with respect to microbes from a common-source outbreak. If an infectious organism arises from a single parent cell, then in order to detect the lineage of the progeny daughter cells that are, for all intents and purposes, genetically identical, a number of detection methods can be used. These include:

- **Multilocus enzyme electrophoresis (MLEE)**: this determines the differential mobility of a set of soluble enzymes (up to 25) using starch gel electrophoresis
- **Pulsed-field gel electrophoresis (PFGE)**: this technique uses restriction endonucleases to cleave microbial DNA into discrete fragments, and these are separated using specialized instruments to generate a restriction profile representing the bacterial/fungal chromosome
- **Restriction fragment length polymorphism (RFLP)**: this combination method uses the number and size of restriction fragments and Southern blot analysis (Chapter 3)
- **Ribotyping**: ribosomal RNA (rRNA) sequences of bacteria are highly conserved; polymorphisms in rRNA genes indicate the ancestral lineage of the organisms, and these can be detected by Southern blot analysis using probes prepared from 16S and 23S rRNA of *Escherichia coli*
- **Pyrosequencing**: pyrosequencing is a DNA sequencing technique that is based on the detection of released pyrophosphate (PPi) during DNA synthesis; it utilizes a cascade of enzymatic reactions, where visible light is generated, which in turn is proportional to the number of incorporated nucleotides; the major advantage of this method is its ability to detect unculturable bacteria; as the role of the latter organisms in oral infections is yet to be unravelled, pyrosequencing—currently very expensive—may not be useful as a laboratory diagnostic technique, at least for the present (see also Chapter 3)

- **Next-generation sequencing (NGS)** or **Second-generation sequencing**: this new technology determines the DNA sequence of a complete bacterial genome very quickly in a single run; information on drug resistance and virulence can also be derived from such data; this technology is mainly used in specialized laboratories due to its complexity and expense (see also Chapter 3)

Immunological Methods

Immunological methods are useful in diagnostic microbiology to identify organisms and to detect antibodies in a patient's body fluids (e.g., serum, saliva), especially when the organism cannot be cultured in laboratory media.

IDENTIFICATION OF ORGANISMS USING IMMUNOLOGICAL TECHNIQUES

Agglutination

Slide Agglutination. Antibodies against the specific serotypes of the organism (e.g., *Salmonella* and *Shigella* species) can be used in identification. When a suspension of the organisms and a few drops of the specific antibody are mixed on a glass slide, visible agglutination (clumping) of the organism indicates a positive reaction.

Latex Agglutination. Here the agglutination of latex beads coated with the specific antibody directed against the unknown organism is used, as in the previous case (e.g., *Neisseria meningitidis*, *Haemophilus influenzae*, the yeast *Cryptococcus neoformans*; Fig. 6.7).

Immunofluorescence

If an organism is exposed to the specific antibody tagged with a fluorescent dye, then the organism binds to the antibody and can be visualized through an ultraviolet microscope. Principles of direct (one-step) and indirect (two-step) immunofluorescence techniques are shown in Fig. 6.8.

Enzyme-Linked Immunosorbent Assay

The **enzyme-linked immunosorbent assay (ELISA)** is a modification of the aforementioned test in which the fluorescent dye tagged to the antibody is replaced by an enzyme. The organism binds to the antibody and the tagged enzyme, and the amount of bound enzyme can then be demonstrated by reaction with the enzyme substrate. This is a highly popular test.

DETECTION OF ANTIBODIES IN A PATIENT'S SERUM

An example of this technique is the serological tests for syphilis. The agent of syphilis, *Treponema pallidum*, does not grow in laboratory media. Hence, serological tests are useful. These are:

- The Venereal Diseases Reference Laboratory (VDRL; nontreponemal) test, in which a cardiolipin, lecithin and cholesterol mixture is used as an antigen. Clumping of the cardiolipin occurs in the presence of antibody to *T. pallidum*. (*Note*: This is a nonspecific test, and, if positive, confirmatory tests must be done.)

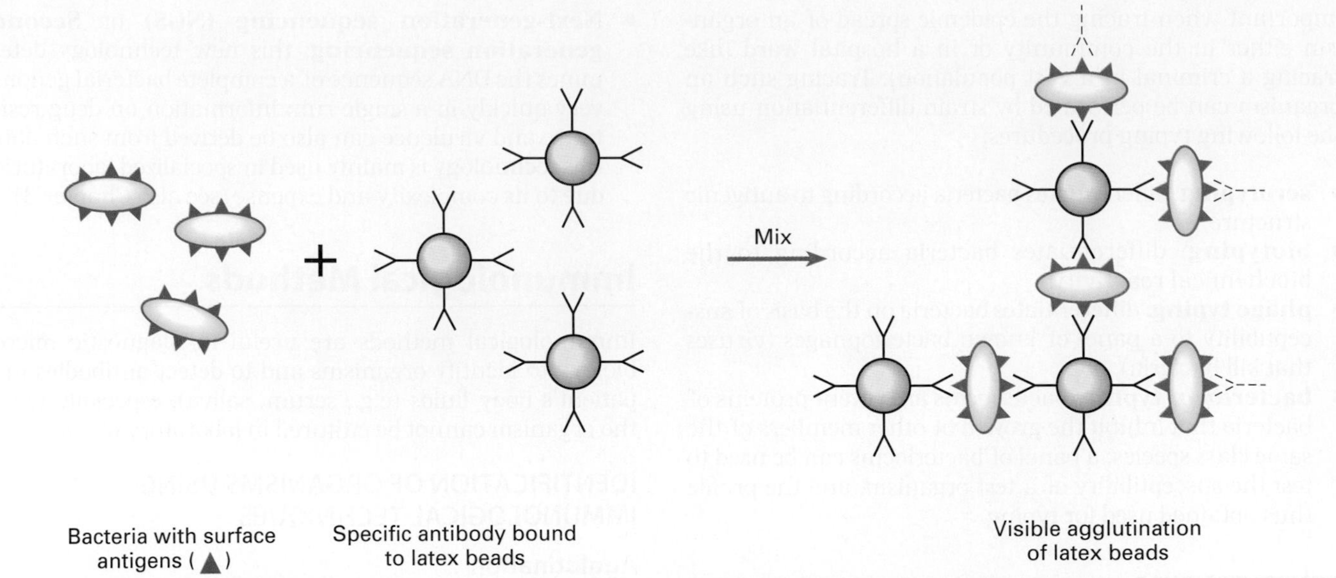

Bacteria with surface   Specific antibody bound   Visible agglutination
antigens (▲)   to latex beads   of latex beads

Fig. 6.7   Latex agglutination test: latex beads coated with a known, specific antibody (e.g., *Haemophilus influenzae*) are mixed with a suspension of the unknown organisms; visible agglutination of the beads occurs instantaneously if the identity is positive.

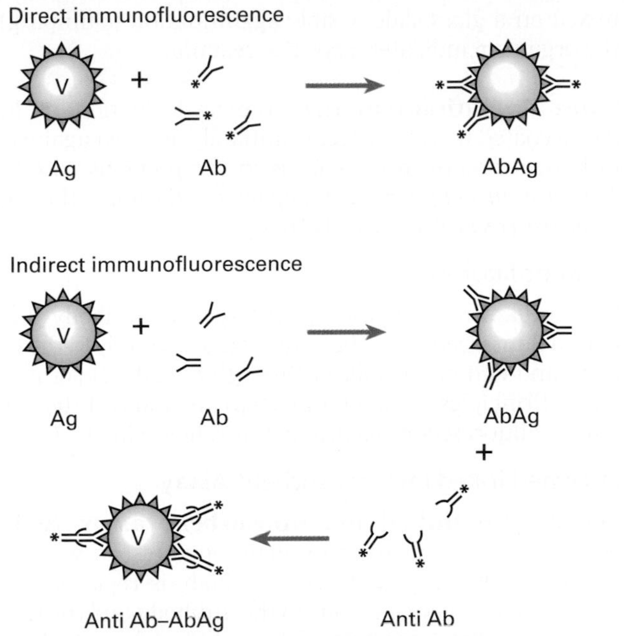

Fig. 6.8   Principles of the direct (one-step) and indirect (two-step) immunofluorescence techniques. This example illustrates the detection of a viral antigen (e.g., herpes simplex). *, Immunofluorescence label; *Ab*, antibody; *Ag*, antigen; *V*, viral antigen.

- The treponemal test, in which nonviable *T. pallidum* is used as the antigen (e.g., fluorescent treponemal antibody absorption test [FTA-ABS]; see Chapter 18).

Laboratory Investigations Related to Antimicrobial Therapy

Once the putative pathogen has been identified from a specimen, its antimicrobial sensitivity can be predicted with some degree of accuracy, based on previous experience and available data. Prescribing in this manner is called **empirical therapy** (e.g., based on the known sensitivity of staphylococci to flucloxacillin). However, it is essential to base **rational therapy** on the results of laboratory antibiotic tests performed on the isolated pathogen.

SUSCEPTIBILITY OF ORGANISMS TO ANTIMICROBIAL AGENTS

In clinical microbiology, a microbe is considered **sensitive** (or **susceptible**) to an antimicrobial agent if it is inhibited by a concentration of the drug normally obtained in human tissues after a standard therapeutic dose. The reverse is true for a **resistant** organism. Organisms are considered **intermediate** in susceptibility if the inhibiting concentration of the antimicrobial agent is slightly higher than that obtained with a therapeutic dose.

LABORATORY TESTING FOR ANTIMICROBIAL SENSITIVITY

The action of an antimicrobial drug against an organism can be measured:

- **qualitatively** (disc diffusion tests)
- **quantitatively** (minimum inhibitory concentration [MIC] or minimum bactericidal concentration [MBC] tests).

A semiquantitative technique, called the **break-point test**, is not described here. These in vitro tests indicate whether the expected therapeutic concentration of the drug given in standard dosage inhibits the growth of a given organism in vivo.

Laboratory results can only give an indication of the activity of the drug in vitro, and its effect in vivo depends on factors such as the ability of the drug to reach the site of infection and the immune status of the host. A strong host defence response may give the impression of 'successful'

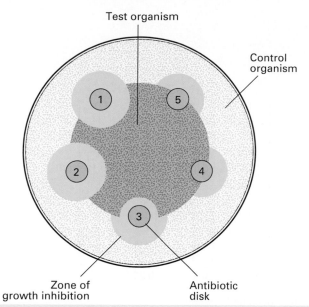

Test organism

Control organism

1   5

2   4

3

Zone of growth inhibition   Antibiotic disk

Fig. 6.9   The antibiotic susceptibility of an organism can be tested by an application of filter-paper discs impregnated with different antibiotics onto a lawn of the organism seeded on an agar plate. After overnight incubation, zones of growth inhibition around discs indicate sensitivity to the antibiotic, whereas growth of the organism up to the disc indicates resistance. In this example, the test organism is sensitive to antibiotics 1 and 2, moderately sensitive to antibiotic 3, and resistant to antibiotics 4 and 5.

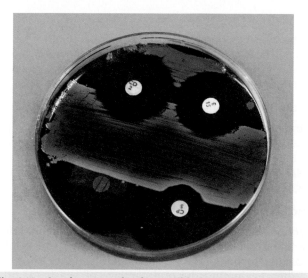

Fig. 6.10   Another example of an antibiotic sensitivity test; here the control organism is inoculated on the polar aspects of the plate and the test organism is inoculated in the middle. In this example, the organism is resistant to ampicillin (AM disc, bottom left) and sensitive to the other three antibiotics. *AM,* Ampicillin; *CD,* clindamycin; *CP,* cephalosporin; *E,* erythromycin.

drug therapy, even though the infecting organism was 'resistant' to a specific drug when laboratory tests were used.

Disc Diffusion Test

The disc diffusion test is the most commonly used method of testing the sensitivity of a microorganism to an antimicrobial agent. Here, the isolate to be tested is seeded over the entire surface of an agar plate, and drug-impregnated filter paper discs are applied. After overnight incubation at 37°C,

zones of growth inhibition are observed around each disc, depending on the sensitivity of a particular organism to a given agent (Figs. 6.9 and 6.10).

Antimicrobial sensitivity tests of this type can be divided into **primary sensitivity** (direct) and **secondary sensitivity** (indirect). A primary test is carried out by inoculating the clinical sample (e.g., pus) directly onto the test zone of the plate. The advantage of this is that the overall sensitivity results for the organisms present in pus will be available after 24- to 48-h incubation (see Fig. 6.2). This is particularly useful when treating debilitated patients with acute infections such as dentoalveolar abscesses. However, because this is a rough estimate, secondary sensitivity tests are therefore performed on a pure culture of the isolated organism, but the results are not available for at least 2–4 days after sampling.

Assessment of MIC and MBC

Determining the MIC and MBC gives a quantitative assessment of the potency of an antibiotic (Fig. 6.11).

Method. A range of twofold dilutions of an antimicrobial agent can be incorporated into a suitable broth in a series of tubes (tube-dilution technique). The broth is inoculated with a standardized suspension of the test organism and incubated for 18 h. The minimum concentration of the drug that inhibits the growth of the test organism in the tube is recorded as the MIC (i.e., the **lowest concentration that will inhibit the visible growth in vitro**). Subsequently, a standard inoculum from each of the tubes in which no growth occurred may be subcultured on blood agar to determine the minimum concentration of the drug required to kill the organism (MBC). The MBC is defined as the **minimum concentration of drug that kills 99.9% of the test microorganisms in the original inoculum**.

These tests are not routinely performed but are useful in patients with serious infections where optimal antimicrobial therapy is essential, for example, to establish sensitivity of streptococci isolated from blood cultures from patients with infective endocarditis, and of bacteria causing septicaemia in immunosuppressed patients.

E-Test. As the routine laboratory method for measuring MIC is rather labour intensive, a simple and quick method to determine the MIC of a drug is to use the commercially available E-test where the MIC may be read directly from the growth inhibition zones associated with a plastic strip carrying varying concentrations of a specific antibiotic (Fig. 6.12).

Appropriate Specimens in Medical Microbiology

See Table 6.3.

APPROPRIATE SPECIMENS FOR ORAL INFECTIONS

Sampling for pathogens within the oral environment poses many problems due to the multitude of indigenous commensal flora that thrive in the oral cavity. Further, many of the pathogens are endogenous in origin and cause disease when an opportunity arises; they are called **opportunistic**

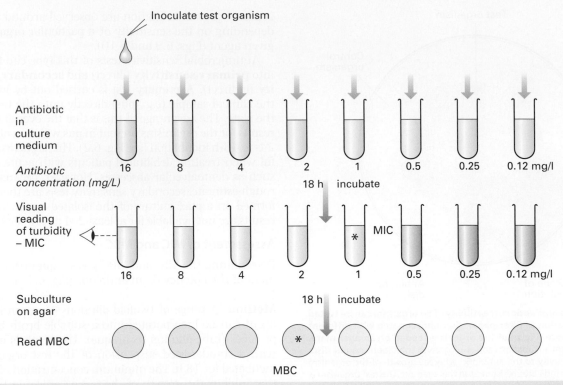

Fig. 6.11 Determination of the minimum inhibitory concentration (MIC) and minimum bactericidal concentration (MBC) of an antibiotic required to inhibit or kill a specific organism. This gives a quantitative estimate of the antibiotic sensitivity of the organism, compared with the disc diffusion method described in Fig. 6.9. (In this example, MIC = 1 mg/l, MBC = 2 mg/l.)

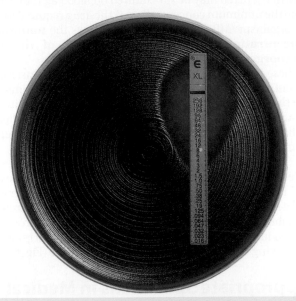

Fig. 6.12 Determination of minimum inhibitory concentration (MIC) using an E-test strip; the MIC can be determined when the edge of the growth inhibition ellipse intersects the side of the antibiotic-infused plastic strip (in this example, the MIC of the culture of *Escherichia coli* to the antibiotic clarithromycin (XL) is 3 μg/ml).

pathogens. In addition obtaining an uncontaminated sample from sites such as the depths of periodontal pockets where disease activity, and hence the numbers of periodontopathogens, is likely to be high is extremely difficult. For these reasons, judicial and appropriate sampling techniques should be used when diagnosing oral infections (Table 6.4).

The specimens submitted to an oral microbiology laboratory can be categorized as those useful for the management of purulent infections, mucosal infections, and periodontal infections and caries.

Purulent Infections

The appropriate specimen is an aspirated sample of pus, if possible. Take care to avoid needle-stick injuries when resheathing the needle cap; drainage of residual pus by incision, after aspiration sampling, is obligatory. The laboratory steps in the diagnosis of a purulent infection are shown in Fig. 6.2.

Mucosal Infections

A common oral mucosal infection is oral candidiasis. Here, the lesion is sampled with a dry swab, and a smear taken immediately thereafter (see Candidal Infections).

When evaluating the oral carriage of yeasts (or other organisms such as Enterobacteriaceae), an **oral rinse** should be collected. This entails requesting the patient to rinse the mouth for 60 s with 10 ml of phosphate-buffered saline and then expectorating the rinse into a container, which is transported to the laboratory for quantification of yeast growth (in terms of CFUs).

Diagnosis of viral infections of the oral mucosa is described in the following section.

Periodontal Infections and Caries

The value of microbiological sampling for the diagnosis of caries and periodontal diseases is limited. In the case of dental caries, salivary counts of lactobacilli and/or *Streptococcus mutans* may be used, and saliva samples should be collected for this purpose (Chapter 32).

Table 6.3 Some appropriate specimens for microbiological investigations

Tissue or System	Specimen	Comments
Skin	Swab	Examine for bacteria and yeasts
	Scrapings	Examine for fungi
	Vesicle fluid	Examine for viruses (electron microscopy and culture)
	Serum	Viral serology
Blood (bacteraemia and septicaemia)	Blood culture	Sterile precautions necessary; multiple specimens required
Gastrointestinal tract	Faeces	Culture for bacteria and viruses; toxin detection for *Clostridium difficile*; light microscopy for parasites and protozoa; electron microscopy for viruses
	Serum	Serological tests for enteric fevers
Urinary tract	Midstream specimen of urine/suprapubic aspirate/catheter specimen of urine (not from a collecting bag)	For quantitative and qualitative bacteriology
Upper respiratory tract	Pernasal, throat and nose swabs; saliva	Culture for *Bordetella pertussis*; culture for β-haemolytic streptococci, other bacteria and viruses
	Throat washings or nose and throat aspirates	Culture and immunofluorescence for viruses
Lower respiratory tract	Sputum	Culture for bacteria, viruses and fungi; fluorescent microscopy for many viruses, *Mycobacterium tuberculosis* and *Legionella* spp.
	Serum	Viral and fungal serology
Meninges	Cerebrospinal fluid	Cell count, microscopy and culture
	Serum	Viral serology
Genital tract	Swab in Amie's or Stuart's transport medium	For bacterial and yeast culture and microscopy for gonococci and *Trichomonas* spp. (wet film)
	Swabs in *Chlamydia* and viral transport medium	Culture of *Chlamydia* and viruses
	Smear of discharge	For detection of gonococci
	Serum	Serological test for syphilis
Abscess	Pus	Aspirates for culture and identification
Wounds	Pus or swab	Avoid contamination from skin; pus preferred
	Tissue	Send small samples in dry sterile containers for homogenization, culture and microscopy
Mucosal lesions	Swab	Avoid contamination with normal flora. Use transport medium if necessary; culture for bacteria, fungi and viruses
	Smear	Fluorescent microscopy; useful for gonococci and yeasts
	Serum	Serological tests for staphylococcal and streptococcal infection and viruses

Modified from Ross, P. W., & Hollbrook, W. P. (1984). *Clinical and oral microbiology*. Blackwell.

Table 6.4 Appropriate Specimens for Microbiological Examination of Oral Infections

Lesion or Site of Lesion	Specimen	Comments
Lips and perioral skin	Moistened swab	Culture for yeasts and bacteria
	Vesicle fluid, swab	Virus culture and electron microscopy
	Aspirate of abscess	Microscopy and culture (see Fig. 6.2)
	Serum	Serological tests for viruses and syphilis
Tongue and oral mucosa	Swab	Culture for bacteria, yeasts and viruses
	Smear of scraping (heat fixed)	Microscopy for yeasts and bacteria
	Vesicle fluid	Microscopy for yeasts and bacteria
	Biopsy tissue	Culture for bacteria and viruses; microscopy for yeasts and suspected tuberculosis
	Serum	Culture for bacteria and viruses; microscopy for yeasts and suspected tuberculosis
Dental abscess or suspected infected cyst	Aspirate	Smear and culture (see Fig. 6.2)
Infected root canal	Paper point or barbed broach	Aseptic collection; use semisolid transport medium; semiquantitative culture
Dental plaque biofilm	Scraping	A variety of sampling tools and procedures available
Gingivae and gingival crevice	Scraping on a sterile sealer	Smear can be diagnostic for fusospirochaetal infection; viral culture possible, DNA tests, BANA tests for periodontopathogens
Severe caries	Saliva	*Lactobacillus/Streptococcus mutans* counts
Prosthesis (dentures)	Swab and smear	In suspected denture stomatitis, examine for yeasts

BANA, *N*-benzoyl-DL-arginine-2-naphthylamide.

The diagnosis of periodontal disease by microbiological means is problematic. A deep gingival smear is useful for the diagnosis of acute necrotizing ulcerative gingivitis, whereas paper-point samples appear useful for DNA analysis of periodontopathic bacteria. However, the latter is not a conclusive test.

Laboratory Isolation and Identification of Viruses

The techniques for isolation and identification of viruses are significantly different from bacteriological techniques. Laboratory procedures for the diagnosis of viral infections are of four main types:

- direct microscopic examination of host tissues for characteristic cytopathological changes and/or for the presence of viral antigens
- isolation and identification of virus from tissues, secretions or exudates
- detection of virus-specific antibodies or antigens in patients' sera
- molecular amplification methods for rapid viral diagnosis.

DIRECT MICROSCOPY OF CLINICAL MATERIAL

Direct microscopy is the quickest method of diagnosis. Virus or virus antigen may be detected in tissues from lesions, aspirated fluid samples or excretions from the patient. The common techniques used are:

- **Electron microscopy**: a common diagnostic tool used in provisional identification of the virus on a morphological basis, although other tests need to be performed to confirm the virus type (e.g., widely used in the examination of stool specimens in infantile diarrhoea).
- **Serology**: tests include immunofluorescence and immunoperoxidase techniques, which commonly employ monoclonal antiviral antibody.

ISOLATION AND IDENTIFICATION FROM TISSUES

Viruses do not grow on inanimate media, and they must be cultivated in living cells. Since no single type of host cell will support the growth of all viruses, a number of different methods of culturing viruses have been developed:

- tissue culture cells: the cheapest and most popular system (e.g., monkey kidney cells, baby hamster kidney cells)
- laboratory animals (e.g., suckling mice): expensive, rarely used.

Tissue Culture

After the inoculation of a **monolayer** of tissue culture with a clinical sample, the culture is examined daily for about 10 days for microscopic evidence of viral growth. Viruses produce different kinds of degenerative changes or **cytopathic effects**, such as rounding of cells and net or syncytial formation, in susceptible cells (Fig. 6.13). The cell type supporting virus growth and the nature of the cytopathic effect help identification of individual viruses (e.g., herpesviruses growing in monkey kidney cells produce fused cells in which nuclei aggregate to form multinucleate giant cells). The time required for the cytopathic effect to be seen can vary from 24 h up to several days, depending on the virus strain and the concentration of the inoculum. Once the virus is cultured, it can be identified by:

- electron microscopy
- haemadsorption: added erythrocytes adhere to the surface of infected cells
- growth neutralization assays using virus-specific antiserum
- immunofluorescence: with standard or monoclonal antibody.

SERODIAGNOSIS OF VIRAL INFECTIONS

Many virus infections produce a short period of acute illness in which viral shedding occurs, and thereafter it is difficult to culture viral samples from clinical specimens. Hence, diagnosis of viral infections by serology is widely used. A diagnosis of a recent viral infection depends on:

- **Demonstration of immunoglobulin M (IgM) antibodies**. These are the earliest antibodies to appear after infection and, if present, indicate unequivocal recent disease. A number of tests are available and include detection of antihuman IgM using ELISA and immunofluorescence techniques.
- **Demonstration of a rising titre of antibody**. For this, the timely collection of a pair of blood samples, one in the **acute** and the other in the **convalescent** phase of the disease, is essential. Acute-phase serum should be collected as early as possible when illness is suspected, whereas convalescent-phase serum is collected when the patient has recovered, usually some 10–20 days after the first specimen has been collected.

Serological test results are interpreted by comparing the antibody titres of the acute and convalescent sera. **Antibody titre** is defined as the reciprocal of the highest serum dilution in a given test that shows antibody activity (e.g., if the patient's serum shows antibody activity when diluted by 1 in 64, then the antibody titre is 64). A greater than fourfold rise in titre between the acute and convalescent samples is considered to be a positive result, indicating that the patient has had an acute illness due to the specific virus.

Serological Tests

A wide array of serological tests is used in virology. The classic and oldest technique of complement fixation is now being supplanted by a number of other tests. These include immunofluorescence (see Fig. 6.8), ELISA and radioimmunoassay. The advantages of the latter methods over the comparison of viral titre in paired sera are that only a single serum sample is needed and results are available quickly. Immunological and tissue culture detection methods have been successfully combined to shorten the time required to identify viral infections. Another method

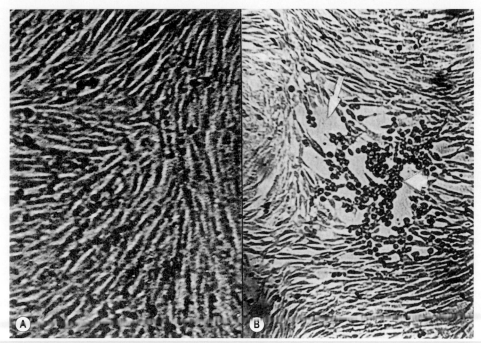

Fig. 6.13 Cytopathic effects caused by herpes simplex virus in baby hamster kidney fibroblasts. (A) Confluent monolayer of cells (control). (B) Cytopathic effect with rounded cells and areas with detached cells (*arrow*).

Table 6.5 Some Applications of Molecular Amplification Methods for Rapid Diagnosis of Infections

Clinical Example	Sample for Direct Examination	Organisms	Comment
Hepatitis C	Serum (frozen)	Hepatitis C virus	Detection of hepatitis C virus RNA by commercial PCR method
HIV-1 and HIV-2 infection	EDTA blood	HIV-1 and HIV-2	Diagnosis of HIV infection in infants or adults when serological tests are difficult to interpret
Tuberculosis	Sputum	*Mycobacterium tuberculosis*	Recommended for sputum smear-positive cases; standard commercial PCR methods, particularly useful for immunocompromised patients or when atypical clinical features of TB present
Leprosy	Tissue biopsy	*Mycobacterium leprae*	PCR method available in reference centre to detect this 'noncultivable' organism

EDTA, Ethylenediaminetetraacetic acid; *HIV*, human immunodeficiency virus; *PCR*, polymerase chain reaction; *TB*, tuberculosis.

frequently used in serodiagnosis of viral infections is haemagglutination.

Serodiagnosis Using Multiple Antigen Systems. Some viruses, such as mumps virus and hepatitis B virus, present with more than a single antigen (and hence antibody), which appear at different periods of the illness. This feature can be exploited to detect the state of illness by using a single sample of serum without waiting for convalescence. A variety of antigens and antibodies used in the detection of various phases of hepatitis B virus infection are described in some detail in Chapter 29.

MOLECULAR AMPLIFICATION METHODS FOR RAPID VIRAL DIAGNOSIS

Molecular methods are increasingly useful and should gradually supplant conventional methods of viral detection, as has already been discussed in Chapter 3. For example, the PCR technique can detect even a few DNA or RNA

molecules of a specific virus in a sample. In addition radioactive virus DNA can detect virus genome or mRNA in tissues by molecular hybridization (Table 6.5).

Diagnosis of Fungal Infections

These principles of diagnosis of fungal diseases are essentially the same as for bacterial and viral infections. Fungal diseases can be diagnosed by:

- examination of specimens by microscopy
- culture and identification of the pathogen
- serological investigations (for both antigen and antibody)
- molecular diagnostic methods.

CANDIDAL INFECTIONS

Smears, swabs and oral rinse samples are the common specimens received in the laboratory for the diagnosis of oral

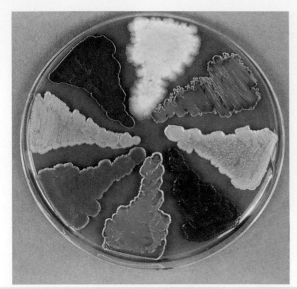

Fig. 6.14 Growth of different *Candida* species on Pagano–Levin agar exhibiting varying colony colours and hues.

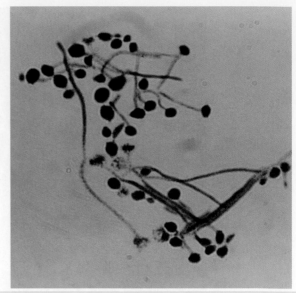

Fig. 6.16 Germ tubes of *Candida albicans* after Gram staining.

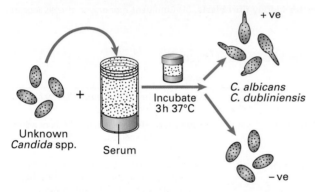

Fig. 6.15 Germ-tube test: *Candida albicans* and *Candida dubliniensis* produce short cylindrical extensions called 'germ tubes' when incubated in serum (3 h, 37°C); other *Candida* species are germ-tube negative and need to be identified by sugar fermentation and assimilation reactions. (+ve, germ tube positive; -ve, germ tube negative).

candidal infections. For this, the lesion is sampled with a dry swab and a smear is taken immediately thereafter (a smear is taken by scraping the lesion with the edge of a flat plastic instrument and transferring the sample to a glass microscope slide). In patients with possible *Candida*-associated denture stomatitis, a smear of the fitting surface of the denture as well as a swab should be taken.

In the laboratory, the smear is stained with the Gram stain or periodic acid-Schiff (PAS) reagent and examined microscopically to visualize the **hyphae** and/or **blastospores** (synonym: blastoconidia, yeast phase) of *Candida*, whose presence in **large numbers** suggests infection. The swabs are cultured on Sabouraud medium and incubated for 48–72 h, when *Candida albicans* appears as cream-coloured large convex colonies. Other species of *Candida* co-infecting with *C. albicans* (e.g., *C. glabrata, C. krusei*) can be identified if the specimen is cultured in commercially available media, such as CHROMagar or Pagano–Levin agar, in which different species produce colonies with varying colours and hues (Fig. 6.14).

Yeasts so derived are speciated by sugar **fermentation and assimilation** tests and the germ-tube test. The latter is a useful quick test to differentiate *C. albicans* and *C. dubliniensis* from the other *Candida* species such as *C. glabrata* and *C. krusei*.

Germ-Tube Test

For a **germ-tube test**, a small inoculum of the isolated yeast is incubated in serum at 37°C for about 3 h and a few drops of the suspension are then examined microscopically. Virtually all strains of *C. albicans* and *C. dubliniensis* produce short, cylindrical extensions termed 'germ tubes', as opposed to the other *Candida* species, which do not exhibit this characteristic (Figs. 6.15 and 6.16).

Histopathology

Incisional and excisional biopsies are useful in the diagnosis of persistent oral white lesions thought to be related to candidal infection. As a significant proportion of *chronic* candidal leukoplakic lesions are premalignant, a biopsy as well as a swab are essential if the lesion does not resolve after antifungal therapy (see Chapter 35).

Other Laboratory Investigations

On occasion, chronic candidal infections are associated with nutritional and haematological abnormalities, and appropriate laboratory investigations (e.g., iron, vitamin levels) should also be carried out.

Key Facts

- The main **stages in the microbiological diagnosis** of an infection are **collection** and **transport** of appropriate specimens, clinical request and **provision of clinical information** to the microbiologist, **laboratory analysis** of the specimen and **interpretation** of these results.
- Always **collect appropriate specimens** and transport them to the laboratory in a fresh state.
- **During collection**, care must be taken to **avoid contamination** of the specimen with normal flora.
- **Methods** used in the laboratory diagnosis of infection can be broadly categorized into **noncultural** (i.e., genomics), **cultural** and **immunological techniques**.
- Some **appropriate specimens** for microbiological examination of important oral infections are aspirates of pus for purulent infections; deep gingival smear for acute ulcerative gingivitis; oral rinse for quantifying oral *Candida* and coliform carnage; and paper-point samples of periodontal pockets for molecular PCR diagnosis of periodontopathic bacterial infections.
- Bacterial species can be divided into subtypes using serotyping, biotyping, phage typing and bacteriocin typing.
- The action of an antimicrobial agent against an organism can be measured either **qualitatively** (disc diffusion tests) or **quantitatively** (minimum inhibitory concentration or minimum bactericidal concentration tests).
- The **minimum inhibitory concentration (MIC)** is the minimum concentration of the drug that will inhibit the visible growth of an organism (in a liquid culture).
- The **minimum bactericidal concentration (MBC)** is defined as the minimum concentration of drug that kills 99.9% of the test microorganisms in the original inoculum.
- The application of nucleic acid probes and PCR techniques is increasingly popular as rapid **diagnostic methods** of microbial infections.
- The major laboratory procedures for **identification** of viruses are (1) **direct microscopy** for **cytopathic effects** or for the presence of **viral antigens**, especially using gene probes; (2) **isolation** and **identification** of viruses grown in tissue culture and (3) detection of virus-specific **antibodies** in the patient's serum.
- *Candida albicans* and *Candida dubliniensis* can be differentiated from other *Candida* species as they are **germ-tube positive**.

Review Questions (Answers on p. 388)

Please indicate which answers are true and which are false.

6.1. When obtaining a microbiological specimen for diagnostic purposes:
  a. the specimen should be obtained prior to the commencement of antibiotics
  b. a swab sample from an abscess is more informative than a sample of aspirated pus
  c. anaerobic transport media are desirable for the diagnosis of oral infections
  d. the patient's name and the clinic number are often adequate in the request form submitted to the laboratory
  e. a blood culture may yield better results if obtained at the height of fever

6.2. Of the common microbiological culture media:
  a. MacConkey's agar is a selective medium for coliform bacteria
  b. blood agar is a nonselective medium
  c. viral transport media are laced with antibiotics
  d. Löwenstein–Jensen medium has malachite green as the selective agent
  e. Mitis Salivarius Agar is the preferred medium for isolating staphylococci

6.3. Match the microbial subtyping methods in the first group (A–E) to the best descriptors in the second group (1–5):
  a. serotyping
  b. biotyping
  c. phage typing
  d. bacteriocin typing
  e. ribotyping
    1. subtypes bacteria according to susceptibility to a panel of viruses

2. subtypes bacteria based on biochemical reactions
3. subtypes bacteria on the susceptibility to known bacterial toxins
4. subtypes bacteria with the aid of ribosomal RNA (rRNA)
5. differentiates bacteria according to antigenic structure

6.4. From the list of infectious disease stated below (A–E), match the most appropriate specimen/s for microbiological analyses in the second group (1–5):
  a. dental abscess
  b. suspected herpetic infection of the lip
  c. lower respiratory tract infection
  d. *Candida*-associated denture stomatitis
  e. bacteraemia
    1. swab for viral culture
    2. aspirate
    3. swabs and smears
    4. blood for culture
    5. serum and sputum

6.5. Which of the following statements on assessment of minimum inhibitory concentration (MIC) and minimum bactericidal concentration (MBC) are true?
  a. MIC is higher than MBC
  b. MIC and MBC need to be routinely carried out for most patients treated for bacterial infections
  c. Once a pure culture is obtained, an additional 48 h are required to assess the MIC of a drug for the pathogen
  d. MBC is defined as the lowest concentration of the drug that inhibits the visible growth in vitro
  e. it provides an indication of the potency of an antimicrobial agent

Further Reading

Goering, R., Dockrell, H., Zuckerman, M., & Chiodini, P. (2018). *Mims' medical microbiology and immunology* (6th ed.). Elsevier.

Procop, G. W., & Koneman, E. W. (2016). *Koneman's color atlas and textbook of diagnostic microbiology* (7th ed.). Wolters Kluwer.

Samaranayake, L. P. (1987). The wastage of microbial samples in clinical practice. *Dental Update, 14,* 53–61.

Scully, C., & Samaranayake, L. P. (1992). Diagnosis of viral infections. In *Clinical virology in oral medicine and dentistry* (Chap. 4). Cambridge University Press.

7 *Antimicrobial Chemotherapy*

Antimicrobial compounds include antibacterial, antiviral, antifungal and antiprotozoal agents. Dentists are known to prescribe 10–15% of all antimicrobials and it is highly likely that a significant proportion of these are unwarranted. Apart from the last group, all of these are prescribed in dentistry. Judicial antimicrobial prescribing by all those who do so is critical to prevent the emergence of drug-resistant microbes, and dentists play a key role in preventing this global emergency. Accordingly, the concept of antibiotic stewardship has been proposed for all those who prescribe antibiotics, including dentists. As described in detail below this comprises the so-called 6Ds of stewardship, viz. the Diagnosis, Drug, Dosage, Duration, Deescalation and Drainage/ Debridement. (Fig. 7.1).

All antimicrobials demonstrate selective toxicity—that is, the drug can be administered to humans with reasonable safety while having a marked lethal or toxic effect on specific microbes. The corollary of this is that all antimicrobials have adverse effects on humans and should therefore be used rationally and only when required.

Antimicrobial therapy aims to treat infection with a drug to which the causative organism is sensitive, so-called **rational antimicrobial therapy**. On the contrary, most antimicrobials in community medical/dental practices are prescribed on a best-guess basis, and this is called **empirical antimicrobial therapy**, which depends on:

- the infectious disease in question
- the most probable pathogen
- the usual antibiotic sensitivity pattern of the pathogen (in the region or the country).

Table 7.1 Cellular Target Sites of Antimicrobial Drugs Commonly Used in Dentistry

Target Site	Drug	Bactericidal/Static	Comments
Cell wall	β-Lactams (e.g., penicillin, ampicillin, cephalosporin, cloxacillin)	Cidal	Interfere with cross-linking of cell wall peptidoglycan molecules
	Bacitracin (topical)	Cidal	Inhibits peptidoglycan formation
Ribosomes	Erythromycin, fusidic acid (topical)	Static[a] or cidal[b]	Interfere with translocation, thus inhibiting protein synthesis
	Tetracycline	Static	Interferes with attachment of transfer RNA, thus inhibiting protein synthesis
Cytoplasmic membrane	Polyenes (e.g., nystatin, amphotericin)	Static	Disrupt yeast cell membrane
Nucleic acid replication	Metronidazole	Cidal	Interferes with DNA replication
	Idoxuridine, aciclovir	Cidal	Interfere with DNA synthesis in DNA viruses

[a]Low concentrations.
[b]High concentrations.

Hence, empirical antibiotic therapy contrasts with rational antibiotic therapy in which antibiotics are administered after the sensitivity of the pathogen has been established by culture and in vitro testing in the laboratory. In general, empirical therapy is undertaken in the majority of situations encountered in dentistry.

Bacteriostatic and Bactericidal Antimicrobial Agents

Antimicrobial agents are classically divisible into two major groups: **bactericidal agents**, which kill bacteria; and **bacteriostatic agents**, which inhibit multiplication without actually killing the pathogen. However, the distinction is rather hazy and is dependent on factors such as the **concentration of the drug** (e.g., erythromycin is bacteriostatic at low concentrations and bactericidal at high concentrations), the **pathogen** in question and the **severity** of infection. Further, host defence mechanisms play a major role in the eradication of pathogens from the body, and it is not essential to use bactericidal drugs to treat most infections. A bacteriostatic drug that arrests the multiplication of pathogens and so tips the balance in favour of the host defence mechanisms is satisfactory in many situations.

MODE OF ACTION OF ANTIMICROBIALS

Antimicrobial agents inhibit the growth of or kill microorganisms by a variety of mechanisms. In general, however, one or more of the following target sites are involved:

- cell wall
- ribosomes
- cytoplasmic membrane
- nucleic acid replication sites.

A summary of the mode of action of commonly used antimicrobials is given in Table 7.1 and 7.2.

Principles of Antimicrobial Therapy

Antimicrobial agents should be prescribed on a rational clinical and microbiological basis. In general, therapy should be

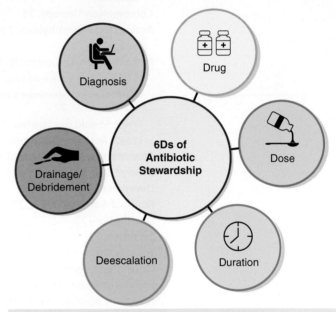

Fig. 7.1   The 6Ds of antibiotic stewardship.

considered for patients when one or more of the following conditions are present (*Note*: this is not an exhaustive list):

- fever and an acute infection
- spreading infection without localization
- chronic infection despite drainage or debridement
- infection in medically compromised patients
- cases of osteomyelitis, bacterial sialadenitis and some periodontal diseases, such as acute ulcerative gingivitis and localized aggressive periodontitis (previously known as 'localized juvenile periodontitis').

CHOICE OF DRUG

The choice of drug is strictly dependent upon the nature of the infecting organisms and their sensitivity patterns. However, in a clinical emergency such as septicaemia or Ludwig angina, antimicrobial agents must be prescribed promptly, and empirically, until laboratory test results arrive. In general, another antimicrobial drug should be prescribed if the patient has had penicillin within the previous month because of the possible presence of penicillin-resistant bacterial populations as a result of being previously exposed to the drug.

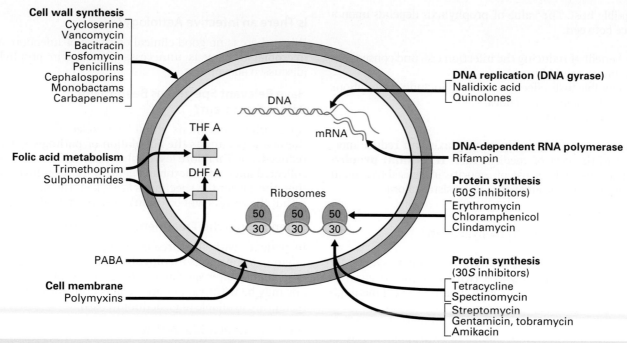

Fig. 7.2   Mode of action of some common antimicrobial agents. *DHF*, dihydrofolic acid; *PABA*, para-aminobenzoic acid (or p-aminobenzoic acid); *THF*, tetrahydrofolic acid.

SPECTRUM OF ACTIVITY OF ANTIMICROBIAL AGENTS

Antimicrobial agents can be categorized as **broad-spectrum** and **narrow-spectrum**, depending on their activity against a range of Gram-positive and Gram-negative bacteria. For example, penicillin is a narrow-spectrum antibiotic with activity mainly against the Gram-positive bacteria, as is metronidazole, which acts almost entirely against strict anaerobes and some protozoa.

Broad-spectrum antimicrobials (e.g., tetracyclines, ampicillins) are active against many Gram-positive and Gram-negative bacteria, and they are often used for empirical or 'blind' treatment of infections when the likely causative pathogen is unknown. This unfortunately leads to 'abuse' of broad-spectrum agents, with the consequent emergence of resistance in organisms that were originally sensitive to the drug. The spectrum of activity of some broad-spectrum and narrow-spectrum antimicrobial agents is shown in Table 7.2.

COMBINATION THERAPY

(*Note:* In dentistry, combination therapy of two or more antibiotics should be avoided as much as possible.)

Whenever possible, a single antimicrobial agent should be used to reduce the:

- incidence of possible side effects
- emergence of resistant bacteria
- drug costs.

However, there are certain clinical situations for which a combination of drugs is valuable, for example, to achieve a high bactericidal level when treating patients with infective

Table 7.2   Spectrum of Activity of Some Commonly Used Antimicrobial Agents

Drug	Spectrum
Phenoxymethylpenicillin (penicillin V)	1. Aerobic Gram-positives (e.g., streptococci, pneumococci, β-lactamase-negative)
	2. Anaerobic Gram-positives (e.g., anaerobic streptococci)
	3. Anaerobic Gram-negatives (e.g., most *Bacteroides*, fusobacteria, *Veillonella*)
Penicillinase-resistant penicillins (e.g., flucloxacillin)	All the above, including β-lactamase-producing staphylococci
Ampicillin	As for penicillin, also includes *Haemophilus* spp.
Cephalosporins	As for penicillin, also includes some coliforms
Erythromycin	Gram-positives mainly but some anaerobes not susceptible at levels obtained by oral administration
Tetracycline	Broad spectrum. Many Gram-positives and -negatives
Metronidazole	All strict anaerobes are sensitive, including some protozoa; of questionable value for facultative anaerobes

endocarditis; the use of gentamicin and metronidazole in the empirical treatment of a patient with serious abdominal sepsis; and combination therapy in the management of tuberculosis.

ANTIMICROBIAL PROPHYLAXIS

Antimicrobial prophylaxis is the use of a drug to prevent colonization or multiplication of microorganisms in a susceptible host. The value of prophylaxis depends upon a balance between:

- the benefit of reducing the infection risk and consequent secondary morbidity
- the possible toxic effects to the host, including alterations of the host commensal flora
- the cost-effectiveness.

When used appropriately, prophylaxis can reduce morbidity and the cost of medical care. **Irrational prophylaxis** leads to a false sense of security, increased treatment cost and the possible emergence of resistant flora.

Aims

The aims of antimicrobial prophylaxis are:

- prevention of host colonization by virulent agents, for example, chemoprophylaxis (with rifampicin) given to close contacts of patients with meningococcal meningitis (see Chapter 25)
- prevention of implantation and/or implanted organisms reaching a critical mass sufficient to produce infection, for example, antimicrobial prophylaxis in infective endocarditis patients before surgical procedures
- prevention of the emergence of latent infection, for example, antifungal agents given either intermittently or continuously to prevent candidal infection in human immunodeficiency virus (HIV)-infected patients.

In dentistry, antibiotics are used as prophylactic agents before dental or surgical treatment of patients who:

- are at risk of infective endocarditis (see Chapter 24)
- have facial fractures or compound skull fractures, and cerebral rhinorrhoea
- are immunocompromised
- have recently received radiotherapy to the jaw (as they succumb to infection as a result of severe ischaemia of the bone caused by radiotherapy)
- have prosthetic hip replacements, ventriculoatrial shunts, insertion of implants or bone grafting.

However, the benefit of prophylactic antimicrobial therapy in most of the aforementioned situations has been recently reviewed and most authorities consider prophylactic antibiotics unnecessary, due to the global threat of the emergence of antibiotic-resistant flora. If prophylactic antibiotics are prescribed, then the advantages and disadvantages must be carefully weighed for each individual clinical situation. In dentistry, there is a continuing ongoing debate on the value of prophylactic antibiotic therapy for patients with a history of infective endocarditis, after third molar surgery, after placement of oral implants and those with orthopaedic implants (Chapter 24).

PRESCRIBING AN ANTIMICROBIAL AGENT

The following should be considered before any antimicrobial agent is prescribed.

Is There an Infective Aetiology?

When there is no good clinical evidence of infection, antimicrobial therapy is unnecessary, except in prophylaxis (discussed above).

Have Relevant Specimens Been Taken Before Treatment?

Appropriate specimens should be collected before drug therapy is begun, as the population of pathogens may be reduced, and therefore less easily isolated, if specimens are collected after antimicrobial agents have been taken. Further, the earlier the specimens are taken, the more likely it is that the results will be useful for patient management.

When Should the Treatment Be Started?

In patients with life-threatening infections (e.g., Ludwig angina), intravenous therapy should generally be instituted immediately after specimen collection. Antimicrobial therapy may be withheld in chronic infections until laboratory results are available (e.g., actinomycosis).

Which Antimicrobial Agent?

Consider the pharmacodynamic effects, including toxicity, when choosing a drug from a number of similar antimicrobial agents that are available to treat many infections (see the following section). An adequate medical history, especially in relation to past allergies and toxic effects, should be taken before deciding on therapy.

Pharmacodynamics of Antimicrobials

DOSAGE

Antimicrobial agents should be given in therapeutic doses sufficient to produce a tissue concentration greater than that required to kill or inhibit the growth of the causative microorganism(s).

DURATION OF TREATMENT

Ideally, treatment should continue for long enough to eliminate all or nearly all of the pathogens, as the remainder will, in most instances, be destroyed by the host defences. Conventionally, this cannot be precisely timed, and standard regimens last for some 3–5 days, depending on the drug. However, a **short-course, high-dose** therapy of certain antibiotics, such as amoxicillin, is as effective as a conventional 5-day course. The other advantages of short courses of antimicrobial agents are good patient compliance and minimal disturbance to commensal flora, leading to an associated reduction in side effects such as diarrhoea.

ROUTE OF ADMINISTRATION

In seriously ill patients, drugs should be given by the parenteral route to overcome problems of absorption from the intestinal tract. All antimicrobial agents given by mouth must be acid stable.

DISTRIBUTION

The drug must reach adequate concentrations at the infective focus. Some antibiotics, such as clindamycin, that penetrate well into bone are preferred in chronic bone infections; in meningitis, a drug that penetrates the cerebrospinal fluid should be given.

EXCRETION

The pathway of excretion of an antimicrobial agent should be noted. For example, drugs metabolized in the liver, such as erythromycin estolate, should not be given to patients with a history of liver disease because they may cause hepatotoxicity, leading to jaundice.

TOXICITY

Most antimicrobials have side effects and the clinician should be aware of these (e.g., see the following section on antibacterial agents).

DRUG INTERACTIONS

Drug interactions are becoming increasingly common owing to the extensive availability and the use of a variety of drugs, as well as the increasing subpopulations of compromised patient groups and the elderly in the community. For instance, antibiotics such as penicillin and erythromycin can significantly reduce the efficacy of some oral contraceptives, and antacids can interfere with the action of tetracyclines. All clinicians should, therefore, be aware of the drug interactions of any antimicrobial they prescribe. The major drug interactions of antimicrobials commonly used in dentistry are given in Table 7.3.

Failure of Antimicrobial Therapy

Consideration should be given to the following potential problems if an infection does not respond to drugs within 48 h:

- inadequate drainage of pus or debridement
- inappropriateness of the antimicrobial agent, including bacterial resistance to the drug, dosage and drug interactions
- presence of local factors such as foreign bodies, which may act as reservoirs of reinfection
- impaired host response, for example, in patients who are immunocompromised by drugs or HIV infection
- poor patient compliance
- possibility of an unusual infection or that the disease has no infective aetiology
- poor blood supply to tissues.

ANTIBIOTIC RESISTANCE IN BACTERIA

Emergence of drug resistance in bacteria is a major problem in antibiotic therapy and depends on the organism and the antibiotic concerned. Whereas some bacteria

Table 7.3 Some Drug Interactions of Antimicrobials Commonly Used in Dentistry

Drug Affected	Drug Interacting	Effect
Penicillins	Probenecid, neomycin	May potentiate the effect of penicillin
		Reduced absorption
Erythromycin	Theophylline	Increase theophylline levels, leading to potential toxicity
Cephalosporins	Gentamicin	Additive effect leading to nephrotoxicity
	Furosemide (Lasix)	Possible increase in nephrotoxicity
Tetracycline	Antacids, dairy products, oral iron, zinc sulphate	Reduced absorption
Metronidazole	Alcohol	'Antabuse' effect
Fluconazole oral (antifungal agent)	Disulfiram, phenobarbital, phenytoin	Reduced effect
	Warfarin	Slows warfarin metabolism and increases warfarin effect

rapidly acquire resistance (e.g., *Staphylococcus aureus*), others rarely do so (e.g., *Streptococcus pyogenes*). Resistance to some antibiotics is virtually unknown (e.g., metronidazole), but strains resistant to others (e.g., penicillin) readily emerge.

Antibiotic resistance develops when progeny of resistant bacteria emerges. As they will be at a selective advantage over their sensitive counterparts, and as long as the original antibiotic is prescribed, the resistant strains can multiply uninhibitedly (e.g., hospital staphylococci with almost universal resistance to penicillin). Such antibiotic resistance can be divided into:

- **primary (intrinsic) resistance:** where the organism is naturally resistant to the drug; that is, its resistance is unrelated to contact with the drug (e.g., resistance of coliforms to penicillin)
- **acquired resistance:** due to either mutation within the same species (chromosomal resistance) or gene transfer between different species via plasmids (extrachromosomal resistance; see Fig. 3.6)
- **cross-resistance:** when resistance to one drug confers resistance to another chemically related drug (e.g., bacteria resistant to one type of tetracycline may be resistant to all other types of tetracycline).

Some mechanisms conferring plasmid mediated antibiotic resistance are shown in Table 7.4.

Inactivation of the Drug. Inactivation of the drug is very common, for example, through production of β-lactamase by staphylococci. The enzyme, which is plasmid coded, destroys the β-lactam ring responsible for the antibacterial activity of penicillins.

Altered Uptake. The amount of drug that reaches the target is either reduced or completely inhibited (e.g., tetracycline resistance in *Pseudomonas aeruginosa*). This can

Table 7.4   Plasmid-Mediated Antibiotic Resistance

Antibiotic	Mechanism of Resistance
β-lactams	β-lactamase breaks down the β-lactam ring to an inactive form
Aminoglycosides	Modifying enzymes cause acetylation, adenylation, phosphorylation
Chloramphenicol	Acetylation of the antibiotic to an inactive form
Erythromycin, clindamycin	Methylation of ribosomal RNA prevents antibiotic binding to ribosomes
Sulphonamides, tetracycline	Alteration of cell membrane decreases permeability to the antibiotic

be either due to altered permeability of the cell wall or to pumping of the drug out of the cell (efflux mechanism).

Modification of the Structural Target of the Drug. Resistance to some penicillins due to loss or alteration of penicillin-binding proteins (PBPs) of the organism (e.g., penicillin resistance in *Streptococcus pneumoniae*).

Altered Metabolic Pathway. This results in bypassing the reactive focus of the drug; for example, a few sulphonamide-resistant bacteria can use preformed folic acid and do not require extracellular *p*-aminobenzoic acid (a folic acid precursor) for the eventual synthesis of nucleic acids.

EMERGENCE OF DRUG-RESISTANT BACTERIA AND A CALL FOR ANTIBIOTIC STEWARDSHIP

Emergence of antibiotic-resistant organisms is now a catastrophic threat of global concern. This is accentuated by the extremely slow discovery of new antimicrobial agents due to the associated massive research and developmental costs, difficulties in conducting extensive clinical trials and a litigious society.

It has been estimated that if new and effective antibiotics are not discovered, the emerging wave of antibiotic-resistant organisms could cause 10 million deaths every year globally by 2050, costing the global economy US$100 trillion.

Antibiotics account for the vast majority of medicines prescribed by dentists. In the UK, for instance, **dentists prescribe between 7% and 11% of all common antibiotics**, which accounts for 7% of all community prescriptions of antimicrobials. Furthermore, it has been estimated that globally approximately one-third of all outpatient antibiotic prescriptions are unnecessary. Hence, dentists must be aware of general principles of minimizing the emergence of drug resistance and rational therapy, which include:

- as far as possible resort to **rational**, rather than empirical, antibiotic therapy (see previous discussion)
- **appropriate dosage** and duration to maintain an adequate level of antibiotic in the tissues to inhibit the offending pathogens and the evolving mutant strains
- **avoidance of polypharmacy**, where two antibiotics with similar properties are prescribed instead of a single antibiotic
- however, in situations not usually encountered in dentistry, such as in the management of tuberculosis, it is imperative to administer two drugs, one of which administered alone will result in the emergence of resistant strains

- usage of proven **traditional drugs as first-line therapy** in preference to newer, more effective and fashionable drugs (e.g., initial use of polyenes for candidal infections instead of triazoles).

THE ERA OF ANTIBIOTIC STEWARDSHIP

As mentioned, dentists prescribe approximately 10% of all antibiotics in global terms, and it has been estimated that 80% of these can be improved upon. Hence, dental professionals have a major role in thwarting the emergence of global antimicrobial resistance. Hence, various organizations have promulgated and approved the importance of antimicrobial stewardship by those who prescribe outpatient antibiotics, **antibiotic stewardship** is defined as coordinated interventions designed to improve and measure the appropriate use of antimicrobial agents by promoting the selection of the optimal antimicrobial drug regimen including dosing, duration of therapy and route of administration. It is therefore critical that dental professionals act as antimicrobial stewards in their daily clinical practice.

An easy to remember framework for remembering this concept has been suggested as the **6Ds of antibiotic stewardship** (Fig 7.1):

- **diagnosis:** making an accurate diagnosis (e.g., bacterial or viral infection)
- **drug:** prescribing the drug of choice as per local antimicrobial guidelines
- **dose:** prescribing the correct dosage (underdosing may lead to emergence of resistant pathogens; overdosing leads to possible toxic events)
- **duration:** shorter duration may lead to emergence of resistant pathogens, and prolongation of illness; unnecessarily long duration needs to possible toxic events
- **deescalation:** reduction in the spectrum of administered antibiotics through the discontinuation of antibiotics or switching to an agent with a narrower spectrum.
- **debridement/drainage:** should be undertaken if prior to antibiotic therapy there is a collection of pus or other necrotic material.

The above *aide-mémoire* summarizes well the action plan and what should be borne in mind whenever antimicrobials are prescribed.

Antimicrobials Commonly Used in Dentistry

Although a large array of antimicrobial agents have been described and are available to medical practitioners, only a limited number of these are widely prescribed by dental practitioners. The following is, therefore, an outline of the major antimicrobials (antibacterials, antifungals and antivirals) used in dentistry.

Antibacterial Agents

PENICILLINS

Penicillins are the most useful and widely used antimicrobial agents in dentistry. A wide array of penicillins have

Table 7.5 Types of Penicillin

Group	Type of Penicillin
Narrow spectrum	Benzylpenicillin
	Phenoxymethylpenicillin
	Procaine penicillin
	Benzathine penicillin
Broad spectrum	Ampicillin
	Amoxicillin
	Esters of ampicillin
Penicillinase resistant	Methicillin
	Flucloxacillin
Antipseudomonal	Piperacillin
	Mezlocillin

been synthesized by incorporating various side chains into the β-lactam ring (Table 7.5). The spectrum of activity and indications for the use of these penicillins vary widely. The more commonly used penicillins, such as phenoxymethyl-penicillin (penicillin V), are described in the following section in some detail. Others, such as the carboxypenicillins (carbenicillin and ticarcillin) and ureidopenicillins (azlocillin and piperacillin), which are active against Gram-negative organisms, are rarely used in dentistry, except for amoxicillin.

The commonly used penicillins are remarkably nontoxic but all share the problem of allergy. Minor reactions such as rashes are common, and although severe reactions are rare, especially anaphylaxis, they can be fatal. Allergy to one penicillin is shared by all the penicillins and, in general, the drug should not be given to a patient who has had a reaction to any member of this group. Some 10% of patients sensitive to penicillin show cross-reactivity to cephalosporins.

Phenoxymethylpenicillin (Penicillin V)

Administration. Oral, as it is acid resistant.

Mode of Action. Bactericidal; inhibits cell-wall synthesis by inactivating the enzyme transpeptidase, which is responsible for cross-linking the peptidoglycan cross-walls of bacteria; an intact β-lactam ring is crucial for its activity.

Spectrum of Activity. Effective against a majority of α-haemolytic streptococci and penicillinase-negative staphylococci. Aerobic Gram-positive organisms, including *Actinomyces*, *Eubacterium*, *Bifidobacterium* and *Peptostreptococcus* spp., are sensitive, together with anaerobic Gram-negative organisms such as *Bacteroides*, *Prevotella*, *Porphyromonas*, *Fusobacterium* and *Veillonella* spp. The majority of *Staphylococcus aureus* strains, particularly those from hospitals, are penicillinase producers and, hence, resistant to penicillin. (A small minority of α-haemolytic streptococci, and some *Aggregatibacter actinomycetemcomitans* strains implicated in aggressive periodontitis are resistant.)

Resistance. Very common, owing to the β-lactamase produced by bacteria, which inactivates the drug by acting on the β-lactam ring.

Indications. As this drug can be administered orally, it is commonly used by dental practitioners in the treatment of acute purulent infections, postextraction infection, pericoronitis and salivary gland infections.

Pharmacodynamics. Phenoxymethylpenicillin is less active than parenteral benzylpenicillin (penicillin G) because of its erratic absorption from the gastrointestinal tract. Therefore, in serious infections phenoxymethylpenicillin could be used for continuing treatment after one or more loading doses of benzylpenicillin, when clinical response has begun.

Toxicity. Virtually nontoxic; may cause severe reactions in patients who are allergic; anaphylaxis may occur very rarely. Other uncommon reactions include skin rashes and fever. Despite these drawbacks, it is one of the cheapest and safest antibiotics.

Benzylpenicillin (Penicillin G)

Administration. Intramuscular, intravenous.

Indications. Useful in moderate to severe infections (e.g., Ludwig angina) as its parenteral administration results in rapid, high and consistent antibiotic levels in plasma.

Toxicity. Chances of allergy developing are increased by injection, and it is obligatory to ascertain the hypersensitivity status of the patient before the drug is administered. Benzylpenicillin may cause convulsions after high doses by intravenous injection or in renal failure.

Broad-Spectrum Penicillins Susceptible to Staphylococcal Penicillinase: Ampicillin and Amoxicillin

Administration. Oral (amoxicillin absorption is better than ampicillin), intramuscular, intravenous.

Spectrum of Activity. Similar to penicillin but effective against a broader spectrum of organisms, including Gram-negative organisms such as *Haemophilus* and *Proteus* spp. Amoxicillin and ampicillin have similar antibacterial spectra.

Resistance. One drawback of amoxicillin is its susceptibility to β-lactamase, but if potassium clavulanate is incorporated with amoxicillin, the combination (co-amoxiclav) is resistant to the activity of β-lactamase (Fig. 7.3).

Indications. Ampicillin is sometimes used in the empirical treatment of dentoalveolar infections when the antibiotic sensitivity patterns of the causative organisms are unknown. In dentistry, amoxicillin is the drug of choice for prophylaxis of infective endocarditis in a restricted group of patients undergoing surgical procedures and scaling (see Chapter 24). A short course of high-dose amoxicillin (oral) has been shown to be of value in the treatment of dentoalveolar infections.

Toxicity. Associated with a higher incidence of drug rashes than penicillin and, hence, should not be administered to patients with infectious mononucleosis (glandular fever) or lymphocytic leukaemia (because of the probability of a drug

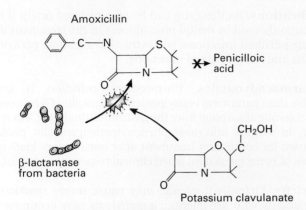

Amoxicillin

β-lactamase
from bacteria

Penicilloic
acid

Potassium clavulanate

Fig. 7.3   Amoxicillin is broken down by β-lactamase of bacteria to penicilloic acid. If potassium clavulanate (a product of *Streptomyces clavuligerus*) is incorporated with amoxicillin, it inhibits the β-lactamase activity. The combination drug is known as co-amoxiclav.

rash). Nausea and diarrhoea are frequent, particularly on prolonged administration; superinfection and colonization with ampicillin-resistant bacteria, such as coliforms and fungi, may also occur. The incidence of diarrhoea is less with amoxicillin.

Isoxazolyl Penicillins: Methicillin, Cloxacillin and Flucloxacillin

Administration. Oral, intramuscular, intravenous.

Spectrum of Activity. Narrow-spectrum antistaphylococcal penicillins relatively resistant to β-lactamase produced by *Staphylococcus aureus*.

Indications. The main use of cloxacillin and flucloxacillin is in the treatment of confirmed infections due to β-lactamase-producing *Staphylococcus aureus*.

Toxicity. These penicillins are safe and nontoxic, even when used in high doses.

Sensitivity. When these antibiotics were introduced, almost all strains of *Staphylococcus aureus* were sensitive to these drugs. However, methicillin-resistant *Staphylococcus aureus* (MRSA) strains are now emerging widely, and hence, these drugs should not be used indiscriminately.

Other Penicillins

Other groups of penicillins, such as carboxypenicillins (e.g., ticarcillin), acylureidopenicillins (e.g., piperacillin) and amidinopenicillins (e.g., mecillinam), are not routinely prescribed in dentistry and, hence, are not described here.

CEPHALOSPORINS, CEPHAMYCINS AND OTHER β-LACTAMS

This group of drugs now includes more than 30 different agents, and newer agents are being manufactured each year. All cephalosporins are β-lactams similar to penicillin but are relatively stable to staphylococcal penicillinase; the degree of stability varies with different cephalosporins. The group includes cephalosporins (cefotaxime, cefuroxime, cephalexin and cephradine), cephamycins (cefoxitin), monobactams (aztreonam) and carbapenems (imipenem and meropenem).

Administration. Cephradine and cephalexin, which can be given by mouth, and cephaloridine belong to the first generation of cephalosporins and are used in dentistry. The vast majority of cephalosporins are given parenterally; hence, they are virtually restricted to hospital use.

Spectrum of Activity. Broad-spectrum; active against both Gram-positive and Gram-negative bacteria, although individual agents have differing activity against certain organisms.

Indications. Few absolute indications. In dentistry, cephalosporins should be resorted to as a second line of defence, depending on culture and antibiotic-sensitivity test results.

Toxicity. Some 10% of penicillin-sensitive patients demonstrate cross-sensitivity; allergic reactions, including urticaria and rashes; possibly nephrotoxicity. Another disadvantage is that oral bacteria, including streptococci, may develop cross-resistance to both penicillins and cephalosporins. Hence, cephalosporins are not suitable alternatives for a patient who has recently had penicillin.

ERYTHROMYCIN

The most popular member of the macrolide group of antibiotics.

Administration. Oral, intravenous.

Mode of Action. Bacteriostatic.

Spectrum of Activity. Similar, though not identical, to that of penicillin and thus the first choice in dentistry for treating penicillin-allergic patients. In addition *Haemophilus influenzae*, *Bacteroides*, *Prevotella* and *Porphyromonas* spp. are sensitive. Erythromycin has the added advantage of being active against β-lactamase-producing bacteria. Not usually used as a first-line drug in oral and dental infections because obligate anaerobes are not particularly sensitive.

Toxicity. A few serious side effects, the main disadvantage being that high doses (given for prophylaxis of infective endocarditis) cause nausea; prolonged use (>14 days) of erythromycin estolate may be hepatotoxic.

CLINDAMYCIN

Administration. Oral, intravenous or intramuscular.

Mode of Action. Inhibits protein synthesis by binding to bacterial ribosomes.

Spectrum of Activity. Similar to that of erythromycin (with which there is partial cross-resistance) and benzylpenicillin; in addition, it is active against *Bacteroides* spp.

Indications. Mainly reserved, as a single dose, for prophylaxis of infective endocarditis in patients allergic to penicillin; particularly effective in penetrating poorly vascularized bone and connective tissue.

Toxicity. Mild diarrhoea is common. Although rare, the most serious side effect of clindamycin, which can sometimes be fatal, is pseudomembranous (antibiotic-associated) colitis, especially in elderly patients and in combination with other drugs. The colitis is due to a toxin produced by *Clostridium difficile*, an anaerobe resistant to clindamycin. Allergy to these drugs is extremely rare, and hypersensitivity to penicillin is not shared by them.

TETRACYCLINES

Formerly one of the most widely used antibiotic groups owing to their very broad spectrum of activity and infrequent side effects. Their usefulness has decreased as a result of increasing bacterial resistance. They remain, however, the treatment of choice for infections caused by intracellular organisms such as chlamydiae, rickettsiae and mycoplasmas, as they penetrate macrophages well. A range of tetracyclines is available, although tetracycline itself remains the most useful for dental purposes.

Administration. Mostly oral.

Mode of Action. Bacteriostatic; interfere with protein synthesis by binding to bacterial ribosomes.

Spectrum of Activity. Have a wide spectrum of activity against oral flora, including *Actinomyces*, *Bacteroides*, *Propionibacterium*, *Aggregatibacter*, *Eubacterium* and *Peptococcus* spp.

Indications. In dentistry, tetracyclines are used with some success as adjunctive treatment in localized aggressive periodontitis (formerly 'localized juvenile periodontitis'); they are effective against many organisms associated with these diseases (see Chapter 33). They are also useful as mouthwashes to alleviate secondary bacterial infection associated with extensive oral ulceration, especially in compromised patients.

Pharmacokinetics. Widely distributed in body tissues, and incorporated in bone and developing teeth (Fig. 7.4); particularly concentrated in gingival fluid. Absorption of oral tetracycline is decreased by antacids, calcium, iron and magnesium salts.

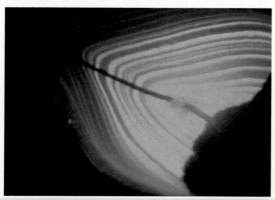

Fig. 7.4   Tetracycline stains in a deciduous tooth visualized by polarizing light microscopy. Each yellow band represents an episode of drug administration.

Toxicity. Because of the deposition of tetracycline within developing teeth, its use should be avoided in children up to 8 years of age and in pregnant or lactating women; otherwise, unsightly tooth staining may occur. Diarrhoea and nausea may occur after oral administration, as a result of disturbance to bowel flora. However, when reduced dosages are used, even for prolonged periods (e.g., for acne), few side effects are apparent. Serious hepatotoxicity may occur with excessive intravenous dosage.

METRONIDAZOLE

The exquisite anaerobic activity of this drug, which was first introduced to treat protozoal infections, makes it exceedingly effective against strict anaerobes and some protozoa.

Administration. Oral, intravenous, rectal (suppositories).

Mode of Action. Bactericidal; it is converted by anaerobic bacteria into a reduced, active metabolite, which inhibits DNA synthesis.

Spectrum of Activity. Active against almost all strict anaerobes, including *Bacteroides* spp., fusobacteria, eubacteria, peptostreptococci and clostridia.

Indications. The drug of choice in the treatment of acute necrotizing ulcerative gingivitis; also used, either alone or in combination with penicillin, in the management of dento-alveolar infections.

Pharmacokinetics. Well absorbed after oral (or rectal) administration; widely distributed and passes readily into most tissues, including abscesses, and crosses the blood–brain barrier into cerebrospinal fluid. The drug is metabolized in the liver.

Toxicity. Minor side effects of metronidazole include gastrointestinal upset, transient rashes and metallic taste in the mouth. Metronidazole interferes with alcohol metabolism and, if taken with alcohol, may cause severe nausea, flushing and palpitations (disulfiram-type effect). It potentiates the effect of anticoagulants and, if used for more than a week, peripheral neuropathy may develop, notably in patients with liver disease; allergenicity is very low.

SULPHONAMIDES AND TRIMETHOPRIM

These drugs interfere with successive steps in the synthesis of folic acid (an essential ingredient for DNA and RNA synthesis). They are widely used in combination because of in vitro evidence of synergism.

Co-trimoxazole

A combination of sulfamethoxazole and trimethoprim in a 5:1 ratio.

Administration. Oral, intramuscular, intravenous.

Mode of Action. Bacteriostatic (see previous text).

Spectrum of Activity. Broad; active against both Gram-positive and Gram-negative bacteria.

Indications. Use now mainly confined to infections in HIV-infected persons.

Pharmacokinetics. A major advantage of sulphonamides is their ability to penetrate into the cerebrospinal fluid; contraindicated in pregnancy or liver disease.

FUSIDIC ACID

A narrow-spectrum antibiotic with main activity against Gram-positive bacteria, particularly *Staphylococcus aureus*. Angular cheilitis associated with *Staphylococcus aureus* is a specific indication for the use of fusidic acid in the form of a topical cream. A small percentage of *Staphylococcus aureus* strains show resistance to fusidic acid.

OTHER ANTIMICROBIAL AGENTS

The foregoing describes the major antimicrobials prescribed by dentists; the student is referred to recommended texts for details of other antibiotics, such as aminoglycosides and antituberculous drugs, and a comprehensive review of this subject.

Antifungal Agents

In contrast to the wide range of antibacterial agents, the number of effective antifungals is limited. This is because selective toxicity is much more difficult to achieve in eukaryotic fungal cells, which share similar features with human eukaryotic cells.

Polyenes and the azoles are the most commonly used antifungals in dentistry. Nystatin and amphotericin are polyene derivatives; miconazole and fluconazole are two examples of a variety of azole antifungals currently available (Table 7.6).

POLYENES

Nystatin

Administration. Too toxic for systemic use; not absorbed from the alimentary canal and, hence, used to prevent or treat mucosal candidiasis; available in the form of pastilles, ready-mixed suspensions, ointments and powder.

Mode of Action. Polyene binds to the cytoplasmic membrane of fungi, altering cell wall permeability, with resultant leakage of cell contents and death; in very low doses, it is fungistatic.

Indications. Widely used in the treatment of oral candidiasis. Patient compliance is superior with the flavoured pastille formulation, as opposed to the bitter-tasting oral suspension or lozenge.

Spectrum of Activity. Nystatin resistance in candidiasis is unknown.

Toxicity. Nausea, vomiting and diarrhoea are rare side effects; no adverse effects have been reported when the topical route is used.

Amphotericin

Amphotericin is the other polyene group antifungal. It is used essentially in the same way as nystatin; lozenges, ointment and oral suspensions are available. As with nystatin, its absorption from the gut is minimal on topical administration. Amphotericin is the drug of choice for the treatment of systemic candidiases and other exotic mycoses (e.g., histoplasmosis, coccidioidomycosis).

AZOLES

Miconazole

Administration. An imidazole available as an oral gel or cream.

Mode of Action. This drug, like other imidazoles, acts by interfering with the synthesis of chemicals needed to form the plasma membrane of fungi, resulting in leakage of cell contents and death.

Indications. Its dual action against yeast and staphylococci is useful in the treatment of angular cheilitis.

Spectrum of Activity. Both fungicidal and bacteriostatic for some Gram-positive cocci, including *Staphylococcus aureus*. Resistance only rarely occurs.

Table 7.6 Common Antifungal Agents Used in Dentistry and Their Activity

Drug Group	Example	Target	Mechanism
Polyenes	Nystatin Amphotericin	Cell membrane function	Bind to sterols in cell membrane, causing leakage of cell constituents and cell death
Azoles	Miconazole Ketoconazole Fluconazole	Cell membrane synthesis	Inhibit ergosterol synthesis

Note: Drugs belonging to echinocandins and terbinafine, the other major antifungal drug groups, are not usually prescribed in dentistry.

Fluconazole

Fluconazole is a triazole drug that is highly popular because of its wide spectrum of activity on yeasts and other fungi. Specifically used to prevent *Candida* infection in HIV-infected individuals as intermittent or continuous therapy.

Administration. Oral; because of its long half-life, it is administered once a day, so patient compliance is good.

Mode of Action. See previous discussion; good concentrations are found in saliva and crevicular fluid.

Indications. As a second-line antifungal for recalcitrant oral *Candida* infections; drug of choice for prophylaxis of oral and systemic candidal infections in HIV-infected patients.

Pharmacokinetics. Weak protein binding, water soluble, long half-life.

Toxicity. Minor: gastrointestinal irritation, allergic rash, elevation of liver enzymes (common to all azoles). Interacts with anticoagulants, terfenadine, cisapride and astemizole.

Itraconazole and Posaconazole

Two other azoles with properties similar to fluconazole; useful for candidiasis in HIV disease.

NEWER ANTIFUNGAL AGENTS

Echinocandins. A class of antifungals that **disrupt cell wall integrity** by inhibiting cell wall polysaccharide synthesis. The intravenous agent, caspofungin, available commercially, belongs to this group and is effective against systemic candidiasis and invasive aspergillosis; no specific role in dentistry.

Terbinafine. A new orally administered, synthetic **allylamine** drug that **blocks fungal ergosterol synthesis**; effective in the management of dermatophyte infections, including nail infections; may be given intermittently with azoles for recalcitrant fungal infections; minimal, if any, role in dentistry.

Antiviral Agents

Few antiviral drugs with proven clinical efficacy are available, in contrast to the great range of successful antibacterial agents. The shortage of antivirals is mainly due to the difficulty of interfering with viral activity within the cell without damaging the host. Most antiviral agents achieve **maximum benefit if given early** in the disease. Immunocompromised patients with viral infections generally benefit from active antiviral therapy, as these infections may spread locally and systemically.

Other problems associated with the therapy of viral infections are:

- The incubation period of most viral infections is short, and by the time the patient shows signs of illness, the virus has already infected the target tissues.

Antiviral Action of Aciclovir

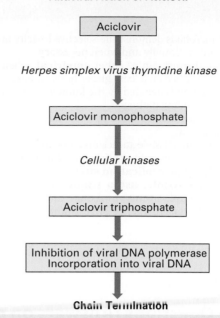

Fig. 7.5   **Mode of action of aciclovir in herpesvirus-infected cells.**

Furthermore, laboratory diagnosis of some viral infections takes several days. However, advances in the rapid viral diagnostic methods using molecular techniques should help overcome this problem.

- Viruses that are latent in cells and not actively replicating (e.g., herpesviruses in the trigeminal ganglion) are immune to antivirals.

Aciclovir is the major antiviral drug prescribed in dentistry.

ACICLOVIR

Aciclovir is an efficient, highly selective antiviral agent useful in the treatment of primary as well as secondary herpetic stomatitis and herpes labialis.

Administration

Topical (cream), oral (tablets, suspensions), intravenous.

Mode of Action. Aciclovir blocks viral DNA production at a concentration of some thousand times less than that required to inhibit host cell DNA production (Fig. 7.5).

Indications. Topical aciclovir (5% cream) can be prescribed for recurrent herpetic ulcers; primary herpetic gingivostomatitis can be treated with either aciclovir cream or tablets. Treatment must be started in the prodromal phase (when there is a local tingling or burning sensation). Application at later stages of infection will correspondingly reduce the length, discomfort and viral shedding period. Aciclovir tablets or oral suspension may be given for severe herpetic stomatitis or herpes zoster.

An alternative agent for herpetic ulcerations is penciclovir cream.

Key Facts

- All antimicrobials demonstrate selective toxicity and should be used only rationally and when necessary.
- Antibiotic therapy can be either **empirical**, when the antibiotic is prescribed on a 'best-guess' basis, or **rational**, when the prescription is dictated by the known antibiotic sensitivity of the offending pathogen.
- Antimicrobials are classified by their target sites and their chemical family.
- There are four possible target areas of antimicrobials: cell wall, ribosomes (protein synthesis), cytoplasmic membrane and **nucleic acid replication sites**.
- **Whenever possible, use a single antimicrobial** drug (and not multiple agents) to reduce the incidence of possible side effects, emergence of resistant bacteria and drug costs.

- **Antibiotic resistance** in bacteria can be either primary (intrinsic) or **acquired**; acquired resistance arises due to either mutation or gene transfer.
- Major mechanisms of antibiotic resistance include the production of drug-destroying enzymes, altering the drug uptake and target site modification.
- An *aide-mémoire*, the **6Ds of antibiotic stewardship**, are **D**iagnosis, **D**rug, **D**ose, **D**uration, **D**eescalation and **D**rainage/**D**ebridement.
- **Selective toxicity** is much more difficult to achieve with antifungal agents because the eukaryotic fungal cells share similar features with human eukaryotic cells.
- The shortage of antiviral agents is mainly due to the difficulty of interfering with the viral activity within the cell without damaging the host cell harboring the virus.

Review Questions (Answers on p. 388)

Please indicate which answers are true and which are false.

7.1. Empirical antimicrobial treatment:
   a. should be reviewed by susceptibility testing whenever possible
   b. can be life-saving
   c. can promote the emergence of resistant species
   d. is superior to rational antibiotic treatment
   e. should be based on the susceptibility and resistance patterns of organisms in the locality

7.2. Antimicrobial prophylaxis:
   a. is often practised in dentistry
   b. dosage and duration are similar as for a treatment regime
   c. does not promote emergence of drug-resistant bacteria
   d. induces changes in the normal flora
   e. may prevent the emergence of latent infections

7.3. Which of the following statements are true?
   a. amoxicillin has a broader antibacterial spectrum than penicillin
   b. amoxicillin is resistant to β-lactamase
   c. amoxicillin is the drug of choice in endocarditis prophylaxis during dental procedures
   d. amoxicillin is effective against methicillin-resistant *Staphylococcus aureus* (MRSA)
   e. amoxicillin is not recommended for the treatment of pharyngitis

7.4. Which of the following statements are true?
   a. tetracycline causes discolouration of developing teeth
   b. tetracyclines have a wide-spectrum activity against oral flora

   c. oral absorption of tetracycline is enhanced by antacids
   d. diarrhoea is a common adverse effect of tetracycline
   e. tetracycline is not recommended for children

7.5. Which of the following statements are true?
   a. metronidazole is bactericidal
   b. metronidazole is effective against anaerobes and facultative anaerobes alike
   c. metronidazole acts on the ribosome
   d. metronidazole is the drug of choice for treating acute necrotizing ulcerative gingivitis
   e. metronidazole synergizes the 'hangover' effect of alcohol

7.6. Which of the following statements are true?
   a. fluconazole is the drug of choice in systemic candidal infections in human immunodeficiency virus (HIV)-infected patients
   b. fluconazole is administered orally
   c. fluconazole acts on the fungal cell membrane
   d. fluconazole is the first-line drug for oral candidal infections
   e. fluconazole may cause hepatotoxicity

7.7. Aciclovir cream in herpes labialis:
   a. is best given during the prodromal stage of the disease
   b. kills latent viruses in neural ganglia
   c. inhibits viral DNA synthesis
   d. local application permanently cures herpetic stomatitis
   e. has reduced patient compliance due to profound adverse effects

Further Reading

Brook, I., Lewis, M. A. O., Sandor, G. K. B., et al. (2005). Clindamycin in dentistry: More than just effective prophylaxis for endocarditis? *Oral Surgery, Oral Medicine, Oral Pathology, Oral Radiology, and Endodontics, 100,* 550–558.

Ellepola, A. N. B., & Samaranayake, L. P. (2000). Oral candidal infections and antimycotics. *Critical Reviews in Oral Biology and Medicine, 11,* 172–198.

Centers for Disease Control and Prevention. (n.d.). *The core elements of outpatient antibiotic stewardship.* https://www.cdc.gov/antibiotic-use/core-elements/outpatient.html.

Government of UK. (2016). Dental antimicrobial stewardship: Toolkit. https://www.gov.uk/guidance/dental-antimicrobial-stewardship-toolkit.

The Joint Commission. 2019. *Antimicrobial stewardship in ambulatory health care.* https://www.jointcommission.org/-/media/tjc/documents/standards/r3-reports/r3_23_antimicrobial_stewardship_amb_6_14_19_final2.pdf.

Samaranayake, L. P., & Johnson, N. (1999). Guidelines for the use of antimicrobial agents to minimise the development of resistance. *International Dental Journal, 49,* 189–195.

Scottish Dental Clinical Effectiveness Programme. (2016). *Drug prescribing for dentistry: Dental clinical guidance* (3rd ed.). efaidnbmnnnibpcajpcglclefindmkaj/https://www.sdcep.org.uk/media/2wleqlnr/sdcep-drug-prescribing-for-dentistry-3rd-edition.pdf.

PART 2

BASIC IMMUNOLOGY

Immunology is a vast and complex subject. What is presented here is a highly abbreviated account of basic immune mechanisms and how they operate when microbes assault the body systems. Students are strongly recommended to consult the books and articles listed at the end of each chapter in order to broaden their understanding of these topics.

- The immune system and the oral cavity
- The immune response
- Immunity and infection

8 The Immune System and the Oral Cavity

THE IMMUNE SYSTEM: GENERAL CONSIDERATIONS

Immunology is the branch of biology concerned with the body's defence reactions. The word 'immunity' is derived from the Latin word *immunis*, meaning 'free of burden'. In essence, the immune system exists to maintain the integrity of the body by excluding or removing the myriad of potentially burdensome or threatening microorganisms that could invade from the environment. Internally derived threats—mutant cells with malignant potential—may also be attacked by the immune system.

There are two kinds of immunological defence:

1. **natural or innate immunity**, comprising mainly pre-existing antigen-nonspecific defences
2. **adaptive or acquired immunity**, during which the immune system responds in an antigen-specific manner to neutralize the threat efficiently, and retains a memory of the threat so that any future encounter with the same threat will result in an accelerated and heightened protective response.

During its development, the immune system must be educated specifically to avoid reacting against all normal components of the body (**tolerance**). Immunology can be considered 'the science of self-nonself discrimination'.

The vital importance of the immune system is evident in the life-threatening infections suffered by patients with immune defects (**immunodeficiency**). In other situations, there may be too much immunity. A by-product of a successful immune response may be damage to normal 'bystander' cells, but this is normally limited by stringent immune regulatory mechanisms. Deficiencies of immunoregulation may be the root causes of **hypersensitivity** diseases such as **autoimmunity** and **allergy**.

These concepts are summarized in Fig. 8.1.

The Innate Immune System

These intrinsic defence mechanisms are present at birth prior to exposure to pathogens or other foreign macromolecules. They are not enhanced by such exposures and are not specific to a particular pathogen.

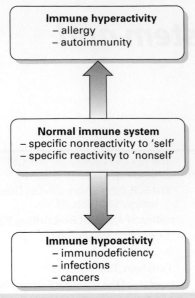

Fig. 8.1   Normal and aberrant immunity.

MECHANICAL AND CHEMICAL BARRIERS

Intact skin is usually impenetrable to microorganisms. Membranous linings of the body tracts are protected by mucus, acid secretions and enzymes such as lysozyme, which breaks down bacterial cell wall proteoglycan. In the lower respiratory tract, the mucous membrane is covered by hair-like protrusions of the epithelial cell membrane called 'cilia.' The movement of cilia can propel mucus-entrapped microorganisms from the tract (mucociliary escalator). Although most pathogens enter the body by binding to and penetrating mucous membranes, several defence mechanisms, including saliva, tears and mucous secretions, are involved in preventing this entry. Apart from acting to wash away potential invaders, these secretions also contain antibacterial or antiviral substances.

DEFENSINS AND CATHELICIDINS

Defensins and cathelicidins are two major families of mammalian antimicrobial proteins. They contribute to host innate antimicrobial defences by disrupting the integrity of the bacterial cell membrane. Further, several members of defensins and cathelicidins have been shown recently to have chemotactic effects on host cells. Their capacity to mobilize various types of phagocytic leukocytes, immature dendritic cells and lymphocytes, together with their other effects, such as stimulating interleukin-8 production and mast cell degranulation, provides evidence for their participation in alerting, mobilizing and amplifying innate and adaptive antimicrobial immunity of the host (Table 8.1). In brief, upon microbial invasion, epithelial cells/keratinocytes and tissue macrophages are induced to produce β-defensins (especially human β-defensin 2 (HBD2) and human β-defensin 3 (HBD3)) and cathelicidin/LI-37. The defensins and cathelicidin form gradients that, in tandem with other chemotactic mediators (e.g., chemokines), lead to extravasation of various types of leukocytes to the site of infection in order to overcome the invading pathogens (Table 8.2).

Table 8.1   Antigen-Nonspecific Defence Chemicals in Oral Secretions

Chemical	Antimicrobial Function(s)	Major Cellular Source(s)
Calprotectin	Divalent cation chelator, restricts microbe nutrition	Oral epithelial cells and neutrophils
Defensins (α and β types)	Membrane pore-forming peptides, cause osmotic lysis	Leukocytes and epithelial cells
Cathelicidins	Lysosomal antimicrobial polypeptides	Macrophages and neutrophils
Saliva	Ig, lysozyme, lactoferrin, peroxidases and GCF	Salivary acinar cells
Lysozyme	Muramidase activity, aggregates microbes and amphipathic sequences	Macrophages, epithelial cells and neutrophils
Peroxidase	Oxidizes bacterial enzymes in glycolytic pathways	Salivary acinar cells, neutrophils, eosinophils
Histatins, Cistatins	Various effects	Salivary acinar cells
SLPI, PRP	Antiviral activities	Various cell types
GCF	Provides blood components	Various cell types
Mucins	Aggregates bacteria, various effects, homotypic and heterotypic complexes	Salivary acinar cells

GCF, Gingival crevicular fluid; *Ig*, immunoglobulin; *PRP*, proline-rich proteins; *SLPI*, secretory leukocyte protease inhibitor.

Table 8.2   Cathelicidin and Defensins, Their Sources and Actions

Peptide	Name(s)	Major Cell and Tissue Sources	Actions
Cathelicidin	LL-37/hCAP18	Neutrophils, mast cells, epithelia (skin, lung, gastrointestinal, urogenital, oral), sweat, seminal fluid	Antimicrobial, chemotactic
α-Defensins	α-Defensins 1–4 (HNP-1 to HNP-4), HD-5, HD-6	Neutrophils	Antimicrobial
β-Defensins	HBD1–HBD4	Neutrophils, epithelia (skin, oral, mammary, lung, urinary, eccrine ducts, ocular)	Antimicrobial, chemotactic; induces histamine release

HBDs, Human β-defensins; *HD*, human defensin; *HNP*, human neutrophil peptide.

PHAGOCYTOSIS

Phagocytosis is a process by which phagocytic cells ingest extracellular particulate material, including whole pathogenic microorganisms. If the mechanical defences are breached, the phagocytic cells become the next barrier. These include polymorphonuclear leukocytes (**polymorphs**) and **macrophages**. The former are short-lived circulating cells, which can invade the tissues, and the latter are the mature, tissue-resident stage of circulating **monocytes**.

Macrophages are found in areas of blood filtration where they are most likely to encounter foreign particles (e.g., liver sinusoids, kidney mesangium, alveoli, lymph nodes and spleen). Phagocytes attach to microorganisms by nonspecific cell membrane 'threat' receptors, after which pseudopodia extend around the particle and internalize it into a phagosome. Lysosomal vesicles containing proteolytic enzymes fuse with the phagosome, and oxygen and nitrogen radicals are generated, which kill the microbe. The phagocytes have several ways of dealing with the phagocytosed material. For example, macrophages reduce molecular oxygen to form microbicidal-reactive oxygen intermediates that are secreted into the phagosome.

PATHOGEN-ASSOCIATED MOLECULAR PATTERNS (PAMPS), PATTERN-RECOGNITION RECEPTORS AND TOLL-LIKE RECEPTORS (TLRS)

Unlike adaptive immunity, innate immunity does not recognize every possible antigen. The cells involved in innate immune responses, such as phagocytes (neutrophils, monocytes, macrophages) and cells that release inflammatory mediators (basophils, mast cells and eosinophils), are designed to recognize only a few highly conserved structures present in many different microorganisms. These cells recognize microbial structures called **pathogen-associated molecular patterns (PAMPs)** in order to activate the innate immune response. PAMPs are molecular components common to a variety of microorganisms but not found as part of eukaryotic cells and include:

- lipopolysaccharide (LPS) from the Gram-negative cell wall
- peptidoglycan, lipoteichoic acids from the Gram-positive cell wall
- mannose (common in microbial glycolipids and glycoproteins but rare in humans)
- bacterial DNA
- N-formylmethionine found in bacterial proteins
- double-stranded RNA from viruses
- glucans from fungal cell walls.

This promotes the attachment of microbes to phagocytes and their subsequent engulfment and destruction. Most defence cells (macrophages, dendritic cells, endothelial cells, mucosal epithelial cells, lymphocytes) have on their surface a variety of receptors called **pattern-recognition receptors (PRRs)** capable of binding specifically to conserved portions of PAMPs so there is an immediate response against invading microbes. These receptors enable

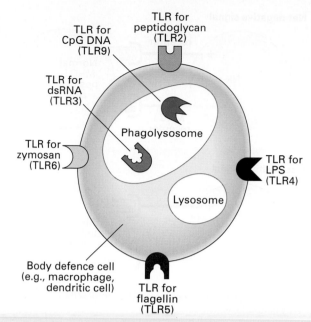

Fig. 8.2   Toll-like receptors (TLRs). *LPS*, lipopolysaccharide.

phagocytes to attach to microbes so they can be engulfed and destroyed by lysosomes. There are two functionally different classes of PRRs:

- endocytic PRRs (mannose receptors, scavenger receptors, opsonin receptors, and N-formyl Met receptors)
- signalling PRRs.

Signalling PRRs bind a number of microbial molecules such as flagellin, pilin, glycolipids, zymosan from fungi and viral double-stranded RNA. A major class of signalling PRRs is **Toll-like receptors (TLRs)**, so named because of their similarity to the protein coded by the Toll gene identified in *Drosophila melanogaster*.

Binding of PAMPs to signalling PRRs promotes the synthesis and secretion of regulatory molecules such as cytokines that are crucial to initiating innate immunity. Various types of TLRs bind different PAMPs and initiate different types of innate immune responses (Fig. 8.2). PAMPs can also be recognized by a series of soluble PRRs in the blood that function as opsonins and initiate the complement pathway.

NATURAL KILLER CELLS

Natural killer (NK) cells are nonphagocytic lymphocytes that account for up to 15% of blood lymphocytes and have a special role in the killing of virus-infected and malignant cells (Fig. 8.3). These cells have two kinds of receptors with opposing action: antigen receptors able to recognize specific molecules on target cells, through which **activation** signals are transmitted, and receptors that recognize self major histocompatibility complex I (MHC I) antigens (see later) through which inactivation signals are transmitted. Activation of NK cells can only occur when there is no **inactivation** signal, so virus-infected and tumour cells with downregulated MHC I antigens are susceptible to NK cytotoxicity, but normal MHC I-positive cells are protected.

Net negative signal

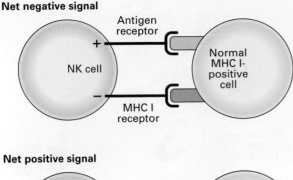

Net positive signal

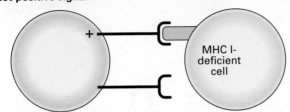

Fig. 8.3 **Killing of major histocompatibility complex (MHC) I-deficient cells by natural killer (NK) cells.**

The killing mechanism is activated by **cytokines** released by virus-infected cells, tissue cells, lymphocytes and NK cells themselves. The NK cells are also important in the adaptive immune response, being the effector cells for killing antibody-coated microorganisms.

ACUTE-PHASE PROTEINS

Acute-phase proteins are serum proteins produced by the liver in response to tissue-damaging infections and other inflammatory stimuli such as cytokines (e.g., interleukin-1 and interleukin-6). Although the physiological role of the acute-phase proteins is not fully understood, it has been recognized to enhance the efficiency of innate immunity. Positive acute-phase proteins increase in plasma concentration in the acute-phase response to inhibit or kill microbes through opsonization, coagulation, antiprotease activity and/or complement activation. Negative acute-phase proteins, including human serum albumin and transferrin, are reduced in concentration in the acute-phase response and act to limit inflammation. Together acute-phase proteins provide immediate defence and enable the body to recognize and react to foreign substances prior to more extensive activation of the immune response. The concentration of the following positive acute-phase proteins in body fluids increases rapidly during tissue injury or infection:

- **C-reactive protein** functions as a soluble PRR and can bind to bacteria to promote their removal by phagocytosis. It is a major acute-phase protein, so named as it binds to the C-polysaccharide cell wall component on a variety of bacteria and fungi. This binding activates the classical complement system, resulting in increased clearance of the pathogen.
- **α_1-Antitrypsin** neutralizes proteases released by bacteria, activated polymorphonuclear leukocytes or damaged tissue to limit damage caused by excessive enzyme activity.

- **Mannose-binding protein** functions as a soluble PRR and activates the lectin complement pathway to promote inflammation and attract phagocytes.

INTERFERON

Interferon, produced by virus-infected cells, comprises a group of cytokines that mediate innate immunity and includes those that protect against viral infection and those that initiate inflammatory reactions that protect against bacterial pathogens.

COMPLEMENT

The complement system is very much involved in the inflammatory response and is one of the key effector mechanisms of the immune system. It consists of at least 30 components—enzymes, regulators and membrane receptors—which interact in an ordered and tightly regulated manner to bring about phagocytosis or lysis of target cells.

Complement components are normally present in body fluids as inactive precursors. The **alternative pathway** of complement activation can be stimulated directly by microorganisms and is important in the early stages of the infection before the production of antibody. It is part of the innate immune system. The **classical pathway** requires antibody, which may take weeks to develop. Both pathways can lead to the lytic or membrane attack pathway. During the course of complement activation, numerous split products of complement components, with important biological effects, are produced.

ALTERNATIVE ACTIVATION

Complement factor C3 is the central component of both the classical and alternative pathways (Fig. 8.4). Products of C3 activation, C3b and inactivated C3b (iC3b) bind to microorganisms and are recognized by complement receptors (CRs) on phagocytes. If any C3b molecules bind to a normal host cell surface, they can then bind the next component in the sequence, factor B. Factor D (the only complement factor present in body fluids as an active enzyme) splits off a small fragment, Ba, leaving an active C3 convertase, C3bBb, on the cell surface. However the normal host cell is able actively to dissociate and inactivate C3bBb. This is achieved by the concerted action of regulatory proteins decay-accelerating factor (DAF), membrane cofactor protein (MCP), β_1H globulin (factor H), CR1 and factor I.

Activator surfaces are those that inhibit the regulatory proteins, allowing C3bBb to remain intact. For example, bacterial endotoxins and LPSs inhibit factor H. The enzyme C3bBb converts C3 into C3a and C3b. The latter is incorporated, along with properdin (factor P), to form PC3bBbC3b. This is a stable enzyme whose substrates are C3 and C5. It amplifies C3b production and activates the membrane attack pathway.

CLASSICAL ACTIVATION

Classical pathway of complement activation (Fig. 8.5) is mainly initiated by complexes of antigen with antibody. Antibodies of the immunoglobulin (Ig) IgG1, IgG2, IgG3

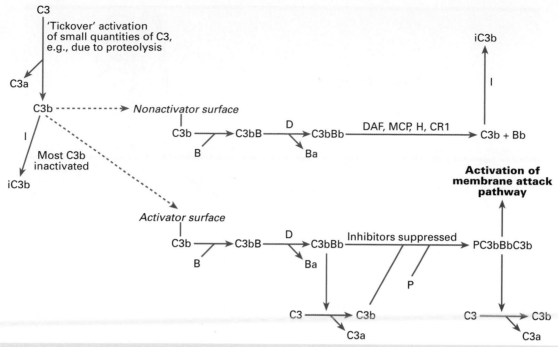

Fig. 8.4 Alternative pathway of complement activation. *B,* Factor B; *CR,* complement receptor; *D,* factor D; *DAF,* decay-accelerating factor; *H,* β₁H-globulin; *I,* C3 inactivator; *MCP,* membrane cofactor protein; *P,* properdin.

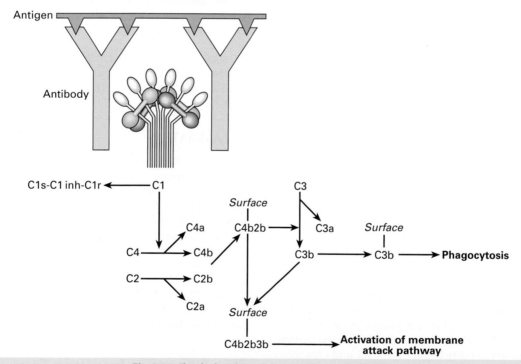

Fig. 8.5 Classical pathway of complement activation.

and IgM classes, but not IgG4, IgA, IgD or IgE, can activate the classical pathway.

The first component of the classical pathway, C1, is actually a complex of C1q, C1r and C1s. This complex can bind very weakly to monomeric IgG, but when IgG complexes with antigen in such a way that adjacent IgG molecules are close together, C1q binds firmly between the two molecules. The C1 complex can bind strongly to a single molecule of pentameric IgM, but only after the conformation of the latter has been altered by binding to antigen.

Activated C1 reacts with fluid-phase C4 and C2, splitting off small peptides C4a and C2a. The resulting C4b2b is deposited on a surface and performs a similar job to C3bBb of the alternative pathway: it can convert C3 into C3a and C3b, and the latter can either opsonize particles for phagocytosis or bind to C4b2b. Cell-bound C4b2b3b is more stable

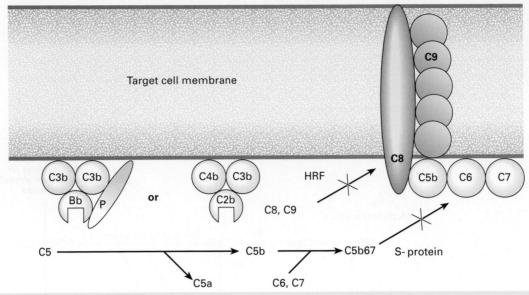

Fig. 8.6   Membrane attack pathway. *HRF,* Homologous restriction factor; *P,* properdin.

than C4b2b, being somewhat protected from the regulatory proteins DAF and C4-binding protein. Like PC3bBbC3b, it activates the membrane attack pathway.

MEMBRANE ATTACK

The peptides Bb and C2b, bound into their respective alternative (PC3bBbC3b) and classical (C4b2b3b) pathway enzymatic complexes, initiate membrane attack (Fig. 8.6) by splitting a small peptide, C5a, from C5 to form C5b. This molecule binds C6 and C7. Cell-bound C5b67 acts as a template for the binding of one molecule of C8 and up to 18 molecules of C9. Normal cells in the body are largely protected from bystander lysis by homologous restriction factor (HRF), which intercepts C8 and C9 before they can be properly assembled into the membrane attack complex (MAC). The MAC, with a molecular weight of $1–2 \times 10^6$, forms transmembrane channels, which permit osmotic influx so that the target cell swells up and bursts.

BIOLOGICAL EFFECTS OF COMPLEMENT ACTIVATION

Probably the most important function of the complement system is to **opsonize** antigen–antibody (immune) complexes, microorganisms and cell debris for phagocytosis (Fig. 8.7). This is achieved by deposition of C3b and iC3b on the particle. Phagocytes bind to the particle via CR1, CR3 and CR4. Also, CR1 is found on erythrocytes, which can bind immune complexes coated with C3b and transport them to the spleen or liver for digestion by macrophages.

The peptides C3a, C4a and C5a are **anaphylatoxins** that cause mast-cell degranulation and smooth-muscle contraction. They increase vascular permeability, which permits cells and fluids to enter the tissues from the circulation. They are regulated by anaphylatoxin inactivator, which splits off the C-terminal arginine so that binding to cellular receptors can no longer occur.

Further important properties of C5a are:

- inducing **adherence** of blood phagocytes to vessel endothelium, following which they are able to migrate into the tissues
- **upregulating** CR1, CR3 and CR4
- attracting phagocytes (**chemotaxis**) towards the site of complement activation.

Certain microorganisms, notably Gram-negative bacteria, can be lysed directly by the MAC. Gram-positive bacteria, however, are protected by their thick peptidoglycan cell walls.

INFLAMMATION

The local inflammatory response is usually accompanied with a systemic response known as the **acute-phase response**. The manifestation of this response includes the induction of fever and increased production of leukocytes, and the production of soluble factors, including acute-phase proteins in the liver. Injured or infected tissues become inflamed in order to direct components of the immune system to where they are needed. The blood supply to the tissues is increased, capillaries become more permeable to soluble mediators and leukocytes, and leukocytes migrate towards the site of infection as a result of the production of chemotactic factors.

The Adaptive Immune System

The defence mechanisms in adaptive immunity can specifically recognize and selectively eliminate pathogens and foreign macromolecules. In contrast to innate immunity, adaptive immune responses are reactions to specific antigenic challenge and display four cardinal features: **specificity, diversity, immunological memory and discrimination of self and nonself**.

Adaptive immune responses are specific for distinct antigens. This unique specificity exists because B and T

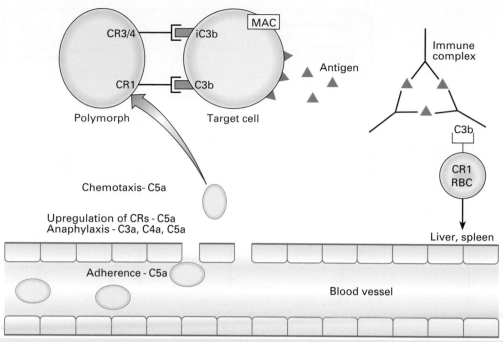

Fig. 8.7 Biological effects of complement. *CR*, Complement receptor; *MAC*, membrane attack complex; *RBC*, red blood cell.

lymphocytes express membrane receptors that specifically recognize different antigens. Importantly, adaptive immunity is not dependent on innate immunity. Through delicately modulated interactions, the two types of defence mechanisms work synergistically to produce more effective immunity.

Cells of the Immune System

All the cells of the immune system (Fig. 8.8) are derived from self-regenerating **haematopoietic stem cells** present in bone marrow and foetal liver. These differentiate along either the **myeloid** or the **lymphoid** pathway. Myeloid precursor cells give rise to mast cells, erythrocytes, platelets, dendritic cells, polymorphs (eosinophils, basophils, neutrophils) and mononuclear phagocytes (monocytes in the blood, macrophages in the tissues). Lymphoid precursor differentiation gives rise to T (thymus-dependent) lymphocytes, B (bone marrow-derived) lymphocytes and NK lymphocytes.

During postnatal life, B-cell genesis takes place in the bone marrow. Each newly formed B cell expresses a unique B-cell receptor (BCR) on its membrane for antigen binding. Although T lymphocytes also arise in the bone marrow, they migrate to the thymus to mature. During its maturation, the T lymphocyte expresses a specific antigen-binding molecule known as the T-cell receptor (TCR) on its membrane.

The B lymphocytes are responsible for secreting Ig antibodies and can also function as highly efficient **antigen-presenting cells (APCs)** for T lymphocytes. The latter are divided into two major subsets: **T-helper cells**, which usually bear the 'cluster of differentiation' marker CD4, and **T-cytotoxic cells**, which usually carry CD8. The T-helper cells are required for activating the effector function of B cells, other T cells, NK cells and macrophages. They do this by transmitting signals via cell-to-cell contact interactions and/or via soluble hormone-like factors called **lymphokines**. The T-cytotoxic cells kill target cells such as virus-infected host cells. Another functional property of some T lymphocytes is to downregulate immune responses. These **T-suppressor cells** are usually CD8-positive. Dendritic cells and monocytes/macrophages play key roles in the immune system as APCs.

THE LYMPHOID ORGANS

The **primary sites** of lymphocyte production are the **bone marrow** and **thymus**. Immature lymphocytes produced from stem cells in the bone marrow may continue their development within the bone marrow (B lymphocytes, NK cells) or migrate to the thymus and develop into T lymphocytes. 'Education' within the primary lymphoid organs ensures that emerging lymphocytes can discriminate self from nonself. They migrate through the blood and lymphatic systems to the **secondary lymphoid organs**—spleen, lymph nodes and mucosa-associated lymphoid tissue (MALT) of the alimentary, respiratory and urogenital tracts. Here, lymphocytes encounter foreign antigens and become activated effector cells of the immune response.

The spleen acts as a filter for blood and is the major site for clearance of opsonized particles. It is an important site for production of antibodies against intravenous antigens. The lymph nodes form a network of strategically placed filters, which drain fluids from the tissues and concentrate foreign antigen onto APCs and subsequently to lymphocytes. Spleen and lymph nodes are encapsulated organs, whereas MALT is nonencapsulated dispersed aggregates of lymphoid cells positioned to protect the main passages by which microorganisms gain entry into the body. **Gut-associated lymphoid tissue (GALT)** includes Peyer's patches

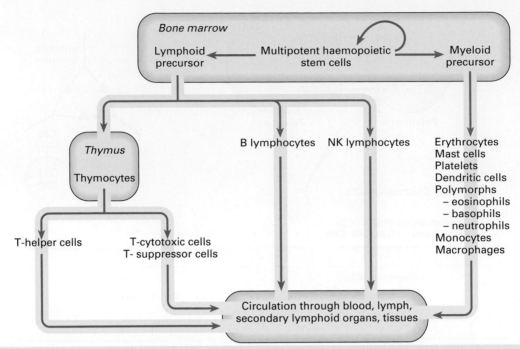

Fig. 8.8   Cells and organs of the immune system. *NK,* Natural killer.

of the lower ileum, accumulations of lymphoid tissue in the lamina propria of the intestinal wall and the tonsils.

Mature lymphoid cells continuously circulate between the blood, lymph, lymphoid organs and tissues until they encounter an antigen, which will cause them to become activated (see Chapter 9).

ANTIGEN RECOGNITION

The T and B lymphocytes are responsible for **specificity** in the immune response. They have cell surface receptors whose purpose is to recognize foreign antigens. Each receptor usually binds only to a single antigen, though there may be a degree of **cross-reactivity** with other antigens of very similar structure. Since all antigen receptors on a given lymphocyte are identical, each B or T cell can usually recognize only one antigen. A single cell, on encountering its specific antigen, must proliferate to form a clone of identical cells able to deal with the offending antigen (clonal selection).

The TCR recognizes linear peptides bound to MHC molecules on the surface of APCs. The BCR binds directly to often nonlinear antigenic determinants (epitopes) and does not require MHC presentation.

Major Histocompatibility Complex

In humans, products of the highly polymorphic MHC genetic loci on chromosome 6 are known as histocompatibility locus antigens (HLAs). Their function is to bind APC-processed short antigenic peptides and present them on the APC surface to T cells. HLA phenotype is responsible for tissue transplant rejection when the recipient and donor are not HLA matched.

There are two classes of HLA molecules:

■ Class I: HLA-A, -B and -C molecules, found on all nucleated cells in the body

■ Class II: HLA-DQ, -DR and -DP molecules, usually only found on monocytes/macrophages, B cells, dendritic cells (i.e., APCs), some epithelial cells and activated T cells.

One HLA-A, -B, -C, -DQ, -DR and -DP antigen is inherited from each parent, so each individual expresses up to six class I and six class II antigens. Each HLA molecule can bind a large number of different antigenic peptides. However, the complement of HLA antigens possessed by an individual will determine the range of antigenic peptides that can be presented by APCs. Class I molecules present peptides to CD8+ T lymphocytes, and CD4+ T cells are restricted to MHC class II.

The TCR and Generation of T-Cell Diversity

The TCR is a two-chain structure comprising polypeptides derived from TCR α and TCR β genes. Less frequently, a subset of T cells will use TCR γ and TCR δ instead. Each chain consists of a variable (V) region and a constant (C) region. The two adjacent V regions make contact with antigenic peptides and the presenting MHC. The genetic template for the α-chain is created by joining one of many Vα genes with one of the more than 40 J (joining) α genes and a single C gene. The β-chain template is similarly created by joining one of the large number of Vβs, one of two D (diversity) βs, one of 2 Jβs and one of the two Cβ genes. The number of different αβ V regions that can be created is high, and the repertoire is further increased by the random addition of small numbers of template-independent nucleotides.

The BCR, Generation of B-Cell Diversity and Isotype Selection

The BCR is a cell membrane–bound form of Ig antibody and recognizes the same antigenic specificity as the antibody that will eventually be secreted by the B-cell. It is a four-chain structure comprising two identical heavy (H) chains, which anchor the receptor in the plasma membrane, and two identical light (L) chains. The whole molecule projects out from the B-cell surface in the shape of a Y. Like TCR chains, each H and L chain consists of V and C regions. The antigen-binding site is created by the juxtaposition of V regions from one H and one L chain, and there are two such sites per BCR. Their tertiary structure creates a pocket that accommodates an epitope with the mirror-image configuration.

The V_L region genetic template is created by rearranging V and J genes, whereas the V_H chain is derived from the recombination of V, D and J genes. Additional diversity is created by n-region additions. Furthermore, point mutations can be introduced into V genes after antigenic stimulation, which tend to increase the strength of binding of an antibody or BCR to its antigen.

There are nine C_H genes on chromosome 14q32 arranged in the order $5'$-μ-δ-$γ_3$-$γ_1$-$α_1$-$γ_2$-$γ_4$-ε-$α_2$-$3'$. The class, or **isotype**, of Ig depends on which C_H gene is used: μ gives IgM, δ IgD, $γ_3$ IgG$_3$, $α_1$ IgA$_1$, ε IgE. Immature B cells use only μ and express IgM, and mature but unstimulated B cells express IgM and IgD. Following stimulation by antigen, B cells can delete $5'$ genes, for example μ, δ, $γ_3$, and express the next most $5'$ C_H gene, in this case $γ_1$ (IgG$_1$). Switching to particular C_H genes is largely under the control of regulatory T cells.

DELETION OF ANTI-SELF REACTIVITIES

Random usage of all the possible TCR and BCR V gene combinations would result in a large fraction of the repertoire being directed against self. This fraction of the repertoire must be purged in order to prevent immune damage to the body. This is achieved largely during late embryonic and early neonatal development. Following seeding of the primary lymphoid organs by lymphoid precursors, differentiation along defined developmental pathways occurs, accompanied by rapid cell proliferation and also massive cell loss due to depletion of anti-self reactivities.

T-Cell Differentiation

The most immature thymocytes are TCR$^-$CD3$^-$CD4$^-$CD8$^-$. These first differentiate into TCR$^-$CD3$^-$CD4$^+$CD8$^+$ and then rearrange TCR αβ or TCR γδ genes and express CD3; TCR$^+$CD3$^+$CD4$^+$CD8$^+$ are then selected for MHC reactivity. Thymocytes with TCRs that bind **weakly** to MHC antigens on thymic cortical epithelial or stromal cells are allowed to survive (**positive selection**); those with no MHC reactivity die 'of neglect'. Thymocytes with strong reactivity against self MHC + self peptides (there will have been little exposure to foreign peptides in utero) expressed on medullary dendritic cells and macrophages are signalled to undergo **programmed cell death (PCD) by apoptosis (negative selection)**.

If the weak reactivity with MHC that results in positive selection is against MHC class I, the T cell, when fully mature, will only respond to peptides presented on class I. It will stop expressing CD4 but continue to express CD8, which itself has the ability to bind to a monomorphic site on MHC I and functions as an important coreceptor to strengthen adhesion between the T cell and the APC. The mature T cell will be TCR$^+$CD3$^+$CD4$^+$CD8$^+$ and function as

a T-cytotoxic or T-suppressor cell. Alternatively, selection on MHC II will produce class II–restricted TCR$^+$CD3$^+$CD4$^+$CD8$^+$ T-helper cells. CD4 strengthens the adhesion between the T cell and the APC by binding to MHC II.

Fewer than 10% of thymocytes survive the selection process. Those that do have the ability to bind weakly to MHC on APCs and the potential to bind strongly to MHC + nonself peptides will leave the thymus and enter the circulation.

B-Cell Differentiation

The process of B-cell development in the bone marrow occurs by the stepwise rearrangements of the V, D and J segments of the Ig H (heavy) and L (light) chain gene loci. During early B-cell genesis, productive IgH chain gene rearrangement leads to assembly of the pre-B-cell receptor (pre-BCR). The pre-BCR, transiently expressed by developing precursor B cells, comprises the Ig γH chain, surrogate light (SL) chains VpreB and δ5, as well as the signal-transducing heterodimer Igα/Igβ. Signalling through the pre-BCR regulates allelic exclusion at the Ig H locus, stimulates cell proliferation and induces pre-B cells that further undergo the rearrangement of the IgL chain genes. Once H and L chains are produced, a complete BCR, consisting of IgM plus Igα and Igδ, will be expressed on the surface of immature B cells.

At this stage, the V genes of the BCR are in **germ-line configuration** (i.e., they have not incorporated any point mutations). Products of germ-line V genes generally have low affinity for antigen and can bind weakly to several different antigens (polyreactivity). Weak binding of antigen plus receipt of signals from T-helper cells induce low-affinity B cells to proliferate. The V gene point mutations introduced at cell division alter the strength of binding to antigen, with retention of B cells with higher-affinity BCRs (affinity maturation).

The need to delete anti-self BCRs is probably less than the need to delete anti-self TCRs, since B cells require T cell help to produce high-affinity antibodies, and deletion of anti-self T-helper cells should be sufficient to prevent activation of anti-self B cells. Furthermore, it is desirable to have low-affinity autoantibodies able to opsonize tissue breakdown products for clearance by phagocytes, which would ensure removal of previously sequestered tissue antigens before they could activate T cells.

Peripheral Tolerance

Thymic deletion of T cells bearing self-reactive TCRs is undoubtedly the most important mechanism for ensuring nonreactivity to self. Nevertheless, not all self-antigens are represented in the thymus, so extrathymic tolerance induction is also needed.

Autoreactive T cells are most likely to encounter extrathymic self peptides on epithelial cells rather than professional APCs. The activation signal through the TCR will therefore not be followed by co-stimulatory signals required for full activation. Such an interaction either may result in apoptosis of the T cell or may become anergic (i.e., it survives but in a nonreactive state, often with downregulated expression of TCR, CD3 and CD4/CD8).

Regulatory T cells can suppress the responses of activated T cells, which are required to regulate anti-self reactions when there is failure of thymic or peripheral tolerance induction. Although their mechanism of action is not fully understood, regulatory T cells appear to operate mainly by producing immunosuppressive cytokines and inhibiting T-helper cells.

DISORDERS OF THE IMMUNE SYSTEM

Hypersensitivity, also called an allergic reaction, is an exaggerated reaction of the immune system to an antigen to which there has been prior exposure (sensitized). Types include:

- anaphylactic reactions (type I)—for example, IgE antibody on basophils and mast cells binds with antigens causing release of histamine, prostaglandins and other effectors; can be localized, respiratory or gastrointestinal related, systemic, or associated with shock
- cytotoxic reactions (type II)—for example, activation of complement and lysis of red blood cells (RBC) (main Ig: IgM), which can involve drugs (haptens) binding to RBC and inducing antibodies against them
- immune complex reactions (type III)—for example, complement fixing antigen–antibody complexes (main Ig: IgA); usually phagocytosed, but if the complexes are too small for phagocytosis, can attach to the basement membrane of blood vessels and trigger inflammation
- cell-mediated reactions (type IV, delayed hypersensitivity)—for example, contact allergy in the skin; involves delayed hypersensitivity T cells and activation of memory cells.

Autoimmune reactions are damaging immunological reactions between the host and its own tissues as a result of breakdown in the mechanisms regulating immune tolerance. Types include:

- type I: mediated by anti-self antibodies, often due to microbial molecular mimicry
- type II: cytotoxic autoimmune reactions, in which antibody reacts with cell surface antigens without cell destruction (e.g., Grave's disease, where the thyroid gland is stimulated to produce large amounts of hormones resulting in an enlarged thyroid, goitre and bulging eyes)
- type III: immune complex autoimmune reactions, where IgG and IgM (and sometimes complement) form immune complexes that cause inflammation (e.g., rheumatoid arthritis, where IgG, IgM and complement immune complexes cause chronic inflammation and severe damage to the cartilage and bone joints)
- type IV: cell-mediated autoimmune reactions, which involve destruction of a particular cell type by T cells (e.g., insulin-dependent diabetes mellitus, where insulin-secreting cells of the pancreas are destroyed by T cells).

Immune deficiency is caused when there is a defect in one or more of the various points along the differentiation pathways of immunocompetent cells. Considering the complex cellular interactions involved in immune responses and the central role of T cells, immune deficiencies primarily involving T cells are also associated with abnormal B-cell function. Immunodeficiency syndromes are associated with unusual susceptibility to infections and often associated with autoimmune disease and cancer. The types of infection occurring in patients with an immune deficiency can often provide the first clue as to the nature of the immune defect. Types include:

- congenital immune deficiency: can involve humoural or cell-mediated immune components and are inherited as recessive traits
- acquired immune deficiency: can involve humoural or cell-mediated immune components and often result from drugs, illness, cancer or viruses.

ORAL DEFENCE MECHANISMS

Innate Immune Mechanisms

As mentioned, innate immunity encompasses all of the antigen-nonspecific defence mechanisms that every person is born with and is the initial response used to eliminate microbes or prevent them from entering the body (Fig. 8.9). This includes:

- anatomical barriers
- mechanical removal
- antigen-nonspecific defence chemicals
- microbial antagonism
- defence cells and their activation
- phagocytosis
- inflammation
- fever
- the acute-phase response
- complement.

Two major mechanisms of innate immunity in the oral cavity are immune exclusion and inflammation. **Immune exclusion** refers to the inactivation and clearance of microbes from the oral mucosal epithelium and enamel surfaces. **Inflammation** occurs when there is a need to remove infectious agents at sites of mucosal penetration, and it encompasses phagocytes, detection of PAMPs by PRRs and various inflammatory mediators. Acquired immune mechanisms are also important in the oral cavity; summaries of both are given in Table 8.3.

The Oral Mucosal Epithelium

The oral mucosa is an anatomical **barrier** that prevents entry of potentially harmful microbes. Oral health depends on the integrity of the mucosal barrier, which also provides a **habitat** for normal oral flora. Continuous sloughing (desquamation) of the oral mucosal epithelium continuously removes microbes that colonize the mucosa, and this minimizes the microbial biomass in the oral cavity. Stable colonization, therefore, requires a continual process of microbial attachment, growth and reattachment to exposed epithelial cells, or growth of microbes in saliva at a rate exceeding the salivary flow or dilution rate. When the oral mucosa is compromised (e.g., during chemotherapy), infections frequently develop. Constituents of the oral mucosa that prevent penetration of microbes into deeper tissues include

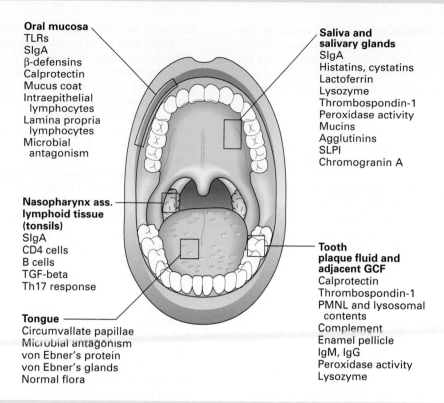

Oral mucosa
TLRs
SIgA
β-defensins
Calprotectin
Mucus coat
Intraepithelial
  lymphocytes
Lamina propria
  lymphocytes
Microbial
  antagonism

**Saliva and
salivary glands**
SIgA
Histatins, cystatins
Lactoferrin
Lysozyme
Thrombospondin-1
Peroxidase activity
Mucins
Agglutinins
SLPI
Chromogranin A

**Nasopharynx ass.
lymphoid tissue
(tonsils)**
SIgA
CD4 cells
B cells
TGF-beta
Th17 response

**Tooth
plaque fluid and
adjacent GCF**
Calprotectin
Thrombospondin-1
PMNL and lysosomal
  contents
Complement
Enamel pellicle
IgM, IgG
Peroxidase activity
Lysozyme

Tongue
Circumvallate papillae
Microbial antagonism
von Ebner's protein
von Ebner's glands
Normal flora

Fig. 8.9 A diagrammatic representation of the natural defence mechanisms of the oral cavity. *Ig,* Immunoglobulin; *PMNL,* polymorphonuclear leukocyte; *TLRs,* Toll-like receptors.

Table 8.3   Nonspecific Host Defence Factors of the Mouth

Defence Factors	Main Function
Epithelial desquamation	Physical removal of microbes
Saliva flow	Physical removal of microbes
Mucin/agglutinins	Physical removal of microbes
Lysozyme	Cell lysis (bactericidal, fungicidal)
Lactoferrin	Iron sequestration (bactericidal, fungicidal)
Apolactoferrin	Iron sequestration (bactericidal, fungicidal)
Sialoperoxidase system	Hypothiocyanite production (neutral pH); hypocyanous acid production (low pH)
Histidine-rich peptides	Antibacterial and antifungal activity
Salivary leukocyte protease inhibitor (SLPI)	Blocks cell surface receptors needed for entry of HIV
Intraepithelial lymphocytes and Langerhans cells	Cellular barrier to penetrating bacteria and/or antigens
Secretory IgA	Prevents microbial adhesion and metabolism
IgG, IgA, IgM	Prevent microbial adhesion; opsonins; complement activators
Complement	Activates neutrophils
Neutrophils/macrophages	Phagocytosis

HIV, Human immunodeficiency virus; *Ig,* immunoglobulin.

saliva, keratin in some areas of the mouth (on the free and attached gingiva, hard palate, areas of the dorsum of tongue); a granular layer, which discharges membrane-coating granules; and a basement membrane that provides barrier function for immune exclusion.

Cells in the oral mucosa also express TLRs for immune surveillance. Resident professional phagocytes as well as circulating cells of the vasculature in the oral mucosal epithelium enable innate defence. Evidence of an intracellular lifestyle of some periodontal pathogens including *Aggregatibacter actinomycetemcomitans* and *Porphyromonas*

gingivalis within buccal epithelial cells suggests that host cells may be used as a protective niche by some microbes to avoid extracellular defences such as antibodies, phagocytes and salivary antimicrobial components, as well as antibiotics.

ANTIGEN-NONSPECIFIC DEFENCE CHEMICALS IN ORAL SECRETIONS

Various antigen-nonspecific defence chemicals (Table 8.3) promote innate immune defence in the oral cavity. These include calprotectin, defensins, saliva (and the enamel pellicle), gingival crevicular fluid (GCF) and mucins. Noncellular mediators of antimicrobial defence help to protect the oral mucosa through potent antibacterial, antiviral and antifungal activities, which can affect oral microbes in several ways:

- they can aggregate or agglutinate microbes
- they can promote or inhibit microbial adhesion
- they can directly kill or inhibit the growth of microbes, and/or
- they can contribute to microbial nutrition.
- **Calprotectin** is a calcium- and zinc-chelating antimicrobial peptide produced by nonkeratinized oral epithelial cells. The chelating activities of calprotectin has an antimicrobial effect as this deprives microbes of essential divalent ions. Calprotectin is present in neutrophils, monocytes, macrophages and probably GCF.
- **Defensins**, in contrast, are a class of pore-forming cationic peptides that insert into the phospholipid bilayer of bacterial membranes causing osmotic instability and cell lysis. Defensins are divided into α- and β-defensins according to their pattern of disulphide bonds and cysteine spacing. Defensins in saliva are also active against fungi and enveloped viruses; cause degranulation of mast cells; and are chemotactic for neutrophils, dendritic cells and memory T cells. Eukaryotic cells resist the lytic action of defensins due to lower phospholipid content in the membranes of these cells. Formation of cell membrane–traversing ring structures by cationic peptides is comparable with the nature of the MAC of the complement cascade.
- **Cathelicidins** are a family of antimicrobial polypeptides found in lysosomes in macrophages and neutrophils that provide innate immune defence against bacteria. These are summarized in Table 8.1.
- **Saliva** contains secretions from the major and minor salivary glands, exfoliated epithelial cells, oral microbes and GCF. The antimicrobial actions of saliva are severalfold; salivary flow combined with the continuous swallowing that cleanses the mouth removes debris and unattached microbes; saliva also replenishes fluids in the oral cavity, which dilutes and clears microbes and acid from plaque; and saliva contains neutrophils as wells as several antigen-nonspecific defence chemicals that kill microbes. These include secretory IgA (S-IgA), IgA, IgG (and sometimes IgM), lysozyme, peroxidases, lactoferrin and chromogranin A (an antifungal protein). These chemicals are synthesized by the salivary glands, the oral epithelium and leukocytes in the gingival crevice/pocket, or they are derived from plasma through the GCF. Saturating levels of calcium and phosphorus in saliva, together with fluoride, help to remineralize white spot lesions and negatively charged salivary molecules, which have a high affinity for the tooth surface, and inhibit the precipitation of calcium phosphate salts.
- The persistent film of saliva that coats the teeth and the oral epithelium as the salivary (enamel) pellicle also helps to maintain a balance between tooth demineralization and remineralization. The pellicle includes many of the defence chemicals found in saliva, as well as proline-rich proteins, albumin, histatins, cystatins, statherin, mucins, amylase and complement component C3. These may serve as receptors for bacteria that adhere to the tooth surface; however, selective attachment of harmless normal resident oral flora probably restricts the attachment of potential pathogens. In conditions of low salivary flow (e.g., Sjögren's syndrome), individuals are more susceptible to colonization with potential pathogens, and severe caries is a frequent outcome of poor salivary protective function.
- **Lysozyme** present in saliva and derived from salivary glands and GCF is similar to lysozyme found in other bodily fluids in that it is bactericidal due to muramidase activity—that is, it splits the β-1,4 glucosidic linkage between NAG (N-acetyl glucosamine) and NAM (N-acetyl muramic acid) in the peptidoglycan of bacterial cell walls causing osmotic lysis. Many oral microbes are resistant to muramidase action, but lysozyme also has other effects: it activates endogenous bacterial enzymes (autolysins) in the cell wall that can kill bacteria, it aggregates oral bacteria to facilitate their removal and it contains amphipathic sequences within the C-terminus that have antimicrobial properties. Lysozyme also synergizes with other defence chemicals including lactoferrin and peroxidase for antimicrobial effect.
- **Peroxidase activity** in saliva comprises peroxidases from salivary glands as well as myeloperoxidase from neutrophils and eosinophil peroxidase. These catalyse the peroxidation of thiocyanate and halides by hydrogen peroxide (from aerobic metabolism of glucose by normal oral flora), which causes the formation of hypothyocyanite. Hypothyocyanite oxidizes bacterial enzymes in glycolytic pathways, and this inhibits the growth of oral microbes. Hydrogen peroxide is also toxic to eukaryotic cells, but its reduction by salivary peroxidases probably helps to protect the oral mucosa. Salivary lactoperoxidase generates toxic superoxide radicals that also kill microbes.
- **Histidine-rich proteins** (histatins) are cationic proteins found in abundance in submandibular/sublingual and parotid saliva. They display various functions, including the initiation of histamine release from mast cells, inhibition of hydroxyapatite crystal growth, neutralization of toxins, protease activity, fungicidal activity and bactericidal activity. Histatins also prevent bacterial coaggregation and serve as competitive inhibitors of certain proteases, which may affect the pathogenesis of periodontitis since it involves extensive proteolytic destruction of host tissues. **Cystatins**, in contrast, are a family of proteins secreted mainly by the submandibular and sublingual salivary glands, which inhibit cysteine proteases. This is considered important for antimicrobial defence because of the beneficial functions of cysteine proteases in many oral microbes. Cystatins also influence inflammation because of their effects on host proteolytic and cytokine activity.
- **Antiviral components** in saliva include the **secretory leukocyte protease inhibitor (SLPI)** and several other proteins that have been demonstrated to possess activity against human immunodeficiency virus (HIV). SLPI is a small, cationic, acid-stable protein produced by serous acinar and epithelial cells. SLPI inhibits viral entry and/or uncoating in host cells and also displays

serine protease inhibitor activity, which would protect the mucosal barrier from neutrophil-derived enzymes secreted during inflammation. SLPI also displays some bactericidal and fungicidal activity. Another class of salivary antiviral proteins is human parotid **proline-rich proteins**, which inhibit HIV activity most likely by interfering with the interactions between virus and host cell surfaces. Finally, **thrombospondin 1** is an extracellular matrix glycoprotein secreted by submandibular and sublingual salivary glands that inhibits viral infection of monocytes and T cells. For HIV, this appears to occur via binding of thrombospondin 1 to viral gp120, which would inhibit the virus interacting with CD4 receptors on T cells.

- **Gingival crevicular fluid (GCF)** is a vehicle by which blood components including leukocytes (estimated to consist of 95% neutrophils, 3% monocytes and 2% lymphocytes) can reach the oral cavity via flow of fluid through the junctional epithelium of the gingivae (gingival margin) into the gingival crevice. Normally, the flow of GCF is low, but flow increases with inflammation to flush oral surfaces that are vulnerable to penetration by microbes. The composition of GCF also changes during inflammation from a transudate to a plasmalike inflammatory exudate, which can be collected from patients with oral disease. Various constituents of innate and acquired immunity reach sites of plaque accumulation from the blood via the GCF, including neutrophils, plasma proteins (e.g., albumin and fibrin), monocytes, T and B lymphocytes and Igs (IgG, IgM and IgA). Signalling molecules and inflammatory mediators—including neutrophil elastase, collagenase-2, prostaglandin E2 and classical and alternative complement pathway components—are also common in GCF. Other enzymes, including lysozyme and proteases (a mixture of host and bacterial), have also been detected in GCF, and these have been shown to inactivate IgA. The functional significance of GCF is related to the antimicrobial properties of its constituents that impact oral microbial colonization and survival.
- The **mucus layer** on intraoral surfaces exists as a sticky, slippery gel-like barrier composed of mucin glycoproteins, which prevent entry of microbes into underlying tissue. Mucus traps microbes and removes them from the oral cavity by sloughing. Mucus is also selectively permeable to allow transition of nutrients and waste products but not microbes. Mucins are derived from salivary glands and include the membrane-bound mucins MUC1 and MUC4, the gel-forming mucin MUC5B (MG1), and MUC7 (MG2). The gelatinous consistency of some mucins (e.g., MUC5B) is due to a threadlike structure rich in carbohydrates (up to 80%) and high molecular mass. In contrast, other mucins display low viscosity due to a smaller mass and relatively simplistic structure (e.g., MUC7); these different physicochemical properties enable distinct functions of different mucins. Mucins are distributed unevenly in the oral cavity—for example, they are rare in parotid secretions. Thus saliva in the areas vestibular to the maxillary molars (derived from the parotid glands) is low in mucins. In contrast, saliva in the areas located vestibular to the upper incisors is derived from submandibular and sublingual glands and is rich in mucins. Similarly, more parotid agglutinin and other serous proteins, such as amylase and proline-rich proteins, are found in maxillary premolar pellicles compared with mandibular anterior pellicles. Unique patterns of mucin distribution probably influence oral microbial communities. Mucins can also aggregate bacteria via interactions between mucin saccharides and bacterial proteins. However, different sugars aggregate different oral bacteria, which may remove some microbes but allow other species to remain. Mucus also contains lysozyme, IgA, lactoperoxidase and lactoferrin to sequester iron from microbes. Mucins can form homotypic complexes (end-to-end oligomers) to enable lubrication properties and heterotypic complexes with S-IgA, lysozyme, cystatins and β-defensin to increase local concentrations of antimicrobial molecules. Low mucin production has been correlated with a higher microbial biomass, suggesting a link between mucins and oral health.

FUNCTIONALITY OF SALIVARY DEFENCE CONSTITUENTS

The functions of individual components in saliva and GCF secretions are **dynamic** and related to **molecular shape** and **enzymatic activity**. The functions of these components may vary under different physicochemical conditions and are sometimes altered following absorption onto surfaces as opposed to in solution. For example, surface-absorbed proline-rich proteins promote bacterial adhesion; however, these molecules do not interact with bacteria when in solution.

Salivary amylase interacts with streptococci, but disruption of its disulphide bonds alters its molecular shape and abates this biological activity. Changes in conformation or epitope structure induced by binding to surfaces are the most likely explanation for divergent function in these components. Multiple overlapping functions are also common among salivary components. This enables redundancy in the activities of many salivary components. **Functional redundancy** may provide more dependable antimicrobial action for circumstances in which host components have been neutralized as a result of microbial activity. For example, agglutination of microbes is a shared function among many salivary components (e.g., mucins, S-IgA, parotid agglutinin, lysozyme, etc.), which would enable agglutination and clearance of microbes from the oral cavity even if one of the components were to be rendered nonfunctional (e.g., inactivation of S-IgA by microbial enzymes).

Amphifunctionality (i.e., both protective and detrimental effects) is also inherent in some salivary components. For example statherin promotes remineralization of the tooth by inhibiting the formation of calcium and phosphate salts; however, when adsorbed to the enamel pellicle, statherin can also promote the adhesion of potentially cariogenic microbes to the tooth. Seemingly contradictory functions should be considered against the background that many salivary and pellicle components must act to promote the harmless normal resident oral flora but must also actively inhibit the adherence and growth of potential pathogens. Functional relationships between different salivary, pellicle and GCF components can be **homotypic** (same molecule) or **heterotypic** (different molecules) as in the case of mucins.

MICROBIAL INTERACTIONS AND THE NORMAL ORAL FLORA

Colonization of the oral mucosal epithelium by normal resident oral flora is an important innate defence mechanism for immune exclusion because it prevents potential pathogens from colonizing the mouth. This is also called **colonization resistance**. The normal flora secretes metabolic by-products such as antibiotics, competes for nutrients and receptors, and may alter the conditions in the microenvironment (e.g., pH, oxygen) to limit the growth of potential pathogens. Components of the normal flora such as LPS may also stimulate nonspecific innate immune defence mechanisms (e.g., activation of phagocytes, synthesis of cross-protective antibodies). When the normal oral flora is depleted (e.g., during broad-spectrum antibiotic therapy), the so called **eubiotic equilibrium** between the oral mucosa and resident flora is disturbed a **dysbiotic** state supervenes, providing an opportunity for potential pathogens to proliferate that may result in oral disease. One example is the infection by the oral fungal pathogen *Candida albicans*, where most of the commensal bacteria are killed by broad-spectrum antibiotics such as tetracycline.

The gingival sulcus, teeth and tongue harbour a normal flora, which includes several species of streptococci and other bacteria, now known to comprise more than 700–1 000 species. Microbial relationships resulting, for example, from coaggregation between different species in mixed biofilms on teeth may encompass:

- **microbial antagonism** (one species harms, and can exclude, the other)
- **synergism** (two species cooperate to benefit both)—for example, cooperation between streptococci and gingivitis pathogens during disease
- **symbiosis** (a close ecological relationship of at least two species where at least one species benefits, the other may be unaffected or harmed)
- **commensalism** (one species benefits, the other is unaffected)
- **mutualism** (both species benefit)
- **parasitism** (one species benefits, the other is harmed).

Adaptive Immunity in Oral Health and Disease

Acquired or adaptive immunity refers to all of the antigen-specific defence mechanisms that take several days to weeks to become protective and are designed to react with and remove specific antigens. Acquired immunity develops throughout one's life and is completely dependent on **T and B lymphocytes**. Acquired immunity in the oral cavity comprises both humoural and cellular mechanisms that involve **GCF Igs** (IgM, IgG and IgA) derived from plasma cells in the gingivae, effector T lymphocytes and, principally, **secretory IgA (S-IgA)**. The normal resident oral flora appears to be important in inducing a self-limiting humoural mucosal immune response that provides defence against potential pathogens. **Mucosa associated lymphoid tissue** (MALT) that lies beneath the oral mucosal epithelium contains phagocytes for killing microbes and APCs, which sample antigens in the oral mucosa and provide the link between innate and acquired immune responses. Lymphoid cells around the basement membrane also help to eliminate any potential pathogens that overcome innate immune exclusion and pass through the intact oral mucosal epithelium.

ORAL LYMPHOID TISSUES

Extraoral lymph nodes and intraoral lymphoid tissues are present in the mouth. Four types of intraoral lymphoid tissues are present:

1. **palatine and lingual tonsils**,
2. **salivary gland lymphoid tissue** (which contributes to S-IgA production),
3. **gingival lymphoid tissue**
4. **submucosal lymphoid cells** scattered in the submucosa

Networks of lymph capillaries and lymph vessels link the oral mucosa, gingivae, and pulp to other structures such as the tongue and drain into submandibular, retropharyngeal and other lymph nodes. Microbes that have overcome innate immune exclusion and penetrated through the oral mucosa may enter the lymphatics directly or be transported into the lymphatics by phagocytes. When microbial antigens reach lymphocytes in the MALT, an immune response is elicited. Activated lymphocytes that have encountered antigen leave the MALT via the efferent lymphatics and enter the circulation, after which they relocate to the lamina propria to drive acquired immune responses. T cells in the lamina propria are predominantly of CD4 and CD8 types, but another type of T cell, termed **intraepithelial lymphocytes (IELs)**, is located between the epithelial cells and basement membrane. These cells appear to be involved in immune surveillance, maintenance of mucosal integrity via synthesis of growth factors and the removal of epithelial cells that become infected. B cells in the lamina propria and associated with acini of the major and minor salivary glands synthesize IgA. Tonsils may also guard the entry into the digestive and respiratory tracts, while the gingival lymphoid tissue may help in the immune response to dental plaque.

S-IGA IN ORAL DEFENCE

S-IgA is the predominant Ig in saliva. It prevents microbes from adhering to mucosal epithelial cells by binding to and agglutinating them, which promotes their removal from the oral cavity. In contrast to the IgA present in plasma that is almost always monomeric (and derived from plasma cells in the bone marrow), S-IgA is composed of an IgA dimer derived from the polymerization of two IgA molecules (derived from plasma cells in the salivary glands) by **joining (J) chain glycoprotein**. Tetramers of S-IgA are also common. Incorporation of a glycoprotein fragment of the polymeric Ig receptor termed the **secretory component** (SC; synthesized by epithelial cells of the salivary acini) into IgA dimers forms a complete S-IgA molecule. **Receptors** for the SC on oral epithelial cells bind to S-IgA, which enables capturing and shedding of opsonized oral microbes, and this contributes to immune exclusion. Antigen-specific inhibition of microbial adherence by S-IgA depends on B-cell clones produced against unique oral microbial antigens. In contrast, S-IgA present in the enamel pellicle may promote attachment of microbes to the tooth surface. S-IgA can also neutralize microbial toxins, enzymes and viruses. However, unlike other Igs, S-IgA does not activate complement and is therefore regarded as a noninflammatory Ig. This unique attribute enables S-IgA to maintain the integrity of the mucosal barrier since complement activation generates potent mediators of inflammation such as C3a and C5a. The SC also makes the normally susceptible hinge region of S-IgA resistant to proteolytic and acidic conditions that exist in the mouth. S-IgA also helps to prevent infection within the salivary glands. It is noteworthy that more IgA (plasma and secretory) is produced each day than is produced by the other four types of Igs combined. Finally, S-IgA also influences innate defence by synergizing with the antimicrobial activities of lysozyme and potentiating the activities of mucins by reducing the negative surface charge and hydrophobicity of oral bacteria (allows the bacteria to be coated with mucins). Some S-IgA displays plurispecific action (polyreactive; i.e., binds a wide range of bacterial and host antigens), which is believed to protect the oral mucosa prior to the induction of highly antigen-specific S-IgA.

Plurispecific S-IgA appears to be derived in a **T-independent** manner against commensal oral microbes, food and host tissue antigens. In contrast, **T-dependent** mechanisms probably impart extremely specific S-IgA through B-cell somatic hypermutation to produce Igs directed against only a single unique antigen. It is notable that some oral pathogens produce proteases that cleave and subvert the function of S-IgA. Heterotypic associations between S-IgA and lactoferrin, and S-IgA and agglutinins have been demonstrated, but their role in oral defence is unclear. Enigmatically, humans with a selective IgA deficiency are not highly susceptible to mucosal infection, and this condition is largely asymptomatic. Functional redundancy of antimicrobial molecules at the oral mucosal surface probably explains this apparent contradiction in the acquired immune response to oral microbes. In many people, selective IgA deficiency correlates with increased transportation of IgM into external secretions, which would compensate for this immune deficiency at mucosal surfaces.

PROGRAMMED CELL DEATH IN RESPONSE TO ORAL MICROBES

Apoptosis, also termed 'programmed cell death' (PCD), is an important physiological mechanism through which the immune system responds to diverse forms of cell damage. PCD occurs normally under many conditions to remove unwanted, damaged or dying host cells—for example, it

removes autoreactive lymphocytes by negative selection, and it regulates the size of T-cell memory pools after resolution of infection. PCD can promote the removal of pathogens by killing the host cells that are infected with them. PCD is controlled by cytoplasmic cysteine-dependent aspartate-directed proteases termed **caspases** that exist in all human cells and direct two pathways of PCD:

1. **Intrinsic pathway:** death receptor-independent deregulation of mitochondrial function
2. **Extrinsic pathway:** activation of death receptors.

End-stage PCD involves cleavage of proteins required for cell integrity, DNA degradation, chromatin condensation, externalization of lipid phosphatidylserine, cell shrinkage and cell disassembly into '**apoptotic bodies**'. Importantly, apoptotic bodies are actively phagocytosed by macrophages to prevent spillage of intracellular contents from dying cells, and this limits inflammation. PCD in gingival epithelial cells has important implications for mucosal barrier function because of effects on immune exclusion, inflammation, antigen processing and presentation, and the acquired regulatory responses of T and B lymphocytes. For example, PCD facilitates antigen presentation to T lymphocytes through MHC I during tuberculosis. A significant group of oral pathogens including *Porphyromonas gingivalis*, *Aggregatibacter actinomycetemcomitans*, *Candida albicans*, and *Treponema denticola* have been shown to modulate PCD pathways in human cells; whether these PCD responses are part of the normal immune response to these microbes and beneficial to oral health is unclear. However, detection of PCD in chronically inflamed gingiva suggests that it may help to maintain homoeostasis in the gingival tissue. On the other hand, induction of PCD by subgingival pathogens may also contribute to local tissue destruction during periodontitis; for example, up to 10% of the total cell population in gingival biopsies from patients with chronic periodontitis has been shown to be apoptotic. PCD in bone-lining cells triggered in the acquired immune response to *P. gingivalis* also appears to contribute to deficient bone formation in periodontitis by reducing the coupling of bone formation and resorption. Finally, delayed PCD in neutrophils during periodontitis has also been observed, suggesting a mechanism of neutrophil accumulation at sites of oral disease.

Some examples of recently discovered cell death responses triggered by oral microbes and substances are given in Table 8.4.

Table 8.4 Examples of Cell Death Responses Triggered by Oral Microbes and Substances

Oral Microbe or Substance	Target Cell Type(s) and PCD Response	Apoptosis Regulatory Molecule
Porphyromonas gingivalis	Epithelial cells, inhibits PCD	Gingipain adhesin peptide A44
Candida albicans	Vascular endothelial cells	Unknown
Streptococcus salivarius	Epithelial cells, no PCD activity, homoeostatic	None detected
Aggregatibacter actinomycetemcomitans	T cells, induces PCD	Leukotoxin
Fusobacterium nucleatum	Human monocyte-derived macrophages, lacks PCD activity	LPS
Fluoride	Various cell types, induces PCD	Unknown
Mastic	Oral polymorphonuclear leukocytes, inhibits PCD; oral squamous cell carcinoma, induces PCD	Unknown

LPS, Lipopolysaccharide; *PCD,* programmed cell death.

Key Facts

- The immune system exists to protect the body against **internal** (e.g. cancer) and **external** threats (e.g. pathogens).
- Various natural or innate defence mechanisms initiate protection, but **specific** or **adaptive responses**, with memory, are required to neutralize fully most threats.
- Deficient immunological function results in increased susceptibility to infection.
- The immune system must learn not to react against 'self components'; otherwise, autoimmune disease results.
- Components of the innate immune system include **phagocytes, natural killer (NK) cells, the alternative complement pathway** and **inflammation**.
- The adaptive immune response requires **antigen-presenting cells** (macrophages, dendritic cells, B cells) to process antigen into peptides displayed on **major histocompatibility complex (MHC)** molecules on the cell surface.
- The T lymphocytes are of two types: **T-helper cells**, which are CD4$^+$ and recognize peptides presented by MHC II molecules, and **T-cytotoxic/suppressor cells**, which are CD8$^+$ and recognize MHC I-peptide complexes.
- Both B cells and T cells recognize antigen through specific receptors. These receptors have variable regions that are derived by selection and recombination of germ-line gene segments.
- Those T cells whose antigen receptors react strongly to self molecules in the thymus are deleted, and those that recognize self molecules outside the thymus are usually made nonreactive.
- In the oral cavity, innate immunity is mediated principally by **immune exclusion** and **inflammation**.

- The oral mucosal epithelium provides a **physical barrier** that, when breached, renders individuals highly susceptible to infection.
- **Antigen-nonspecific defence chemicals** important in the oral cavity are calprotectin, defensins, salivary constituents, lysozyme, peroxidases, histidine-rich proteins and cystatins.
- **Antiviral components** in saliva include the secretory leukocyte protease inhibitor (SLPI), parotid proline-rich proteins and thrombospondin 1.
- Gingival crevicular fluid (GCF) is a plasma-like inflammatory exudate containing neutrophils, plasma proteins, monocytes, lymphocytes and immunoglobulins (IgG, IgM and IgA), which collectively impede microbial colonization, persistence and survival.
- **Functional redundancy** provides dependable antimicrobial action in the oral cavity and is related to the dynamic nature of enzymatic activity and shape of individual molecules.
- **Amphifunctionality** (i.e., both protective and detrimental effects) is inherent in some salivary components.
- Intraoral **lymphoid tissues** are palatine and lingual tonsils, salivary gland lymphoid tissue, gingival lymphoid tissue and scattered submucosal lymphoid cells.
- **S-IgA**, the predominant immunoglobulin in saliva, prevents microbes from adhering to mucosal epithelial cells and can display pluri- or highly antigen-specific actions.
- **Apoptosis** in gingival epithelial cells and leukocytes has important implications for mucosal barrier function, acquired immunity and disease pathogenesis in the oral cavity.

Review Questions (Answers on p. 388)

Please indicate which answers are true and which are false.

8.1. Lymphocyte populations do not include:
 a. B lymphocytes
 b. phagocytes
 c. CD4$^+$ helper T cells
 d. natural killer cells
 e. CD8$^+$ cytotoxic T cells

8.2. Innate immune mechanisms do not include:
 a. mechanical barriers
 b. phagocytosis
 c. acute-phase proteins
 d. antibody-mediated neutralization
 e. complement activation

8.3. Which of the following is not a molecular event occurring during cell development in bone marrow?
 a. immunoglobulin heavy-chain gene rearrangement
 b. immunoglobulin light-chain gene rearrangement
 c. μ heavy-chain expression in precursor B cells
 d. expression of IgE on B-cell surface
 e. pairing of μ heavy chain with light chain to form IgM molecule

8.4. During T-cell development in the thymus:
 a. CD4$^+$CD8$^+$ cells differentiate into CD4$^-$CD8$^-$ cells
 b. positive selection takes place after negative selection
 c. CD4$^-$CD8$^-$ cells are located in the thymic medulla
 d. mature, functional T cells are either CD4$^+$CD8$^-$ or CD4$^-$CD8$^+$ cells
 e. thymocytes undergo extensive immunoglobulin gene rearrangements

8.5. Two major mechanisms of innate immunity in the oral cavity are:
 a. gingival crevicular fluid (GCF) and salivary agglutinins
 b. mucins and peroxidases
 c. calprotectin and lysozyme
 d. complement and S-IgA
 e. immune exclusion and inflammation

8.6. Which of the following oral mucosa constituents prevent microbial penetration?
 a. saliva
 b. keratin
 c. granular layer
 d. basement membrane
 e. resident professional phagocytes

8.7. Antimicrobial actions of antigen-nonspecific defence chemicals in oral secretions include but are not limited to:
   a. aggregation of microbes
   b. agglutination of microbes
   c. promotion of microbial adhesion
   d. inhibiting the growth of microbes
   e. contributing to microbial nutrition

8.8. Defensins in oral secretions are:
   a. pore-forming peptides that cause osmotic instability in microbes
   b. divided into α and γ types according to disulphide bond patterns
   c. active against bacteria, fungi and some enveloped viruses
   d. chemotactic for eosinophils and basophils
   e. comparable in mode of action to the membrane attack complex

8.9. In addition to the defence chemicals normally found in saliva, the salivary pellicle contains which of the following defence chemicals?
   a. proline-rich proteins
   b. histatins and cystatins
   c. calprotectin
   d. complement component C3
   e. cathelicidins

8.10. Antiviral components in saliva include:
   a. complement component C5
   b. peroxidases
   c. lactoferrin
   d. secretory leukocyte protease inhibitor
   e. parotid proline-rich proteins

8.11. Constituents of acquired immunity that reach sites of plaque accumulation from the blood via the GCF include:
   a. IgA
   b. neutrophils
   c. T and B lymphocytes
   d. alternative complement pathway components
   e. IgG and IgM

8.12. Mucins:
   a. are distributed evenly in the oral cavity
   b. aggregate bacteria via interactions between mucin proteins and bacterial saccharides
   c. form homotypic complexes to enable lubrication
   d. form heterotypic complexes to concentrate antimicrobial molecules locally
   e. (production) has been correlated with lower microbial biomass

8.13. Which of the following statements regarding the functions of salivary and GCF antimicrobial components are true?
   a. changes in conformation or epitope structure induced by binding to surfaces do not explain divergent function in relation to antimicrobial action
   b. amphifunctionality refers to antimicrobial components with either protective or detrimental effects towards microbes
   c. functional redundancy provides more wide-ranging antimicrobial activity for the control of many different classes of microbes
   d. functional relationships between GCF antimicrobial components are always heterotypic
   e. functions of salivary antimicrobial components are related to molecular shape and enzymatic activity

8.14. A microbial relationship between streptococci and fusobacteria leading to plaque biofilm formation can be regarded as:
   a. microbial antagonism
   b. microbial synergism
   c. microbial symbiosis
   d. microbial commensalism
   e. microbial parasitism

8.15. Adaptive immunity in the oral environment:
   a. encompasses nonantigen-specific defence mechanisms that take several days to weeks to become protective
   b. is mediated largely by S-IgA
   c. influences innate defence in the oral cavity by synergizing with lysozyme and mucins
   d. utilizes immunoglobulin to neutralize microbial toxins, enzymes and viruses
   e. inhibits microbial adherence using S-IgA produced against oral microbial antigens

8.16. Which of the following statements on programmed cell death in response to oral microbes are true?
   a. it is controlled by cytoplasmic cysteine-dependent arginine-directed proteases termed caspases
   b. it occurs normally in the oral cavity to remove unwanted, damaged or dying host cells
   c. two pathways of programmed cell death are the intrinsic and the extrinsic pathways
   d. apoptotic bodies promote inflammation in response to oral microbes
   e. programmed cell death may be beneficial to oral health but may also contribute to local tissue destruction during periodontitis

Further Reading

Diamond, G., Beckloff, N., Weinberg, A., et al. (2009). The roles of antimicrobial peptides in innate host defense. *Current Pharmaceutical Design, 15*(21), 2377–2392.

Gorr, S. U. (2009). Antimicrobial peptides of the oral cavity. *Periodontology, 51*, 152–180.

Janeway, Jr., C. A., Travers, P., Walport, M., et al. (2001). *Immunobiology* (5th ed.). Garland Publishing.

Lamster, I. B., & Ahlo, J. K. (2007). Analysis of gingival crevicular fluid as applied to the diagnosis of oral and systemic diseases. *Annals of the New York Academy of Sciences, 1098*, 216–229.

Macpherson, A. J., McCoy, K. D., Johansen, F. E., et al. (2008). The immune geography of IgA induction and function. *Mucosal Immunology, 1*(1), 11–22.

Mestecky, J., Lamm, M. F., McGhee, J. R., et al. (2005). *Mucosal immunology* (3rd ed.). Elsevier.

Roitt, I. M. (1997). *Roitt's essential immunology* (9th ed.). Blackwell.

Roitt, I., Brostoff, J., & Male, D. (1998). *Immunology* (5th ed.). Mosby.

Staines, N., Brostoff, J., & James, K. (1994). *Introducing immunology* (2nd ed.). Mosby.

Ulett, G. C., & Adderson, E. E. (2006). Regulation of apoptosis by Gram-positive bacteria: Mechanistic diversity and consequences for immunity. *Current Immunology Reviews, 2,* 119–141.

9 The Immune Response

Chapter 8 described the development of B- and T-cell repertoires. At birth, the immature immune system consists of B cells selected for low-affinity antibody production, while the T-cell repertoire consists of T-cell antigen receptors (TCRs) potentially able to recognize foreign but usually not self-peptides presented by major histocompatibility complex (MHC) molecules on antigen-presenting cells (APCs). The latter must also provide co-stimulatory signals for full T-cell activation.

During the vulnerable few months following birth, while immune system maturation is continuing, the infant receives protection against pathogens from the mother's 'experienced' immune system. Maternal immunoglobulin G (IgG) antibodies cross the placenta and provide **passive immunity**. The IgA antibodies in mother's milk protect the infant's digestive system. By the age of 9 months, all maternal IgG antibodies will have been catabolized and suckling may have been terminated. The infant must now be able to mobilize its own adaptive immune response mechanisms to fight off potential pathogens.

Antibodies

Antibodies, or immunoglobulins (Igs), are the secreted products of B lymphocytes which have become activated following binding of antigen to their B-cell receptors (BCRs). The specificity for antigen of the secreted antibody is the same as that of the BCR, so they will bind to the same antigen that induced their production. The formation of the antigen–antibody complex may result in:

- neutralization of the antigen (e.g., soluble toxins, viruses)
- removal of the complex by phagocytic cells which bind via **Fc receptors (FcRs)** to the Ig constant region
- killing of antigen-bearing cells by the membrane attack complex of complement or by natural killer (NK) cells, monocyte/macrophages or granulocytes, which bind antibody-coated cells via FcRs.

The basic Y-shaped, four-chain structure of the antibody molecule is shown in Fig. 9.1. Antigen-binding specificity is provided by the combined variable (V) regions of heavy (H) and light (L) chains. Since the basic Ig unit has two such pairings, the molecule can bind two identical epitopes (i.e., it is bivalent). The Ig heavy-chain constant region, particularly domains 2 and 3, which make up the Fc region, largely determines the biological activity of the molecule.

There are five distinct classes of Ig (IgG, IgA, IgM, IgD, IgE), four subclasses of IgG (IgG1, IgG2, IgG3, IgG4) and two subclasses of IgA (IgA1, IgA2). These are derived from usage of different heavy-chain genes, as described in Chapter 8. The different structures and properties of Ig molecules are summarized in Fig. 9.2.

Cytokines

Cytokines are low-molecular-weight hormone-like glycoproteins secreted by leukocytes and various other cells in response to a number of stimuli, which are involved in communication between cells, particularly those of the immune system. Lymphocyte-derived cytokines are known as **lymphokines**, those produced by monocyte/macrophages as **monokines**. Many of the cytokines are referred to as **interleukins (ILs)**, a name indicating that they are secreted by some leukocytes and act upon other leukocytes. They are required for the initiation and regulation of all stages of the immune response, from stem cell differentiation to effector cell activation. Their action is mediated by binding to specific receptors on target cells; often the receptor may be released from the target cell in soluble form so that it may intercept the cytokine and act as an inhibitor. There are also other forms of cytokine inhibitors responsible for keeping these molecules under tight regulation. Each cytokine has several different activities (**pleiotropy**), and the same activity may be produced by

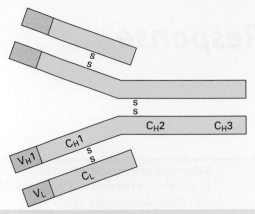

Fig. 9.1 Structure of the immunoglobulin molecule. *C*, Constant region; *H*, heavy chain; *L*, light chain; *C_H_1*, *C_H_2*, *C_H_3* are globular domains with different biological properties; *V*, variable region.

several different cytokines (**redundancy**). The response of a cell to an individual cytokine depends on the context in which it receives the signal (e.g., its state of differentiation and activation and the presence of other cytokines in the microenvironment).

Chemokines are a family of low-molecular-weight, structurally related cytokines that promote adhesion of cells to endothelium, chemotaxis and activation of leukocytes. They are involved in leukocyte trafficking, providing specific signals for lymphocyte entry into lymphoid and other tissue.

Table 9.1 outlines the main sources and activities of cytokines. The table is not exhaustive, and new cytokines and activities are undoubtedly awaiting discovery. The exciting field of cytokine research has led to the isolation of genes for cytokines and their receptors and inhibitors and the ability to manufacture these molecules by recombinant DNA

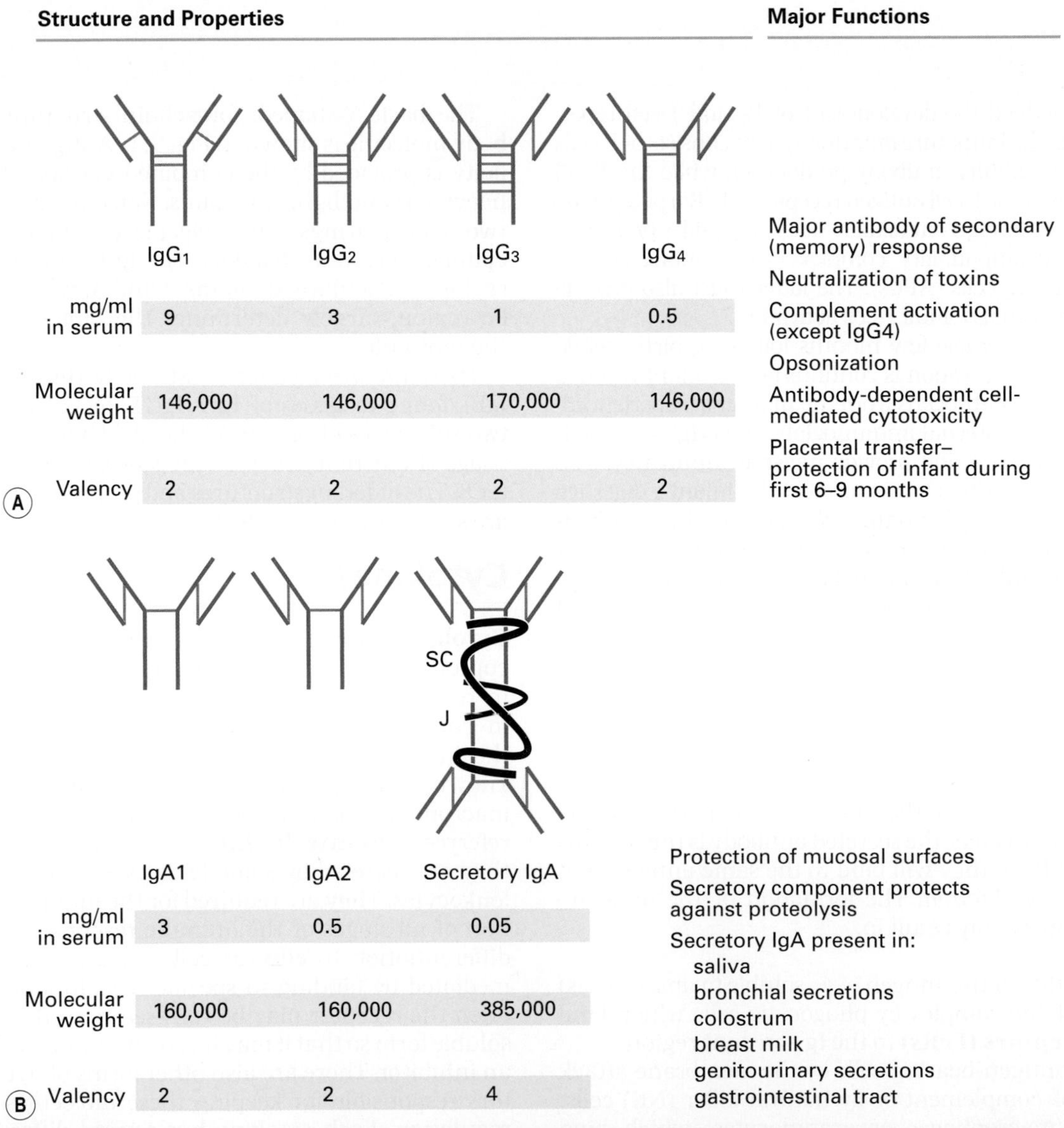

Structure and Properties				Major Functions
IgG₁	IgG₂	IgG₃	IgG₄	Major antibody of secondary (memory) response
				Neutralization of toxins
mg/ml in serum 9	3	1	0.5	Complement activation (except IgG4)
				Opsonization
Molecular weight 146,000	146,000	170,000	146,000	Antibody-dependent cell-mediated cytotoxicity
Valency 2	2	2	2	Placental transfer–protection of infant during first 6–9 months

(A)

			Major Functions
IgA1	IgA2	Secretory IgA	Protection of mucosal surfaces
mg/ml in serum 3	0.5	0.05	Secretory component protects against proteolysis
Molecular weight 160,000	160,000	385,000	Secretory IgA present in: saliva, bronchial secretions, colostrum, breast milk, genitourinary secretions, gastrointestinal tract
Valency 2	2	4	

(B)

Fig. 9.2 Structure, properties and functions of different classes of immunoglobulins (Igs). *BCR*, B cell receptor; *J*, joining chain; *SC*, secretory component.

Structure and Properties   **Major Functions**

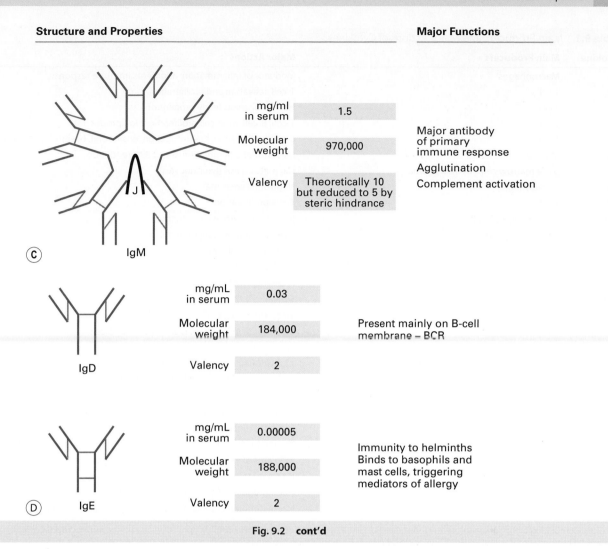

mg/ml in serum	1.5	
Molecular weight	970,000	Major antibody of primary immune response
Valency	Theoretically 10 but reduced to 5 by steric hindrance	Agglutination Complement activation

© IgM

mg/mL in serum	0.03	
Molecular weight	184,000	Present mainly on B-cell membrane – BCR
Valency	2	

IgD

mg/mL in serum	0.00005	
Molecular weight	188,000	Immunity to helminths Binds to basophils and mast cells, triggering mediators of allergy
Valency	2	

Ⓓ IgE

Fig. 9.2   cont'd

technology. There is optimism that therapeutic use of these reagents will, in the near future, benefit patients with infections, autoimmunity, allergy and other immunologically mediated diseases.

B Cell Activation

B cells are highly efficient APCs. They receive signal 1 for activation by binding antigen, often concentrated on the surface of follicular dendritic cells within lymph node germinal centres, to the BCR, and then proceed to internalize antigen and process peptides onto MHC II molecules for presentation to T-helper cells (Fig. 9.3). They are then induced to express co-stimulatory B7 and can therefore provide signal 2 for T-helper cell activation through CD28. Activated T-helper cells are induced to express CD40L for binding to B cell CD40. Interaction between these two molecules induces B cell activation, Ig production and isotype switching.

IL-12 is not usually the dominant cytokine at the site of B–T_H interaction, so T-helper cells induced by B-APC will generally be of the T_H2 type, secreting IL-4, IL-5 and IL-10. These lymphokines further promote B-cell proliferation, activation and isotype switching.

Antigen Processing and Presentation

The T lymphocytes use their TCRs to recognize short antigenic peptides bound to MHC class I or class II molecules. This requires that protein antigens be processed and directed to the site of MHC assembly within an MHC-expressing cell. Although virtually any cell type can process peptides onto MHC I molecules, 'professional' APCs (monocyte/macrophages, dendritic cells, B lymphocytes) are usually the only cell types to present MHC II + peptide (Fig. 9.4).

APCs express a variety of adhesion molecules that bind to counterstructures on T cells during engagement of the TCR. This maintains the necessary intercellular contact for transfer of activation signal 1. Adhesion molecules include intercellular adhesion molecules ICAM-1 (CD54) and ICAM-2 (CD102) and leukocyte function-associated antigen LFA-3 (CD58) on APCs and LFA-1 (CD11a/CD18), which binds ICAM-1 or -2, and LFA-2 (CD2), which binds LFA-3, on T cells.

Professional APCs also express the B7.1 (CD80) and B7.2 (CD86) co-stimulator molecules, which both interact with CD28 and cytotoxic T-lymphocyte-associated antigen

Table 9.1   Main Producers and Major Actions of Cytokines

Cytokine	Main Producers	Major Actions
IL-1	Macrophages	Mediator of inflammation; augments immune response
IL-2	T cells	T-cell activation and proliferation
IL-3	T cells	Haematopoiesis (early progenitors)
IL-4	T cells	T-cell, B-cell, mast cell proliferation; IgE production
IL-5	T cells	B-cell proliferation; IgA production; eosinophil, basophil differentiation
IL-6	Macrophages, T cells	Mediator of inflammation; B-cell differentiation
IL-7	Bone marrow cells, thymic stroma	Haematopoiesis (lymphocytes)
IL-8	Macrophages	Neutrophil chemotaxis
IL-9	T cells	T-cell proliferation
IL-10	Macrophages, T cells	Inhibitor of cytokine production
IL-11	Bone marrow stromal cells	Haematopoiesis (early progenitors)
IL-12	Macrophages	T-cell differentiation
IL-13	T cells	Similar to IL-4
IL-14	T cells	Proliferation of activated B cells
IL-15	Stromal cells	Similar to IL-2
IL-16	T cells	T-cell chemotaxis
IL-17	T cells	Mediator of inflammation and haematopoiesis
IL-18	Macrophages	Similar to IL-12
IFN-α	Leukocytes	Activation of macrophages, NK cells; upregulation of MHC expression; protection of cells against virus infection
IFN-β	Fibroblasts	
IFN-γ	T cells, NK cells	
LT	T cells	Mediator of inflammation; killing of tumour cells; inhibition of tumour growth
OSM	Macrophages, T cells	
TGF-β	Macrophages, lymphocytes, endothelial cells, platelets	Wound healing; IgA production; suppression of cytokine production
TNF-α	Macrophages, T cells	Mediator of inflammation; killing of tumour cells
gCSF	Macrophages	Haematopoiesis (granulocytes)
mCSF	Monocytes	Haematopoiesis (monocyte/macrophages)
gmCSF	T cells	Haematopoiesis (granulocytes, monocyte/macrophages)

CSF, Colony-stimulating factor; *g*, granulocyte; *Ig*, immunoglobulin; *IFN*, interferon; *IL*, interleukin; *LT*, lymphotoxin; *m*, monocyte/macrophage; *MHC*, major histocompatibility complex; *NK*, natural killer; *OSM*, oncostatin M; *TGF*, transforming growth factor; *TNF*, tumour necrosis factor.

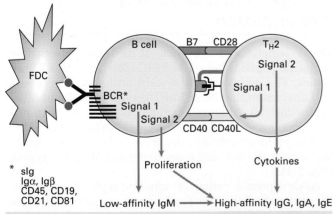

Fig. 9.3   Activation of B cells. *BCR*, B-cell receptor; *FDC*, follicular dendritic cell; *L*, ligand; *sIg*, surface immunoglobulin.

(CTLA-4) on T cells. While CD28 transmits activation signal 2 to the responding T cell, CTLA-4 appears to be involved in termination of activation. Interaction between CD40 on APC and CD40 ligand (CD40L, CD154) on responding T cells is another important signal 2 for activation. Cells other than professional APCs, despite expression of MHC

I + peptide, cannot usually stimulate T cells because they lack B7 and CD40.

The MHC + peptide, adhesion molecules and co-stimulator molecules on APCs interact with clusters of TCRs and ligands on T cells, forming an organized interface termed the **immunological synapse**. It is the overall strength of this multipoint interaction that determines the strength of the activation signal received by the T cell. Strong signals lead to full activation, whereas weak signals may induce partial or no activation.

There are two separate pathways of antigen processing for endogenous and exogenous antigens. Endogenous antigens are usually processed onto MHC I and presented to CD8+ cytotoxic T cells; exogenous antigens are processed onto MHC II and presented to CD4+ T-helper cells.

PROCESSING OF ENDOGENOUS ANTIGENS

Cellular cytoplasmic proteins, including cell surface molecules, which are recycled to the cytoplasm, undergo proteolysis to small peptides in the **proteosome**, and the peptides are then taken to the endoplasmic reticulum, which is the site of production of MHC I molecules, by the **transporter associated with antigen processing**

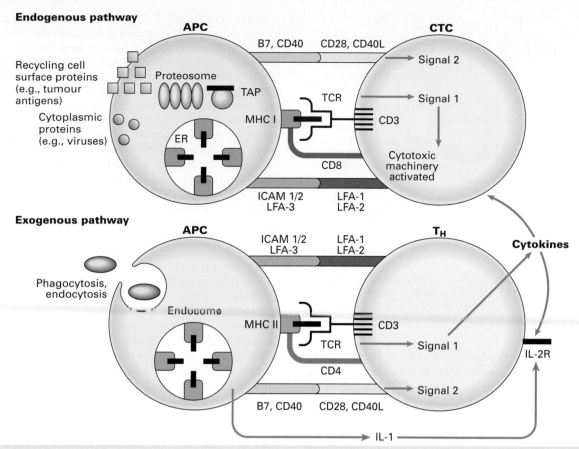

Fig. 9.4   Antigen processing and presentation to cytotoxic T cells (CTC) and T-helper cells (T$_H$). *APC*, Antigen-presenting cell; *ER*, endoplasmic reticulum; *ICAM*, intercellular adhesion molecule; *IL*, interleukin; *LFA*, leukocyte function-associated antigen; *MHC*, major histocompatibility complex; *R*, receptor; *TAP*, transporter associated with antigen processing; *TCR*, T-cell receptor.

(TAP). The assembly of the complete class I molecule, α-chain + β_2-microglobulin, requires the introduction of an 8- to 11-amino acid peptide into the peptide-binding groove. 'Empty' MHC molecules are highly unstable. Once assembled, MHC I + peptide is transported to the cell surface.

Endogenous antigen presentation leads to expression of a target structure recognizable only by CD8$^+$ T cells, since recognition of MHC I and CD8 expression are co-selected in the thymus (see Chapter 8). The CD8 molecule binds to MHC I and helps to generate an intracellular signal of TCR engagement. Endogenous processing of intracellular pathogens thus leads to activation of cytotoxic effector cells able to destroy the infected cell.

PROCESSING OF EXOGENOUS ANTIGEN

Phagocytic or endocytic uptake of exogenous antigens such as extracellular pathogens results in proteolysis within the endosomal compartment. Here, peptides encounter MHC II molecules consisting of α- and β-chains held together by the **invariant chain**. Peptides of 15–18 amino acids can replace the invariant chain. MHC II + peptide is transported to the cell surface to be 'seen' by the TCR of a CD4$^+$ T-helper cell. Engagement of the TCR induces signal 1 for T-cell activation, interaction of adhesion molecules and of CD4 with MHC II helps to transfer this signal to the nucleus, and B7-CD28 and/or CD40–CD40L interaction generates

signal 2. A clone of activated T-helper cells is produced, each member of which can recognize the original MHC II + peptide and is able to secrete various lymphokines for activation of other immune effector mechanisms.

T-Helper Subsets

The nature of the immune effector response is largely determined by the range of lymphokines secreted by activated T-helper cells. Upon initial stimulation, an activated T-helper cell will secrete a wide range of lymphokines (T$_H$0 phenotype), but, depending on the type of APC and the environment in which T-helper activation is taking place, the lymphokine secretion profile will usually polarize towards production of either IL-2, interferon-γ (IFN-γ) and lymphotoxin (LT) (T$_H$1) or IL-4, IL-5 and IL-10 (T$_H$2). While T$_H$1 lymphokines stimulate mainly macrophage and dendritic cell activation, T$_H$2 lymphokines stimulate B-cell activation and antibody production (Fig. 9.5).

If the APC is a macrophage or dendritic cell, it will normally be stimulated to produce IL-12 during T-helper cell activation. Neighbouring NK cells and possibly other cell types respond to IL-12 by producing IFN-γ, which stimulates the T$_H$1 and suppresses the T$_H$2 secretion profile. If the APC is a non-IL-12-producing cell, such as a B cell, or if T$_H$0 activation takes place in an environment containing

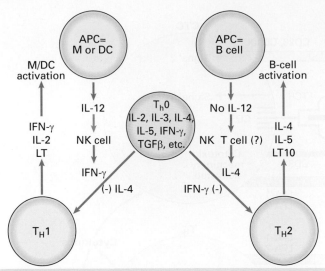

Fig. 9.5   Secretion profiles of T$_H$0, T$_H$1 and T$_H$2 cells. *APC,* Antigen-presenting cell; *DC,* dendritic cell; *IFN,* interferon; *IL,* interleukin; *LT,* lymphotoxin; *Mφ,* macrophage; *NK,* natural killer; *NKT,* natural killer T cell; *TGF,* transforming growth factor.

IL-4-secreting cells (possibly NK-T cells, a poorly understood population of lymphocytes bearing both NK and T cell markers), IL-4 will be the dominant early lymphokine. IL-4 stimulates production of T$_H$2- and suppresses T$_H$1-type lymphokines.

Recent studies have identified IL-17-producing CD4$^+$ T cells (Th17) as a distinct effector T-helper subpopulation. With their own set of lineage-specific developmental genes, Th17 cells have been recognized as main proinflammatory CD4$^+$ effector T cells involved in autoimmune pathogenesis.

Target Cell Killing

Cytotoxic T cells carrying CD8, activated via the endogenous antigen presentation pathway, are able to recognize and kill target cells, such as virus-infected cells, expressing MHC I + foreign peptide (Fig. 9.6). Both CD8 and various adhesion proteins are important in enhancing and maintaining target cell–effector cell contact.

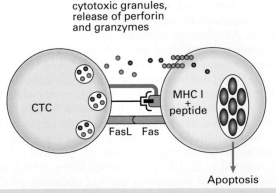

Fig. 9.6   Target cell killing. *CTC,* Cytotoxic T cell; *L,* ligand; *MHC,* major histocompatibility complex.

When a cytotoxic T cell makes contact with its specific target, cytoplasmic granules polarize to the contact point and are released into the narrow gap between the cells. Cytotoxic granules contain perforin and granzymes. **Perforin** is related to complement C9, with which it shares the ability to polymerize on the target cell surface, forming transmembrane channels. **Granzymes** are granular proteases, which gain entry into the target cell through perforin pores. Granzymes activate the target cell's suicide programme (**apoptosis**), which leads to nuclear fragmentation and packaging of products of nuclear disintegration into apoptotic bodies, which are efficiently removed by phagocytosis.

Target cell apoptosis can also be induced by binding of Fas ligand (FasL), induced during activation of cytotoxic effector T cells, with the death receptor Fas (CD95) on target cells.

NK cells and γδ T cells also employ perforin and granzymes to kill target cells. The γδ TCR can apparently receive signal 1 for activation without participation of classical MHC I or II molecules, and γδ T cells are either CD8$^-$ or express CD8αα rather than the usual CD8αβ. The γδ T cells are important in defence against infection, and experimental animals' depleted of γδ T cells eliminate microbes inefficiently.

NK cells are apparently responsible for killing target cells that express lower-than-normal levels of MHC I molecules, such as some malignant or virus-infected cells (see Fig. 8.3). Cells deficient in MHC I cannot be attacked by cytotoxic T cells; however, production of IFN-γ by activated NK cells will promote the expression of MHC I on target cells and permit the more efficient T-cell cytotoxicity to proceed. The recent molecular characterization of the surface receptors mediating NK-cell activation or inactivation have shed new light on how NK cells function. MHC class I-specific inhibitory and activating receptors are now recognized to be responsible for innate recognition of foreign, abnormal or virally infected cells by NK cells.

Certain cells that possess cytotoxic potential express membrane receptors for the Fc region of the antibody molecule. When antibody binds specifically to a target cell, these FcR-bearing cells such as NK cells, macrophages and neutrophils can bind to the Fc portion of antibody and thus to the target cells. Subsequently, these cytotoxic cells cause lysis of the target cell via a process called **antibody-dependent cell-mediated cytotoxicity (ADCC)**.

Activation of Macrophages

Macrophages receive activation signal 1 when they bind pathogens to threat receptors (Fig. 9.7). When they present MHC II + peptide and provide activation signals 1 and 2 for T-helper cells, they also receive a second signal for their own activation. Macrophage-derived IL-12 induces T-helper cells of the T$_H$1 phenotype. IFN-γ released by T$_H$1 induces macrophages to express receptors for tumour necrosis factor-α (TNF-α). These can bind membrane-bound TNF-α expressed by T$_H$1, inducing the activated state. Activated macrophages secrete autocrine TNF-α for maintaining this state, along with the inflammatory cytokines IL-1 and IL-6.

Following activation, macrophages express increased levels of Fc and complement receptors and thereby have higher

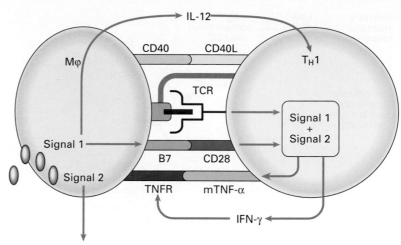

Fig. 9.7 Activation of macrophages. *CR,* Complement receptor; *FcR,* Fc receptor; *IFN,* interferon; *IL,* interleukin; *Mφ,* macrophage; *R,* receptor; *TNF,* tumour necrosis factor.

- induction and secretion of IL-1, IL-6, TNF-α – inflammation
- ↑FcR, C'R, – phagocytosis
- ↑MHC II, adhesion molecules – antigen presentation
- ↑proteolytic enzymes, oxygen radicals, no – microbial killing

phagocytic capability. They also increase expression of MHC and adhesion molecules, increasing the efficiency of antigen presentation. Their ability to kill pathogens increases as a result of raised levels of intracellular and secreted enzymes. Most importantly, powerful microbicidal mechanisms involving generation of reactive oxygen intermediaries (OH, O, O_2^-, H_2O_2) and nitric oxide (NO) are induced.

Regulation of the Immune Response

The specific immune response involving activation and clonal expansion of B cells and T cells brings into play a variety of nonspecific effector mechanisms involving complement, cytokines, granulocytes, macrophages and mast cells. These have the potential to damage normal host tissues, so it is crucial that the specific immune response be swiftly curtailed once the initiating foreign invader has been effectively neutralized.

ANTI-IDIOTYPIC ANTIBODY

The variable regions, or **idiotypes (ids)**, of antibodies, BCRs and TCRs represent novel molecules not previously experienced by the immune system. Tolerance will not have been induced against them and, if present in sufficient quantity, as occurs during a clonally expanded immune response, they will be immunogenic and induce **anti-idiotypic antibodies (anti-ids)**.

Secreted antibody may be recognized by B cells bearing BCRs with anti-id reactivity. This usually takes place on the surface of follicular dendritic cells and transmits activation signal 1 to the anti-id B cell. Further activation signals are received following processing of the id and presentation of its peptides to a specific T_H2 cell. The fully activated anti-idiotypic B cell undergoes clonal expansion and secretes anti-id. This will form immune complexes with circulating id, which will be removed by phagocytes.

Anti-id will also bind to id (BCR) on the surface of B cells. This will lead to cross-linking of BCRs and FcRs, which generates an inactivation signal.

The TCR on clonally expanded activated T cells can also lead to the generation of anti-id, which could induce tolerogenic signals when it binds to cell-bound TCR, perhaps by inducing activation signal 1 in the absence of signal 2.

REGULATORY T CELLS

Activation of immune effector mechanisms involving B cells, cytotoxic T cells, macrophages or NK cells all require participation of T-helper cells and their secreted lymphokines. Termination of a successful immune response could therefore be effectively achieved by silencing the driving T-helper cells.

Although the phenomenon of T-helper inactivation by **T-suppressor cells** has long been observed, its mode of action is still not fully understood. As T-helper cells recycle their TCRs and process TCR id peptides onto MHC I, CD8+ T cells with appropriate anti-id TCRs might bind to and inactivate the T-helper cell by a cytotoxic mechanism or by transmitting 'off signals' through membrane interactions.

An important mechanism of immune suppression is induction of a different cytokine profile from the one driving the ongoing reaction, for example, suppression of cell-mediated immunity by type 2 cytokines or suppression of humoral immunity by type 1 cytokines (**immune deviation**). A T-regulatory cell, a population of suppressor T cell, is functionally defined as a T cell that inhibits an immune response by controlling the activity of another cell type. T-regulatory cells are a minor population of thymus-derived CD4+ T cells that co-express the CD25 antigen (IL-2R α-chain), which constitute 5–10% of the peripheral naïve CD4+ T cell repertoire of normal mice and humans. Unlike conventional T-helper cells, regulatory T cells express Foxp3, a transcription factor essential for the development and function of regulatory T cells. Several types of T-regulatory cell populations including CD8+ regulatory T cells have

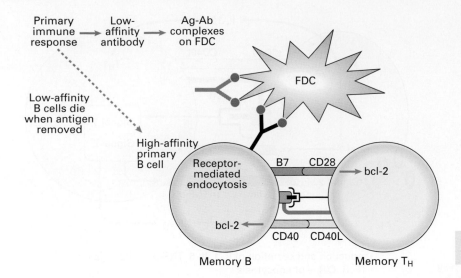

Fig. 9.8 Induction of memory cells. *Ag–Ab,* Antigen–antibody; *FDC,* follicular dendritic cell; *L,* ligand.

been identified, each with a specific surface phenotype and cytokine production potential. After activation, T-regulatory cells secrete mainly transforming growth factor-β and/or IL-10 and mediate peripheral tolerance by suppressing cytokine-dependent immune reactions.

Immunological Memory

The initial encounter with foreign antigen leads to an immune response that evolves slowly over days or weeks and eventually neutralizes and eliminates the invader. Although effector mechanisms are switched off once they are no longer required, the original antigenic experience is not forgotten. Long-lived T and B memory cells are selected for survival and mount an accelerated and enhanced response on encountering the antigen for a second time (Fig. 9.8).

MEMORY B CELLS

The primary B-cell response leads to the production of mainly low-affinity IgM antibodies, but some responding B cells undergo heavy-chain class-switching and V-region somatic mutation to produce higher-affinity IgG, IgA or IgE antibodies. Memory B cells are selected from this latter population because their BCRs can interact with antigen–antibody complexes formed during the primary response. These remain for long periods on the surface of follicular dendritic cells within germinal centres of secondary lymphoid tissue. High-affinity BCRs compete successfully with the lower-affinity antibody within the complex and bind antigen. Signalling between B cell CD40 and CD40L on activated T cells also appears to be required for memory B-cell survival. This interaction induces activation of the *bcl-2* oncogene, an inhibitor of programmed cell death.

When memory B cells reencounter their specific antigen, they rapidly produce high-affinity IgG, IgA or IgE.

This requires fewer T-helper cells and lower levels of lymphokines than the primary response. Recent studies have demonstrated that some antibody-secreting plasma cells localized in the bone marrow are long-lived and maintain high antibody titres for years upon repeated immunization with same antigen. Thus, these long-lived plasma cells are responsible for maintaining humoral antibody memory.

MEMORY T CELLS

Memory T cells cannot be distinguished from naïve T cells on the basis of isotype switch or affinity maturation because TCRs do not undergo these processes. Memory and naïve T cells, at least those of the CD4+ T-helper subset, can at present best be distinguished by expression of different isoforms of the common leukocyte antigen CD45: CD45RO on the former and CD45RA on the latter. The two isoforms of CD45 are also segregated on subsets of CD8+ cells.

While CD4+CD45RO+ memory T cells provide help for B-cell activation, CD4+CD45RA+ naïve cells preferentially induce T-suppressor cells. This may be related to the different lymphokine secretion profiles of the two subsets, with naïve T cells producing mainly IL-2 and memory T cells producing multiple lymphokines.

Memory T cells express higher levels of various adhesion and co-stimulatory molecules than naïve T cells and are much more efficient at interacting with other cell types.

As with memory B cells, long-term survival of memory T cells is triggered by re-exposure to the same antigen. Antigen is retained in the body for prolonged periods, mainly in the form of immune complexes on the surface of follicular dendritic cells, and is only available to the high-affinity BCRs of memory B cells. Therefore selection of memory T cells probably requires recognition, processing and presentation of MHC II + peptide by memory B cells.

Key Facts

- **Antibodies**, the secreted products of B lymphocytes, neutralize antigens, induce killing of target cells by complement and natural killer cells and opsonize particles for phagocytosis.
- **Cytokines** and **chemokines** mediate intercellular communication within the immune system, being required for initiation and regulation of all stages of the immune response. **Type 1 cytokines** induce mainly macrophage activation, while **type 2 cytokines** induce mainly antibody secretion.
- B cells are activated when they present antigen to T-helper cells and receive both a first signal through the B-cell receptor (BCR) and a second signal from CD40L binding to CD40. Type 2 cytokines, including interleukin-4 (IL-4), stimulate clonal proliferation, antibody secretion, affinity maturation and isotype switching of antibody.
- T cells and B cells require two signals for activation, the first through the T-cell receptor (TCR)/BCR, the second through B7-CD28 or CD40-CD40L interaction. Receipt of only the first signal usually results in anergy or cell death.
- **Cytotoxic T cells** become activated when they encounter endogenous antigen processed onto major histocompatibility complex I (MHC I) and are stimulated by signal 1, signal 2 and type 1 cytokines. They kill by secreting perforin and granzymes towards the target cell or by inducing apoptosis of Fas-expressing cells.
- **Macrophages** are activated when they process exogenous antigen onto MHC II and present peptides to T-helper cells. The latter become activated and secrete type 1 cytokines, including interferon-γ, a powerful macrophage activator. Activated macrophages secrete inflammatory cytokines and are highly efficient at phagocytosis, antigen presentation and microbial killing.
- Termination of the immune response is essential to prevent widespread damage to healthy tissues. **Anti-idiotypic antibodies** bind to BCRs and TCRs and switch off activated cells. Regulatory T cells can switch off the responses of activated T-helper cells. Type 1 cytokine production can be suppressed by the induction of type 2 cytokines, and vice versa.
- At the end of an immune response, responding high-affinity B cells and T cells survive in a resting state for long periods and respond rapidly and efficiently on reencountering the same antigen (**immunological memory**).

Review Questions (Answers on p. 389)

Please indicate which answers are true, and which are false.

9.1. Features of immunoglobulin (Ig) structure include:
   a. typical Y-shaped antibody consisting of two polypeptide chains, one heavy chain and one light chain
   b. Ig heavy chains have both constant region and variable region
   c. Ig light chains have no constant region
   d. the antigen-binding site is located in the Fc portion of Ig molecule
   e. the constant regions form the antigen-binding site

9.2. The functions of antibodies include:
   a. neutralization
   b. opsonization
   c. complement activation
   d. recognizing specific antigens only when peptides are bound to major histocompatibility complex (MHC) molecule
   e. enhancing phagocytosis

9.3. Which of the following statements on B cell differentiation and maturation are true?
   a. the first Ig molecule expressed by a B cell is IgE
   b. mature B cells can develop into memory cells after antigenic stimulation
   c. plasma cells differentiate into memory B cells
   d. B cell receptor is expressed by natural killer cells
   e. B cell activation usually does not need a signal from T-helper cells

9.4. Which of the following is/are not involved in cytotoxic T cell killing?
   a. granzymes
   b. perforin
   c. MHC II
   d. Fas ligand
   e. MHC I

Further Reading

Janeway, C. A., Jr., Travers, P., Walport, M., et al. (2001). *Immunobiology* (5th ed.). Garland Publishing.
Mims, C., Playfair, J., Roitt, I., et al. (1998). *Vaccination.* In *Medical microbiology* (2nd ed., Chapter 15). Mosby Year Book.

Roitt, I. M. (1997). *Roitt's essential immunology* (9th ed.). Blackwell.
Roitt, I., Brostoff, J., & Male, D. (1998). *Immunology* (5th ed.). Mosby.

10 Immunity and Infection

Bacterial, viral, parasitic and fungal infections are major causes of morbidity and mortality worldwide, especially in poorer societies with greater exposure to infectious agents, poorer nutrition and less access to medicines and vaccines. Infectious and parasitic diseases were responsible for 29.6% of the world's disease burden in 1999, according to the World Health Organization (WHO) (Table 10.1). In a recent review, the authors estimated that, out of 13.7 million infection-related deaths in 2019, 7.7 million deaths were associated with 33 bacterial pathogens. At the time of this writing (September 2023), over 6.9 million have died due to the recent COVID-19 pandemic caused by SARS-CoV-2.

All of the immunological mechanisms described in the previous two chapters are called upon to limit and eliminate the foregoing infectious agents. However, pathogens have developed a remarkable variety of strategies to evade the host's immune defences, and the immune response itself may damage host tissues.

Immunity to Bacteria

SUMMARY OF DEFENCE MECHANISMS

- The bacterial cell wall proteoglycan can be attacked by lysozyme.
- **Bacteria release peptides**, which are chemotactic for polymorphs.
- **Polymorphs and macrophages use receptors** for bacterial sugars to bind and slowly phagocytose them.
- Bacteria induce macrophages to release inflammatory cytokines such as **interleukin-1 (IL-1) and interleukin-6 (IL-6) and tumour necrosis factor-α (TNF-α)**.

- Bacterial lipopolysaccharides (LPS) or **endotoxins activate the alternative complement pathway**, generating opsonizing C3b and iC3b on the bacterial surface. The **membrane attack complex (MAC)** can lyse Gram-negative but not Gram-positive bacteria.
- Bacterial polysaccharides (e.g., pneumococcal) with multiple repeated epitopes may activate B cells independently of T-helper cells because of their ability to cross-link B-cell receptors (BCRs). The resultant mainly immunoglobulin M (IgM) antibodies efficiently agglutinate bacteria and activate the classical complement pathway.
- Exogenous processing of phagocytosed bacteria by macrophages results in presentation of peptide epitopes in the context of **major histocompatibility complex (MHC) II to T_H1 cells**. These induce macrophage activation for efficient bacterial killing.
- Processing of **bacterial antigens** by B cells **induces T_H2 responses** and high-affinity antibody production: IgG antibodies neutralize soluble bacterial products such as toxins; IgA antibodies protect mucosal surfaces from bacterial attachment. Immune complexes activate the classical complement pathway. Phagocytic uptake of bacteria coated with C3b/iC3b and antibody is rapid and efficient.

BACTERIAL EVASION STRATEGIES

Many bacteria **have developed ways of interfering with phagocytosis. Encapsulated bacteria do not display sugar molecules for recognition by receptors** on phagocytes. They are only phagocytosed when coated with antibodies, so they can proliferate in nonimmune individuals in the first few days after infection. Even when taken up

Table 10.1 Leading Causes of Infectious Diseases Worldwide (in decreasing order of importance)

Infectious Disease	Cause
Acute respiratory infections including deaths dues to COVID-19 (mostly pneumonia)	Bacterial or viral
Diarrhoeal diseases	Bacterial or viral
Tuberculosis	Bacterial
Hepatitis B	Viral
Malaria	Protozoan
Acquired immune deficiency syndrome (AIDS)	Viral
Measles	Viral
Neonatal tetanus	Bacterial
Pertussis (whooping cough)	Bacterial

Modified from World Health Organization (WHO). (1999). *The World Health Report.* Geneva: WHO. (In decreasing order of importance).

by phagocytes, many encapsulated bacteria resist digestion (e.g., *Haemophilus influenzae, Streptococcus pneumoniae, Klebsiella pneumoniae, Pseudomonas aeruginosa*) or can even kill phagocytes (e.g., streptococci, staphylococci, *Bacillus anthracis*). Mycobacteria, listeria and *Brucella* spp. are able to survive within the cytoplasm of nonactivated macrophages and can only be killed by a cell-mediated immune response driven by T_H1 macrophage-activating lymphokines.

DAMAGE CAUSED BY IMMUNE RESPONSES TO BACTERIA

Group A β-haemolytic streptococci cause sore throat and scarlet fever, which resolve on induction of specific antibody. Certain components of some strains of streptococci contain **epitopes**, which are **cross-reactive with epitopes present on heart tissue**. Antibodies that eliminate the infecting bacteria can bind to heart tissue and cause complement-mediated lysis and **antibody-dependent cellular cytotoxicity** (e.g., leading to rheumatic heart disease). Furthermore, **circulating immune complexes** can deposit in

synovia and glomeruli, causing complement-mediated **joint pain and glomerulonephritis**, respectively. Induction of cross-reacting anti-heart antibody by group A streptococci is illustrated in Fig. 10.1 (see also Fig. 23.2).

Persistent infection of macrophages, for example, with *Mycobacterium tuberculosis* or *Mycobacterium leprae*, provokes a chronic, local, **cell-mediated immune reaction** due to continuous release of antigen. **Lymphokine production** causes large numbers of macrophages to accumulate, many of which give rise to **epithelioid cells** or fuse to form **giant cells (syncytia)**. These giant cells release high concentrations of **lytic enzymes**, which destroy the surrounding tissue. Incorporation of fibroblasts also occurs, and the persisting pathogen becomes walled off inside a **fibrotic, necrotic granuloma**. Because the macrophages in a granuloma are activated, this mechanism also enhances the activation of T-helper cells. Granulomas may replace extensive areas of normal tissue—for example, in the lungs of tuberculosis patients.

Immunity to Viruses

Viruses cannot proliferate outside a host cell. The infectious virion must attach to a suitable cell via a specific membrane receptor and enter the cell cytoplasm. Viral replication may or may not destroy the host cell. Viral genes may become incorporated within the host cell genome and remain in a state of **latency** for long periods (Chapter 5). In some cases, integrated viral genes **activate cellular oncogenes** and induce malignant transformation.

SUMMARY OF DEFENCE MECHANISMS

■ Viral proliferation induces infected cells to produce **interferons (IFNs) α and β**, which protect neighbouring cells from productive infection. **Interferons induce enzymes** that inhibit messenger RNA translation into proteins and degrade both viral and host-cell messenger RNA, effectively preventing the host cell from supporting replication of the virus or replicating itself.

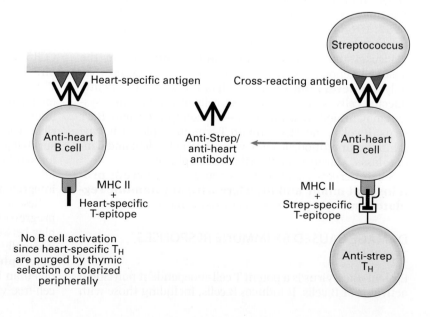

Fig. 10.1 Induction of anti-heart antibodies by group A streptococci.

- Some viruses, notably Epstein–Barr virus, bind Cl and **activate the classical complement pathway**, resulting in MAC-induced lysis.
- Macrophages readily take up viruses nonspecifically and kill them. Some viruses, however, are able to survive and multiply in macrophages. Viruses do not usually induce macrophages to release inflammatory cytokines.
- Processing of viral antigens by B cells and presentation to T_H2 cells induces **high-affinity antibody production**. Antibodies are effective against free rather than cell-associated viruses. Antibody-coated viruses may be destroyed by the classical complement activation pathway or may be taken up by phagocytes bearing Fc or complement receptors.
- Intracellular viral antigens are processed by the **endogenous pathway**, and viral peptides presented on MHC I molecules can be recognized by **CD8⁺ T cytotoxic cells**. These effector cells efficiently destroy virus-infected cells and provide long-term protection against subsequent infection with the same virus.
- Free virions taken up by macrophages and processed by the exogenous pathway stimulate specific T_H1 cells to **release IFN-γ**, which, like IFN-α and IFN-β, protects neighbouring cells from productive infection.
- Virally infected cells may downregulate MHC molecules and become susceptible to killing by **natural killer (NK) cells. IFN-γ activates the killing mechanism of NK cells**, but paradoxically induces reexpression of MHC antigens on the target cells and suppression of NK cytotoxicity. However, such target cells would then be susceptible to T cell cytotoxicity.

VIRAL EVASION STRATEGIES

Certain viruses can modify the structure of components that are targets for the immune response (**antigenic variation**). Point mutations in the genes encoding viral antigens cause minor structural changes (**antigenic drift**), while exchange of large segments of genetic material with other viruses changes the whole structure of the antigen (**antigenic shift**). Antigenic drift of influenza A virus haemagglutinin occurs before each winter's minor influenza epidemic, whereas major epidemics, such as those of 1918, 1957, 1968 and 1977, were the result of antigenic shift of haemagglutinin and/or neuraminidase.

Viruses that can **integrate their genes** within the host cell genome, such as human herpesviruses, provoke only **low-level immunity**, which fails to clear the latently infected cells. Viruses that infect cells of the immune system may inhibit their function—for example, Epstein–Barr virus (B cells); measles, human T-lymphotropic virus type I, human immunodeficiency virus (HIV) (T cells); and dengue, lassa, Marburg–Ebola, HIV (macrophages).

Some herpesviruses and poxviruses can **secrete proteins that mimic and interfere with key immune regulators** such as cytokines and cytokine receptors.

DAMAGE CAUSED BY IMMUNE RESPONSES TO VIRUSES

Epstein–Barr virus is a potent T cell-independent polyclonal activator of B cells. It induces B cells, including those with anti-self BCRs, which are normally inactive due to purging of the corresponding anti-self T-helper cells, to secrete antibodies. Several viruses, notably hepatitis B virus, can cause chronic autoimmune disease due to release of previously sequestered (i.e., nontolerogenic) self-antigens following tissue damage. **Complexes of antivirus antibodies with antigen can activate complement** in the blood vessels, joints and glomeruli, causing vasculitis, arthritis and glomerulonephritis. Cytotoxic T cells may destroy essential host cells displaying viral antigens, for example, coxsackievirus (myocarditis), mumps virus (meningoencephalitis) and viruses causing damage to the myelin nerve sheath (postviral polyneuritis).

HIV AND AIDS

By the end of 2022, approximately 86.5 million people worldwide had become infected with HIV and approximately 40.4 million had died of the acquired immune deficiency syndrome (AIDS; see also Chapter 30). The virus causes **depletion of CD4⁺ T-helper lymphocytes** over many years. Globally 39.5 million are living with HIV with the help of retroviral therapy which keeps the virus in check. Some patients eventually succumb to opportunistic infections (*Pneumocystis carinii*, *Mycobacterium tuberculosis*, atypical mycobacteria, *Histoplasma*, *Coccidioides*, *Cryptococcus*, *Cryptosporidium* and *Toxoplasma* spp., herpes simplex, cytomegalovirus) and may develop Kaposi's sarcoma, B-cell lymphomas and other malignancies. Infection of the brain by HIV can cause dementia and encephalitis.

The major route of transmission of HIV is by unprotected **sexual intercourse**: male to female, female to male and male to male. It can also be transmitted from mother to fetus across the placenta, during delivery or by breastfeeding. Direct injection into the blood stream (e.g., by multiple use of needles and syringes for injection of drugs) also transmits HIV.

The life cycle of HIV is shown in Fig. 10.2. The virus gains entry into target cells by binding its surface gp120 molecule (glycoprotein of 120 kDa) to CD4 on T-helper cells and a subset of macrophages. The latter can also take up opsonized HIV via Fc or complement receptors. A coreceptor is also required for infection of target cells: CXCR4, also known as fusin or LESTR, is the receptor for the chemokine SDF-1 and is the coreceptor for infection of T cells by HIV; CCR5, the receptor for chemokines RANTES, MIP-1α and MIP-1p, is the coreceptor for infection of macrophages. Viral gp41 causes fusion with the cell membrane and injection into the target cell of two strands of viral genetic information, which is RNA. One strand is destroyed by viral ribonuclease H and viral reverse transcriptase converts the surviving strand into a DNA copy. This forms the template for synthesis of the complementary second strand by cellular DNA polymerase. The double-stranded DNA is then integrated into host-cell DNA by viral integrase.

Research into the pathogenic process that underlies the progression of HIV to AIDS has revealed a dynamic interplay between the virus and the immune system. The virus is usually **transmitted from person to person within macrophages** (infected macrophages are more numerous than infected T-helper cells in genital secretions) or as cell-free virus. Infected macrophages contain HIV virions

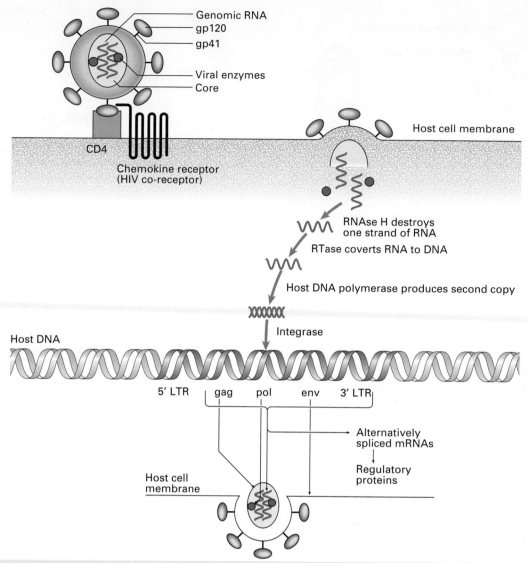

Fig. 10.2 **Life cycle of human immunodeficiency virus (HIV).** *LTR,* Long terminal repeat; *mRNA,* messenger RNA; *RNAse,* ribonuclease; *Rtase,* reverse transcriptase.

within cytoplasmic vacuoles; probably IL-6 and TNF-α produced in response to phagocytic uptake induce constant slow production of virions from integrated proviral DNA. When infected macrophages enter the new host, they are destroyed, releasing HIV. Dendritic cells transport HIV to draining lymph nodes where they infect CD4⁺ cells.

Proliferation of HIV within lymph nodes occurs throughout the long period of clinical latency, even though the patient remains well and is not deficient in T-helper cells. Eventually the lymph node architecture becomes damaged and generalized release of HIV causes rapid destruction of T-helper cells.

Budding of HIV from an infected T-helper cell **destroys the integrity of the cell membrane**. In addition to this direct form of killing of infected cells, HIV can apparently destroy or inactivate uninfected T-helper cells by various indirect mechanisms, most of which remain theoretically possible rather than of proven clinical relevance. These possible pathogenic mechanisms are shown in Figs. 10.3, 10.4, 10.5, 10.6 and 10.7.

Throughout the period of clinical latency there is massive infection, **destruction and replacement of CD4⁺ T cells**, with billions of new cells being infected and killed every day. Ultimately the processes leading to replacement of T-helper cells become exhausted, the cell number drops and immune function deteriorates. The virus may reduce replenishment of T cells from haematopoietic stem cells following infection of the bone marrow. Furthermore, destroyed CD4⁺ cells can be replaced by CD4⁺ or CD8⁺ T cells with equal likelihood, so the representation of the latter gradually increases compared with the former, and **immune suppressor activity will come to dominate over helper activity**. Virus-infected macrophages are deficient in IL-12 production and, therefore, cannot induce T_H1 responses. Instead, the dominant T_H2 response leads to hypergammaglobulinaemia and production of autoantibodies and B-cell lymphomas.

Newly available, highly active drug combinations interfere with virus proliferation and T-cell destruction and delay disease progression. The prototype of the drugs that interfere with reverse transcription is zidovudine, or

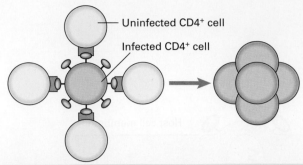

Fig. 10.3 Giant cell formation induced by human immunodeficiency virus (HIV). Glycoprotein gp120 present on the surface of HIV-infected cells binds to CD4 on uninfected cells; gp41 induces fusion of adjacent cells and production of nonfunctional, infected giant cells (syncytia). Thus, HIV can pass from cell to cell without being exposed to the host's immune response.

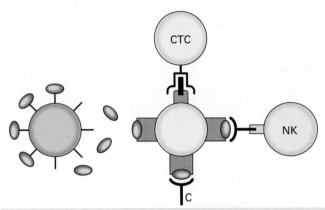

Fig. 10.4 Release of soluble gp120. Glycoprotein gp120 released from human immunodeficiency virus *(HIV)*-infected cells can bind to CD4 of uninfected cells, which can then be destroyed by antibody-dependent complement or natural killer *(NK)* cell cytotoxicity after binding of anti-gp120 antibody. Processing of gp120 onto MHC I forms a target structure for cytotoxic T cells *(CTC)*.

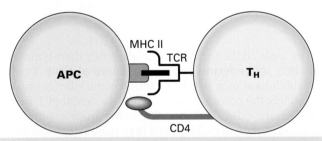

Fig. 10.5 Inhibition of T-helper cell (T$_H$) activation: gp120 inhibits CD4–MHC II and TCR–MHC II–peptide interaction. *APC,* Antigen-presenting cell; *MHC II,* major histocompatibility complex II; *TCR,* T cell receptor.

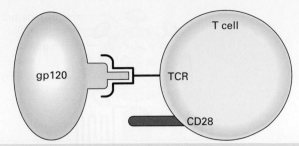

Fig. 10.6 Inactivation of T cell: gp120 has sequence homology with major histocompatibility complex II *(MHC II)* and can bind to T-cell receptors *(TCRs)*. Transmission of signal 1 without signal 2 *(B7-CD28)* inactivates the cell or induces apoptosis.

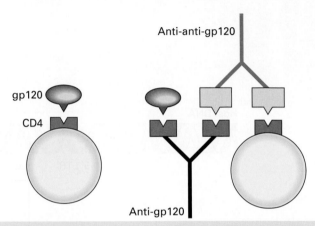

Fig. 10.7 Induction of anti-CD4 antibody. Antiidiotypic antibody against anti-gp120 cross-reacts with CD4. Antibody-coated CD4-positive cells are destroyed by antibody-dependent complement or cellular cytotoxicity.

azidothymidine (AZT). Current treatment for AIDS is a combination therapy, using regimens designated **highly active antiretroviral therapy (HAART**; see Chapter 30).

CORONAVIRUSES, SARS AND COVID-19

In the past few decades, newly evolved coronaviruses such as SARS-CoV-1 (agent of SARS), MERS virus (agent of Middle East Respiratory Syndrome) and SARS-CoV-2 (agent of COVID-19) have posed a threat to public health with millions of deaths worldwide.

A healthy immune response is essential to control and eliminate these coronavirus infections. However, a **dysregulated immune response** may result in immunopathology and impaired pulmonary gas exchange, leading to pneumonia in most patients as well as acute respiratory distress syndrome (ARDS) in 15% of cases and death.

ARDS is one of the leading causes of death in patients with COVID-19 and is mainly triggered by **elevated levels of proinflammatory cytokines**, referred to as a **cytokine storm** and defined as acute overproduction and uncontrolled release of proinflammatory markers, both locally and systemically. Interleukins, such as 1L-1, IL-6, IL-17, and tumour necrosis factor-alpha (TNF-α) play a key role in lung damage in ARDS patients through the impairments of the respiratory epithelium.

Another *rare* syndrome called **multisystem inflammatory syndrome in children (MIS-C)** may be seen in those **children** infected with COVID-19. This is also due to immune dysregulation after SARS-CoV-2 infection. The blood vessels, digestive system, skin or eyes become swollen and dysfunctional in MIS-C. Similarly, multisystem inflammatory syndrome in adults (MIS-A) can occur after COVID-19 vaccination in a previously infected patient and can manifest as respiratory distress. This too is extremely rare.

Immunity to Parasites

SUMMARY OF DEFENCE MECHANISMS

- **Protozoan parasites** such as *Plasmodium* (malaria), *Leishmania* (leishmaniasis) and *Trypanosoma* (Chagas disease, sleeping sickness) **induce macrophages** to release inflammatory IL-1, IL-6 and TNF-α.
- Protozoa that survive within macrophages (e.g., *Trypanosoma cruzi, Leishmania*) can be killed following macrophage activation by T_H1 cells.
- **IgG and IgM antibodies are effective against parasites** that circulate freely in blood (e.g., *Trypanosoma brucei*, plasmodium sporozoite and merozoite stages) and against parasite-infected cells that display parasite antigens on the surface. Complement activation leads to target cell lysis and opsonization for phagocytosis.
- **IgE antibodies** are of major importance against helminths such as *Schistosoma, Trichinella, Strongyloides* and *Wucheria*. T_H2 cells produce IL-4 and IL-5 in response to helminth antigens presented by B cells. IL-4 stimulates switching to IgE production, whereas IL-5 induces eosinophilia. IgE binds to mast cell or basophil Fcε receptors, and cross-linking of IgE by parasite antigens leads to release of eosinophil chemotactic factor. Eosinophils attracted to the parasite release **eosinophil cationic protein and major basic protein**, which damage the tegument of the parasite.

PARASITE EVASION STRATEGIES

Trypanosoma brucei possesses variant surface glycoproteins (VSGs). There are several genes for different VSGs, only one of which is expressed at any given time. After antibodies have been produced against one VSG, it is shed from the surface and a new VSG gene is expressed (**antigenic variation**). *Leishmania* cap off their surface antigens when exposed to antibody (**antigenic modulation**). Schistosomes synthesize **host-like antigens such as α₂-macroglobulin** to mask their own foreignness and also adsorb host molecules, such as red blood cell antigens, MHC antigens, complement factors and immunoglobulins, onto their surface (**antigenic disguise**).

Parasites have various **immune suppressor capabilities**: *Trypanosoma brucei* induces T-suppressor cell activation. *Plasmodium* and *Leishmania* release soluble antigens that intercept antiparasite antibodies and saturate phagocytes. *T. cruzi* produces molecules that inhibit or accelerate the decay of C3 convertases. *Leishmania* downregulates MHC II expression on parasitized macrophages, reducing their ability to present antigenic peptides to CD4⁺ T cells. *Toxoplasma* prevents fusion of phagocytic vacuoles with lysosomes. *Leishmania* inhibits the respiratory burst of macrophages. Schistosomes release peptidases that cleave bound immunoglobulin, and other factors that inhibit T-cell proliferation, release of IFN-γ and eosinophil activation.

DAMAGE CAUSED BY IMMUNE RESPONSES TO PARASITES

Helminths induce not only parasite-specific IgE but also **polyclonal IgE**, which can give rise to **manifestations of allergy** such as urticaria and angioedema. Sudden release of large amounts of parasite antigen can trigger **fatal anaphylactic shock**.

Parasite antigens that cross-react with host antigens (e.g., *Trypanosoma cruzi* antigens cross-reactive with cardiac antigens) and parasites coated with host antigens can induce **autoimmune attack** against host tissues (see Fig. 10.1).

Circulating immune complexes containing parasite antigens cause some of the tissue damage seen in malaria, trypanosomiasis and schistosomiasis. Portal fibrosis and pulmonary hypertension in schistosomiasis are due to T cell-mediated granulomatous responses to schistosome eggs.

Immunity to Fungi

Fungal infections may be **superficial** (e.g., ringworm caused by *Trichophyton rubrum*, oral thrush and vulvovaginitis caused by *Candida albicans*), **subcutaneous** (e.g., abscesses and ulceration caused by *Sporothrix schenckii*) or **systemic** (e.g., histoplasmosis, coccidioidomycosis, systemic candidiasis, cryptococcosis, aspergillosis).

In healthy individuals, and even in immunodeficient patients with defects in antibody production, fungal infections generally remain localized and resolve rapidly. By contrast, patients with T-cell or neutrophil defects may suffer chronic infections, indicating that these are the important effector cells in immunity to fungi.

Production of antifungal antibodies may result in **IgE-mediated allergic disease**, for example, allergic bronchopulmonary aspergillosis, or IgG-mediated immune complex disease (e.g., when *Aspergillus* grows to form an aspergilloma in preexisting lung cavities). *Histoplasma, Coccidioides* and *Cryptococcus* can induce granuloma formation in the lungs.

Vaccination

Natural infection often produces lifelong protection, with development of memory T and B cells able to respond rapidly on subsequent challenges with the same agent. Many infections cause severe clinical symptoms and even death, which could be **prevented by inducing memory cells** *before* **exposure to pathogens** occurs (Fig. 10.8).

PASSIVE IMMUNIZATION

Passive transfer of **maternal antibodies during pregnancy** and breast-feeding provides limited protection for the newborn baby, but following catabolism of these antibodies, protection is lost. Vaccination to induce memory B cells is not successful during the neonatal period because maternal antibodies neutralize vaccine antigens, although induction of memory T cells can be achieved at this time.

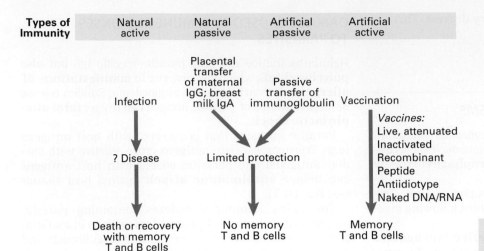

Fig. 10.8 Natural and artificial immunization. *Ig,* Immunoglobulin.

Short-term protection can also be achieved later in life by **passive transfer of immune globulin**. Short-term passive immunization using hyperimmune globulin or monoclonal antibodies can be useful as postexposure prophylaxis (e.g., following exposure to rabies virus).

ACTIVE IMMUNIZATION

Memory T and B cells can be induced most successfully using **live vaccines** containing microorganisms that have been attenuated to reduce their virulence. A single dose is usually sufficient to induce both systemic and mucosal immunity. Immunocompromised patients must not be given live vaccines because of the danger of disseminated infection.

Inactivated vaccines consist of killed whole organisms, products of organisms or subunits of organisms. Because there is no replication of the organism to provide immune stimulation over several days, inactivated vaccines must be given in multiple doses in the presence of an **adjuvant**. The most widely used adjuvant for human vaccines is alum, which forms a precipitate with protein antigens from which the antigens are slowly released to the immune system.

Toxoids consist of bacterial exotoxins rendered harmless by treatment with formaldehyde. Antigenicity can be increased by combination with suspensions of other bacteria containing endotoxins, for example, diphtheria–tetanus–pertussis triple vaccine (see also Chapter 36). Vaccination with the toxoid induces antitoxoid antibodies that are capable of binding to the toxin and neutralizing its effect.

Vaccines currently available for active immunization are shown in Table 10.2, and recommended vaccination schedules are shown in Table 10.3.

NEWER VACCINES AND CURRENT APPROACHES TO VACCINE DEVELOPMENT

Proven, effective vaccines are still not available against many of today's leading killers, notably malaria, parasitic diseases and HIV. Even the vaccines in regular use cannot be considered 100% effective. Most of them induce

Table 10.2 Currently Available Active Immunizing Agents

Vaccine	Formulation*
Anthrax	Inactivated *Bacillus anthracis*
Bacille Calmette–Guérin (BCG)[a]	**Live attenuated *Mycobacterium bovis***
Cholera	Inactivated *Vibrio cholerae*
Diphtheria[a]	**Toxoid**
Haemophilus influenzae	Capsular polysaccharide conjugated to protein
Coronavirus Disease – 2019[a]	Viral vector, attenuated whole virus
Influenza[a]	**Inactivated virus**
Measles[a]	**Live attenuated virus**
Meningococcus	Capsular polysaccharide
Mumps[a]	**Live attenuated virus**
Pertussis[a]	Killed whole *Bordetella pertussis*
Plague	Inactivated *Yersinia pestis*
Pneumococcus	Capsular polysaccharide of *Streptococcus pneumoniae*
Polio[a]	**Inactivated or live attenuated virus**
Rabies	Inactivated virus
Rubella[a]	**Live attenuated virus**
Tetanus[a]	**Toxoid**
Typhoid	Inactivated or live attenuated *Salmonella typhi*
Yellow fever	Live attenuated virus

[a]Vaccines available/recommended for dental care workers (in bold).
*Although a single formulation is given here, newer vaccines developed on various new platforms are available for some of these infections (see also Table 10.4).

antibody effectively but are less able to stimulate cell-mediated immunity. It has even been suggested that current vaccines given early in life polarize cytokine production towards type 2 rather than type 1 responses and that the increasing prevalence of asthma and allergies could be partly a consequence of immunization with IL-4-inducing vaccines. However, new approaches to vaccine development promise greater control of infectious diseases in the not-too-distant future.

Table 10.3   Recommended Immunization Schedules (*for guidance only*; some authorities may recommend variations of these schedules)

Age	BCG	Polio	HBV	Haem	DTP	DT	Tet	MMR	Rub	Pneu	Flu	COVID-19[b]
Birth	√		√									
1 month			√									
2–4 months		√		√	√							√
3–5 months		√	√	√	√							
4–6 months		√		√	√							√
12 months								√				√
18 months				√	√							
5–6 years						√		√				
10–14 years	√[a]					√			√			
15–18 years		√					√+					
50 years										√	√	
65 years											√	√

[a]If negative by Mantoux skin test. + Repeat every 10 years.
Note: These immunization schedules are relatively standard, although minor geographic variations in policy exist due to disease prevalence.
[b]Vaccination schedules for COVID-19 depend on the type of vaccine; the periodicity of the booster doses is yet unclear but likely to be annual for health care workers; these COVID-19 vaccine recommendations may change eventually, and the readers should keep abreast of new developments due to this dynamic scenario.
BCG, Bacille Calmette–Guérin; *DT,* diphtheria–tetanus; *DTP,* diphtheria–tetanus–pertussis; *Flu,* influenza; *Haem, Haemophilus influenzae; HBV,* hepatitis B virus; *MMR,* measles–mumps–rubella; *Pneu,* pneumococcus; *Polio,* poliomyelitis; *Rub,* rubella; *Tet,* tetanus.

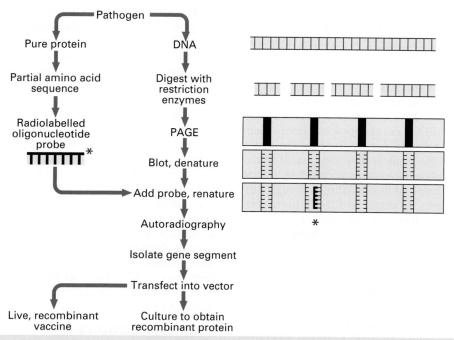

Fig. 10.9   Recombinant vaccines. *PAGE,* Polyacrylamide gel electrophoresis.

One way of improving the efficacy of inactivated vaccines would be to develop more effective **adjuvants**. **Freund's Complete Adjuvant**, which contains oil, detergent and mycobacteria, stimulates powerful B-cell and T-cell responses in experimental animals, but it is too toxic for human use. The active principal of mycobacteria, muramyl dipeptide, strongly enhances macrophage activity, is nontoxic, and may become useful in human vaccines. Immunostimulating complexes (ISCOMs), prepared from saponin, cholesterol and phosphatidylcholine, provide a vehicle for presenting proteins to the immune system and induce T- and B-cell memory.

Inactivated vaccines made from whole microorganisms may contain proteins that stimulate both protective and nonprotective—or even suppressive—immune responses. Subunit vaccines containing only protection-inducing proteins should be much more effective than cruder preparations.

Modern subunit vaccines are now being produced by **recombinant DNA technology** (Fig. 10.9). Candidate protein antigens must first be identified and purified so that a partial amino acid sequence can be determined. An oligonucleotide probe consisting of the corresponding nucleotide sequence is then constructed and labelled with a radioisotope.

Next, DNA is extracted from the pathogen, digested with restriction enzymes and the DNA fragments separated by polyacrylamide gel electrophoresis (PAGE). After blotting onto nitrocellulose, the DNA is denatured by heating. The probe is added and binds to its complementary sequence when the temperature is lowered, thereby identifying the relevant gene segment. Autoradiography reveals its position on the blot and the original polyacrylamide gel can be sliced to obtain the gene. This is then transfected into the DNA of suitable host cells (bacterial, yeast, insect or human). When the host cells are cultured, recombinant as well as host proteins are synthesized.

This technology is particularly useful for producing antigenic proteins from viruses that are difficult to culture, and a highly effective recombinant hepatitis B vaccine is already in routine use. DNA vaccines offer advantages over many of the existing vaccines because the encoded protein is expressed in its natural form in the host. DNA vaccines cause prolonged expression of the antigen that generates significant immunological memory.

Synthetic peptide vaccines containing only **relevant epitopes of the antigenic protein** have also been produced and shown to be effective in animal models. In theory it should be possible to construct vaccines containing both B-cell and T-cell epitopes on a carrier molecule such as poly-L-lysine. For pathogens that undergo antigenic variation, notably HIV, it might be possible to construct peptide vaccines containing sufficiently large arrays of peptides to protect against most variants of the pathogen. Because peptides are usually not as immunogenic as proteins, adjuvants and conjugates have been used to assist in raising protective immunity to synthetic peptides.

Live recombinant vaccines also hold considerable promise. Gene segments coding for pathogen proteins can be inserted into attenuated vectors such as vaccinia, bacille Calmette–Guérin (BCG) or adenovirus. Immunizing pathogen proteins are released during the time the vector replicates in the host. Live, replication-incompetent microorganisms can be engineered for use as vaccines by removing some of the genes involved in replication, though later reversion to full pathogenicity would be difficult to rule out.

Antiidiotypic antibodies can be used as vaccines instead of pathogen proteins. The **protein antigen (X)** is used to raise monoclonal antibodies in mice; V regions of anti-X are then used to immunize a second mouse. The resultant monoclonal anti-anti-X has similar antigenic properties to X itself (Fig. 10.10). By isolating the V genes from the hybridoma producing anti-anti-X, antiidiotypic vaccines can be produced using recombinant DNA technology.

Recent progress in production of **genetic vaccines** using RNA or DNA coding for specific pathogen proteins has revolutionized the field of vaccinology. Of these, particular mention must be made of the **mRNA vaccines** that were first successfully introduced to curb the COVID-19 pandemic. Millions of doses of mRNA vaccine together with other generic vaccines, essentially modified the dynamics of the COVID-19 pandemic and brought it under control (Fig. 10.11).

mRNA vaccines: Mechanisms of action (Fig. 10.11). mRNA vaccine induces immunity to SARS-CoV-2 as follows. The vaccine containing mRNA of SARS-CoV-2 with the code for either the spike (S) protein or the receptor-binding domain (RBD) proteins of the virus, contained within lipid particles are administered to the vaccinee. Once injected, the lipid particles are 'ingested' by vaccinees' cells. The protein-making machinery in these cells is instructed

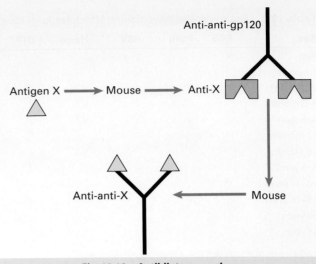

Fig. 10.10   Antiidiotype vaccines.

to produce viral proteins (i.e., S or RBD antigens), which are displayed on the cell surface of antigen-presenting cells (APCs). APCs then recruit T cells that are activated to kill SARS-CoV-2-infected cells. APCs also recruit B cells that are primed to produce neutralizing antibodies to the viral S and RBD proteins, preventing viral attachment to host cells and stopping the infection. Long-lived memory B and T cells (light brown) are also produced simultaneously that can patrol the body for any incoming viruses for months/years and rekindle an identical B- and T-cell response.

On the other hand, in the case of the **DNA vaccines** when injected intramuscularly, the genetic information remains unintegrated in muscle cells but gives long-term expression of properly folded and glycosylated immunogenic protein and strong cell-mediated, as well as humoral, immunity. In mice, DNA vaccines have been shown to induce protective cell-mediated immunity against leishmaniasis, tuberculosis and malaria. A trial of a DNA vaccine against malaria in humans showed induction of malaria-specific cytotoxic T cells. Recombinant DNA technology, coupled with the identification of viral and bacterial epitopes for T- and B-cell responses, will lead to vaccines of the future that are safe, easy to administer and affordable to a vast majority of the world population, especially in developing nations.

Vaccines for COVID-19

The recent COVID-19 pandemic revitalized the vaccine industry with various new approaches for novel vaccine development and their delivery (Table 10.4). For instance, mRNA vaccine development was at a fledgling stage when the COVID-19 pandemic struck the world, but these vaccines are now considered the most effective for curbing COVID-19 spread. Various vaccine developmental approaches that were undertaken in the wake of the COVID-19 infection together with their modes of action are shown in Table 10.4.

Incidentally, nasal (delivered as puffs) and oral (delivered as drops of the vaccine) COVID-19 vaccines are currently in the final trial stages of development and should be available soon. These will obviate the current, unpleasant injectable vaccinations that are not very popular among children and some adults. Hopefully, these new delivery modes, which are simple to administer (without

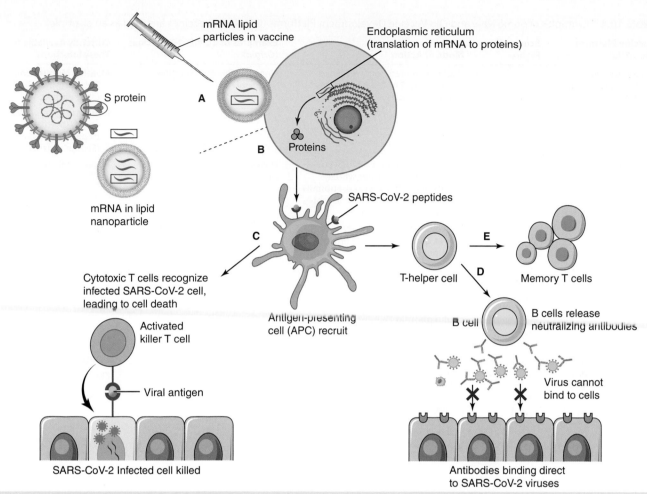

Fig 10.11   A simplified representation of how mRNA vaccine works. (A) The vaccine containing mRNA of SARS-CoV-2 with the code for either the spike *(S)* protein or the receptor-binding domain *(RBD)* proteins, within lipid particles are administered to the vaccinee. (B) Once injected, the lipid particles are 'ingested' by vaccinees' cells. The protein-making machinery in these cells is instructed to produce viral proteins (i.e., S or RBD antigens), which are displayed on the cell surface of antigen-presenting cells (APCs) *(purple)*. (C) APCs then recruit T cells *(green)* that are activated to kill SARS-CoV-2-infected cells (lower left panel). (D) APCs also recruit B cells *(blue)* that are primed to produce neutralizing antibodies to the viral S and RBD proteins, preventing viral attachment to host cells and stopping the infection *(lower right panel)*. (E) Long-lived memory B and T cells *(light brown)* are also produced simultaneously and can patrol the body for any incoming viruses for months/years and rekindle an identical B- and T-cell response.

a physician) and effective, will assist in the not-too-distant future the global eradication of not only COVID-19 but also other killer infections such as malaria.

'-omics' Developments Impacting Oral Immunology

Many recent developments in approaches to advanced genomics, transcriptomics, proteomics and metabolomics have enabled a deeper understanding of immunity to infection, cancer and disease in the context of the oral cavity. These applications of '-omic' technologies to better understand oral immunology and host–pathogen interactions encompass multiple cutting-edge methodologies.

GENOMICS AND TRANSCRIPTOMICS

Most notably, among recent applications of '-omic' technologies are **next-generation sequencing (NGS)** methods that have revolutionized studies of genomics and transcriptomics. Various types of NGS have evolved in recent years for unprecedented speed, read length, accuracy, throughput and cost in sequence analysis. NGS is so powerful that it has been used to define elements of host immunity and pathogen virulence in the ancient human oral cavity. One type of NGS that is particularly prominent is the technique of RNA sequencing (RNA-seq) that involves mass parallel sequencing of complementary DNA (cDNA). This technique is being used to enable the discovery and quantification of novel RNA transcripts in human and microbial cells and for shedding new light on the nature of the immune response in oral health and disease.

As described in Chapter 3, NGS technology has revolutionized the identification of nonculturable organisms from the oral cavity, providing new insights on the oral microbiota. These include hitherto unknown, newer bacterial and fungal phylotypes that inhabit the oral microbiome.

Table 10.4   Examples of Some New and Old Vaccine Development Platforms (COVID-19 vaccines are used as an example)

Vaccine Platform (*New/Old*)	Schematic Figure	Mode of Action	Examples of COVID-19 Vaccines (*Origin*)	Currently Available for These Infections
Inactivated or attenuated virus (*Old*)		Vaccines created from weakened SARS-CoV-2 or those attenuated with chemicals.	Sinovac – Biotech, Sinopharm (*China*)	**Measles, Mumps, and Rubella (MMR), Varicella (chickenpox),** **Influenza;** Whooping cough (pertussis); Hepatitis A, Polio (Sabine variant)
Subunit /Protein-based vaccines (*New*)		Vaccines that contain SARS-CoV-2 proteins only, either whole protein, or fragmented, subunits. Some pack many of these molecules in nanoparticles.	Novavax (*India*) Sanofi; GlaxoSmithKline (*USA*)	**Hepatitis B,** Acellular Whooping Cough vaccine (aP)
mRNA Vaccines (*New*)		Delivers one or more of SARS-CoV-2 RNA genes into cells to provoke an immune response.	Moderna (*USA*); Cominarty – Pfizer/BioNTech (*Germany*)	**COVID-19**
DNA Vaccines (*New*)		Delivers SARS-CoV-2 DNA genes into cells, with the help of a plasmid ('a jumping gene' found in bacteria) to provoke an immune response.	INO-4800 Inovio (*USA*)	Veterinary infections
Replicating or non-replicating Viral Vector Vaccines (*Old*) (vector examples: chimpanzee adenovirus; vaccinia virus)		Viruses engineered to carry coronavirus genes (Trojan horse principle), but nonreplicating, enter receptive cells and instruct them to make viral proteins or slowly replicate, carrying coronavirus proteins on their surface.	AstraZeneca (*UK*); Johnson & Johnson (*USA*); Sputnik V – Gamaleya Research Institute (*Russia*)	**COVID-19** Ebola infection

Note: Viral vaccines currently recommended for dental care workers are in bold (last column on right).

PROTEOMICS AND METABOLOMICS IN IMMUNOLOGY

Proteomics approaches utilize methods to analyze the total protein component of a biological system. Methodologies that enable the analysis of total protein expression profiles include liquid chromatography (LC) and high-throughput mass spectrometry (MS). LC–MS/MS is an MS-based approach being used to identify, quantify and characterize the salivary proteome and associated immune responses in oral-cavity squamous cell carcinoma. **Metabolomics** methods are being used to understand the role of specific metabolites in oral biofilms, oral cancers and other periodontal diseases. Further development of '-omic' technologies will offer new unique insights into oral immunology and may lead to new approaches to diagnose, treat and prevent various diseases.

Key Facts

- **Infectious diseases** are responsible for **30%** of the world's disease burden.
- All of the immunological mechanisms described in the previous two chapters are involved in defence against pathogens.
- Microorganisms have developed various strategies to avoid host defences.
- The **immune response** against pathogens may secondarily **cause damage to host** tissues.
- **Natural infection *may* produce lifelong protection against reinfection** with the same pathogen, with induction of memory T and B lymphocytes.
- Some, but by no means all, infectious diseases can be prevented by **vaccination in childhood** with a variety of vaccines produced by older and newer technologies.

- Currently available vaccines are better at inducing **type 2 rather than type 1 cytokines**, and hence induce humoral immunity but often little cell-mediated immunity.
- **mRNA vaccines** have played a major role in curbing the COVID-19 pandemic, although periodic repeat vaccination is required to rejuvenate the immune response.
- New approaches are required to produce stronger vaccines against today's leading killer infections. **Genetic or DNA vaccines** appear to offer promise in this regard, inducing powerful cell-mediated as well as humoral immune responses in animal and human studies.
- **'-omic' technologies** of next-generation sequencing for genomics and transcriptomics, proteomics and metabolomics are offering unprecedented insight into oral immunobiology.

Review Questions (Answers on p. 389)

Please indicate which answers are true and which are false.

10.1. Which of the following statements are true?
a. polymorphs and macrophages bind to sugar molecules on bacterial cell walls prior to phagocytosing them
b. some antibodies that eliminate the infecting bacteria may cause antibody-dependent cellular cytotoxicity
c. interferons induce enzymes that inhibit messenger RNA translation into proteins
d. viruses usually induce macrophages to release inflammatory cytokines
e. antigenic shift in the influenza virus can result in pandemic disease

10.2. Which of the following statements are true?
a. the bacterial cell wall proteoglycan can be destroyed by lysozyme present in saliva
b. *Streptococcus pneumoniae* resists phagocytic digestion by virtue of its capsule
c. human herpesviruses have the ability to integrate their genes into the host cell genome and evade host defences

d. highly active antiretroviral therapy (HAART) can prevent HIV infection
e. in fungal infections, the production of antifungal antibodies may lead to IgE-mediated allergic diseases

10.3. Which of the following statements on vaccines are true?
a. memory T and B cells can be induced successfully using live (rather than inactivated) vaccines
b. toxoidable vaccines contain antibodies to the specific toxin
c. immunocompromised patients should not be given live vaccines
d. flu vaccine should be provided for all dental health care workers
e. BCG vaccine is effective for preventing *Mycobacterium tuberculosis* infection

Further Reading

Delves, P. J., Martin, S. J., Burton, D. R., & Roitt, I. M. (2017). *Roitt's essential immunology* (13th ed.). Blackwell.

Janeway, C. A., Jr., Travers, P., Walport, M., et al. (2001). *Immunobiology* (5th ed.). Garland Publishing.

Li, G, Fan, Y, Lai, Y, et al. (2020). Coronavirus infections and immune responses. *Journal of Medical Virology, 92*, 424–432. https://doi.org/10.1002/jmv.25685.

Mikkonen, J. J., Singh, S. P., Herrala, M., et al. (2016). Salivary metabolomics in the diagnosis of oral cancer and periodontal diseases. *Journal of Periodontal Research, 51*, 431–437.

Moon, J. H., & Lee, J. H. (2016). Probing the diversity of healthy oral microbiome with bioinformatics approaches. *BMB Reports, 49*, 662–670.

Salisbury, D. M., & Begg, N. T. (1996). *Immunisation against infectious disease*. HMSO.

Samaranayake, L. P., Seneviratne, C. J., & Fakhruddin, K. S. (2021, May). Coronavirus disease 2019 (COVID-19) vaccines: A concise review. *Oral Diseases, 28*(suppl. 2), 2326–2336. https://doi.org/10.1111/odi.13916.

Samaranayake, L. P., & Fakhruddin, K. S. (2021). COVID-19 vaccines and dentistry. *Dental Update, 48*, 76–81.

Warinner, C., Rodrigues, J. F., Vyas, R., et al. (2014). Pathogens and host immunity in the ancient human oral cavity. *Nature Genetics, 46*, 336–344.

Washio, J., & Takahashi, N. (2016). Metabolomic studies of oral biofilm, oral cancer, and beyond. *International Journal of Molecular Sciences, 17*, E870.

Winck, F. V., Prado Ribeiro, A. C., Ramos Domingues, R., et al. (2015). Insights into immune responses in oral cancer through proteomic analysis of saliva and salivary extracellular vesicles. *Scientific Reports, 5*, 16305.

PART 3

MICROBES OF RELEVANCE TO DENTISTRY

This section outlines the characteristic features of important microbes that are particularly relevant to dentistry. The information given here relates intimately to the diseases described in the rest of the book: the chapters in this section should therefore be reviewed in conjunction with those on systemic and oral diseases in Parts 4 and 5.

- Streptococci, staphylococci and enterococci
- Lactobacilli, corynebacteria and propionibacteria
- Actinomycetes, clostridia and *Bacillus* species
- Neisseriaceae, *Veillonella*, parvobacteria and *Capnocytophaga*
- Enterobacteria
- Vibrios, campylobacters and *Wolinella*
- *Bacteroides*, *Tannerella*, *Porphyromonas* and *Prevotella*
- Fusobacteria, *Leptotrichia* and spirochaetes
- Mycobacteria and legionellae
- Chlamydiae, rickettsiae and mycoplasmas
- Viruses of relevance to dentistry
- Fungi of relevance to dentistry

11 Streptococci, Staphylococci and Enterococci

Streptococci comprise a diverse group of Gram-positive cocci which continuously undergo taxonomic revision. They are distributed widely in humans and animals, mostly forming part of their normal flora. A few species cause significant human morbidity. The **oral streptococci**, which include the cariogenic **mutans group**, are important members of the genus. There is also an accumulating database to indicate that enterococci, particularly *Enterococcus faecalis* (commonly found as gut microbes), are a pathogen of significance in endodontic (root canal) infections. Another common group of cocci, the **staphylococci**, live on the skin but are infrequently isolated from the oral cavity and are significant agents of many pyogenic (pus-producing) human infections.

Streptococci

GENERAL PROPERTIES

Characteristics

Streptococci are **catalase-negative**, **Gram-positive** spherical or oval cocci in pairs and chains, 0.7–0.9 μm in diameter.

Chain formation is best seen in liquid cultures or pus. Cell division in this genus occurs along a single axis; thus they grow in chains or pairs, and hence the name: from Greek *streptos*, meaning 'easily bent or twisted', like a chain.

Culture

These cocci grow well on blood agar, although enrichment of media with glucose and serum may be necessary. Typical haemolytic reactions are produced on blood agar (Fig. 11.1):

- **α-haemolysis**: narrow zone of partial haemolysis and green (viridans) discolouration around the colony—for example, viridans streptococci
- **β-haemolysis**: wide, clear, translucent zone of complete haemolysis around the colony—for example, *Streptococcus pyogenes*
- **no haemolysis** (γ-haemolysis)—for example, nonhaemolytic streptococci.

Serology

The carbohydrate antigens found on the cell walls of the organisms are related to their virulence. Hence,

127

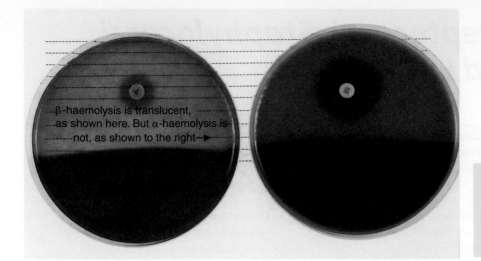

β-haemolysis is translucent, as shown here. But α-haemolysis is not, as shown to the right→

Fig. 11.1 α- and β-haemolysis: β-haemolytic colonies (e.g., *Streptococcus pyogenes*) produce complete translucence of blood agar, whereas α-haemolytic colonies (e.g., *Streptococcus pneumoniae*) do not. Note also the sensitivity of *Streptococcus pneumoniae* to a disc impregnated with optochin.

serogrouping, termed **Lancefield grouping**, is useful in the identification of the more virulent β-haemolytic species. Currently, 20 Lancefield groups are recognized (A–H and K–V), but not all are equally important as human pathogens. The following are worthy of note:

- **group A** includes the important human pathogen *Streptococcus pyogenes*, the agent of scarlet fever, and many other infections. It is estimated that infections caused by this group of streptococci are currently responsible for more than 500 000 deaths annually worldwide.
- **group B** contains one species, *Streptococcus agalactiae*, an inhabitant of the female genital tract; it causes infection in neonates
- **group C** mainly causes diseases in animals
- **group D** includes the enterococci (*Enterococcus faecalis*, an endodontic pathogen) and ranks next to group A in causing human disease.

STREPTOCOCCUS PYOGENES (GROUP A)

Habitat and Transmission

The normal habitat of this species is the human **upper respiratory tract and skin**; it may survive in dust for some time. Spread is by airborne droplets and by contact.

Characteristics

It is found as a commensal in the nasopharynx of a minority of healthy adults, but more commonly (about 10%) in children. It grows well on blood agar, with a characteristic halo of **β-haemolysis**. Some strains produce mucoid colonies as a result of having a hyaluronic acid capsule. This may contribute to virulence by offering resistance to phagocytosis.

Exotoxins and Enzymes. Produces a large number of biologically active substances, such as:

- **streptokinase (fibrinolysin)**: a proteolytic enzyme that lyses fibrin
- **hyaluronidase**: attacks the material that binds the connective tissue, thereby causing increase in permeability (hence called the 'spreading factor')

- **DNAases** (streptodornases): destroy cellular DNA
- **haemolysins** (streptolysins, leukocidins): phage mediated and are responsible for the characteristic erythematous rash in scarlet fever; also cause the translucency around colonies in blood agar due to breakdown of haemoglobin (Fig. 11.1)
- **pyrogenic exotoxins (erythrogenic toxin)**: associated with streptococcal toxic shock syndrome and scarlet fever.

(*Note*: not all these products are produced by every strain; the combined synergistic action of enzymes and toxins contributes to the pathogenicity.)

Culture and Identification

Culture on blood agar yields characteristic **β-haemolytic** colonies (lysis of blood due to streptolysins O and S). A Gram-stained smear may show characteristic cocci in chains (Fig. 11.2); these are more developed in liquid than in solid media. The isolate can be presumptively identified as *Streptococcus pyogenes* if it is **sensitive to bacitracin**.

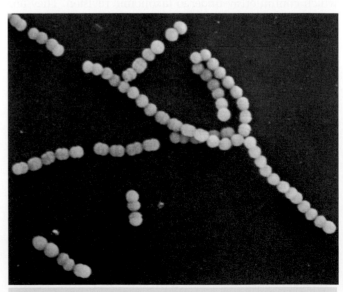

Fig. 11.2 Scanning electron micrograph of a chain of streptococci.

If rheumatic fever is suspected, then testing the **patient's antistreptolysin O** (ASO) antibody titre will demonstrate previous exposure to *Streptococcus pyogenes*.

Pathogenicity

Streptococcus pyogenes causes a number of spreading infections with minimal local suppuration; the most notable are:

- tonsillitis and pharyngitis
- necrotizing fasciitis (streptococcal gangrene; so-called disease of 'flesh-eating bacteria')
- scarlet fever
- mastoiditis and sinusitis
- otitis media (middle-ear infection)
- wound infections leading to cellulitis and lymphangitis
- impetigo and erysipelas (a brawny, massive skin infection).

Complications

After an episode of infection, particularly scarlet fever, some patients develop complications, such as rheumatic fever, glomerulonephritis and erythema nodosum, which may have long-lasting effects. Early diagnosis and management of scarlet fever are important to prevent its aforementioned inflammatory sequelae. Note that:

- in cellulitis, hyaluronidase (spreading factor) mediates the subcutaneous spread of infection
- erythrogenic toxin causes the rash of scarlet fever
- poststreptococcal infection, manifesting as **rheumatic fever**, is caused by immunological cross-reaction between bacterial antigen and human heart tissue, and **acute glomerulonephritis** is caused by immune complexes bound to glomeruli (see Chapter 23).

Treatment and Prevention

Penicillin is the drug of choice; erythromycin and clindamycin are suitable for patients hypersensitive to penicillin. No vaccine is available.

STREPTOCOCCUS AGALACTIAE (GROUP B)

This species is increasingly recognized as a human pathogen, especially as a cause of **neonatal meningitis and sepsis**.

Habitat and Transmission

Streptococcus agalactiae is found in the human vagina; sometimes anorectal carriage occurs. Babies acquire infection from the colonized mother during delivery or during nursing.

Characteristics

Gram-positive cocci in chains.

Culture and Identification

Gram-stained smear and culture yielding **β-haemolytic colonies** on blood agar; colonies on blood agar are generally larger than *Streptococcus pyogenes*. Lancefield group is determined by antiserum against cell wall polysaccharide.

Pathogenicity

No toxins or virulence factors have been identified. This species causes neonatal meningitis and septicaemia; it is also associated with septic abortion and gynaecological sepsis.

Treatment and Prevention

Penicillin is the drug of choice; erythromycin is suitable for patients hypersensitive to penicillin. Prophylactic antibiotics may be given to neonates if the mother is culture-positive.

ORAL STREPTOCOCCI

Oral streptococci, which live principally in the oropharynx, are a mixed group of organisms with variable characteristics. New typing techniques, particularly those based on molecular biology, have revealed the complex nature of the origin and taxonomy of this group. Hence, the nomenclature of oral streptococci is in a constant state of flux. This pathogen typically shows **α-haemolysis** on blood agar, but this is not a constant feature as some strains are nonhaemolytic and others β-haemolytic. Oral streptococci can be divided into four main **species groups** as follows:

- *mutans* group
- *salivarius* group
- *anginosus* group
- *mitis* group.

Each of these groups comprises a number of species (Table 11.1). See also Chapter 31 for further details of oral streptococci.

Habitat and Transmission

Streptococci make up a large proportion of the **resident oral microbiota**. It is known that roughly one-quarter of the total cultivable flora from supragingival and gingival plaque and half of the isolates from the tongue and saliva are streptococci. They are vertically transmitted from mother to child. Infective endocarditis caused by these organisms (loosely termed *viridans* streptococci) in specific susceptible patient groups is generally a result of their entry into the blood stream (bacteraemia) during intraoral surgical procedures (e.g., tooth extraction) and sometimes even during tooth brushing.

Culture and Identification

Gram-positive cocci in chains; α-haemolytic; catalase-negative. Growth **not inhibited by bile or optochin**

Table 11.1 Some Recognized Species of Oral Streptococci

Group	Species
mutans group	*S. mutans*, serotypes c, e, f
	S. sobrinus, serotypes d, g
	S. cricetus, serotype a
	S. rattus, serotype b and others
salivarius group	*S. salivarius*
	S. vestibularis
anginosus group	*S. constellatus*
	S. intermedius
	S. anginosus
mitis group	*S. sanguinis*
	S. gordonii
	S. parasanguinis
	S. oralis and others

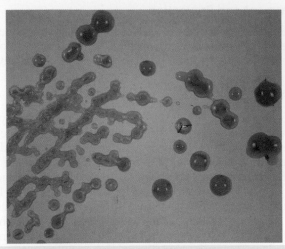

Fig. 11.3   Gelatinous colonies of *mutans* streptococci mainly comprising extracellular polysaccharides.

(ethylhydrocupreine hydrochloride), in contrast to pneumococci. Commercially available kits are highly useful in laboratory identification of these organisms.

Pathogenicity

The *mutans* group of streptococci are the major agents of dental caries (but in the absence of predisposing factors, such as sucrose, they cannot cause caries). They have a characteristic ability to produce voluminous amounts of **sticky, extracellular polysaccharides** in the presence of dietary carbohydrates (Fig. 11.3); these help tenacious binding of the organisms to enamel and to each other.

They are also important agents of **infective endocarditis**, and some 60% of cases are due to this organism. Usually, bacteria released during dental procedures settle on damaged heart valves, causing infective endocarditis (see Chapter 24).

Treatment and Prevention

In patients at risk of infective endocarditis (e.g., those with damaged or prosthetic heart valves), prophylactic antibiotic cover should always be given before dental procedures (see Chapter 24).

See Chapter 32 for caries.

STREPTOCOCCUS MUTANS

Streptococcus mutans gained notoriety in the 1960s when it was demonstrated that caries could be experimentally induced and transmitted in animals by oral inoculation with the organism. The name *mutans* results from its frequent transition from coccal phase to coccobacillary phase. Currently, seven distinct species of human and animal *mutans* streptococci and eight serotypes (*a–h*) are recognized, based on the antigenic specificity of cell wall carbohydrates. The term *Streptococcus mutans* is limited to human isolates belonging to **three serotypes (*c, e* and *f*).**

Other Oral Gram-Positive Cocci

A group of oral organisms previously classified as **nutritionally variant streptococci** (*Streptococcus adjacens*,

Streptococcus defectivus) and isolated under appropriate environmental conditions has been assigned to a new genus called *Granulicatella*. Their role in oral disease is not well characterized. (See Chapter 31 for further details.)

STREPTOCOCCUS PNEUMONIAE (PNEUMOCOCCUS)

This organism causes a number of common diseases, such as **pneumonia and meningitis** in adults and **otitis media and sinusitis** in children.

Habitat and Transmission

A normal commensal in the human upper respiratory tract; up to 4% of the population carry this bacteria in small numbers. Transmission is via respiratory droplets.

Characteristics

Gram-positive 'lancet-shaped' cocci in pairs (diplococci) or short chains; cells are often capsulate; α-haemolytic on blood agar; catalase-negative; facultative anaerobe (i.e., grows under both aerobic and anaerobic conditions).

Culture and Identification

Forms **α-haemolytic** colonies. After incubation for 2 days, the colonies appear typically as 'draughtsmen' because of their central indentation (a result of spontaneous autolysis of older bacteria in the centre of the colony). The species is differentiated from other α-haemolytic streptococci by its sensitivity to optochin and solubility in bile (Fig. 11.1). Observation for the capsular swelling with type-specific antiserum (quellung reaction) confirms the identity and is the standard reference method. The latex agglutination test (see Fig. 6.7) for capsular antigen in spinal fluid can be diagnostic.

Pathogenicity

Although no exotoxins are known, this organism induces an inflammatory response. The substantive polysaccharide capsule retards phagocytosis. **Vaccination with antipolysaccharide vaccine** helps provide type-specific immunity. Viral respiratory infection predisposes to pneumococcal pneumonia by damaging the mucociliary lining of the upper respiratory tract (*mucociliary escalator*). Other common diseases caused by pneumococci include lobar pneumonia, acute exacerbation of chronic bronchitis, otitis media, sinusitis, conjunctivitis, meningitis and, in splenectomized patients, septicaemia.

Treatment and Prevention

Penicillin or erythromycin is very effective. However, resistance to penicillin is rapidly emerging as a global concern.

GRAM-POSITIVE ANAEROBIC COCCI

Gram-positive anaerobic cocci (GPAC) all belonged to the genus *Peptostreptococcus* until recently. However, they now comprise three genera: *Peptostreptococcus*, *Micromonas* and *Finegoldia*. The representative species are *Peptostreptococcus anaerobius*, *Finegoldia magnus* (previously *Peptostreptococcus magnus*) and *Micromonas micros* (previously *Peptostreptococcus micros*).

These GPAC can often be isolated from dental plaque and the female genital tract. They are also found in carious dentine, subgingival plaque, dentoalveolar abscesses and in advanced periodontal disease, usually in mixed culture. Their pathogenic role is still unclear.

Staphylococci

Staphylococci are also Gram-positive cocci, but in contrast to streptococci, they divide along multiple axes and generate **grapelike clusters** of cells. The *Staphylococcus* genus contains more than 15 different species, of which the following are of medical importance: *Staphylococcus aureus*, *Staphylococcus epidermidis* and *Staphylococcus saprophyticus*.

Staphylococci cause a variety of both common and uncommon infections, such **as abscesses of many organs, endocarditis, gastroenteritis (food poisoning) and toxic shock syndrome**. They are not infrequent isolates from the oral cavity. Higher proportions of *Staphylococcus aureus* are found in the saliva of healthy subjects older than 70 years.

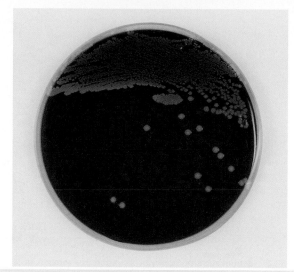

Fig. 11.4   **Golden-yellow colonies of *Staphylococcus aureus*.**

STAPHYLOCOCCUS AUREUS

Habitat and Transmission

The habitat is the human skin, especially the anterior nares and the perineum. Domesticated animals also carry staphylococci. Higher carriage rates are seen in hospital patients and staff. These bacteria are disseminated through air and dust and are always present in the hospital environment. The usual transmission route is via the hands and fingertips.

Characteristics

Gram-positive cocci in clusters (cluster formation is due to their ability to divide in many planes); nonsporing, nonmotile; some strains are capsulate.

Culture and Identification

Grows aerobically as yellow or gold colonies on blood agar (Fig. 11.4); catalase-positive (this differentiates them from the catalase-negative streptococci).

Other tests used to differentiate the more virulent *Staphylococcus aureus* from the less pathogenic *Staphylococcus epidermidis* include the following.

Coagulase Test. *Staphylococcus aureus* coagulates dilute human serum or rabbit plasma (i.e., it is coagulase-positive), whereas *Staphylococcus epidermidis* does not (coagulase-negative). This test could be done either in a test tube (the tube test), which requires overnight incubation (Fig. 11.5), or on a slide (the slide test), which is a rapid test.

Protein A: Latex Agglutination Test. Protein A, synthesized by almost all strains of *Staphylococcus aureus*, has a special affinity to the Fc fragment of immunoglobulin G (IgG). Hence, when latex particles coated with IgG (and fibrinogen) are mixed with an emulsified suspension of *Staphylococcus aureus* on a glass slide, visible agglutination

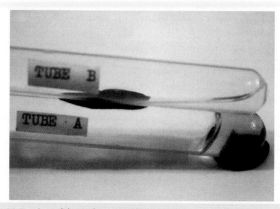

Fig. 11.5   **A positive tube coagulase test for *Staphylococcus aureus* (tube A); tube B: bacteria-free control with uncoagulated plasma**.

of the latex particles occurs; no such reaction is seen with *Staphylococcus epidermidis* (Fig. 11.6).

Other Tests. These include the phosphatase test, DNAase test and mannitol fermentation test (most strains of *Staphylococcus aureus* form acid from mannitol, whereas few *Staphylococcus epidermidis* do so).

Typing of *Staphylococcus aureus*

Typing is important to determine the source of an outbreak of infection. This was commonly done by the pattern of susceptibility to a set of more than 20 bacteriophages: **phage typing** and **serotyping**. These methods are currently supplanted by molecular typing techniques. Antibiotic-susceptibility patterns are also helpful in tracing the source of outbreaks.

Pathogenicity

A variety of enzymes and toxins are produced by *Staphylococcus aureus*, although no one strain produces the whole range listed in Table 11.2. The two most important are **coagulase** and **enterotoxin**. Coagulase is the best correlate of pathogenicity. Some of the diseases caused by *Staphylococcus aureus* are:

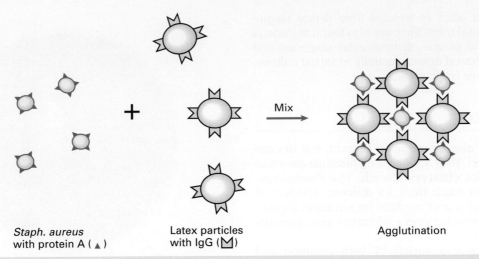

Staph. aureus
with protein A (▲)

Latex particles
with IgG (⋈)

Agglutination

Fig. 11.6 Identification of *Staphylococcus aureus*. Protein A of *Staphylococcus aureus* has a special affinity for immunoglobulin G (IgG); when latex particles coated with IgG are mixed with a suspension of the organism, visible agglutination of latex particles occurs.

Table 11.2 Toxins and Enzymes Produced by *Staphylococcus aureus*

Toxin/Enzyme	Activity
Toxins	
Cytotoxins (α, β, γ, δ)	Cell lysis
Leukocidin	Kills leukocytes
Epidermolytic toxin	Exfoliation and splitting of epidermis
Toxic shock syndrome toxin	Shock, rash, desquamation
Enterotoxin (A–E)	Induces vomiting and diarrhoea
Enzymes	
Coagulase	Clots plasma
Catalase	Affects bactericidal activity of polymorphs
Hyaluronidase	Connective tissue breakdown
DNAase (nuclease)	DNA hydrolysis
Lipase	Breaks lipids of cell membranes
Penicillinase	Breaks down β-lactam drugs
Protein A	Antiphagocytic

- **superficial infections**: common agent of boils, carbuncles, pustules, abscesses, conjunctivitis and wound infections; rarely causes oral infections; may cause angular cheilitis (together with the yeast *Candida*) at the angles of the mouth
- **food poisoning** (vomiting and diarrhoea) caused by enterotoxins
- **toxic shock syndrome**, also caused by an enterotoxin
- **deep infections**: osteomyelitis, endocarditis, septicaemia, pneumonia.

Predisposing factors for infection are minor and major breaks in the skin, foreign bodies such as sutures, low neutrophil levels and injecting drug abuse.

Treatment and Prevention

The vast majority (>80%) of strains are resistant to β-lactam drugs, and some to a number of antibiotics. The latter phenomenon (**multiresistance**) is common, particularly in strains isolated from hospitals; these cause hospital (**nosocomial**) infection. Penicillin resistance is due to the production of β-lactamase encoded by plasmids. The enzyme destroys the efficacy of antibiotics with a β-lactam ring (i.e., the penicillin-group drugs).

Antibiotics active against *Staphylococcus aureus* include penicillin for sensitive isolates, flucloxacillin (stable against β-lactamase), erythromycin, fusidic acid (useful for skin infections), cephalosporins and vancomycin.

Cleanliness, hand-washing and aseptic management of lesions reduce the spread of staphylococci.

ANTIBIOTIC RESISTANCE IN STAPHYLOCOCCI

This is a global problem of immense concern and falls into several classes:

- resistance to β-lactam drugs (see earlier discussion)
- resistance to methicillin (and to nafcillin and oxacillin) independent of β-lactamase (The spread of methicillin-resistant *Staphylococcus aureus* (**MRSA**) worldwide is posing problems in many community and hospital settings.)
- resistance to vancomycin, one of the last-line defences against staphylococci and the emergence of vancomycin-resistant *Staphylococcus aureus* (**VRSA**) (The mechanism of resistance here is due to alterations in the cell wall.)
- 'tolerance', where the organism is inhibited but not killed by the antibiotic (i.e., there is a large difference between minimum inhibitory concentration and minimum bactericidal concentration), leading to prolonged course of infections (e.g., staphylococcal infective endocarditis).

STAPHYLOCOCCUS EPIDERMIDIS

Habitat and Transmission

This species is found on the skin surface and is spread by contact.

Culture and Identification

Grows on blood agar as white colonies, hence the earlier name *Staphylococcus albus*; catalase-positive; coagulase-negative;

biochemically characterized by commercially available kits (e.g., API STAPH).

Pathogenicity

Being a normal **commensal of the skin**, this bacterium causes infection only when an opportunity arises (it is an opportunist pathogen). Common examples are **catheter-related sepsis, infection of artificial joints and urinary tract infections.**

Treatment

Staphylococcus epidermidis exhibits resistance to a number of drugs (multiresistance), including penicillin and methicillin. It is sensitive to vancomycin.

STAPHYLOCOCCUS SAPROPHYTICUS

This organism causes urinary tract infections in women, an infection especially associated with intercourse. It has the ability to colonize the periurethral skin and mucosa. The organism can be differentiated from *Staphylococcus epidermidis* (both grow on blood agar as white colonies) by the mannitol fermentation reaction and other biochemical tests.

Enterococci

Habitat and Transmission

Normal constituents of the gut microbiota; *Enterococcus faecalis* is the most virulent species.

Commonly isolated from **endodontic infections**, and difficult to eradicate due to persistence within dentinal tubules where access to antibiotics or antiseptics is limited. Why enterococci preferentially colonizes dentine and

how these organism are transmitted to infected pulp is yet unknown.

Culture and Identification

Grows well on blood agar even with 6.5% NaCl; usually nonhaemolytic but are occasionally α-haemolytic. Enterococci are pyridoxine positive, grow in the presence of bile and hydrolyse esculin (bile esculin positive).

Pathogenicity

In general, enterococci are among the most **frequent causes of nosocomial infections**, particularly in intensive care units, where they are selected due to constant antibiotic exposure. *E faecalis* is common in pulpal infection and is commonly associated with treatment failure in endodontic infections (see Chapter 34).

Treatment

Enterococci can be very resistant to antibiotics and antiseptics. For instance, they are more resistant to penicillin G than the streptococci, and rarely β-lactamase positive; many are vancomycin resistant.

Micrococci

Micrococci are catalase-positive organisms similar to staphylococci. They are coagulase-negative and usually grow on blood agar as white colonies, although some species are brightly pigmented: pink, orange or yellow.

Stomatococcus mucilaginous, formerly classified in the genus *Micrococcus*, is found in abundance on the lingual surface. This species has the ability to produce an extracellular slime, which correlates with its predilection for the lingual surface. Its role in disease, if any, is unknown.

Key Facts

- Streptococci are **Gram-positive** and appear as **spherical** or oval cocci in **chains and pairs**.
- Streptococci can be **classified** according to (1) the **degree of haemolysis** on blood agar (α, mild; β, complete; γ no haemolysis) and (2) the cell wall carbohydrate antigens into the 20 **Lancefield groups**.
- **Lancefield group A** contains the important human pathogen *Streptococcus pyogenes*; the latter infection leads to rheumatic fever and rheumatic carditis, which makes the endocardium susceptible to future episodes of infection.
- **Oral streptococci** are a mixed group of organisms and typically show α-**haemolysis** on blood agar.
- Oral streptococci can be divided into **four main 'species groups'**, and of these the *mutans* group bacteria are the major agents of dental caries.

- **Staphylococci** resemble streptococci in appearance but are arranged in **grapelike clusters** and are all **catalase-positive** (all streptococci are catalase-negative).
- *Staphylococcus aureus* is a common pathogen causing localized skin infections and serious systemic infections; it produces numerous toxins and enzymes as virulence factors.
- Antibiotic resistance in staphylococci, a problem of worldwide concern, has led to the emergence of methicillin-resistant *Staphylococcus aureus* (**MRSA**), vancomycin-resistant *Staphylococcus aureus* (**VRSA**) and **antibiotic-'tolerant'** isolates.
- Enterococci are normal constituents of the gut microbiota, and *Enterococcus faecalis* is the most virulent species.
- *Enterococcus faecalis*, a common isolate form pulpal infection, is associated with **endodontic treatment failure**.

Review Questions (Answers on p. 389)

Please indicate which answers are true and which are false.

11.1. Which of the following statements on streptococci are true?
   a. some are Gram-positive and anaerobic
   b. can be primarily differentiated by their haemolytic reactions on blood agar
   c. can cause caries in the absence of sucrose
   d. *mutans* group streptococci cause caries
   e. oral streptococci typically show β-haemolysis on blood agar

11.2. *Staphylococcus aureus* can be differentiated from *Staphylococcus epidermidis* by:
   a. the coagulase test
   b. protein A latex agglutination test
   c. mannitol fermentation test
   d. Gram stain
   e. oxidase test

11.3. An 18-year-old male patient has a facial abscess from which a β-lactamase-positive *Staphylococcus aureus* strain was cultured. This organism:
   a. is resistant to penicillin
   b. is coagulase-positive
   c. is β-haemolytic
   d. may possess the ability to cause diarrhoea
   e. may cause rheumatic carditis

11.4. Common staphylococcal infections include:
   a. suppurative skin infections
   b. food poisoning
   c. toxic shock syndrome
   d. osteomyelitis
   e. pharyngitis

Further Reading

Beighton, D., Hardie, J., & Whiley, R. A. (1991). A scheme for the identification of viridans streptococci. *Journal of Medical Microbiology, 35,* 367–372.

Brooks, J. F., Carroll, K. C., Butel, J. S., et al. (Eds.). (2013). The staphylococci. In *Jawetz, Melnick and Adelebergs's medical microbiology* (26th ed., pp. 199–206, 209–225). Lange McGraw Hill.

Jone, D., Board, R. G., & Sussman, M. (1990). Staphylococci. *Society for Applied Microbiology Symposium Series No. 19.* Blackwell Scientific.

Matsubara, V. H., Christoforou, J., & Samaranayake, L (2023). Recrudescence of scarlet fever and its implications for dental professionals. *International Dental Journal, 73*(3), 331–336.

Murdoch, D. A. (1993). Gram-positive anaerobic cocci. *Clinical Microbiology Reviews, 11,* 81–120.

12 Lactobacilli, Corynebacteria and Propionibacteria

Lactobacilli

Lactobacilli are saprophytes in vegetable and animal material (e.g., milk). Some species are common animal and human commensals inhabiting the oral cavity and other parts of the body. They have the ability to tolerate acidic environments and hence are believed to be associated with human and animal caries.

The taxonomy of lactobacilli is complex. They are characterized into two main groups: **homofermenters**, which produce mainly lactic acid (65%) from glucose fermentation (e.g., *Lactobacillus casei*); and **heterofermenters**, which produce lactic acid as well as acetate, ethanol and carbon dioxide (e.g., *Lactobacillus fermentum*). *L. casei* and *L. rhamnosus*, *L. acidophilus* and the newly described species, *L. oris*, are common in the oral cavity.

Habitat and Transmission

Lactobacilli are found in the oral cavity, gastrointestinal tract and female genital tract. In the oral cavity, they constitute less than 1% of the total flora. Transmission routes are unknown.

Characteristics

Gram-positive coccobacillary forms (mostly bacillary), α- or nonhaemolytic, are facultative anaerobes. These organisms ferment carbohydrates to form acids (i.e., they are **acidogenic**) and can survive well in acidic milieu (they are **aciduric**); they may be **homofermentative or heterofermentative**. The question as to whether they are present in carious lesions because they prefer the acidic environment or whether they generate an acidic milieu and destroy the tooth enamel has been debated for years (the classic 'chicken and egg' argument). Lactobacilli are also major constituents of the vaginal flora and help maintain its low pH equilibrium.

The beneficial role of lactobacilli in maintaining the homoeostasis of the intestinal microbiome has been recognized, and 'lactobacillus-laced' food items, sold as **probiotics**, have gained popularity among the health-conscious public (see Chapter 26).

Culture and Identification

Lactobacilli grow under microaerophilic conditions in the presence of carbon dioxide and at acidic pH (6.0). Media enriched with glucose or blood promote growth. A special selective medium, tomato juice agar (pH 5.0), promotes the growth of lactobacilli while suppressing other bacteria. Identification is by biochemical reactions.

Pathogenicity

Lactobacilli are frequently isolated from deep carious lesions where the pH tends to be acidic, and they are commonly isolated from the advancing front of the dentinal caries lesions. Indeed, early workers believed that lactobacilli were the main cariogenic agent (a theory that has been disproved), so much so that the number of lactobacilli in saliva (the **lactobacillus count**) was taken as an indication of an individual's caries activity. Although this test is not very reliable, it is useful for monitoring the dietary profile of a patient because the level of lactobacilli correlates well with the intake of dietary carbohydrate and the number of acidic niches in the oral cavity.

Corynebacteria

The genus *Corynebacterium* contains many species that are widely distributed in nature. These Gram-positive bacilli demonstrate pleomorphism (i.e., coccobacillary appearance) and are nonsporing, noncapsulate and nonmotile. In common with *Mycobacterium* and *Nocardia* spp., they have a cell wall structure containing **mycolic acid**. A number of species are important human pathogens and commensals. The sometimes-fatal upper respiratory tract infection of childhood, **diphtheria**, is caused by *Corynebacterium diphtheriae*. It is important to distinguish this and other pathogens within the genus from commensal corynebacteria.

CORYNEBACTERIUM DIPHTHERIAE

Habitat and Transmission

Human throat and nose, occasionally skin; patients carry toxigenic organisms up to 3 months after infection. Transmission is via respiratory droplets.

Characteristics

Pleomorphic, Gram-positive, club-shaped (tapered at one end) bacilli, 2–5 μm in length, arranged in palisades. They divide by 'snapping fission' and hence are arranged at angles to each other, resembling Chinese characters. The rods have a beaded appearance, with the beads comprising an intracellular store of polymerized phosphate. The granules stain **metachromatically** with special stains such as Neisser methylene blue stain (i.e., the cells are stained with blue and the granules in red).

Culture and Identification

A nonfastidious, facultative anaerobe that grows well at 37°C. Grows on blood agar but selective media are helpful for isolation from clinical specimens. In **blood tellurite agar**, commonly used for this purpose, corynebacteria produce distinctive **grey–black colonies** after 48-h incubation at 35°C. Preliminary identification is helped by the shape and size of the colonies on tellurite agar. Specific identification is by biochemical reactions and demonstration of toxin production.

The test for toxin production is important as some corynebacteria are nontoxigenic (and hence nonvirulent) and are normal skin or throat commensals.

Toxin Production

The **exotoxin** responsible for virulence can be demonstrated by the gel precipitation test, which uses the **Elek plate**. In this test, a filter paper soaked in diphtheria antitoxin is incorporated into serum agar before it has set; the test strain of C. diphtheriae under investigation is then streaked on to the agar at right angles to the filter-paper strip and incubated at 37°C. After 24 h, white lines of precipitation will be visible as a result of the combination of the antitoxin and the antigen (i.e., the toxin) if the strain is a toxigenic isolate (Fig. 12.1). Although this is the traditional method for toxin detection, enzyme-linked immunosorbent assays (**ELISAs**) and immunochromatographic strips are now available for quick detection of the exotoxin from the cultured isolates.

A rapid diagnostic test based on **polymerase chain reaction** (PCR) for the **toxin gene** (*tox*) is another new direct assay of patient specimens, prior to culture and isolation of the organism.

Diphtheria Toxin. This exotoxin—produced by strains carrying bacteriophages with the ***tox* gene**—inhibits protein biosynthesis in all eukaryotic cells. The toxin has two components: *subunit A*, which has adenosine diphosphate ribosylating activity; and *subunit B*, which binds the toxin to cell surface receptors. Essentially, the toxin blocks protein synthesis of host cells by inactivating an elongation factor.

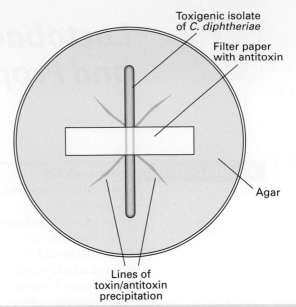

Fig. 12.1   Elek test for toxin-producing *Corynebacterium diphtheriae*. A filter paper impregnated with diphtheria antitoxin is incorporated into agar and the unknown (test) and the known (control) toxin-producing *C. diphtheriae* are streaked at right angles; after 24-h incubation, white lines of precipitation are produced due to the combination of the antigen (toxin) and the antibody. (Only the test inoculum is shown.)

Macroscopically, its action on the respiratory mucosa results in the production of a grey, adherent **pseudomembrane** comprising bacteria, fibrin and epithelial and phagocytic cells. This may obstruct the airway, and the patient may die of asphyxiation. When the toxin permeates into the blood stream, it acts systemically, affecting motor nerves of the myocardium and the nervous system.

The toxin can be converted to a **toxoid** (i.e., made nontoxic but still antigenic) by treatment with formaldehyde; the toxoid can then be used for prophylactic immunization: the first component of the **diphtheria–tetanus–pertussis (DTP) vaccine**.

Antitoxin, produced by injecting the toxin into horses, neutralizes the toxin (see below).

Pathogenicity

C. diphtheriae is the agent of **diphtheria**; it usually affects the mucosa of the upper respiratory tract, and sometimes the skin. Cutaneous infections are especially seen in the tropics and are usually mixed infections with *Staphylococcus aureus* and/or *Streptococcus pyogenes*. Serious systemic manifestations are the result of the absorption of the exotoxin.

Treatment and Prevention

In the acute phase, supportive therapy to maintain the airway is critical. Antitoxin is given to neutralize the toxin and penicillin to kill the organisms. Antibiotics have little effect once the toxin has spread, but they will eliminate the toxigenic focus of bacteria. In epidemic outbreaks, carriers are given either penicillin or erythromycin.

Immunization is highly effective in preventing diphtheria. A special test (the **Schick test**) is used to demonstrate immunity. Here, the circulating level of antibody after immunization (or clinical/subclinical infection) is assessed by inoculating a standardized dose of the toxin.

OTHER CORYNEBACTERIA

Corynebacterium ulcerans is responsible for diphtheria-like throat lesions, but it does not cause toxaemia.

Corynebacterium (formerly *Bacterionema*) *matruchotti* is the only true coryneform organism in the oral cavity. It resembles a whip (whip-handle cell), with a short, fat body and a long filament at one end.

Diphtheroids

Bacilli that morphologically resemble diphtheria bacilli are called **diphtheroids** (e.g., *Corynebacterium hofmannii*, *Corynebacterium xerosis*). They are normal inhabitants of the skin and conjunctiva and are occasional opportunistic pathogens in compromised patients (e.g., endocarditis in prosthetic valves).

Propionibacteria

Propionibacteria are obligate anaerobic, Gram-positive rods, sometimes called **diphtheroids** for the aforementioned reasons. *Propionibacterium acnes* is part of the normal skin flora and may also be isolated from dental plaque. The pathogenesis of **facial acne** is closely related to the lipases produced by *P. acnes*, hence the name.

A new member of this genus is *Propionibacterium propionicum* (formerly *Arachnia propionica*), morphologically similar to *Actinomyces israelii* (except for the production of propionic acid from glucose by the former).

Key Facts

- Lactobacilli are **acidogenic and aciduric**.
- Lactobacilli are common constituents of the oral flora and are regular isolates from dentinal caries lesions.
- The numbers of lactobacilli in saliva correlate positively with caries activity.
- **Toxigenic strains** of *Corynebacterium diphtheriae* are responsible for diphtheria, the sometimes fatal upper respiratory tract infection of childhood.

- The diphtheria toxin is **toxoidable** and is a component of the **triple vaccine** (diphtheria–tetanus–pertussis or DTP).
- *Propionibacterium acnes* (loosely termed 'diphtheroids') strains are a significant component of the normal skin flora and associated **facial acne** lesions.

Review Questions (Answers on p. 389)

Please indicate which answers are true and which are false.

12.1. Lactobacilli:
   a. are saprophytic
   b. are mostly homofermenters
   c. are aciduric and acidogenic
   d. are best grown in strict anaerobic conditions
   e. count in a saliva sample is by far the best indicator of cariogenic activity

12.2. Corynebacterium diphtheriae:
   a. are Gram-positive club-shaped spore-bearing rods
   b. contains metachromatic granules
   c. produces a toxin that is similar to endotoxin
   d. causes pharyngeal and skin infections
   e. is transmitted by airborne droplets

12.3. Toxin produced by *C. diphtheriae*:
   a. is mediated by a lysogenic phage
   b. is similar to endotoxin
   c. is a polypeptide
   d. inhibits protein synthesis
   e. causes neurological symptoms

12.4. Propionibacteria:
   a. are Gram-negative coccobacilli
   b. are the members of 'diphtheroids'
   c. are facultatively anaerobic
   d. are exclusive to the oral cavity
   e. are frequently associated with dental caries

Further Reading

Brooks, J. F., Carroll, K. C., Butel, J. S., et al. (Eds.) (2013). Aerobic non-spore-forming Gram-positive bacilli: *Corynebacterium, Listeria, Erysipelothrix, Actinomycetes*, and related pathogens. In *Jawetz, Melnick & Adelberg's medical microbiology* (26th ed., pp. 187–195). McGraw Hill.

Grange, J. M. (2003). Streprococci and staphylococci. In D. Greenwood, R. Slack, & J. Peutherer (Eds.), *Medical microbiology* (16th ed., Chap. 18). Churchill Livingstone.

13 Actinomycetes, Clostridia and Bacillus Species

Actinomycetes

Actinomycetes, which were formerly thought to be fungi, are true bacteria with long, branching filaments analogous to fungal hyphae. The two important genera of this group are *Actinomyces* and *Nocardia*. The chemical structure of the cell wall of these organisms is similar to that of corynebacteria and mycobacteria, and some are acid-fast. *Actinomyces* spp. are microaerophilic or anaerobic organisms; *Nocardia* spp. are aerobic organisms.

ACTINOMYCES SPP.

Although most *Actinomyces* are soil organisms, the potentially pathogenic species are oral commensals in humans and animals. They are a major **component of dental plaque**, particularly at approximal sites of teeth, and are known to increase in numbers in gingivitis. An association between root surface caries of teeth and *Actinomyces* has been described. Other sites colonized are the female genital tract and the tonsillar crypts.

A number of *Actinomyces* spp. are isolated from the oral cavity. These include *A. israelii*, *A. gerencseriae*, *A. odontolyticus*, *A. naeslundii* (genospecies 1 and 2), *A. meyeri* and *A. georgiae*. A close relationship between *A. odontolyticus* and the earliest stages of enamel demineralization and the progression of small caries lesions have been reported. The most important human pathogen is *A. israelii*.

ACTINOMYCES ISRAELII

Habitat and Transmission

This organism is a commensal of the mouth and possibly of the female genital tract. It is a major agent of human **actinomycosis**.

Characteristics

Gram-positive filamentous branching rods. Nonmotile, nonsporing and nonacid-fast. Clumps of the organisms can be seen as yellowish '**sulphur granules**' in pus discharging from sinus tracts, or the granules can be squeezed out of the lesions. (Strains belonging to *A. israelii* serotype II are now a separate species called *A. gerencseriae*. The latter is a common but minor component of healthy gingival flora).

Culture and Identification

Grows slowly under anaerobic conditions, on blood or serum glucose agar at 37°C. After about a week, it appears as small, creamy-white, adherent colonies on blood agar. The colonies resemble **breadcrumbs** and the appearance resembles the surfaces of 'molar' teeth (Fig. 13.1). Because of the exacting growth requirements and the relatively slow growth, isolating this organism from clinical specimens is difficult, particularly because the other, faster-growing bacteria in clinical (mainly pus) specimens tend to obscure the slow-growing actinomycetes. '**Sulphur granules**' in lesions are a clue to their

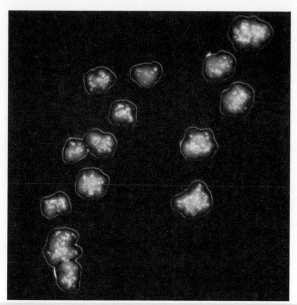

Fig. 13.1 Molar tooth-shaped colonies of *Actinomyces israelii* on blood agar.

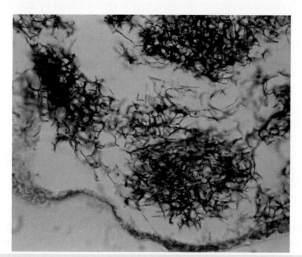

Fig. 13.2 A histopathological section from an actinomycetic lesion of the mandible showing a branching filamentous mass of *Actinomyces* spp. infiltrating the bony cortex.

presence. When possible, these granules should be crushed, Gram-stained and observed for Gram-positive, branching filaments and also cultured in preference to pus.

Once a pure culture of the organisms is isolated, commercial identification kits could be used to speciate the isolate, although these may yield equivocal data. Hence, more sophisticated 16S ribosomal RNA (rRNA) gene sequence analysis technology is now frequently used for their identification.

Pathogenicity

Most (70–80%) actinomycotic infections are **chronic, granulomatous, endogenous infections** of the orofacial region (Fig. 13.2). Typically, the lesions present as a chronic abscess, commonly at the angle of the lower jaw, with multiple external sinuses. There is usually a history of trauma, such as a tooth extraction or a blow to the jaw.

Actinomycetes are also isolated from infections associated with intrauterine devices, but their pathogenic role is unclear.

While the majority of the lesions (60–65%) are in the **cervicofacial** region, some 10–20% are **abdominal** (usually ileocaecal) and others are in the lung (**thoracic**) or skin. Although most infections are **monomicrobial** in nature (i.e., with *Actinomyces* alone causing the disease), a significant proportion of infections could be **polymicrobial**, with other bacteria such as *Aggregatibacter actinomycetemcomitans*, *Haemophilus* spp. and anaerobes acting as co-infecting agents.

Treatment and Prevention

Sensitive to penicillin, but **prolonged courses up to 6 weeks are necessary** for chronic intrabony infections where there is limited drug access. Oral penicillins such as amoxicillin are now popular. Recalcitrant lesions respond well to tetracycline because of its good bone penetration. Surgical intervention may be necessary in chronic jaw lesions.

Prevention of these infections is difficult because of their endogenous nature.

Nocardia

Nocardia species are soil saprophytes and cause nocardiosis in humans, especially in immunocompromised patients. These organisms are aerobic, Gram-positive rods which form thin, branching filaments. *Nocardia asteroides* causes the most common form of human nocardiosis, which is essentially a pulmonary infection that progresses to form abscesses and sinus tracts.

Clostridia

Clostridia comprise many species of Gram-positive, anaerobic spore-forming bacilli (but spores are not found in infected tissues); a few are aerotolerant. They are an important group of pathogens widely distributed **in soil and in the gut of humans** and animals. There are four medically important species (*Clostridium tetani*, *C. botulinum*, *C. welchii* and *C. difficile*) that cause significant morbidity and mortality, especially in developing countries. The major diseases caused by these organisms are listed in Table 13.1.

Table 13.1 Common *Clostridium* Species Associated With Human Disease

Clostridium spp.	Disease
C. welchii	Gas gangrene, food poisoning, bacteraemia, soft-tissue infections
C. tetani	Tetanus
C. botulinum	Botulism (foodborne, infant, wound)
C. difficile	Pseudomembranous colitis, antibiotic-associated diarrhoea
Other species (e.g., C. septicum, C. ramosum, C. novyi, C. bifermentans)	Bacteraemia, gas gangrene, soft-tissue infections

CLOSTRIDIUM SPP.

Habitat

Soil, water, decaying animal and plant matter, and human and animal intestines.

Characteristics

Gram-positive rods, but older cultures may stain irregularly. All species form characteristic endospores, which create a bulge in the bacterial body—for instance, the **drumstick-shaped C. tetani** (this shape is useful in laboratory identification of the organisms). Some species are motile with peritrichous flagella (e.g., *C. tetani*), whereas others (e.g., *C. welchii*) have a capsule.

Culture and Identification

Grow anaerobically on blood agar or Robertson's cooked meat medium (liquid culture). Although *C. tetani* and *C. novyi* are strict anaerobes, *C. histolyticum* and *C. welchii* can grow in the presence of limited amounts of oxygen (aerotolerant). The saccharolytic, proteolytic and toxigenic potentials of the organisms are useful in identification.

CLOSTRIDIUM WELCHII

Habitat and Transmission

Spores are found in the soil, and vegetative cells are normal flora of the colon and vagina. This bacterium causes two discrete diseases, due to either exogenous or endogenous infection:

- **gas gangrene** (myonecrosis) resulting from infection of dirty ischaemic wounds (e.g., war injuries)
- **food poisoning** due to ingestion of food contaminated with enterotoxin-producing strains.

Characteristics

A short, fat bacillus. Spores are not usually found as they are formed under nutritionally deficient conditions. More tolerant of oxygen than other clostridia. *C. welchii* is divided into five types (A-E) on the basis of the toxins they produce; type A is the major human pathogen.

Toxins. A variety of toxins (at least 12), including collagenase, proteinase and hyaluronidase, are formed, the most notable of which is the **α-toxin**, which lyses the phospholipids of eukaryotic cell membranes (i.e., a phospholipase). (*Note:* these phospholipases are the active ingredients of snake venom.)

Culture and Identification

Grows well on blood agar under anaerobic conditions, producing β-haemolytic colonies; some are nonhaemolytic. The saccharolytic characteristic is used for identification purposes as it ferments litmus milk, producing acids and gases responsible for the so-called stormy-clot reaction.

Nagler's Reaction. The neutralization of the α-toxin of the organism growing on agar plates by a specific antitoxin is useful in identification. In this test, the organism is streaked on an agar plate containing egg yolk (which contains high concentrations of phospholipase), half of the

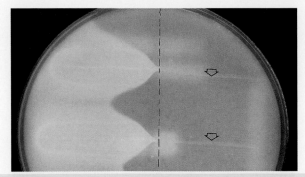

Fig. 13.3 Nagler's reaction: when *Clostridium welchii* is grown in a medium containing egg yolk (lecithin), the enzyme (lecithinase) activity can be detected as opacity around the line of growth. On the right of the plate, no opacity develops, as antitoxin previously applied to this half of the plate has neutralized the toxin. A positive control (*top arrow*) and a test sample, which is also positive (*bottom*), are shown.

plate having been spread with antitoxin; an opaque reaction develops, surrounding the growth of *C. welchii* in the untreated half of the plate, whereas in the other half, no such reaction occurs as the toxin is neutralized by the antitoxin (Fig. 13.3).

Pathogenicity

Causes gas gangrene and food poisoning.

Gas Gangrene (Myonecrosis). Wounds associated with traumatized tissue (especially muscle) may become infected with *C. welchii* and other clostridia, with severe, life-threatening spreading infection. Activity of the bacillus in injured tissue results in toxin enzyme and gas production, allowing the organism to establish and multiply in the wound. Characteristic signs and symptoms include pain, oedema and crepitation produced by gas in tissues.

Food Poisoning. Some strains of *C. welchii* produce an **enterotoxin** that induces **food poisoning**. This is due to the ingestion of large numbers of vegetative cells from contaminated food, which then sporulate in the gut and release enterotoxin. The disease is characterized by watery diarrhoea with little vomiting.

Treatment and Prevention

Gas Gangrene. Rapid intervention with:

- extensive **debridement** of the wound
- **antibiotics** (penicillin or metronidazole)
- **anti-α-toxin** administration.

Food Poisoning. Symptomatic therapy only; no specific treatment.

CLOSTRIDIUM TETANI

Habitat and Transmission

C. tetani is present in the intestinal tract of herbivores, and spores are widespread in soil. Germination of spores is promoted by poor blood supply and necrotic tissue and debris in wounds.

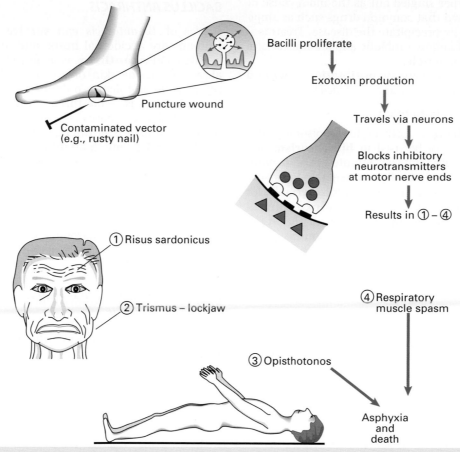

Bacilli proliferate

Exotoxin production

Travels via neurons

Blocks inhibitory
neurotransmitters
at motor nerve ends

Results in ① – ④

Puncture wound

Contaminated vector
(e.g., rusty nail)

① Risus sardonicus

② Trismus – lockjaw

④ Respiratory
muscle spasm

③ Opisthotonos

Asphyxia
and
death

Fig. 13.4   Pathogenesis of tetanus and its sequelae. *Risus sardonicus* – `grinning face` due to sustained contraction of facial muscles; *trismus* – due to sustained contraction of masseter muscle complex; *opisthotonos* – due to hyperextension of spine and sustained contraction of thoracic muscle complexes; *asphyxia* – due to sustained contraction of respiratory muscles.

Characteristics

Long, thin bacilli with terminal spores giving the characteristic 'drumstick' appearance. An extremely potent neurotoxin, **tetanospasmin**, is produced by vegetative cells at the wound site. Another less powerful toxin, **tetanolysin**, is haemolytic in nature.

Culture and Identification

Grows on blood agar, anaerobically, as a fine spreading colony. Identification in vitro is by a toxin neutralization test on blood agar, or in vivo by inoculation of culture filtrate into mice. The two-mouse model is used: one animal is protected with antitoxin and the other is unprotected; the latter dies with typical tetanic spasms.

Pathogenicity

The agent of tetanus (**lockjaw**), which is a typical toxin-mediated disease. The powerful, heat-labile **neurotoxin (tetanospasmin)** is produced at the wound site and released during cell lysis (Fig. 13.4). It is retrogradely carried via the peripheral nerves (intra-axonally) to the central nervous system where it blocks inhibitory mediators at spinal synapses. This causes sustained muscle spasm and the characteristic signs of spasm of jaw muscles (lockjaw, **trismus**) and facial muscles (**risus sardonicus**), and arching of the body (**opisthotonos**). Toxin genes are plasmid coded. *C. tetani* also produces an oxygen-labile **haemolysin** (**tetanolysin**); the clinical significance of this enzyme is not clear.

Treatment and Prevention

Antitoxin (hyperimmune human α-globulin) administered with or without toxoid, depending on the immunization history of the patient. Prevention is by tetanus toxoid (a component of the **diphtheria–tetanus–pertussis (DTP) vaccine**) with boosters every 10 years (see Chapter 37). Proper wound **debridement** and **administration of penicillin** (to inhibit clostridial growth and secondary infection) are other important management measures.

CLOSTRIDIUM DIFFICILE

Found in the faeces of 3–6% of adults and almost all healthy infants, *C. difficile* is the agent of **antibiotic-associated colitis**, which may lead to sometimes lethal **pseudomembranous colitis**. It multiplies in the gut under the selective pressure of antibiotics. Although clindamycin was earlier singled out as the main cause of colitis, it is now known that common drugs such as ampicillin may occasionally precipitate the disease. Treatment is to withhold the offending antibiotic and administer oral vancomycin or metronidazole.

As much as 25% of the common **antibiotic-associated diarrhoea** is considered to be due to *C. difficile.*

A Note on *Clostridium botulinum*

The agent of **botulism**, a form of food poisoning, has powerful toxins that can be used in **bioterrorism** and **biological warfare**. By contrast, minute doses of botulinum toxin, injected periodically, are popular in beauty therapy as facial muscle relaxants to minimize wrinkles for a youthful appearance and as so-called **botox** treatment utilized in cosmetic dentistry in some parts of the world. Botox is now therapeutically used for conditions as varied as chronic migraine and back pain to excessive sweating and twitching eyelids.

Bacillus

The genus *Bacillus* comprises nearly 50 species of sporing, Gram-positive, chain-forming bacilli. Most are soil saprophytes. Two species, *B. anthracis* and *B. cereus*, cause significant morbidity.

BACILLUS ANTHRACIS

Spores of *B. anthracis* can survive in soil for years. Humans are accidental hosts, and infection due to the bacillus, called **anthrax**, is acquired when spores enter abrasions on the skin or are inhaled. Infection causes septicaemia and death; pulmonary anthrax (**woolsorters' disease**) is a life-threatening pneumonia caused by inhalation of spores. The polyglutamic acid capsule of the organism is antiphagocytic. Recently, the organism has received much attention due to the likelihood of the use of anthrax spores in **biological warfare and bioterrorism**.

BACILLUS CEREUS

B. cereus causes food poisoning, especially when contaminated rice is reheated and eaten (particularly in restaurants serving rice-based dishes).

BACILLUS SEAROTHERMOPHILUS AND BACILLUS SUBTILIS

These are used as **biological indicators to test the sterilization efficacy** of autoclaves, ethylene oxide and ionizing radiation (see Chapter 38).

Key Facts

- *Actinomyces* spp. are **potentially pathogenic commensals** and are frequent isolates from dental plaque.
- They cause **cervicofacial** (most common), **ileocaecal and thoracic** actinomycoses, which are essentially chronic, granulomatous infections.
- 'Sulphur granule' production (a tangled mass of filamentous organisms and debris) is a hallmark of actinomycosis.
- A prolonged course of antibiotics (up to 6 weeks) may be necessary to manage chronic actinomycosis.
- **Clostridia** are Gram-positive, anaerobic, spore-forming bacilli, although spores are not found in infected tissues.
- **Pathogenic clostridia** produce powerful **exotoxins** that are responsible for most disease symptoms.

- Spore-bearing *Clostridium tetani* cells are characterized by their **drumstick shape**.
- **Tetanospasmin** and **tetanolysin** are toxins produced by *C. tetani*, the agent of tetanus.
- **Tetanus** causes **sustained muscle spasm** (including the masticatory muscles) resulting in lockjaw **(trismus)**, **risus sardonicus** and arching of the body **(opisthotonos)**.
- Tetanus toxin (tetanospasmin) can be attenuated to form a toxoid. The latter is a component of the diphtheria–tetanus–pertussis **(DTP)** vaccine.
- The **spores** of *Bacillus stearothermophilus* and *Bacillus subtilis* are used as **biological indicators to test the sterilization efficacy** of autoclaves, ethylene oxide and ionizing radiation.

Review Questions (Answers on p. 389)

Please indicate which answers are true and which are false.

13.1. Which of the following statements on clostridia are true?
   a. they are Gram-positive nonspore-forming rods
   b. they are commonly found in soil
   c. they are strict anaerobes
   d. they produce powerful endotoxins that cause nerve damage
   e. they are commensals in mammalian intestines

13.2. With regard to gas gangrene:
   a. *Clostridium welchii* is the primary causative organism
   b. it is common in agricultural and warfare injuries
   c. high doses of penicillin and metronidazole alone are sufficient for the treatment
   d. Gram-positive spore-bearing rods are often isolated from the infected sites
   e. vascular damage facilitates the infections

13.3. Which of the following statements on *Bacillus anthracis* are true?
   a. it bears a polyglutamic acid capsule that is antiphagocytic
   b. it is anaerobic
   c. it could be used in germ warfare
   d. it causes pulmonary and cutaneous infections and food poisoning
   e. humans are the only known hosts

13.4. Which of the following statements on actinomycetes are true?
   a. it is a eukaryote
   b. it causes chronic granulomatous infections
   c. it infrequently causes actinomycoses of the jaws after tooth extractions
   d. infections are often sensitive to penicillins
   e. infections are difficult to eradicate because of the endogenous nature

13.5. Which of the following statements on tetanus toxin/toxoid are true?
   a. tetanus toxin is an endotoxin
   b. tetanus toxoid is derived from hyperimmune human gamma globulin
   c. tetanus toxoid booster should be given once every 10 years
   d. tetanus toxoid is a component of the diphtheria–tetanus–pertussis (DTP) vaccine
   e. tetanus toxin causes trismus

Further Reading

Brooks, J. F., Carroll, K. C., Butel, J. S., et al. (Eds.). (2013). Infections caused by anaerobic bacteria. In *Jawetz, Melnick & Adelberg's medical microbiology* (26th ed., pp. 295–302). McGraw Hill.

Greenwood, D., Slack, R., & Peutherer, J. (Eds.). (2003). *Medical microbiology* (16th ed.). Churchill Livingstone.

Könönen, E., & Wade, W. G. (2012). *Actinomyces* and related organisms in human infections. *Clinical Microbiology Reviews, 28,* 419–442.

Neisseriaceae, Veillonella, Parvobacteria and Capnocytophaga

Neisseriaceae

The Neisseriaceae family of bacteria includes the genera *Neisseria* and *Moraxella*. Two species of *Neisseria* are human pathogens:

- *Neisseria gonorrhoeae* (the gonococcus)
- *Neisseria meningitidis* (the meningococcus).

There are a number of nonpathogenic species, such as *N. sicca*, *N. mucosa* and *N. lactamica*, which are members of the indigenous flora, including the oral mucosa. Hence it is important to differentiate these from the pathogenic species isolated from oral samples.

N. gonorrhoeae is the agent of **gonorrhoea**, the most frequently diagnosed venereal disease in Western Europe and the United States. Gonococci frequently cause **pelvic inflammatory disease (PID)** and **sterility** in women, in addition to arthritis and sometimes septicaemia. *N. meningitidis* is the aetiological agent of **meningococcal meningitis**, a highly contagious disease associated with a mortality rate approximating 80% when untreated.

GENERAL CHARACTERISTICS

Nonmotile, Gram-negative cocci ranging from 0.6–1.0 μm in diameter. On microscopy, the cocci are seen as pairs with concave adjacent sides (bean shaped); tetrads, short chains and clusters are occasionally seen, but all show the characteristic pairing.

Pathogenic *Neisseria* species are **nutritionally fastidious**, especially on initial isolation from clinical specimens; the nonpathogenic species are less so. Though aerobic, most strains of *N. gonorrhoeae* are **capnophilic** (they require increased carbon dioxide for growth); haemolysed blood and solubilized starch enhance growth.

Members of this genus grow optimally at 36–39°C, although the nonpathogenic species can grow at temperatures below 24°C.

NEISSERIA GONORRHOEAE

Habitat and Transmission

The human urogenital tract is the usual habitat; oral, nasopharyngeal and rectal carriage in healthy individuals is not uncommon. Spread is by both homosexual and heterosexual intercourse or intimate contact.

Characteristics

Nonmotile, Gram-negative, noncapsulate diplococci.

Culture and Identification

Specimens are usually inoculated onto an enriched medium (**lysed blood or chocolate agar** normally) and incubated under 5–10% carbon dioxide (as the species is capnophilic). Small, grey, oxidase-positive colonies initially become large and opaque on prolonged incubation. Subsequent staining by fluorescent antibody techniques, and the production of acid from glucose but not from maltose or sucrose, confirm the identification. Gram-stained smears (of urethral exudate from men and the cervix in women) usually reveal Gram-negative, **kidney-shaped intracellular cocci** in pairs. Additionally, several reliable, and sensitive, nucleic acid amplification assays are available for direct detection of *N. gonorrhoeae* in genitourinary specimens.

Pathogenicity

Gonococci possess a number of virulent attributes:

- **pili** allow gonococci to adhere and colonize epithelial surfaces and thus cause infection
- **immunoglobulin A (IgA) proteases** produced by some gonococci break the heavy chain of IgA, thereby inactivating it (IgA is a major defence factor universally present on mucosal surfaces)
- some isolates of *N. gonorrhoeae* produce **β-lactamase**, which is plasmid mediated (β-lactamase breaks down β-lactam group antibiotics such as penicillin)
- a **tracheal cytotoxin** damages the ciliated cells of the fallopian tube, leading to scarring and sterility.

Treatment and Prevention

The majority of gonococci are resistant to β-lactam drugs and hence the choice is **β-lactamase-stable cephalosporins**. Prevention of gonorrhoea requires the practice of 'safe sex', health education and contact tracing.

NEISSERIA MENINGITIDIS

Habitat and Transmission

The main reservoir is the nasopharynx in healthy individuals (10–25%). Droplet spread is the most common transmission mode.

Characteristics

This organism resembles the gonococcus, but *N. meningitidis* cells are capsulate.

Culture and Identification

As for *N. gonorrhoeae*, presumptive identification is made by observing Gram-negative cocci in pairs in nasopharyngeal discharge, cerebrospinal fluid or blood smears. Selective media are not required as the organism is found pure in cerebrospinal fluid. Identified by the carbohydrate utilization test or newer PCR based tests: produces acid from the oxidation of glucose and maltose. Serology is useful.

Pathogenicity

In susceptible individuals, meningococci spread from the nasopharynx into the blood stream (septicaemia), and then to the meninges. Septicaemia is accompanied by a rash. Eventual death may be due to meningitis or adrenal haemorrhage (Waterhouse–Friderichsen syndrome). The antiphagocytic properties of the capsule help dissemination, whereas the toxic effects are mainly due to the meningococcal endotoxin.

Treatment and Prevention

Penicillin or preferably ceftriaxone (or equivalent cephalosporin) due to wide prevalence of penicillin-resistant strains worldwide.

COMMENSAL *NEISSERIA* SPECIES

Commensal *Neisseria* species are common in the oral cavity, nose and pharynx, and sometimes in the female genital tract. The Human Oral Microbiome Database (HOMD) currently identifies **25 oral species**. The three main species are **Neisseria subflava**, **N. mucosa** and **N. sicca**. The main difference between these and the pathogenic *Neisseria* species is the ability of the commensal species to grow on ordinary agar at room temperature in the absence of carbon dioxide supplements.

Oral Neisseriaceae are **essentially nonpathogenic** and are almost always found in oral specimens contaminated with saliva or mucosa. *Neisseria* species are among the earliest colonizers of a clean tooth surface. They consume oxygen during early plaque biofilm development, thus facilitating the subsequent colonization of the biofilm by facultative and obligate anaerobic **late colonizers.**

MORAXELLA

Moraxella (formerly *Branhamella*) are Gram-negative cocci closely related to the nonpathogenic *Neisseria* species, but asaccharolytic and nonpigmented. They are commensals of the human respiratory tract and are recognized opportunistic pathogens causing meningitis, endocarditis, otitis media, maxillary sinusitis and chronic obstructive pulmonary disease. As the majority of strains produce β-lactamase, they may indirectly 'protect' other pathogens and thus complicate antibiotic therapy.

Veillonella

Veillonella species are obligate anaerobic, Gram-negative cocci frequently isolated from oral samples. Three oral species are recognized: *V. parvula* (the type species), *V. dispar* and *V. atypica*.

VEILLONELLA PARVULA

Gram-negative, small anaerobic cocci. Found in the human oral cavity, mostly in dental plaque biofilm, they are considered to be **'benevolent organisms'** in relation to dental caries as they metabolize the lactic acid produced by cariogenic bacteria into weaker acids (acetic and propionic) with a reduced ability to solubilize enamel. No known pathogenic potential.

Parvobacteria

Parvobacteria are so called because of their size (Latin *parvus*: small). They are a miscellaneous, heterogeneous group of small, Gram-negative bacilli that cause a number of different diseases. They include the following genera:

- *Haemophilus*
- *Brucella*
- *Bordetella*
- *Pasteurella* (includes *Aggregatibacter* species)
- *Francisella*
- *Gardnerella*
- *Eikenella*.

Of these, *Haemophilus* and *Bordetella* spp. are of particular interest, as the former causes significant morbidity in the general population and the latter is the agent of **whooping cough**. Additionally, *Haemophilus* spp. and *Aggregatibacter* spp. are common inhabitants of the oral cavity, the latter being an important periodontopathogen.

Haemophilus Species

The genus *Haemophilus* is composed of tiny, nonmotile, aerobic, Gram-negative coccobacilli; some are capsulated. One of its major distinguishing features is the requirement of two growth factors:

- **X factor:** haematin present in blood
- **V factor:** nicotinamide adenine dinucleotide (NAD) or NAD phosphate (NADP), a vitamin obtained from yeast and vegetable extracts or a metabolic product of most bacteria, including *Staphylococcus aureus*.

Haemophilus species cause a variety of diseases, as shown in Table 14.1.

HAEMOPHILUS INFLUENZAE

Habitat and Transmission

An upper respiratory tract commensal of humans and associated animals, *Haemophilus influenzae* is a major aetiological agent of upper respiratory tract infections and acute exacerbations of chronic bronchitis. Although not the cause, *H. influenzae* is a common secondary colonizer of the respiratory tract after a bout of influenza (the agent of which is the influenza virus).

Characteristics

Small, Gram-negative, nonsporing, nonmotile rods; predominantly coccobacillary in nature with a few long bacilli

Table 14.1   Some Characteristics of *Haemophilus* Spp.[a]

Species	Factor Requirement	Diseases Caused
H. influenzae	X and V	Acute exacerbation of chronic bronchitis, epiglottitis, meningitis, sinusitis, otitis media, osteomyelitis, arthritis
H. parainfluenzae	V	Commensals of the oral cavity and upper respiratory tract; rarely cause disease
H. parahaemolyticus	V	
H. haemolyticus	X and V	
H. aegyptius	X and V	Conjunctivitis
H. ducreyi	X	Chancroid (a sexually transmitted disease; a soft sore)

[a]*H. aphrophilus* has been recently renamed as *Aggregatibacter aphrophilus*, hence it is not included here, although it is a frequent oral commensal.

and filamentous forms. Virulent strains (e.g., isolated from the cerebrospinal fluid in meningitis) are capsulated.

Culture and Identification

Requires both V factor (NADP) and X factor (haematin) for growth on nutrient agar, but grows on blood-enriched media containing these nutrients. Typically forms large colonies around colonies of other organisms that secrete the V factor, a phenomenon called **satellitism**. For example, if a blood agar plate (containing the X factor) seeded with *H. influenzae* is streaked with *S. aureus* (which secretes the V factor) and incubated overnight at 37°C, the former will grow as large colonies adjacent to the streak of *S. aureus* (Fig. 14.1).

Pathogenicity

H. influenzae causes four major infections, often accompanied by septicaemia, especially in children and the elderly:

- meningitis
- acute epiglottitis
- osteomyelitis
- arthritis

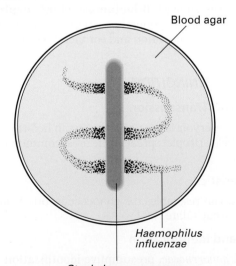

Blood agar

Haemophilus influenzae

Staphylococcus aureus

Fig. 14.1 Satellitism of *Haemophilus influenzae* (zigzag streak); enhanced growth adjacent to *Staphylococcus aureus* (vertical streak), which supplies the V factor.

The most important virulence factor of *H. influenzae* is the **polysaccharide capsule**. An **IgA protease** and a factor that causes slowing and incoordination of (respiratory tract) ciliary beating are produced; the outer membrane and **endotoxin** may contribute to the pathogenesis; there are no known exotoxins. Noncapsulated strains cause exacerbation of chronic bronchitis.

Treatment and Prevention

All strains are susceptible to the third-generation cephalosporins, and intramuscular cefotaxime gives excellent results. Prevention by **haemophilus b conjugate vaccine** against invasive *H. influenzae* type b infection is recommended in some countries. Close contacts of meningitis patients should be given rifampicin as a prophylactic measure.

Bordetella

There are three species in the genus *Bordetella*, of which *Bordetella pertussis*, the agent of whooping cough, is the most important.

BORDETELLA PERTUSSIS

Habitat and Transmission

Found in the human respiratory tract in diseased individuals; healthy carriage is not known. Spread is by the airborne route.

Characteristics

Short, sometimes oval, Gram-negative rods; fresh isolates may be capsulated. Fastidious growth requirements.

Culture and Identification

Requires a special enriched medium for growth—that is, **Bordet–Gengou medium or blood-charcoal agar** supplemented with antibiotics. On incubation for 3–5 days at 35°C, under high humidity, iridescent colonies resembling mercury drops appear on Bordet–Gengou medium. Identification is confirmed serologically. Currently, a polymerase chain reaction (PCR)–based technique is the most sensitive and rapid method to confirm the identity.

Pathogenicity

Causes whooping cough, especially in preschool children (severe in those under 12 months). The characteristic symptom is the bout of **paroxysmal coughs** followed by the 'whoop' of rapid inhalation after coughing. Virulence factors identified are tracheal cytotoxin, fimbrial antigen and endotoxin.

Treatment and Prevention

Erythromycin is the drug of choice for patients and close contacts, but antibiotics have little effect on the course of infection, although they may reduce spread and minimize superinfection.

Prevention is by immunization with whole cell–inactivated vaccine, a component of the diphtheria–tetanus–pertussis (DTP) vaccine of childhood. New acellular, subunit vaccines appear effective.

AGGREGATIBACTER ACTINOMYCETEMCOMITANS

This relatively new genus *Aggregatibacter* (formerly called *Actinobacillus*) includes species isolated from humans and mammals. (Latin *aggregare*: to come together, aggregate; *bacter*: bacterial rod; *Aggregatibacter*: rod-shaped bacterium that aggregates with others.)

The only species of this genus routinely isolated from the oral cavity is *Aggregatibacter actinomycetemcomitans* (acronym: Aa), so named because it is frequently isolated with *Actinomyces* spp. from actinomycotic lesions. The reason for this association is unknown. Multiple biotypes and **up to six serotypes (*a–e*)** have been described. This species is a major infective agent in particularly **aggressive forms of periodontal disease** in adolescents and rapidly destructive periodontal disease in adults.

Habitat and Transmission

Primary habitat is unknown but is likely to be subgingival sites of humans and mammals. Infection is endogenous.

Characteristics

Small, short (0.4–1 μm), straight or curved rods with rounded ends. Electron microscopic studies have revealed bleb-like structures on the cell surface, which appear to be released from the cells. Fresh isolates possess fimbriae (lost on subculture).

Culture and Identification

Grows as white, translucent, smooth, nonhaemolytic colonies on blood agar; grows best aerobically with 5%–10% carbon dioxide. Selective media are available for identification; the tryptone–soy–serum–bacitracin–vancomycin agar yields white, translucent colonies with a **star-shaped or crossed cigar-shaped internal structure** on first isolation, but this is not a consistent finding (Fig. 14.2). There are two phenotypes: smooth and rough. The latter phenotype is related to fimbriation and to the production of hexosamine-containing exopolysaccharide. Cells from rough colonies grow in broth as granular, autoaggregated cells that adhere to the glass and leave a clear broth. Identified by sugar fermentation and assimilation reactions and acid end-products of carbohydrate metabolism.

Pathogenicity

A number of virulence factors—including **lipopolysaccharide** (endotoxin), a **leukotoxin**, **collagenase**, **cytolethal distending toxin** (cdt), **epitheliotoxin-bone resorption inducing factor** and a **protease**-cleaving IgG—have all been isolated from *A. actinomycetemcomitans*. The leukotoxin, in particular, is thought to play a significant role in subverting the host immune response in the gingival crevice. It also has the potency to invade epithelial and vascular endothelial cells in vitro, and buccal epithelial cells in vivo. Together with other coagents, *A. actinomycetemcomitans* is involved in **localized aggressive periodontitis in adolescents and destructive periodontal disease in adults**. Also isolated from cases of infective endocarditis, and from brain and subcutaneous abscesses.

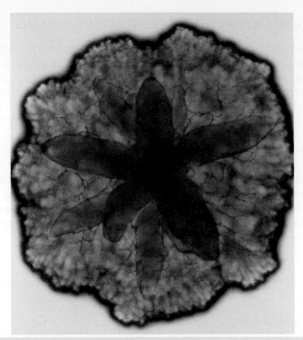

Fig. 14.2 A star-shaped colony of *Aggregatibacter actinomycetemcomitans* in TSSBV agar (see text).

Treatment

This species is sensitive to **tetracycline**.

EIKENELLA

Members of the genus *Eikenella* resemble *Haemophilus* species and are commensals of the human oral cavity and the intestine. Although in the past their presence was linked to periodontal diseases, this has now been disproved. The type species is *Eikenella corrodens*. These organisms are capnophilic, Gram-negative, short coccobacillary forms that are asaccharolytic. When grown on nonselective media,

they corrode the agar surface (hence the name *corrodens*). Human infection usually results from predisposing factors, such as trauma to a mucosal surface, which allow the organism access to the surrounding tissues; thus, they may cause extraoral infections, including brain and abdominal abscesses, peritonitis, endocarditis, osteomyelitis and meningitis. Also **associated with human bites or fist-fight injuries**.

CAPNOCYTOPHAGA

The genus *Capnocytophaga* was created for fusiform species isolated from periodontal pockets, which, unlike *Fusobacterium* and *Bacteroides* spp., grow under capnophilic conditions. They have a characteristic ability to glide over routine blood agar (compare 'swarming' of *Proteus* spp.). Species recognized include *C. ochracea* (type species), *C. sputigena*, *C. gingivalis*, *C. granulosa* and *C. haemolytica*.

Habitat

The primary ecological niche is the subgingival area.

Characteristics

Long, thin fusiform organisms that demonstrate gliding motility seen on bright-field microscopy.

Culture and Identification

Facultative anaerobes, but most strains require carbon dioxide for growth. Colonies spread over the agar surface with uneven edges and may be pink, yellow or white. Identification is by gliding characteristic, cell morphology, biochemical reactions and acid end-products.

Pathogenicity

Opportunistic pathogens, sometimes associated with gingivitis and other systemic infections in immunocompromised patients; some strains produce an IgAl protease.

Key Facts

- All *Neisseria* species are kidney shaped, **Gram-negative cocci** usually arranged in pairs, and are **oxidase-positive**.
- Pathogenic *Neisseria* have fastidious growth requirements, unlike the nonpathogenic species, which are often part of the normal flora.
- *Neisseria gonorrhoeae* (the gonococcus) is the agent of the common sexually transmitted disease **gonorrhoea** and its complications.
- *Neisseria meningitidis* (the meningococcus) is an important cause of **meningitis** in children and young adults.
- *Veillonella* spp. present in plaque are considered '**benevolent organisms' in relation to dental caries** as they metabolize lactic acid produced by cariogenic bacteria into weaker acids.
- The generic name *Haemophilus* is derived from their requirement of blood or blood products to support growth.
- *Haemophilus influenzae* causes **meningitis, acute epiglottitis, osteomyelitis and arthritis**, often accompanied by septicaemia, especially in children and the elderly.
- *Bordetella pertussis* is the agent of **whooping cough (pertussis)**, prevented by the whole-cell vaccine incorporated in the childhood diphtheria–tetanus–pertussis (DTP) vaccination programme.
- *Aggregatibacter actinomycetemcomitans* is a coagent of **localized aggressive periodontitis** (formerly localized juvenile periodontitis) and **destructive periodontal disease** in adults (also an agent of infective endocarditis, and brain and subcutaneous abscesses).
- *Eikenella* and *Capnocytophaga* species are **oral commensals** and their role in oral disease is unclear.

Review Questions (Answers on p. 389)

Please indicate which answers are true and which are false.

14.1. Which of the following statements on Neisseriaceae are true?
a. they possess a capsule
b. they are commensals of the oral cavity
c. they demonstrate motility
d. *Neisseria gonorrhoeae* causes syphilis
e. most gonococci are resistant to penicillin

14.2. Which of the following statements on *Haemophilus* are true?
a. it needs coagulation factors X and V for growth
b. it is a causative agent of periodontal disease
c. some are capsulated
d. it causes sexually transmitted diseases
e. it forms spores under harsh environmental conditions

14.3. Virulence factors of *Haemophilus influenzae* include:
a. the polysaccharide capsule
b. immunoglobulin A (IgA) protease
c. an exotoxin
d. an endotoxin
e. a pyrogenic factor causing influenza

14.4. Which of the following statements on *Aggregatibacter actinomycetemcomitans* are true?
a. it is a key pathogen in localized aggressive periodontitis
b. it possesses an IgG protease
c. it can cause deep-seated abscesses
d. it can be presumptively identified by star-shaped colonies in selective media
e. it is susceptible to tetracycline

14.5. *Eikenella* spp.:
a. are Gram-positive coccobacilli
b. are commensals of the oral cavity
c. are implicated in human bite (clench-fist) injuries
d. are known to cause endocarditis
e. are closely associated with severe periodontitis

14.6. *Capnocytophaga* spp.:
a. are isolated from periodontal pockets
b. are fusiform bacilli
c. frequently cause co-infections with *Actinomyces* species
d. require carbon dioxide for growth on blood agar
e. demonstrate gliding motility on agar media

Further Reading

Brooks, J. F., Carroll, K. C., Butel, J. S., et al. (Eds.). (2013). The neisseriae. In *Jawetz, Melnick & Adelberg's medical microbiology* (26th ed., pp. 285–293). McGraw Hill.

Haffajee, A. D., & Sockransky, S. S. (1994). Microbial aetiological agents of destructive periodontal diseases. *Periodontology 2000, 5*, 78–111.

Kachlany, S. C. (2010). *Aggregatibacter actinomycetemcomitans* leukotoxin: From threat to therapy. *Journal of Dental Research, 89*, 561–570.

Periasamy, S., & Kolenbrander, P. E. (2010). Central role of the early colonizer *Veillonella* sp. in establishing multispecies biofilm communities with initial, middle, and late colonizers of enamel. *Journal of Bacteriology, 192*, 2965–2972.

Most of the commensal Gram-negative rods that inhabit the normal gastrointestinal tract, and sometimes cause disease, belong to the family **Enterobacteriaceae**. They are also colloquially termed **coliforms**. All species belonging to this family are **Gram-negative, facultative anaerobes that ferment glucose**. The major medically important species are listed in Table 15.1.

General Characteristics of Enterobacteria

Habitat

Found in the human gut, at a density of approximately **10⁹ cells per gram of faeces**. The predominant species in the gut is *Bacteroides*. Up to 15% of the population may harbour enterobacteria in the oral cavity, mostly as transient commensals. Their oral carriage rate may increase in old age, and in states leading to reduced salivary flow (xerostomia).

Characteristics

Rapidly growing cells 2×0.4 μm in size; may appear coccobacillary. Many species are motile and possess a capsule, especially on initial isolation. All species are endotoxigenic because of the lipopolysaccharide outer cell wall. They also possess **pili** and **flagella**, which mediate adhesion and locomotion, respectively (Fig. 15.1).

Culture and Identification

Grow well on ordinary media (e.g., blood agar, MacConkey's agar), producing characteristic circular, convex and glistening/mucoid colonies. Some motile species form swarming patterns on agar cultures. Most species are nonpigmented; a few produce red, pink, yellow or blue pigment.

Enterobacteriaceae ferment a large number of carbohydrates. This property, together with other biochemical tests, is used to identify and differentiate species.

Lactose Fermentation. Growth on indicator media is used for the initial categorization of Enterobacteriaceae into two groups: **lactose fermenters** and **lactose nonfermenters**. Several selective media, such as **MacConkey's and cystine–lactose–electrolyte-deficient (CLED) media**, are available for this purpose. On MacConkey's agar, the lactose fermenters appear as pink colonies, whereas on CLED medium, the colour of lactose fermentation is yellow.

Other Biochemical Tests. Commercially available kit systems are routinely used to identify species of enterobacteria. The commonly available test systems are based on 10 (API 10E) or 20 (API 20E, Rapid E) biochemical tests (Fig. 15.2).

Serological Tests. Serological tests are based on the antigens of the organisms. All species have the **somatic** (O) antigen, and most have the **flagellar** (H) antigen. The

Table 15.1 Enterobacteria Commonly Causing Human Disease

Genus	Representative Species (no. of species)	Disease
Escherichia	E. coli (5)	Gastroenteritis, wound and urinary tract infection
Shigella	S. dysenteriae	Dysentery
	S. flexneri	
	S. boydii	
	S. sonnei	
Salmonella	S. typhi	Enteric fever (typhoid)
	S. typhimurium (7 subgroups)	Food poisoning
Klebsiella	K. pneumoniae (7)	
Morganella	M. morganii (2)	Urinary tract infection and other types of sepsis
Proteus	P. mirabilis (4)	
Providencia	P. stuartii (5)	
Yersinia	Y. pestis (11)	Plague, septicaemia, enteritis, etc.
Citrobacter	C. freundii (4)	Low pathogenicity, opportunistic infections
Enterobacter	E. cloacae (13)	
Serratia	S. marcescens (10)	

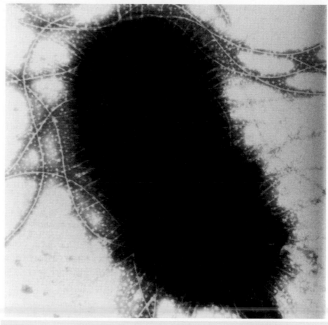

Fig. 15.1 A scanning electron micrograph of *Escherichia coli* showing short fimbriae and longer flagellae (×10,000).

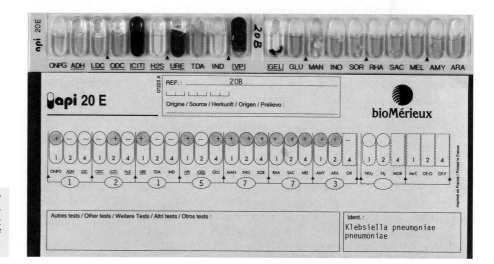

Fig. 15.2 Commercial identification kit for Enterobacteriaceae. This plate illustrates a colour reaction profile obtained after overnight incubation of the organism. The identity of the organism is *Klebsiella pneumoniae*.

capsular (K) antigen is seen in some species. The antigens are useful in the classification of species and invaluable for epidemiological investigation of outbreaks of disease. Identification of strains within a species can also be done by bacteriophage typing, bacteriocin typing, plasmid analysis and polypeptide analysis.

Pathogenicity

All Enterobacteriaceae are potentially pathogenic. Patients who are immunosuppressed, undergoing mechanical or medical manipulation, and have underlying disease are most susceptible to infection.

Endotoxin Shock. Endotoxin shock can be precipitated in humans by lipopolysaccharide (the major constituent of the cell walls of all Gram negative bacteria), which all Enterobacteriaceae release when they are destroyed. Toxic lipopolysaccharide comprises **lipid A**, the core polysaccharide and the **O antigen**; the lipid A is responsible for most of the symptoms associated with **endotoxic shock**. The toxic effects of lipopolysaccharide are many and include fever, hypotension, intravascular coagulation and effects on the immune system. Large doses of endotoxin may cause death.

Treatment

The antibiotic sensitivity patterns of enterobacteria are complex as they readily acquire resistance-coding plasmids. A spectrum of antibiotics are used, including ampicillin/amoxicillin, cephalosporins, aminoglycosides, trimethoprim, chloramphenicol and ciprofloxacin.

Eschericheae

The tribe Eschericheae includes five genera: *Escherichia*, *Salmonella*, *Shigella*, *Edwardsiella* and *Citrobacter*. The most important human pathogens in this group, *Escherichia coli* and the *Salmonella* and *Shigella* species, are described here.

ESCHERICHIA COLI

Habitat and Transmission

Indigenous commensal of the human intestinal tract; transmission is either endogenous or exogenous.

Characteristics

Gram-negative rods, motile, sometimes capsulate, facultative anaerobe, bile tolerant.

Culture and Identification

Grows well on blood agar; ferments lactose (hence pink colonies on MacConkey's agar and yellow on CLED agar). Commercial kits, such as API 20E, are used in identification (Fig. 15.2). Biotyping systems are useful for strain delineation.

Pathogenicity

Escherichia coli is a major agent of sepsis; it causes the following diseases.

Urinary Tract Infection. Young women and elderly adults are the most susceptible. The disease varies from simple urethritis to serious pyelonephritis.

Diarrhoeal Diseases. These range from simple diarrhoea to severe disease leading to excessive fluid loss and dehydration, which may be fatal in malnourished infants and elderly debilitated adults. Many strains of enteropathogenic *Escherichia coli* have powerful toxins and other mechanisms by which they cause diarrhoea:

- **Enterotoxins**: mainly two types, both coded by plasmids, one is **heat-labile (LT)** and is similar in action to the cholera toxin, and the other is **heat-stable (ST)**.
- **Enteroinvasiveness**: some strains have the ability to invade intestinal epithelial cells and cause inflammation.
- **Adhesive factors** are produced by some strains enabling adhesion to mucosae; termed 'colonization factor antigens', these are mediated by plasmid-coded pili.
- **Vero cytotoxicity** is caused by strains that have the ability to induce cytopathic effects on Vero cells (grown in tissue culture). Verotoxin (VT) producers can cause diarrhoea with haemorrhagic symptoms (e.g., *Escherichia coli* O157).

Based on the above, diarrhoea-producing *Escherichia coli* can be divided into five types:

- enteropathogenic *Escherichia coli* (EPEC)
- enteroinvasive *Escherichia coli* (EIEC)
- enterotoxigenic *Escherichia coli* (ETEC)
- enterohaemorrhagic *Escherichia coli* (EHEC)
- enteroaggregative *Escherichia coli* (EAEC).

Neonatal Meningitis and Septicaemia. Other infections *Escherichia coli* may cause include neonatal meningitis, septicaemia and wound infection, particularly after surgery of the lower intestinal tract.

Salmonellae

The genus *Salmonella* has a bewildering spectrum of more than 2 000 species living in the intestinal tract of humans, domesticated animals and poultry. *Salmonella typhi* and *Salmonella paratyphi* differ from others in that humans are the only known natural host.

SALMONELLA SPECIES

Habitat and Transmission

Leading sources of salmonella infection are poultry products (i.e., flesh and eggs) and pet turtles (in the US). **Occupational salmonellosis** affects veterinary and slaughterhouse workers. Infection is by ingestion of contaminated food, or person-to-person via the faecal–oral route. The carrier state, which develops in some after infection, is an important source of organisms.

Characteristics

Gram-negative, motile, nonsporing rods. All except *Salmonella typhi* are noncapsulate; facultative anaerobes.

Culture and Identification

Culture on MacConkey's medium or deoxycholate citrate agar yields non-lactose-fermenting colonies. A combination of biochemical tests and serotyping is required for full identification. The latter is complex as salmonellae have a variety of antigens; notable are the **somatic (O)** and the **flagellar (H)** antigens; virulent strains, notably *Salmonella typhi*, have a capsular polysaccharide antigen designated the **virulence (Vi)** antigen. There are more than 1 700 serotypes of *Salmonella enteritidis*.

Pathogenicity

The major types of salmonellosis (diseases due to *Salmonella*) are enteric fever, gastroenteritis and septicaemia.

Enteric Fever (Typhoid Fever). Caused by *Salmonella typhi* or *Salmonella paratyphi* A, B or C (see Chapter 26).

Gastroenteritis. The most common form of salmonellosis, can be due to any of the *Salmonella enteritidis* serotypes. Symptoms appear 10–24 h after ingestion of highly contaminated food or beverage. Nausea, vomiting, abdominal cramps, headache and diarrhoea are common.

Septicaemia. Frequently caused by *S. dublin* or *S. choleraesuis*; a fulminant, sometimes fatal disease independent of intestinal symptoms. Pneumonia, meningitis and osteomyelitis may result from haematogenous spread of the bacteria.

Treatment and Prevention

Proper cooking of foods derived from animal sources. Typhoid vaccine, a killed suspension of *Salmonella typhi*, is available for those travelling to or living in areas where typhoid fever is endemic.

Shigellae

Shigella species cause bacillary dysentery. The genus is divided into four species (*S. dysenteriae*, *S. sonnei*, *S. flexneri* and *S. boydii*) and a variety of serotypes.

SHIGELLA SPECIES

Habitat and Transmission

The only reservoir is the human intestine. Infection is spread by the faecal–oral route under crowded conditions. A minute dose of the organism is adequate to cause disease.

Characteristics

Gram-negative, nonmotile rods (compare salmonellae); noncapsulate.

Culture and Identification

All species grow well on ordinary media and are non-lactose fermenters (except *Shigella sonnei*, a slow lactose fermenter). Commercial kits are used in identification.

Pathogenicity

Although shigellae do not invade systemically like salmonellae, they locally invade the intestinal epithelium (ileum and colon). The resultant intense inflammatory response is characterized by **bloody, mucopurulent diarrhoea (dysentery)**. Although no enterotoxin is produced, the exotoxin of *Shigella* species is neurotoxic.

Treatment and Prevention

Severe dysentery is managed by fluid and electrolyte replacement. Antibiotics should be avoided as many strains are resistant to multiple antibiotics. Spread can be controlled by improving sanitation and personal hygiene to interrupt faecal–oral transmission; hand hygiene is critical.

Klebsielleae

A number of species belonging to this tribe, namely *Klebsiella*, *Enterobacter* and *Serratia*, are indigenous to the human intestinal and respiratory tracts. They are also occasionally isolated from the oral cavity and hence are considered transient oral commensals. They cause serious disease in immunocompromised patients, especially in hospital environments **(nosocomial infection)**.

KLEBSIELLA PNEUMONIAE

As the name indicates, *Klebsiella pneumoniae* may sometimes cause a severe destructive pneumonia. It also causes nosocomial urinary tract infection. The virulence of the organism is mainly due to its large **antiphagocytic capsule**. This species is isolated from the oropharynx or gastrointestinal tract of about 5% of healthy people, and the isolation rate is higher in the hospitalized.

ENTEROBACTER SPECIES

Enterobacter species are indigenous to the intestinal tract but can be found on plants and as free-living saprophytes. They may cause nosocomial urinary tract infection and very rarely a primary infection. *E. cloacae* and *E. aerogenes* are the most frequently isolated as transients in the oral cavity.

SERRATIA SPECIES

Serratia marcescens grows as characteristic magenta-coloured colonies. It may occasionally cause fatal disease in neonates, and in immunosuppressed and debilitated individuals.

Pseudomonads

Pseudomonas species are not enterobacteria, but they are included in this chapter for convenience as they are Gram-negative rods with somewhat similar properties. The genus contains a large number of species, but only a few are human pathogens. They are widely distributed in the environment and may cause disease, especially in hospital settings. *Pseudomonas aeruginosa* is the most important species to cause such infection and is a special problem in **burn patients**.

PSEUDOMONAS AERUGINOSA

Habitat and Transmission

Colonizes the human intestine in a few healthy individuals and in a large proportion of hospitalized patients. **Colonizes environmental surfaces**, especially under moist conditions. Thus they are found in dental unit water lines as harmless saprophytes.

Characteristics

Aerobic, Gram-negative rods, motile by means of polar flagella. Grow over a very wide temperature range, including room temperature.

Culture and Identification

Grow easily on routine media, producing irregular, moist, iridescent colonies with a characteristic 'fishy' aroma. Identified using commercial kits.

Pathogenicity

Virulence factors identified include lipopolysaccharide endotoxin, an exotoxin, extracellular proteases and elastases, and an extracellular 'slime' that prevents phagocytosis.

Treatment and Prevention

Although this species is resistant to most antimicrobials, it is sensitive to aminoglycosides and certain β-lactams (e.g., acylureidopenicillins), cephalosporins and polymyxin. Prevention is by good asepsis in hospitals and rational antibiotic therapy (to prevent emergence of resistant isolates).

Key Facts

- **Enterobacteriaceae** are short **Gram-negative rods, facultative anaerobes** that ferment glucose and usually live in the intestinal tract.
- They are an extensive group of bacteria that are classified according to their **somatic (O) antigen** (cell wall lipopolysaccharide), **flagellar (H) antigen** and **capsular (K) antigen**.
- Most, if not all, possess **pili**; **capsules** and **flagella** may be present.
- **All** produce **endotoxin**, and **some** produce powerful **exotoxins**.
- *Escherichia coli* is the predominant facultative inhabitant of the human intestinal tract.
- **Diarrhoea-producing** *Escherichia coli* can be divided into **enteropathogenic (EPEC), enteroinvasive (EIEC), enterotoxigenic (ETEC), enterohaemorrhagic (EHEC)** and **enteroaggregative (EAEC)** types.

- Salmonellae and shigellae are responsible for a variety of gastrointestinal disorders.
- *Shigella* is the cause of most **dysentery** in the West.
- Hundreds of species of **Salmonella** have been identified; they are the **agents of typhoid fever**, **gastroenteritis** and septicaemia.
- **Klebsiella**, **Enterobacter** and **Serratia**, together with *Escherichia coli*, are indigenous to the human intestinal and respiratory tracts but are also occasionally isolated from the oral cavity; hence, they are considered to be **transient oral commensals**.
- The latter groups may cause serious disease in hospital environments **(nosocomial infection)**, particularly in compromised patients; these infections are often resistant to many antimicrobials.

Review Questions (Answers on p. 389)

Please indicate which answers are true and which are false.

15.1. Enterobacteria:
   a. are frequently implicated in periodontal infections
   b. are Gram-variable
   c. are an important cause of hospital-acquired infections
   d. are found in the oral cavity of up to 25% of the population
   e. are associated with ventilator-associated pneumonia

15.2. *Escherichia coli*:
   a. produces a heat-labile and a heat-stable enterotoxin
   b. causes neonatal meningitis
   c. is a major pathogen causing nosocomial infections
   d. strain O157 causes a diarrhoeal disease similar to cholera
   e. can cause food poisoning

15.3. Which of the following organisms has a polysaccharide capsule?
   a. *Shigella sonnei*
   b. *Klebsiella pneumoniae*
   c. *Escherichia coli*
   d. *Salmonella paratyphi*
   e. *Bacillus anthracis*

15.4. *Pseudomonas aeruginosa*:
   a. is an important agent of nosocomial infections
   b. is resistant to most antimicrobial agents
   c. colonies produce a 'fruity' smell
   d. in dental unit water lines cause significant morbidity
   e. produces an extracellular slime that resists phagocytosis

Further Reading

Brooks, J. F., Carroll, K. C., Butel, J. S., et al. (Eds.). (2013). Enteric Gram negative rods (Enterobacteriaceae). In *Jawetz, Melnick & Adelberg's medical microbiology* (26th ed., pp. 229–244).

Sedgley, C., & Samaranayake, L. P. (1994). Oropharyngeal prevalence of Enterobacteriaceae in humans: A review. *Journal of Oral Medicine and Oral Pathology, 23*, 104–113.

16 Vibrios, Campylobacters and Wolinella

Bacteria belonging to the *Vibrio, Campylobacter* and *Wolinella* genera (together with others such as the genus *Helicobacter*) are morphologically similar, being Gram-negative curved bacilli. They are **enteric pathogens of humans or part of the normal flora**. Because of their unusual growth requirements (formate and fumarate needed), they have to be cultured in special media.

Vibrios

The genus *Vibrio* includes two important human pathogens, but their natural habitat is water. *Vibrio cholerae* causes cholera, whereas *Vibrio parahaemolyticus* causes a less severe diarrhoea. The main symptom of cholera is watery diarrhoea that can be fatal as a result of severe dehydration, water and electrolyte loss.

VIBRIO CHOLERAE

Habitat and Transmission

The habitat is water contaminated with **faeces of patients or carriers**; there is no animal reservoir. A life-threatening, watery diarrhoea (rice-water stools) is the characteristic disease.

Characteristics

Gram-negative slender bacilli, comma-shaped with pointed ends. Highly motile by means of a single polar flagellum. May be seen directly in stool samples by dark-field microscopy.

Culture and Identification

Grows in alkaline conditions (pH 8.5–9.2 approximately): selective media for culture such as **thiosulphate citrate–bile salts–sucrose** (TCBS) agar medium is based on this property. This, together with biochemical tests and serology, helps identification. Serotyping is based on the somatic O antigens. All diarrhoea-producing strains of *V. cholerae* are designated as O1 and are subdivided into three major serotypes: the Ogawa, Inaba and El Tor strains.

Pathogenicity

V. cholerae has the ability to colonize the intestinal tract in very high numbers, and about 10^8 cells per millilitre are seen in patients' faeces. The cells attach to but do not invade the intestinal mucosa. Pathogenicity is due to secretion of an **enterotoxin**, which binds to ganglioside receptors on mucosal cells. After a lag period of 15–45 min, adenylate cyclase is activated and the cyclic adenosine monophosphate concentration inside the intestinal cells increases. This in turn leads to **excretion of electrolytes and water and subsequent diarrhoea**, leading to severe dehydration. Watery diarrhoea and vomiting are the major symptoms.

Treatment and Prevention

Intravenous administration of **fluids and electrolytes** is essential for recovery. Oral administration of a solution containing glucose and electrolytes (oral rehydration therapy) is successful, but the patient must be capable of consuming the liquid by mouth. Severely ill patients are generally too weak to ingest fluids. Antibiotics (usually tetracycline) do not affect the disease outcome once the enterotoxin attaches to the intestinal cells, but they prevent subsequent attacks by reducing the number of toxin-producing *V. cholerae* cells in the intestine.

An inactivated as well as an attenuated vaccine for cholera is available for those travelling to affected areas. The vaccine (two doses given 1–6 weeks apart) as a drink provides protection for up to 2 years.

VIBRIO PARAHAEMOLYTICUS

This vibrio requires a relatively high salt concentration for growth and is distributed worldwide in marine environments, for example in Southeast Asia. A common agent of acute enteritis associated with the consumption of **improperly cooked seafood**, it accounts for about half of all cases of food poisoning in Japan.

There is no specific treatment for diarrhoea. The best control measure is the consumption of only thoroughly cooked seafood.

Campylobacters

The genus *Campylobacter* contains medically important species that are important human pathogens, once classified as vibrios. *Campylobacter jejuni* is the major human pathogenic species; *Campylobacter rectus* has been isolated from active periodontal disease sites and has been implicated as a periodontopathogen.

CAMPYLOBACTER SPECIES

Habitat and Transmission

The natural reservoir is animals. Organisms are acquired from contaminated food and milk.

Characteristics

Curved, seagull-shaped, Gram-negative rods; mobile with a single polar flagellum.

Culture and Identification

C. jejuni grows best under **microaerophilic** (i.e., an environment of 10% oxygen and 10% carbon dioxide) and **thermophilic** (a temperature of 43°C) conditions in an enriched medium. Further identification is by biochemical tests and antibiotic-susceptibility patterns.

Pathogenicity

Gastroenteritis, especially in children, is the most common human infection caused by *Campylobacter* species. It resembles dysentery and is usually self-limiting, but it may last for several days. The heat-labile enterotoxin of *Campylobacter fetus* is implicated. Campylobacters may occasionally cause bacteraemia, meningitis, endocarditis, arthritis and urinary tract infection. *C. jejuni* has been implicated as the aetiological agent of Guillain-Barré

syndrome. Some strains of *C. rectus* isolated from periodontal disease sites produce a cytotoxin similar to that of *Aggregatibacter actinomycetemcomitans* and stimulate human gingival fibroblasts to produce interleukin-6 and interleukin-8.

Treatment and Prevention

No specific therapy is necessary for the mild diarrhoea. Good food and hand hygiene are important.

HELICOBACTER PYLORI

This organism (previously classified as a campylobacter) causes a significant proportion of gastritis and duodenal ulcers in humans; it plays a major role in the development of **gastric cancer**. Antimicrobial therapy eradicates the bacteria from the stomach and resolves many of the ulcers that were formerly thought to be due to gastric acidity. A few studies have demonstrated the presence of this organism, albeit in small numbers, in human supragingival plaque.

Wolinella

Members of the genus *Wolinella* are curved or helical Gram-negative motile rods. Its darting motility is due to a polar flagellum; they are anaerobes and require formate and fumarate for growth. The main species is *Wolinella succinogenes*.

Habitat

These organisms are frequently isolated from the oral cavity, especially the gingival sulcus.

Culture and Identification

A selective medium is available for culturing the organism from plaque samples. Identification is by colonial characteristics (dry, spreading or corroding colonies), whole-cell protein profiles and serology.

Pathogenicity

Although some studies have shown a high correlation between periodontal disease activity and isolation of *Wolinella* spp., the pathogenic role is not clear. The organisms can induce alveolar bone loss in gnotobiotic rats. A possible periodontal pathogen.

Key Facts

- **Vibrios** are small, **comma-shaped**, **Gram-negative**, **oxidase-positive** bacteria that prefer an alkaline growth environment.
- **Vibrio cholerae** is the major pathogen in the genus and is **responsible for cholera epidemics**, especially in the developing world.

- *Campylobacter jejuni* is a thermophilic, microaerophilic vibrio that causes human diarrhoeal illness.
- *Helicobacter pylori* causes a significant proportion of **gastritis and duodenal ulcers** in humans and may play a role in gastric cancer.

Review Questions (Answers on p. 390)

Please indicate which answers are true and which are false.

16.1. *Vibrio cholerae*:
   a. are Gram-negative, highly motile slightly curved rods
   b. grow well in alkaline media
   c. pathogenicity is by means of invasion of the intestinal mucosa
   d. cause dysentery
   e. whole-cell vaccine is effective in preventing the disease

16.2. *Wolinella* spp.:
   a. are often isolated from plaque biofilms
   b. are major periodontal pathogens
   c. are implicated in gastritis
   d. require folate and fumarate for growth
   e. form dry spreading colonies

16.3. *Campylobacter* spp.:
   a. are implicated in food poisoning
   b. are isolated from active sites of periodontal infection
   c. grow best under strict anaerobic conditions
   d. are thermophilic
   e. are Gram-negative curved bacilli

Further Reading

Brooks, J. F., Carroll, K. C., Butel, J. S., et al. (Eds.). (2013). Enteric Gram negative rods (Vibrios, Campylobacters, Helicobacter and associated bacteria). In *Jawetz, Melnick & Adelberg's medical microbiology* (26th ed., pp. 255–263). McGraw Hill.

Macuch, P. J., & Tanner, A. C. (2000). *Campylobacter* species in health, gingivitis, and periodontitis. *Journal of Dental Research, 79*, 785–792.

17 Bacteroides, Tannerella, Porphyromonas *and* Prevotella

The genera described in this chapter are obligately anaerobic, short Gram-negative rods or coccobacilli. Historically, only the *Bacteroides* genus was known, but the application of new taxonomic techniques has resulted in the definition of three additional genera: *Tannerella, Porphyromonas* and *Prevotella*. Together, they comprise a substantial proportion of the microflora of dental plaque, the intestine and the female genital tract (Table 17.1)

- *Bacteroides* spp. are mainly restricted to species found **predominantly in the gut** and are the most common agents of serious anaerobic infections; *Bacteroides fragilis* is the main pathogen.
- *Tannerella* spp. are **black-pigmented**, anaerobic rods, strongly implicated as a major pathogen of periodontal disease. *Tannerella forsythia* (formerly *Bacteroides forsythus* and *Tannerella forsythensis*) is frequently isolated with *Porphyromonas gingivalis*, indicating an ecological relationship between them.
- *Porphyromonas* spp. are asaccharolytic pigmented species and form part of the normal oral flora. They are agents of periodontal disease and hence considered as **periodontopathic** organisms.
- *Prevotella* spp. include saccharolytic oral and genitourinary species; some species are periodontopathic.

Collectively, *Tannerella, Porphyromonas* and *Prevotella* species are referred to as **black-pigmented anaerobes**, as some organisms from these genera form a characteristic brown or black pigment on blood agar (Fig. 17.1).

Bacteroides

BACTEROIDES FRAGILIS

Habitat and Transmission

Bacteroides species are the most predominant flora in the intestine (10^{11} cells per gram of faeces), far outnumbering *Escherichia coli*. They cause serious anaerobic infections such as intraabdominal sepsis, peritonitis, liver abscesses, brain abscesses and wound infection.

Characteristics

Strictly anaerobic, Gram-negative, nonmotile, nonsporing bacilli, but may appear pleomorphic. The polysaccharide capsule is an important virulence factor.

Culture and Identification

These organisms have stringent growth requirements; they demonstrate slow growth on blood agar and appear as grey to opaque, translucent colonies. They grow well in Robertson's cooked meat medium supplemented with yeast extract.

Identified by biochemical tests, growth inhibition by bile salts, antibiotic resistance tests and gas–liquid chromatographic analysis of fatty acid end-products of glucose metabolism.

Pathogenicity

Mainly the result of its **endotoxin** and **proteases**. No exotoxin has been reported. Other organisms, such as coliforms,

Table 17.1 Anaerobic Gram-Negative Bacilli of Clinical Interest

Organism	Main Colonization Sites
BACTEROIDES	
B. fragilis group	Intestine
B. fragilis	Intestine
B. ovatus	Intestine
B. vulgatus	Intestine
B. distasonis	Intestine
B. capillosus	Intestine, oropharynx
B. ureolyticus	Oropharynx, intestine, genitourinary tract
TANNERELLA	
T. forsythia	Oropharynx
PORPHYROMONAS	
P. gingivalis	Oropharynx
P. endodontalis	Oropharynx
PREVOTELLA	
P. intermedia	Oropharynx
P. nigrescens	Oropharynx
P. melaninogenica	Oropharynx
P. loescheii	Oropharynx
P. pallens	Vagina, oropharynx
P. corporis	Vagina, oropharynx

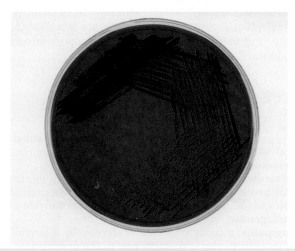

Fig. 17.1 Black-pigmented colonies of periodontopathogen *Porphyromonas gingivalis* on blood agar. The pigment is thought to be related to breakdown products of the blood.

are commonly associated with sepsis. The latter facultative anaerobes utilize oxygen in the infective focus and facilitate the growth of the anaerobic *Bacteroides* strains. Consequently, many *Bacteroides* infections are **polymicrobial** in nature.

Treatment and Prevention

Sensitive to metronidazole and clindamycin. Resistant to penicillins, first-generation cephalosporins and aminoglycosides. Penicillin resistance is due to **β-lactamase** production. As *Bacteroides* spp. are normal gut commensals, infections are **endogenous** and diseases are virtually impossible to prevent.

Tannerella

TANNERELLA FORSYTHIA

(Formerly *Bacteroides forsythus* and *Tannerella forsythensis*.)

Habitat and Transmission

Both supragingival and subgingival sites but more common in the latter; the degree of isolation strongly related to increasing pocket depth and, increasingly, recovered from sites that converted from periodontal health to disease and sites with periodontal breakdown, hence considered a **consensus periodontal pathogen**. Indeed, *Tannerella forsythia, Treponema denticola* and *Porphyromonas gingivalis* are considered the three agents of *red complex* bacteria almost always associated with periodontal disease (see Chapter 33). A number of other epithets have been given to this group of pathogens such as **pathobionts, keystone pathogens** and **inflammophilic bacteria**. As these bacteria are always present in inflamed regions of the periodontium, they are thought to have coevolved not only to endure inflammation but also to take advantage of it. Inflammatory by-products drive the selection and enrichment of these pathogenic communities by providing a source of nutrients in the form of tissue breakdown products (e.g., degraded collagen peptides and haeme-containing compounds).

Characteristics

Nonmotile, pleomorphic, spindle-shaped Gram-negative rods.

Culture and Identification

Grows anaerobically but sometimes requires up to 14 days for visible growth. Growth enhanced by co-cultivation with *Fusobacterium nucleatum*. Media supplemented with N-acetylmuramic acid enhances growth.

Pathogenicity

Periodontal pathogen in both human and animals; induces apoptotic cell death; invades epithelial cells in vitro and in vivo. Its endotoxin, fatty acid and methylglyoxal production are considered virulence factors; increased levels found in ligature-induced periodontitis and peri-implantitis in dogs.

Porphyromonas

PORPHYROMONAS GINGIVALIS

Habitat and Transmission

Found almost solely at subgingival sites, particularly in advanced periodontal disease: considered a **consensus periodontal pathogen or periodontopathogen**. As mentioned, *Porphyromonas gingivalis, Tannerella forsythia* and *Treponema denticola* are considered the three agents of 'red complex', inflammophilic (i.e., inflammation-loving) bacteria almost always associated with periodontal disease (see Chapter 33). *Porphyromonas gingivalis* is occasionally recovered from the tongue and tonsils. *Porphyromonas endodontalis* is mainly isolated from endodontic infections, whereas *Porphyromonas catoniae* is found in healthy gingivae or shallow pockets.

Characteristics

Nonmotile, asaccharolytic, short, pleomorphic, capsulate, Gram-negative coccobacilli. Six serotypes are recognized.

Culture and Identification

Grows anaerobically, with dark pigmentation, on media containing lysed blood (Fig. 17.1); identified by biochemical characteristics using commercially available kits (e.g., AnIdent); DNA and molecular probes are now used to identify these organisms directly from plaque samples.

Pathogenicity

An **aggressive periodontal pathogen** in both humans and animals (e.g., guinea pig, monkey, dog [beagle]); its fimbriae mediate adhesion and the capsule defends against phagocytosis. Produces a range of virulence factors including collagenase, endotoxin, fibrinolysin, phospholipase A, many proteases that destroy immunoglobulins, gingipain, a fibroblast-inhibitory factor, complement and haeme-sequestering proteins, and a haemolysin.

Gingipains, a family of proteases secreted by *P. gingivalis* are thought to play a potential role in the development of Alzheimer disease, although conclusive evidence is yet to come.

Prevotella

This genus includes a number of pigmented as well as non-pigmented species that are moderately saccharolytic; all produce acetic and succinic acid from glucose. *Prevotella melaninogenica* is the type species (Table 17.1).

PREVOTELLA SPECIES

Habitat and Transmission

The predominant ecological niche of all *Prevotella* species appears to be the **human oral cavity**. Strains of *Prevotella intermedia* are associated more with periodontal disease, whereas *Prevotella nigrescens* is isolated more often from healthy gingival sites.

Culture and Identification

Nonmotile, short, round-ended, Gram-negative rods; brown-black colonies on blood agar (when pigmented). Molecular techniques are required to differentiate some species.

Pathogenicity

Prevotella intermedia is closely associated with periodontal disease and shares a number of virulence properties exhibited by *Porphyromonas gingivalis*. These organisms are classified as belonging to the ***orange complex*** bacteria associated with the developmental stages of periodontal disease, and precede the arrival of the *red complex* group of bacteria (see Chapter 33). The pathogenicity of other subdivided species awaits clarification. Oral nonpigmented species such as *Prevotella buccae*, *Prevotella oralis* and *Prevotella dentalis* are isolated occasionally from healthy sub-gingival plaque. Some of the latter are associated with disease, and increase in numbers and proportions during periodontal disease.

Key Facts

- ▪ ***Tannerella***, ***Porphyromonas*** and ***Prevotella*** form a substantial proportion of the microflora of **dental plaque,** the **intestine** and the **female genital** tract.
- ▪ *Bacteroides* spp. are the **predominant** flora **in the intestine**.
- ▪ Collectively, *Tannerella*, *Porphyromonas* and *Prevotella* species are referred to as **black-pigmented anaerobes**.
- ▪ *Tannerella forsythia* is a key periodontopathogen and induces apoptotic cell death.
- ▪ *Tannerella forsythia*, *Treponema denticola* and *Porphyromonas gingivalis* are considered the three agents of **'red complex' bacteria** almost always associated with periodontal disease.

- ▪ *Porphyromonas gingivalis* is found almost **solely at subgingival sites** and is a key periodontopathic organism (i.e., a **periodontopathogen**).
- ▪ The **virulence** of *Porphyromonas gingivalis* is partly due to its many **proteases** (which destroy immunoglobulins, complement and haeme-sequestering proteins), a **haemolysin** and a **collagenase**.
- ▪ **Gingipains**, a family of proteases secreted by *P. gingivalis*, are thought to play a potential role in the development of Alzheimer's disease.
- ▪ Strains of *Prevotella intermedia* are associated more with periodontal disease, whereas *Prevotella nigrescens* is isolated more often from **healthy gingival sites**.

Review Questions (Answers on p. 390)

Please indicate which answers are true and which are false.

17.1. *Bacteroides* spp. are:
  a. facultative anaerobes
  b. outnumbered by Escherichia spp. in the intestine
  c. spore formers
  d. capsulated
  e. capable of growing in a media rich in bile salts

17.2. *Porphyromonas gingivalis*:
  a. are Gram-negative pleomorphic rods
  b. are noncapsulated
  c. form dark colonies on lysed blood
  d. are aggressive periodontal pathogens
  e. are isolated from many extraoral sites

17.3. Which of the following organisms is/are likely to be isolated from a subgingival plaque sample cultured anaerobically?
a. *Fusobacterium nucleatum*
b. *Escherichia coli*
c. *Pseudomonas aeruginosa*
d. *Aggregatibacter actinomycetemcomitans*
e. *Haemophilus influenzae*

Further Reading

Holt, S. C., & Ebersole, J. L. (2005). *Porphyromonas gingivalis, Treponema denticola* and *Tannerella forsythia*: The 'red complex', a prototype poly-bacterial pathogenic consortium in periodontitis. *Periodontology 2000, 38*, 72–122.

Marsh, P., Lewis, M., Williams, D., et al. (Eds.). (2009). The resident oral microflora. In *Oral microbiology* (5th ed., pp. 24–44). Churchill Livingstone.

Mohanty, R., Asopa, S. J., Joseph, M. D., Singh, B., Rajguru, J. P., Saidath, K., & Sharma, U. (2019). Red complex: Polymicrobial conglomerate in oral flora: A review. *Journal of Family Medicine and Primary Care, 8*(11), 3480–3486. doi:10.4103/jfmpc.jfmpc_759_19.

Shah, H. N., Mayrand, D., & Genco, R. J. (Eds.). (1993). *Biology of the species Porphyromonas gingivalis*. CRC Press.

Tanner, A. C. R., & Izard, J. (2006). *Tannerella forsythia*, a periodontal pathogen entering the genomic era. *Periodontology 2000, 42*, 88–103.

18 *Fusobacteria, Leptotrichia and Spirochaetes*

Fusobacteria are nonsporing, anaerobic, nonmotile, non- or weakly fermentative, spindle-shaped bacilli (with fused ends: hence, the name). They are normal inhabitants of the oral cavity, intestine and female genital tract and are sometimes isolated from pulmonary and pelvic abscesses. **Fusospirochaetal infections**, which they cause in combination with spirochaetes, are noteworthy. *Fusobacterium nucleatum* (the type species), *Fusobacterium periodonticum* and *Fusobacterium simiae* are isolated mainly from periodontal disease sites, and others such as *Fusobacterium alocis* and *Fusobacterium sulci* are sometimes found in the healthy gingival sulcus. Nonoral species include *Fusobacterium gonidiaformans*, *Fusobacterium russii* and *Fusobacterium ulcerans*.

Although not a component of oral microbiota, it is noteworthy that *Fusobacterium necrophorum* is the cause of **Lemierre's disease,** characterized by acute jugular vein septic thrombophlebitis and subsequent systemic metastatic abscesses.

Fusobacteria

FUSOBACTERIUM NUCLEATUM

Habitat and Transmission

Several subspecies of *F. nucleatum* have been identified in different habitats. These include *F. nucleatum* subsp. *polymorphum*, found in the healthy gingival crevice, and *F. nucleatum*
subsp. *nucleatum*, recovered mainly from periodontal pockets. A third subspecies is *F. nucleatum* subsp. *vincentii*. Infections are almost invariably **endogenous**.

Characteristics

Gram-negative, strictly anaerobic, cigar-shaped bacilli with pointed ends (Fig. 18.1). Cells often have a central swelling. A Gram-stained smear of deep gingival debris obtained from a lesion of acute ulcerative gingivitis is a simple method of demonstrating the characteristic fusobacteria, together with spirochaetes and polymorphonuclear leukocytes (Fig. 18.2). These, together with the clinical picture, confirm a clinical diagnosis of acute ulcerative gingivitis.

Culture and Identification

Grows on blood agar as dull, granular colonies with an irregular, rhizoid edge. Biochemical reactions and the acidic end-products of carbohydrate metabolism help identification. As fusobacteria can remove sulphur from cysteine and methionine to produce **odoriferous hydrogen sulphide and methyl mercaptan,** they are thought to be associated with **halitosis.**

Pathogenicity

The endotoxin of the organism appears to be involved in the pathogenesis of periodontal disease. It possesses remarkable adherence properties and the fusobacterium **adhesin A (FadA),** which confers this property, has recently been isolated. *F. nucleatum* is usually isolated from polymicrobial infections; it is rarely the sole pathogen. Thus in

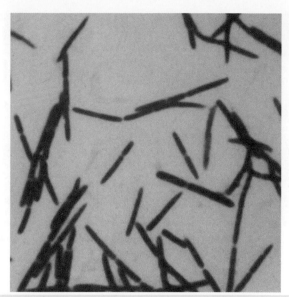

Fig. 18.1   A photomicrograph of fusobacteria showing characteristic Gram-negative, cigar-shaped cells with pointed ends.

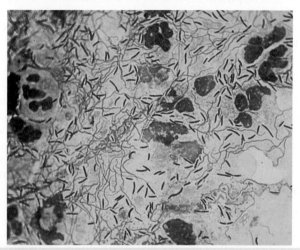

Fig. 18.2   A Gram-stained smear obtained from deep gingival plaque of a patient with acute ulcerative gingivitis (see also Fig. 33.6) showing the fusospirochaetal complex. (*Note:* The large cells are polymorphs.)

combination with oral spirochaetes (*Treponema vincentii* and others), it causes the classic **fusospirochaetal infections.** These are:

- **acute (necrotizing) ulcerative gingivitis** or trench mouth, so called because it was first described in soldiers 'in the trenches' of the World War I (see Chapter 33)
- **Vincent's angina**, an ulcerative tonsillitis causing tissue necrosis, often due to extension of acute ulcerative gingivitis
- **cancrum oris or noma**, a sequela of acute ulcerative gingivitis with resultant gross tissue loss of the facial region.

As fusobacteria coaggregate with most other oral bacteria, they are believed to be important **bridging organisms** between early and late colonizers during plaque formation (see Fig. 31.2).

Antibiotic Sensitivity and Prevention

Fusobacteria are uniformly sensitive to penicillin and, being strict anaerobes, are sensitive to metronidazole. Regular oral hygiene and antiseptic mouthwashes are the key to prevention of oral fusobacterial infections in susceptible individuals.

Leptotrichia

Leptotrichia spp. are oral commensals previously thought to belong to the genus *Fusobacterium*. They are Gram-negative, strictly anaerobic, slender, filamentous bacilli, usually with one pointed end. *Leptotrichia buccalis*, present in low proportions in dental plaque, is the sole representative of this genus.

Spirochaetes

Spirochaetes are a diverse group of spiral, motile organisms comprising five genera. Of these, three genera are human pathogens:

- **Treponema** causes syphilis, bejel, yaws, pinta and, in the oral cavity, acute necrotizing ulcerative gingivitis (together with fusobacteria)
- **Borrelia** causes relapsing fever and Lyme disease
- **Leptospira** causes leptospirosis.

Spirochaetes are motile, helical organisms with a central protoplasmic cylinder surrounded by a cytoplasmic membrane (Fig. 18.3). The cell wall is similar to Gram-negative bacteria but stains poorly with the Gram stain. Underneath the cell wall run three to five **axial filaments** that are fixed to the extremities of the organism. Contractions of these filaments distort the bacterial cell body to give it its helical shape. The organism moves either by rotation along the long axis or by flexion of cells. Because of their weak refractile nature, dark-ground microscopy is used to visualize these organisms in the laboratory, although immunofluorescence is more useful for identification purposes. All spirochaetes are strictly anaerobic or microaerophilic.

Treponema

The coils of *Treponema* are regular, with a longer wavelength than that of *Leptospira* (Fig. 18.3). A number of species and subspecies are recognized, some of which are important systemic pathogens, whereas others are oral inhabitants implicated in periodontal disease.

TREPONEMA PALLIDUM

Habitat and Transmission

Lesions of Primary and Secondary Syphilis. Transmission is by direct contact with lesions, body secretions, blood, semen and saliva, usually during sexual contact, and from mother to foetus by placental transfer.

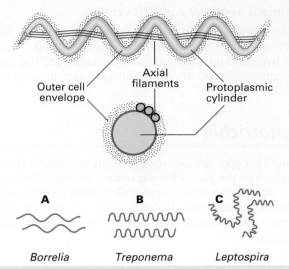

Fig. 18.3 Structure of a spirochaete (*top*) and the morphology of the three major genera of spirochaetes.

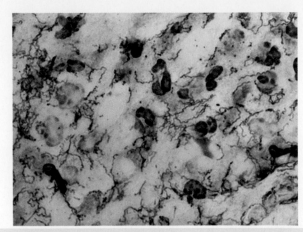

Fig. 18.4 *Treponema pallidum* spirochetes in a tissue fluid sample from a secondary clinical lesion stained with a silver stain. (Courtesy Professor Dr. Willie Van Heerden, University of Pretoria, South Africa.)

Characteristics

Slender, corkscrew-shaped cells with 6–12 evenly spaced coils, 6–14 × 0.2 μm; too slender to visualize by light microscopy but can be seen by silver impregnation (Fig. 18.4) or immunofluorescent techniques; strictly anaerobic and extremely sensitive to drying and heat, hence dies rapidly outside the body.

Culture and Identification

Cannot be cultured in vitro, but can be propagated in the testes of rabbits; *Treponema pallidum* thus harvested can be used as antigens to detect specific antibody in the patient's serum.

Dark-ground microscopy of tissue fluid from primary and secondary clinical lesions helps identification, but serological tests are the mainstay of diagnosis.

Pathogenicity

Causes **syphilis**, a sexually transmitted disease with protean manifestations (see Chapter 27). The virulence factors of *Treponema pallidum* are not well characterized. Immunopathology plays a significant role in disease manifestations, especially in the late (tertiary and quaternary) stages of the disease. The syphilis spirochete's well-recognized capacity for early dissemination and immune evasion has earned it the designation **'the stealth pathogen'**.

Antibiotic Sensitivity and Control

Penicillin is the drug of choice; for allergic patients, tetracycline is an alternative. Prevention of syphilis is based on early detection, contact tracing and serological testing of pregnant women.

TREPONEMA PALLIDUM SUBSPECIES PERTENUE

The agent of **yaws**, characterized by chronic, ulcerative, granulomatous lesions of skin, mucosae and bone. The disease, widespread in the tropics, is spread by direct contact.

TREPONEMA CARATEUM

The agent of **pinta**, a nonvenereal skin infection characterized by depigmented and hyperkeratotic skin. The disease affects mainly dark-skinned natives of Central and South America and the West Indies.

ORAL TREPONEMES

All oral spirochaetes are classified in the genus *Treponema*. Although many species have been described, only four have been cultivated and maintained reliably: *Treponema denticola*, *Treponema vincentii*, *Treponema pectinovarum* and *Treponema socranskii*. In another classification, they are categorized according to cell size as **small, medium and large spirochaetes.**

Habitat and Transmission

Predominantly the oral cavity of humans and primates, at the gingival margin and crevice in particular. Transmission routes are unknown. Infections are endogenous.

Characteristics

Motile, helical rods, 5–15 × 0.5 μm, with irregular (three to eight) spirals, which are less tightly coiled than, for instance, *Treponema pallidum* (Figs. 18.3 and 18.5). Cell walls are Gram-negative but stain poorly. The size is variable and can be used as a basis for classification (large, medium or small).

Culture and Identification

In contrast to *Treponema pallidum*, oral spirochaetes can be grown *in vitro*. They are strict anaerobes, slow-growing in **oral treponema isolation** (OTI) medium. Subspecies can be differentiated by fermentation reactions and serology (agglutination).

Suspect lesions of **acute necrotizing ulcerative gingivitis** or advanced periodontitis can be examined by obtaining a Gram-stained smear of deep gingival plaque and visualizing the characteristic **fusospirochaetal complex** under light microscopy (see Fig. 18.2); alternatively, dark-ground microscopy may be used.

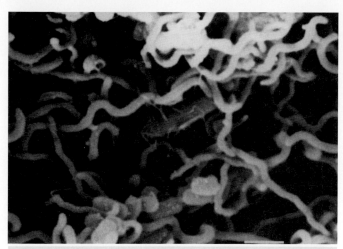

Fig. 18.5 Scanning electron micrograph of the radicular surface of a tooth affected by advanced periodontal disease showing numerous spirochaetes.

Pathogenicity

These organisms are a component of the fusospirochaetal complex of acute necrotizing ulcerative gingivitis and **Vincent's angina,** and they are a co-agent of advanced periodontal disease. *Treponema denticola*, in particular, is a consensus periodontopathogen and member of the triad of red-complex bacteria (together with *Tannerella forsythia* and *Porphyromonas gingivalis*) implicated in the pathogenesis of chronic periodontal diseases.

Their ability to travel through viscous environments enables oral spirochaetes to migrate within the gingival crevicular fluid and to penetrate sulcular epithelial linings as well as gingival connective tissue. Virulence factors are little known; endotoxin is possibly contributory to disease. *Treponema denticola* is more proteolytic than other species and degrades collagen and dentine.

Antibiotic Sensitivity and Control

Sensitive to penicillin and metronidazole. Prevention of infection is achieved by good oral hygiene practices.

Borrelia

BORRELIA BURGDORFERI

Habitat and Transmission

Found in ticks and small mammals, particularly deer. Transmission is by a tick vector.

Characteristics

This species is a helical spirochaete, 0.18–0.25×4.3 μm. Gram-negative, it grows under microaerophilic conditions at $34°C$. Identification is by serology and immunofluorescence or enzyme-linked immunosorbent assay (ELISA).

Pathogenicity

The agent of **Lyme disease**, a generalized infection with neurological and cardiac manifestations as well as Lyme arthritis. One of the earliest and most common neurological manifestations is unilateral **facial palsy**.

Antibiotic Sensitivity

Sensitive to tetracycline and amoxicillin.

Other *Borrelia* Species

These include *Borrelia recurrentis* and *Borrelia duttonii*, agents of **louse-borne and tick-borne relapsing fever,** respectively, seen in parts of Africa, Asia and South America.

Leptospira

Leptospira biflexa and *Leptospira interrogans* are the recognized species, each of which comprises a number of serogroups.

These organisms are found in damp environments such as stagnant water and wet soil. The kidneys of some rodents and domestic animals act as a reservoir for *Leptospira interrogans*. The urine of these animals serves as a vehicle of transmission of human leptospirosis, the symptoms of which vary from mild febrile illness to fatal attacks of jaundice and renal failure.

Key Facts

- Fusobacteria are nonsporing, anaerobic, spindle-shaped bacilli inhabiting the oral cavity, intestine and female genital tract.
- The type species ***Fusobacterium nucleatum*** and ***Fusobacterium periodonticum*** are isolated mainly from periodontal disease sites and, hence, considered to be **periodontopathic bacteria**.
- Fusospirochaetal infections caused by fusobacteria in combination with spirochaetes are acute ulcerative gingivitis, Vincent's angina and cancrum oris (or noma).
- **Spirochaetes** are **long, slender, coiled** and highly **mobile** bacteria that do not take up the Gram stain.

- Spirochaetes comprise three genera: ***Treponema, Borrelia*** **and *Leptospira.***
- ***Treponema pallidum***, the agent of syphilis, cannot be cultivated in vitro and is uniformly **sensitive to penicillin**.
- All oral spirochaetes are classified in the genus *Treponema* (type strain: ***Treponema denticola***).
- *Treponema denticola* is a coagent of **fusospirochaetal infection and advanced periodontal disease**.
- *Treponema denticola*, *Tannerella forsythia* and *Porphyromonas gingivalis* are considered the three agents of red complex bacteria almost always associated with periodontal disease.

Review Questions (Answers on p. 390)

Please indicate which answers are true and which are false.

18.1. Which of the following statements on acute (necrotizing) ulcerative gingivitis (ANUG) are true?
a. ANUG is a polymicrobial infection
b. ANUG is a complication of advanced periodontal disease
c. a sequela of ANUG may be gross facial tissue loss
d. metronidazole is the antimicrobial of choice for ANUG
e. ANUG is often preventable with good oral hygiene

18.2. Spirochaetes:
a. possess cell walls similar to that of mycobacteria
b. are best viewed using dark-ground or fluorescence microscopy
c. are implicated in Vincent's angina
d. are found in the oral cavity and can be grown in vitro
e. are generally sensitive to penicillin

18.3. Spirochaetal infections:
a. are a cause of human Lyme disease
b. if systemic, are traditionally diagnosed using serology
c. can lead to liver failure and renal failure
d. may cause facial palsy
e. induce lifelong immunity

Further Reading

Duerden, B. I., & Drasar, B. S. (Eds.). (1991). *Anaerobes in human disease.* Edward Arnold.

Greenwood, D., Slack, R., & Peutherer, J. (Eds.). (2003). *Medical microbiology* (16th ed., Chaps. 37 & 38). Churchill Livingstone.

Holt, S. C., & Ebersole, J. L. (2005). *Porphyromonas gingivalis, Treponema denticola,* and *Tannerella forsythia*: The "red complex", a prototype polybacterial pathogenic consortium in periodontitis. *Periodontology 2000, 38,* 72–122.

Radolf, J. D., Deka, R. K., Anand, A., Šmajs, D., Norgard, M. V., & Yang, X. F. (2016). Treponema pallidum, the syphilis spirochete: Making a living as a stealth pathogen. *Nature Reviews Microbiology, 14*(12), 744–759. doi:10.1038/nrmicro.2016.141.

19 *Mycobacteria and Legionellae*

Mycobacteria

According to the World Health Organization (WHO), nearly 2 billion people, **one-third of the world's population**, have disease caused by mycobacteria, particularly **tuberculosis**. Mycobacteria are widespread both in the environment and in animals and cause two major human diseases: tuberculosis and leprosy. They are aerobic, acid-fast bacilli (not stained by the Gram stain because of the high lipid component of the cell wall). The major medically important pathogens are:

- *Mycobacterium tuberculosis*, the agent of **tuberculosis**; one of the top three infectious diseases affecting humans globally
- *Mycobacterium bovis*, which causes tuberculosis in humans as well as in cattle
- *Mycobacterium africanum*, which also causes human tuberculosis
- *Mycobacterium leprae*, the agent of **leprosy**, a disease affecting millions in Asia and Africa
- **Mycobacteria other than tuberculosis (MOTT)**, such as *Mycobacterium avium–intracellulare* complex and *Mycobacterium kansasii*, which cause frequent disease in human immunodeficiency virus (HIV)-infected patients.

MYCOBACTERIUM TUBERCULOSIS

Habitat and Transmission

Found in infected humans, mainly in the lungs; in the body, it resides primarily in the cells of the reticuloendothelial system; transmission is mainly by droplet spread via coughing.

Characteristics

Acid- and alcohol-fast, slender, beaded bacilli; nonsporing. As the organisms do not take up the Gram stain because of the long-chain fatty acids (**mycolic acid**) in the cell wall, a special stain (the **Ziehl-Neelsen stain**) is required to visualize them (Fig. 19.1). However, fluorescent microscopy, with auramine stain, is now used commonly for this purpose.

Culture and Identification

This species does not grow on ordinary media and requires **Löwenstein-Jensen medium** for growth (constituents: whole egg, asparagine, glycerol, malachite green). Slow growing (2–3 weeks; sometimes up to 6 weeks) at 37°C. They grow as '**rough, tough and buff**' colonies: rough due to dry, irregular growth; tough due to difficulty in lifting the colony from the surface; and buff due to the pale yellow colour (Fig. 19.2).

Identification of mycobacteria is classically based on their rate of growth, optimum temperature requirements and pigment production in the presence or absence of light, together with biochemical tests. However, these slow procedures are being supplanted by more efficient nucleic acid amplification (polymerase chain reaction (PCR) tests. Combination of nucleic acid tests together with a smear of sputum or the lesion with acid- and alcohol-fast bacilli is confirmatory of the disease.

Pathogenicity

This organism is the agent of tuberculosis: a **chronic, granulomatous, slowly progressive infection**, usually of the lungs; eventually, many other organs and tissues may be affected. A pandemic disease, tuberculosis is especially common in the developing world owing to HIV infection (15–20% of individuals with HIV disease may have tuberculosis). The oral cavity is affected secondary to primary disease elsewhere (see Chapter 35). The hallmark of the disease is **granulomas**, which have a concentric structure with a necrotic centre of **caseation** surrounded by a zone of multinucleated giant cells, monocytes and

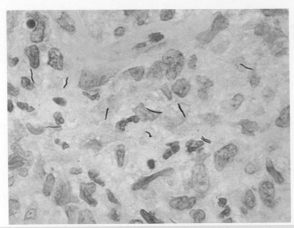

Fig. 19.1 A sputum sample from a patient with tuberculosis stained with Ziehl-Neelsen stain showing the pink-staining, slender, acid- and alcohol-fast bacilli. (Courtesy Professor Dr. Willie Van Heerden, University of Pretoria, South Africa.)

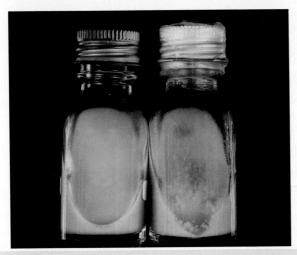

Fig. 19.2 Growth of *Mycobacterium tuberculosis* on Löwenstein-Jensen medium: the bottle on the left is uninoculated; the bottle on the right shows 'rough, tough and buff' colonies of the organism.

histiocytic cells with an outer ring of fibrosis, a consequence of cell-mediated immune reactivity. No exotoxins or endotoxins.

Antibiotic Sensitivity and Control

Long-term (6–9 months) **combination therapy** with antituberculous drugs (isoniazid, rifampicin, pyrazinamide, ethambutol and streptomycin) is the cornerstone of treatment. Tubercle bacilli are resistant to a number of antituberculous drugs, and **multidrug-resistant tuberculosis (MDR-TB)** and **extensively drug-resistant tuberculosis (XDR)** are major worldwide concerns. Hence, regimentation of drug delivery is critical for managing the disease and is achieved by a global programme termed **directly observed therapy (DOT)**.

Prevention is by **bacille Calmette-Guérin (BCG) vaccination** containing **live attenuated organisms**, in childhood. Pasteurization of milk and general improvement of living standards have played a valuable role in prevention.

Table 19.1 Comparison of the Different Types of Leprosy

	Tuberculoid	Lepromatous
Cell-mediated immunity	Predominant	Uncommon or absent
Antibody response	Absent	Predominant
Widespread lesions	Absent	Common
Numbers of *Mycobacterium leprae* in lesions	Uncommon	Predominant

MYCOBACTERIUM BOVIS

Mycobacterium bovis **infects cattle**. Humans become infected by ingesting *M. bovis*-contaminated milk. Infection is rarely seen in the West owing to eradication of the disease in cattle. The organism specifically causes the childhood disease **scrofuloderma**, characterized by enlarged, caseous cervical lymph nodes. *M. bovis* is similar in many respects to *M. tuberculosis*; in the laboratory, it can be distinguished from the latter by its poor growth on Löwenstein-Jensen medium and ready infection of rabbits.

MYCOBACTERIUM LEPRAE

Habitat and Transmission

M. leprae is the agent of leprosy, and some 10 million cases of leprosy exist, mainly in Asia. Humans are the only known hosts of *M. leprae*, which resides mainly in the skin and nerves. Prolonged contact is thought to be the mode of transmission.

Characteristics

Aerobic, acid-fast bacilli (they are not alcohol-fast, i.e., decolourized by alcohol); no known toxins.

Culture and Identification

Cannot be cultured in vitro but grows on the **footpads of mice or armadillos**, yielding chronic granulomas at the inoculation site.

Pathogenicity

The leprosy bacillus causes a slow, progressive, chronic disease that mainly affects the skin and the nerves; the lesions are predominantly seen in the cooler parts of the body. Two forms of leprosy are recognized (Table 19.1).

Lepromatous Leprosy. The **cell-mediated immune response is depressed or absent**; *M. leprae* bacilli are usually seen in large numbers in the lesions and in blood; commonly involves mucosae, especially the nose (Fig. 19.3); leads to much disfigurement.

Tuberculoid Leprosy. Associated with an intense **cell-mediated immune response** to the organisms; principally involves the nerves, with resultant anaesthesia and paraesthesia. Hence, damage to extremities is caused, with resultant loss of fingers and toes (see Chapter 35 for oral manifestations).

Antibiotic Sensitivity and Control

Antileprotic drugs are dapsone, rifampicin and clofazimine; several years of therapy are essential. As drug resistance is a

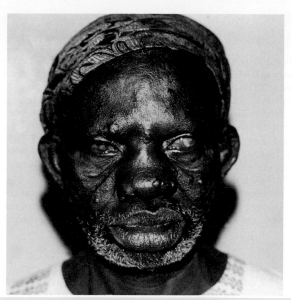

Fig. 19.3 A patient with lepromatous leprosy. Note the saddle nose and associated general disfigurement and blindness.

growing problem, **combination therapy**, as in tuberculosis, is always given. No vaccine is available. Family contacts may be given dapsone.

MYCOBACTERIA OTHER THAN TUBERCULOSIS (MOTT)

MOTT is a collective name given to a group of mycobacteria of low human pathogenicity. These species include *Mycobacterium avium, Mycobacterium intracellulare, Mycobacterium kansasii, Mycobacterium marinum, Mycobacterium fortuitum* and others.

Habitat and Transmission

Isolated from soil, water, birds and animals.

Culture and Identification

Grow on **Löwenstein-Jensen** medium but differ from 'pathogenic' mycobacteria in the colour of pigment produced and temperature requirements. Some species produce pigments in the dark (scotochromogens), others after exposure to light **(photochromogens)**, and still others are nonchromogenic.

Pathogenicity and Antibiotic Sensitivity

In the main, MOTT cause pulmonary infection, often with *M. tuberculosis*; infections are especially seen in compromised individuals (e.g., in those with HIV disease). These mycobacteria are thought to be passengers in the disease process. They are usually sensitive to the normal antituberculous drugs.

M. marinum, associated with the keeping of tropical fish, causes skin ulcers.

Legionella

There are currently some 39 recognized species belonging to the genus *Legionella*, but *Legionella pneumophila*, the species first described, is the most important human pathogen. It causes an **atypical pneumonia** in both community dwellers and hospitalized patients.

LEGIONELLA PNEUMOPHILA

Habitat and Transmission

Ubiquitous organisms found in soil and water, including air-conditioning units, domestic and hospital water supplies, and sometimes in **dental unit water systems**. More than 50 species are known. They survive well within biofilms and free-living amoebae. Spread is known to occur by contaminated aerosols.

Characteristics

Gram-negative slender rods, which stain faintly with the standard Gram stain.

Culture and Identification

Does not grow on ordinary media; grows slowly (3 weeks) in a special medium (cysteine–charcoal–yeast extract agar) under 5% carbon dioxide. Identification is by direct immunofluorescence.

Pathogenicity

The portal of entry is the respiratory tract, and infection results in **legionnaires disease**, a severe form of pneumonia. Patients at risk for infection include the immunocompromised, older men who smoke in excess and have chronic lung disease and diabetics. The clinical picture is variable, ranging from mild influenza-like illness to severe pneumonia with mental confusion, diarrhoea, haematuria and proteinuria. A less severe form of pneumonia **(Pontiac fever)** may be produced by some legionellae.

As there has been some concern that *Legionella* forms biofilms in **stagnant dental unit water lines** and because of the possibility of dental patients acquiring legionellosis through aerosols, dental unit water line hygiene must be maintained at all times (see Chapter 38).

Antibiotic Sensitivity and Control

Erythromycin is the drug of choice and may be combined with rifampicin or ciprofloxacin.

It is impossible to eradicate the organism from water supplies as it is ubiquitous, but protective measures include increasing chlorine concentration and the temperature of hospital water supplies; aerosolization of water should be minimized.

Key Facts

- Mycobacteria are **acid-fast**, beaded bacilli and resist decolourization with strong acids. Hence, a special stain, the **Ziehl-Neelsen stain**, is used to visualize them.
- The aforementioned property is due to the **high lipid content** (40–60%) of the cell wall (mycolic acid), which is also an effective defence mechanism resisting phagocytosis.
- Mycobacterial infections are **chronic**, **granulomatous** (leads to granuloma formation) and insidious.
- *Mycobacterium tuberculosis*, the agent of tuberculosis, is a long, slender, nonsporing, beaded bacillus.
- *M. tuberculosis* grows slowly (up to 6 weeks) in **Löwenstein-Jensen medium** as **'rough, tough and buff'** colonies.
- Humans acquire tuberculosis through inhalation of infested droplet nuclei.

- The increasingly common **multidrug-resistant tuberculosis (MDR-TB)** and **extensive drug-resistant tuberculosis (XTB)** are a global concern.
- **Leprosy**, a disfiguring, chronic illness, is caused by *Mycobacterium leprae*.
- Up to 39 species belonging to the genus *Legionella* are recognized; *Legionella pneumophila* is the most important human pathogen.
- Legionellae are Gram-negative slender rods, but they stain faintly with the standard Gram stain.
- *L. pneumophila* causes **legionnaires disease**, a condition that may range from a mild influenza-like illness to severe pneumonia with mental confusion, especially in the elderly.

Review Questions (Answers on p. 390)

Please indicate which answers are true and which are false.

19.1. Which of the following statements of tuberculosis are true?
   a. *Mycobacterium tuberculosis* is the organism solely responsible for human disease
   b. Pathogenesis is characterized by granuloma formation and multiorgan involvement
   c. tuberculosis is commonly seen in human immunodeficiency virus (HIV) disease
   d. tuberculosis of the oral cavity is often the primary lesion
   e. tuberculosis needs multiple drugs for effective treatment

19.2. Tuberculosis can be diagnosed:
   a. by culturing the organism in Löwenstein-Jensen medium
   b. by the Mantoux test
   c. by using polymerase chain reaction–based tests
   d. by demonstrating acid- and alcohol-fast bacilli in a sputum sample
   e. by isolating the organism from blood cultures

19.3. Leprosy:
   a. may cause facial disfigurement
   b. is caused by *Mycobacterium marinum*
   c. is associated with HIV disease
   d. may lead to deformed extremities
   e. bacillus can be cultured in footpads of mice

19.4. *Legionella pneumophila*:
   a. is a Gram-positive slender rod
   b. causes a debilitating pneumonia in the elderly and alcoholics
   c. are infrequently isolated from dental unit water lines
   d. grows well in routine culture media
   e. is often susceptible to erythromycin

Further Reading

Bagg, J. (1996). Tuberculosis: A re-emerging problem for health care workers. *British Dental Journal, 180,* 376–381.

Bayani, M., Raisolvaezin, K., Almasi-Hashiani, A. et al. (2023). Bacterial biofilm prevalence in dental unit waterlines: a systematic review and meta-analysis. BMC Oral Health 23, 158. https://doi.org/10.1186/s12903-023-02885-4.

Ricci, M. L., Fontana, S., Pinci, F., et al. (2012). Pneumonia associated with a dental unit waterline. *Lancet, 379,* 684.

Sanyaolu, A., Schwartz, J., Roberts, K., Evora, J., Dhother, K., Scurto, F., Lamech, S., Rungteranoont, T., Desai, V., Dicks, C., Dimarco, C., & Patel, S. (2019). Tuberculosis: A review of current trends. *Epidemiology International Journal, 3*(2), 000123. doi:10.23880/eij-16000123.

20 | Chlamydiae, Rickettsiae and Mycoplasmas

Chlamydiae, rickettsiae and mycoplasmas are a miscellaneous group of organisms with properties common to both bacteria and viruses. Although they are categorized together in this chapter for the sake of convenience, they differ markedly from each other and cause divergent human diseases. A comparison of bacteria, chlamydiae, rickettsiae, mycoplasmas and viruses is given in Chapter 2, Table 2.1.

Chlamydiae

The chlamydiae are a group of microorganisms **related to Gram-negative bacteria.** However, unlike bacteria, they are unable to grow on inanimate culture media. They are therefore **obligatory intracellular parasites**. Their main characteristics include the following:

- **larger than most viruses** and hence visible by light microscopy
- both DNA and RNA are present
- **obligate intracellular parasites** with a complex growth cycle
- sensitive to tetracycline, erythromycin, sulphonamides. There are three species in the genus *Chlamydia*:
- *Chlamydia trachomatis*—an agent of many diseases (see below)
- *Chlamydia pneumoniae*—causes acute respiratory tract infection, including sore throat, mild pneumonia and fever in humans
- *Chlamydia psittaci*—primarily causes disease **(psittacosis)** in birds such as pet parrots and budgerigars, from which humans contract the infection; the human infection, also known as psittacosis, takes the form of a **primary atypical pneumonia.**

CHLAMYDIA TRACHOMATIS

Causes a spectrum of diseases:

- **ocular infections**: neonatal conjunctivitis (blennorrhoea), keratoconjunctivitis, blindness (trachoma); trachoma is a major cause of blindness in the developing world
- **genital infections**: nonspecific urethritis, the most common sexually transmitted disease in the UK; causes lymphogranuloma venereum in the tropics
- **pneumonia**: in neonates.

Culture and Diagnosis

Identified by **tissue culture** (e.g., HeLa cells), **serology** (complement fixation test) and **fluorescent antibody staining** of smears from the lesion. Nucleic acid amplification tests (NAATs) are now the choice for genital *Chlamydia trachomatis* infections.

Antibiotic Sensitivity

Tetracycline is effective for all chlamydial infections.

Rickettsiae

Rickettsiae are pleomorphic coccobacilli **smaller but similar to Gram-negative bacteria** resembling them structurally and metabolically; they do not stain with Gram stain. They, like *Chlamydia* and viruses, are **obligate intracellular parasites**. The best-known human rickettsial disease is **typhus**, which spreads wildly in conditions of malnutrition and poverty. Rickettsiae are:

- coccobacilli, with a multilayered outer cell wall resembling that of Gram-negative bacteria
- obligate intracellular parasites that replicate by binary fission
- **visible by light microscope** when special stains are used (e.g., Giemsa)
- able to infect many species, including arthropods, birds and mammals; members of the genus are transmitted to humans via bites of infected arthropods
- sensitive to tetracycline and chloramphenicol.

There are two genera within the Rickettsiae: *Rickettsia* and *Coxiella*.

RICKETTSIA

Rickettsial diseases include:

- **typhus**, an acute febrile illness, now rare, with a maculopapular rash transmitted by the rat flea; the fatality rate is frequently high as a result of haemorrhagic complications
- **spotted fevers**: Rocky Mountain spotted fever and other tickborne fevers.

COXIELLA

Coxiella burnetii, an organism closely resembling rickettsiae, causes **Q fever**, a typhus-like illness. Usually Q fever presents as a 'nonbacterial' pneumonia, but lesions may be seen in the brain and other organs, including the heart, with resultant infective endocarditis.

Culture and Diagnosis

- grows well in all culture lines and yolk sac
- serology: rising titre of antibody in paired sera
- molecular identification methods are now common.

Antibiotic Sensitivity

Tetracycline or doxycycline.

Mycoplasmas

Mycoplasmas are the **smallest prokaryotes capable of binary fission,** and they grow, albeit slowly, on inanimate media. There are more than 200 species of these cell wall–free bacteria considered to be parasites living within eukaryotic cells. They **do not possess a peptidoglycan cell wall** and are bound by a plasma membrane consisting of lipids and sterols (including cholesterol derived from the host cell). Hence, they are highly **pleomorphic**. They cause both human and animal diseases and are normal commensals of human mucous membranes, including the oral cavity.

The most important species of the genus *Mycoplasma* is *Mycoplasma pneumoniae*, which causes:

- a common pneumonia, **atypical pneumonia**
- **mucocutaneous eruptions,** including the oral mucosa
- **haemolytic anaemia.**

MYCOPLASMA PNEUMONIAE

Primary Atypical Pneumonia

Primary atypical pneumonia takes the form of fever, nonproductive cough, severe headache, weakness and tiredness; it is an important cause of community-acquired pneumonia. The acute illness lasts for about 2 weeks but, in a majority, the symptoms last longer.

Mucocutaneous Eruptions

M. pneumoniae may cause skin rashes and ulcerations of both the **oral and vaginal mucosae**. These appear as maculopapular, vesicular or erythematous eruptions. The skin lesions, which often affect the extremities, have a target or iris appearance (**target lesions**). In the oral mucosa, erythematous patches may appear first, quickly becoming bullous and erosive. This leads to extensive blood encrustations, especially the labial lesions. When the oral ulceration is associated with the skin rash and conjunctivitis, it is called **Stevens-Johnson syndrome**.

Culture and Diagnosis

Mycoplasma can be cultured in special media but is a slow grower (about 10 days); the colonies have a characteristic **'fried-egg'** appearance. Immunofluorescence of colonies transferred to glass slides is useful (as they do not take up the Gram stain well).

Serology is useful as the culture results are delayed. Complement fixation testing for *M. pneumoniae* antibodies is diagnostic. Nucleic acid amplification tests (NAATs) are increasingly being employed for laboratory diagnosis.

Antibiotic Sensitivity

Tetracycline for adults and erythromycin for children.

ORAL MYCOPLASMAS

Mycoplasmas have been isolated from saliva, oral mucosa, periodontal pockets and plaque biofilm, both in health and disease, but their **significance is not clear.** Estimates of the oral carriage of mycoplasma vary from 6–32%, and they appear to exist as oral commensals in some adults. The oral species are poorly characterized and include *Mycoplasma buccale*, *Mycoplasma orale* and *Mycoplasma salivarium*. The latter two species have been isolated from salivary glands and are thought to play a role in salivary gland hypofunction. Based on the consistent demonstration of Mycoplasma in oral leukoplakia, some have suggested a causal role for *M. salivarium* in oral leukoplakia.

Key Facts

- **Chlamydiae** are obligatory **intracellular parasites** related to Gram-negative bacteria.
- *Chlamydia trachomatis* causes **ocular** (neonatal conjunctivitis, keratoconjunctivitis, blindness: trachoma), **genital** (nonspecific urethritis, lymphogranuloma venereum) and **respiratory** tract (pneumonia) infections.
- Rickettsiae are tiny coccobacilli resembling Gram-negative bacteria and, like chlamydiae, are obligatory intracellular parasites.
- All members of the genus *Rickettsia* **are transmitted** to humans **by bites** of infected **arthropods.**
- **Rickettsial diseases** include **typhus**, an acute febrile illness (frequently fatal) with a maculopapular rash.
- **Mycoplasmas** are the **smallest prokaryotes** capable of binary fission and exist as **pleomorphic** morphological forms (as they lack a peptidoglycan cell wall).

- *Mycoplasma pneumoniae* is an important human pathogen and causes atypical pneumonia, haemolytic anaemia and mucocutaneous eruptions.
- Mucocutaneous eruptions often affect the extremities and have a target or iris appearance (target lesions).
- The **oral mucosal lesions** of *M. pneumoniae* appear erythematous at first and quickly become **bullous** and **erosive**, leading to extensive **blood encrustations.**
- **Oral mycoplasmas** (*Mycoplasma buccale, Mycoplasma orale, Mycoplasma salivarium*) have been **isolated from saliva, oral mucosa, periodontal pockets** and **plaque biofilm**, but their significance in either health or disease is unclear.

Review Questions (Answers on p. 390)

Please indicate which answers are true and which are false.

20.1. Chlamydial infections:
   a. may cause primary atypical pneumonia
   b. can lead to blindness
   c. are the commonest cause of nongonococcal urethritis
   d. are diagnosed by culturing the organism on selective agar media
   e. are treated by tetracycline

20.2. Rickettsiae:
   a. are obligatory intracellular parasites
   b. commonly have an arthropod vector
   c. cause spotted fevers
   d. infections are often diagnosed by serological tests
   e. infections are best treated with cephalosporins

20.3. Mycoplasma:
   a. are highly pleomorphic obligatory intracellular parasites
   b. cause oral mucosal ulcerations
   c. skin lesions have characteristic target appearance
   d. cannot be grown in vitro
   e. infections in children are treated by erythromycin

Further Reading

Brooks, J. F., Carroll, K. C., Butel, J. S., et al. (Eds.). (2013). *Chlamydia* spp. In *Jawetz, Melnick & Adelberg's medical microbiology* (26th ed., pp. 359–368). McGraw Hill.

Brooks, J. F., Carroll, K. C., Butel, J. S., et al. (Eds.). (2019a). *Mycoplasma* and cell wall-defective bacteria. In *Jawetz, Melnick & Adelberg's medical microbiology* (28th ed., pp. 341–345). McGraw Hill.

Brooks, J. F., Carroll, K. C., Butel, J. S., et al. (Eds.). (2019b). *Rickettsia* and related genera. In *Jawetz, Melnick & Adelberg's medical microbiology* (28th ed., pp. 349–356). McGraw Hill.

Vyhnalova, T., Danek, Z., Gachova, D., & Linhartova, P. B. (2021, July). The role of the oral microbiota in the etiopathogenesis of oral squamous cell carcinoma. *Microorganisms*, 9(8), 1549. doi:10.3390/microorganisms9081549.

21 Viruses of Relevance to Dentistry

DNA Viruses

This chapter gives an outline of the viruses that are of special relevance to dentistry. The DNA viruses are described first, followed by the RNA viruses (see Table 4.1).

PAPOVAVIRUSES

These DNA viruses infect both humans and animals; however, human disease is infrequent.

Human Papillomavirus

Human papillomavirus (HPV) is one of the **most common sexually transmitted viruses** causing transient or persistent infection (see Chapter 37). The majority of HPV infections are asymptomatic and resolve spontaneously, though persistent infections can develop into **anogenital or oropharyngeal cancers**.

The oral cavity is considered a reservoir of the virus. Intraoral lesions caused by HPV include oral papillomas, oral verrucous carcinomas and focal epithelial hyperplasia. **Over 200 different genotypes** of HPV have been identified, some of which are more closely associated with lesions (both benign and cancerous) than others. HPV commonly causes skin warts (verrucae).

Skin Warts

- **Clinical features**: warts typically are benign epithelial tumours. Specific serological types of HPV are associated with anogenital warts (condylomata acuminata) and are seen in all cervical biopsies that show precancerous change.

- **Epidemiology**: warts are generally more common in children than in adults. The virus is likely to be transmitted by direct contact or autoinoculation.

Oral Infections With HPV. Over 40% of healthy individuals have HPV in the normal oral mucosa sometime over their lifetime, suggesting that the **oral mucosa is a reservoir** of the virus. A number of HPV genotypes preferentially colonize the oral mucosa, and some of these—such as **HPV-16, HPV-18 and HPV-31**—can cause oral precancers or cancers (Fig. 21.1).

Oral Squamous Papillomas and Warts

- **Clinical features**: most are single, small (1 cm), pedunculated, exophytic lesions (Fig. 21.2). They rarely, if ever, progress to carcinomas.
- **Epidemiology**: occur mainly in the third to fifth decades of life, with a male preponderance.

Verrucous Carcinoma. There is evidence to indicate that HPV is associated with human carcinomas, on the basis of:

- the frequent malignant change in virus-induced warts in **epidermodysplasia verruciformis**
- the frequent association of **HPV-16, -18 and -31** with invasive cervical cancer
- development of cancer in vulvar warts in women with lymphoma

Prevention. Vaccination prevents HPV infection, benefitting both the vaccinated person and their future sex partners by preventing the spread of HPV. HPV transmission can be reduced, but not eliminated, with the consistent and correct use of physical barriers such as condoms.

A highly efficacious HPV vaccine is now available. It is administered as a two- or three-dose series, depending on age at initiation and the medical condition of the recipient.

ADENOVIRUSES

These DNA viruses induce **latent infections** of the tonsils, adenoids (hence the name *adenoviruses*) and other lymphoid tissues of humans. However, most infections caused by adenoviruses are acute and self-limiting.

Adenoviral Diseases

Acute respiratory disease is the most common adenovirus infection. It is an influenzalike illness seen commonly in military training camps. Clinically, the main symptoms are **pharyngitis and conjunctivitis**. Although self-limiting, acute respiratory disease may be complicated by pneumonia in some cases. Other infections caused by these viruses include pharyngoconjunctival fever (a disease of infants and children), epidemic keratoconjunctivitis, pneumonia and gastroenteritis.

Epidemiology. Adenoviruses are ubiquitous, and human beings are the only known reservoir for the human strains. The infections are spread from person to person by

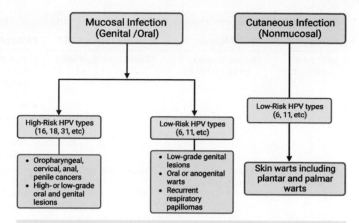

Fig. 21.1 **Broad categorization of human papillomavirus infections and the associated virus types.**

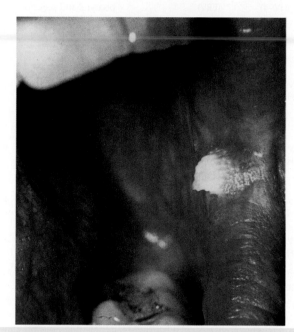

Fig. 21.2 **A papilloma at the angle of the mouth.**

respiratory and ocular secretions. Adequate chlorination of pools may help decrease the spread of pharyngoconjunctival fever.

HERPESVIRUSES

There are a range of different human herpesviruses (HSVs), currently numbered 1–8 (Table 21.1). All of them are structurally similar (enveloped, icosahedral with double-stranded DNA) and infect both humans and animals. They are the **most common causes of human viral infections**. All have the important property of remaining **latent**, with the ability to **reinfect the host** a variable period after the primary infection. Important human pathogens include herpes simplex virus types 1 and 2 (HSV-1 and HSV-2), varicella-zoster virus (VZV), Epstein-Barr virus (EBV) and cytomegalovirus (CMV; see Chapter 4). **Dental science**

Table 21.1   Human Herpesvirus (HHV) Classification and Clinical Epidemiology[a]

Name	Trivial Name	Primary Target Cell	Pathophysiology	Site of Latency	Means of Spread
HHV type 1 (HHV–1)	Herpes simplex virus-1 (HSV-1)	Mucosal and epithelial	Predominantly orofacial (above the belt infections); occasionally genital or other herpes simplex infections ■ *Primary oral infection:* herpetic gingivostomatitis ■ *Reactivation/recurrent oral infection:* herpes labialis (cold sores/ fever blisters)	Neurone	Close contact (oral or sexually transmitted infection)
HHV type 2 (HHV–2)	Herpes simplex virus-2 (HSV-2)	Mucosal and epithelial	Predominantly genital (below-the-belt infections); occasionally orofacial or other herpes simplex infections	Neurone	Close contact (oral or sexually transmitted disease)
HHV type 3 (HHV–3)	Varicella-zoster virus (VZV)	Mucosal and epithelial	Primary infection: ■ Chickenpox (varicella) ■ Reactivation/recurrent infection: shingles (herpes zoster)	Neurone	Respiratory and close contact (including sexually transmitted disease)
HHV type 4 (HHV–4)	Epstein-Barr virus (EBV)	Epithelial cells of oro-pharynx and parotid gland; B cells	■ Infectious mononucleosis ■ Burkitt lymphoma and other B cell lymphomas ■ Nasopharyngeal carcinoma ■ Oral hairy leukoplakia ■ Posttransplant lymphoproliferative diseases	B cell	Close contact, transfusions, tissue transplant and congenital
HHV type 5 (HHV–5)	Human cytomegalovirus (HCMV)	Monocyte, lymphocyte and epithelial cells of the respiratory tract, salivary glands and kidneys	May infect foetus during pregnancy leading to neurological sequelae, such as deafness and mental retardation	Monocyte, lymphocyte and possibly other cells	Saliva, urine, blood, breast milk
HHV type 6 (HHV–6)	*Roseolovirus*, herpes lymphotropic virus	T cells and possibly other cells	■ Sixth disease (roseola infantum or exanthem subitum) ■ Mononucleosis with cervical lymphadenopathy	T cells and possibly other cells	Possibly respiratory and close contact
HHV type 7 (HHV–7)	Nil	T cells and possibly other cells	Possibly associated with roseola infantum or exanthem subitum as HHV-6	T cells and possibly other cells	Yet unknown
HHV type 8 (HHV–8)	Kaposi sarcoma–associated herpesvirus (KSHV)	Lymphocytes and other cells	Kaposi sarcoma, primary effusion lymphoma, some types of multicentric Castleman disease	B cell	Close contact (sexual), possibly saliva

[a]Please also refer to Table 4.3.

students should be thoroughly conversant with the **herpes group of viruses**, as the majority of them either cause oral infection or are intimately associated with orofacial tissues and saliva.

Structure

See Chapter 4.

HUMAN HERPESVIRUSES 1 AND 2

There are two types of HSV: **human herpesvirus type 1 (HSV-1) and type 2 (HSV-2)**. They can be differentiated by serotyping, by DNA homology and, to some extent, by clinical disease pattern.

Clinical Disease

Disease due to HSV can be either a **primary infection**, due to first encounter with the virus, or a **reactivation** or **recurrent infection**, due to activation of the latent virus.

Primary Infection. There is an incubation period of 2–20 days, depending upon the infected site and the infecting strain of virus. The lesions include:

■ **primary gingivostomatitis** with lesions on the lips and mouth; very common (see Chapter 35)
■ **genital herpes**: vesicular eruption of the genitalia, mostly due to HSV-2 (but up to one-third of the cases may be due to HSV-1)
■ **herpetic whitlow**: infection of the fingers, acquired by dentists and nurses as a result of contamination of the hands by virus-laced saliva or other secretions (Fig. 21.3)
■ **conjunctivitis and keratitis**: less commonly, HSV infections involve the eyes, sometimes leading to blindness
■ **encephalitis**: a result of either primary or recurrent infection; may lead to permanent defects or death.

Recurrent Infections. Recurrence or reactivation of HSV entails activation of the noninfectious form of the latent

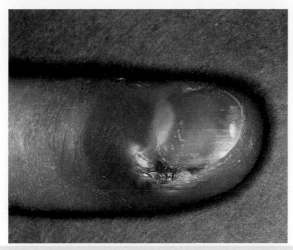

Fig. 21.3   A herpetic whitlow in a dentist caused by herpes simplex virus.

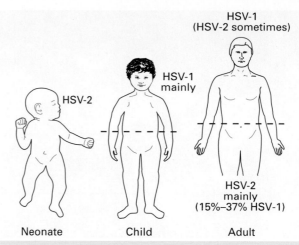

Fig. 21.5   Predominant distribution of infection with herpes simplex virus types 1 and 2 (HSV-1 and HSV-2, respectively), in different age groups.

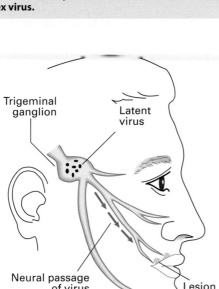

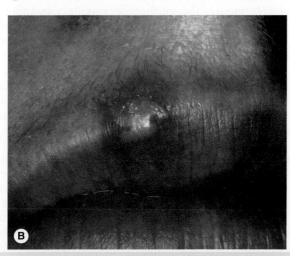

Fig. 21.4   Herpes labialis: (A) recurrence of facial herpes infection due to reactivation of the latent virus in the trigeminal ganglion; (B) clinical presentation of herpes labialis on the mucocutaneous junction of the upper lip.

virus residing in **the neurons of either the trigeminal ganglion** (Fig. 21.4) or the **sacral ganglia**. Reactivation is provoked by menstruation, stress, sunlight (possibly ultraviolet rays), and local trauma; the lesions tend to recur at the site of the primary lesion. HSV has been implicated in **Bell palsy**.

Epidemiology. Humans are the only known reservoir for HSV-1 and HSV-2; experimental infection can be induced in animals and cell cultures. As the virus is highly labile, most primary infections are acquired through **direct contact with a lesion or contaminated secretions**. In general, HSV-1 causes orofacial lesions or lesions 'above the belt', whereas HSV-2 causes lesions 'below the belt'—that is, genital herpes (Fig. 21.5). However, because of sexual promiscuity or for other reasons, this may not be always true. HSV-1 is acquired early in life, whereas HSV-2 appears after the onset of sexual activity.

As recurrent infection is common in the presence of high antibody titres, circulating antibodies appear to be unhelpful in controlling HSV infection. One reason for this may be the contiguous cell-to-cell spread of the virus, which cannot be prevented by antibody. Reactivation is not accompanied by a rise in herpes antibody titre.

Diagnosis. Diagnosis is usually achieved clinically; laboratory diagnosis is useful to confirm infection, especially in compromised patients. This entails:

■ performing **polymerase chain reaction (PCR)** assays, which are sensitive, and specific assays that are now commonly used for diagnosis; the most reliable diagnostic method

The traditional and more cumbersome techniques, now out of favour, are:

■ direct demonstration of **viral antigens** in vesicular fluid or scrapings by electron microscopy or immunofluorescence (Fig. 21.6)

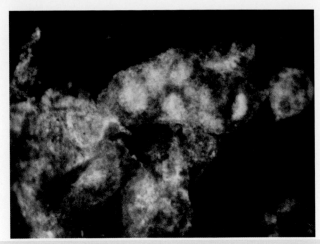

Fig. 21.6 Positive immunofluorescence of a smear taken from the lip lesion shown in Fig. 21.3(B) (stained with antiherpes antibody tagged to a fluorescing chemical), indicating that the patient has herpes labialis.

- demonstration of characteristic **multinuclear giant cells** in scrapings from lesions—simple but not always successful
- **propagation** of virus in tissue culture.

Prevention. Control is difficult because of the high frequency of asymptomatic infection. It is important to routinely wear gloves to avoid contact with acute herpetic lesions and contaminated body fluid (e.g., saliva). No vaccine is available.

Treatment. The course of primary infection can be altered significantly with drugs that interfere with viral DNA synthesis, such as **aciclovir** and **vidarabine**, but these should be administered in the early prodromal phase of the disease for best results (see also Chapter 35).

VARICELLA-ZOSTER VIRUS (HUMAN HERPESVIRUS 3)

This organism causes both **varicella** (chickenpox) and **herpes zoster** (shingles): two different diseases due to an identical organism. Chickenpox is the primary infection, and herpes zoster is the reactivation of illness.

Clinical Disease

Varicella. A common childhood fever, varicella is mild and self-limiting. The disease is more severe if contracted in adulthood. After a 2-week incubation period, fever develops, followed by a papular rash of the skin and mucous membranes, including the oral mucosa. The papules rapidly become vesicular and itchy but painless (in contrast to the rash in zoster).

Zoster (Shingles). Zoster (shingles) occurs primarily as a reactivation of the virus in dorsal root or cranial nerve (usually trigeminal) ganglia (Fig. 21.7). The disease usually affects adults, and the virus is reactivated despite circulating antibodies. Zoster is triggered by trauma, drugs, neoplastic disease or immunosuppression.

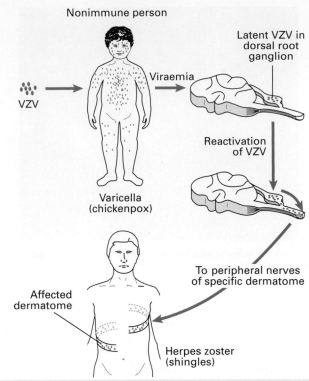

Fig. 21.7 Pathogenesis and sequelae of varicella-zoster virus (VZV) infection.

The virus remains latent in ganglionic nerve cells and, after activation, travels back along the nerve fibre to the skin. Thoracic nerves supplying the chest wall are most often affected, and the lesion presents as a unilateral, painful vesicular rash, which extends in a horizontal strip from the middle of the back around the side of the chest wall ('belt of roses from hell'). Fever and malaise accompany the lesion. The rash may last for 2–4 weeks, with pain (**postherpetic neuralgia**) persisting for weeks or months.

The **trigeminal nerve** is affected in about 15% of cases, with involvement of the ophthalmic, maxillary and mandibular divisions (in that order of precedence). Severe localized oral pain precedes the rash and may be easily confused with toothache (see Chapter 35). Involvement of the ophthalmic nerve may lead to eye lesions and sometimes blindness.

Ramsay Hunt syndrome is a rare manifestation of zoster, with a vesicular rash on the tympanic membrane and the external auditory canal, together with unilateral facial nerve palsy.

Epidemiology. Shingles is primarily a disease of older adults and immunocompromised persons; it is rare in children. The incidence increases with advancing age and with decreasing degree of immunocompetence. It is a highly contagious infection in a host not previously exposed to the virus. Transmission occurs by direct contact with skin lesions or droplet infection from infectious saliva.

Diagnosis. The clinical picture is pathognomonic, as the lesion distribution overlaps and accurately maps the

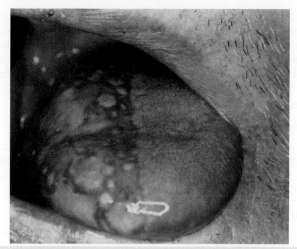

Fig. 21.8 Herpes zoster infection of the tongue in an elderly patient: note the sharp midline demarcation of the lesion (due to reactivation of the virus travelling via the lingual branch of the right trigeminal nerve).

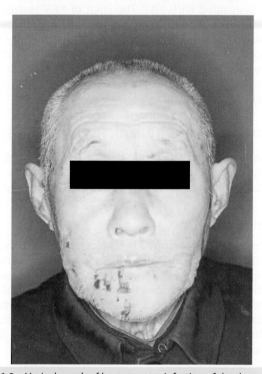

Fig. 21.9 Vesicular rash of herpes zoster infection of the dermatome of the right mandibular division of the trigeminal nerve in an elderly patient. Note the sharp demarcation of skin infection accurately reflecting the distribution of the nerve, a feature pathognomonic of herpes zoster infection.

distribution of the sensory nerve (Figs. 21.8 and 21.9). Laboratory diagnostic methods include:

- sensitive and specific **PCR**
- **serology**, if needed, that entails detecting a fourfold rise in antibody titre in paired sera (compare herpes simplex reactivation, where antibody rise is not significant)
- cytopathology investigations that include staining (Tzanck smear) a scraping from the base of vesicles for the presence of multinucleated giant cells.

Treatment. Chickenpox is self-limiting and requires symptomatic treatment, if any. Disseminated zoster in immunocompromised patients requires antiviral drugs (e.g., aciclovir, vidarabine), which interfere with herpesvirus DNA replication. VZV is less sensitive to aciclovir than is HSV, and hence a higher dosage is required; therapy should start within 72 h of onset. Systemic aciclovir may reduce the duration of the early infective phase and the associated pain. In addition it may reduce the prevalence of postherpetic neuralgia.

Prevention. Passive immunization with varicella-zoster immune globulin (VZIG) may be indicated for persons at high risk of severe infection. A vaccine for chickenpox and zoster, which is extremely effective against developing severe disease, is now available. The vaccine could also be administered with the measles–mumps–rubella (MMR) vaccine as a combined vaccine (MMRV vaccine).

The vaccine regimes for adults and children are different.

EPSTEIN-BARR VIRUS (HUMAN HERPESVIRUS 4)

Epstein-Barr virus (EBV) is widespread in humans. Up to 20% of healthy adults will yield virus-positive **throat washings**, and most adults have antibody to the virus; it is present in the saliva of many immunosuppressed patients. The virus persists in latent form within lymphocytes after primary infection (**lymphotropic**, unlike HSV and VZV, which are neurotropic). The genome resides in a latent form in B cells; latent EBV infection is common in the population. It is the aetiological agent of a number of diseases:

- infectious mononucleosis (glandular fever)
- Burkitt lymphoma and other B cell lymphomas
- nasopharyngeal carcinoma (especially in southern Chinese populations)
- oral hairy leukoplakia
- posttransplant lymphoproliferative diseases.

Infectious Mononucleosis

An **acute infection** affecting lymphoid tissue throughout the body, infectious mononucleosis is commonly seen in teenagers, with a peak incidence at 15–20 years of age. The organism is present in saliva and is thought to be transmitted during kissing, and hence it is called the **'kissing disease'**.

Incubation Period. Incubation is 4–7 weeks, possibly shorter (10–40 days) in young children.

Signs and Symptoms. Low-grade fever with generalized lymphadenopathy and **abnormal lymphocytes** in the blood (note that a similar illness, a glandular feverlike syndrome, develops during the first fortnight after infection with human immunodeficiency virus (HIV)). Fever, tonsillitis and fatigue are common, and many patients have splenomegaly. Lymphocytosis is a characteristic feature, hence the term 'mononucleosis'; some 10% of the lymphocytes are atypical, with enlarged misshapen nuclei and increased cytoplasm (Fig. 21.10).

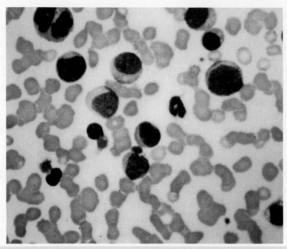

Fig. 21.10 Infectious mononucleosis: characteristic blood film with many mononuclear cells. Note the enlarged dark staining nuclei and misshapen cells.

Chronic, Persistent or Reactivated EBV Infection

This may take many clinical forms and is less common than acute mononucleosis (previously described). The syndrome is characterized by persistent fatigue, with or without physical or laboratory findings.

Epidemiology. The virus is ubiquitous, and humans are its only known host. Spread of EBV is via respiratory secretions, primarily through oral contact. Those from lower socioeconomic classes are exposed to EBV at an early age and typically develop asymptomatic infections, whereas in higher socioeconomic classes, particularly in developed countries, primary infection is usually delayed to adolescence or young adulthood.

Diagnosis. As EBV cannot be easily propagated in culture, serological diagnosis is common:

- **PCR** assays have supplanted traditional virus isolation techniques.
- **Indirect immunofluorescence** is used to detect EBV-specific immunoglobulin M (IgM); the antibody is directed against both the capsid antigen and a noncapsid early antigen.
- **Haematology**: a blood film is useful for demonstrating **atypical lymphocytosis** in infectious mononucleosis.
- **Serology: heterophile antibody** (nonspecific): infectious mononucleosis is characterized by the appearance of heterophile (*hetero*: other, *phile*: liking) antibodies in the patient's serum, which agglutinate sheep or horse red blood cells. This property is made use of in the **Paul-Bunnell diagnostic test**.

Treatment. Infectious mononucleosis is generally mild and self-limiting; hence, therapy is usually symptomatic.

Burkitt Lymphoma

Burkitt lymphoma is a highly **malignant tumour** that spreads rapidly, with widespread metastases; it is particularly common in African children. The disease is especially common in areas of Africa with endemic malaria. Hence, it is thought that the effect of the malarial parasite on the reticuloendothelial system could cause an abnormal response to infection with EBV. Under these conditions, the EBV may become frankly **oncogenic**, producing a malignant transformation in lymphoid tissue (lymphoma) instead of the benign proliferation seen in infectious mononucleosis.

Nasopharyngeal Carcinoma

A tumour with a remarkable geographic and probably racial distribution, it is particularly common among the southern Chinese. EBV DNA is regularly present in the malignant epithelial cells of the tumour.

Hairy Leukoplakia

The term 'hairy leukoplakia' is given to raised, white areas of thickening, particularly on the lateral border of the tongue (see Fig. 30.3). Although this new clinical entity was first described in HIV-infected patients, other immunosuppressed patients may develop the lesion, which is very closely associated with EBV. The DNA of EBV is present in the epithelial cells of hairy leukoplakia. The lesion is **nonmalignant**, but about one-third of HIV-infected individuals who develop hairy leukoplakia may develop acquired immune deficiency syndrome (AIDS) in 3–5 years. Demonstration of **EBV in biopsy tissue** of hairy leukoplakia is essential for a definitive diagnosis.

CYTOMEGALOVIRUS (HUMAN HERPESVIRUS 5)

Cytomegalovirus (CMV) rarely causes disease unless other precipitating factors, such as immunocompromising states, are present. However, it can infect the foetus during pregnancy.

Clinical Disease

Symptomless Infection. The majority of **infants** show no signs of infection, and **diagnosis is made by serology**. Although a large proportion of the infants are unharmed, a significant number of neonates with congenital infection show neurological sequelae, such as **deafness and mental retardation**, later in life. A minority develop a severe, often fatal illness associated with infection of the salivary glands, brain, kidneys, liver and lungs.

Postnatal Infection. Later in life, CMV may be activated by pregnancy, multiple blood transfusions or immunosuppression. Infection in immunocompromised patients can be severe and involve many organs, such as the lungs, liver, gastrointestinal tract and eyes.

Epidemiology. Infection appears to increase during the **perinatal period** and during early adulthood; patients with **neoplastic disease or AIDS and transplant recipients** often have local and disseminated CMV disease. The route of CMV transmission is not clear.

Diagnosis and Treatment. Diagnosis is by viral isolation in human embryonic fibroblast tissue cultures; it is confirmed using immunofluorescence and DNA hybridization.

There are no proven regimens for therapy and prevention of CMV infections.

HUMAN HERPESVIRUS 6 (ROSEOLA VIRUS; HERPES LYMPHOTROPIC VIRUS)

A DNA virus closely related to CMV, human herpesvirus 6 (HHV-6) was originally isolated from peripheral blood cells of immunocompromised patients, such as those with AIDS. The virus shows affinity for T and B cells in particular. Infection with HHV-6 is common in childhood, and most **primary infections are asymptomatic** followed by latency. The pathogenicity of HHV-6 is as yet unclear. Recently, it has been found in active plaques in patients with multiple sclerosis.

Exanthem Subitum (Roseola Infantum)

This common childhood disorder characterized by **mild fever and a facial rash** appears to be associated with HHV-6 infection. The disease exanthema subitum is also called roseola infantum ('roseola of children') or **'sixth disease'**.

Mononucleosis With Cervical Lymphadenopathy

This is a febrile illness in adults with bilateral cervical lymphadenopathy, somewhat like glandular fever; it is thought to be a primary infection with HHV-6.

HHV-6 and the Oral Cavity

The virus is present in the saliva of most healthy adults, and it can also be demonstrated in ductal and alveolar epithelium of major salivary glands. There are **no specific oral lesions reported for HHV-6**, though erythematous papules seen in soft palate and uvula (**Nagayama spots**) and in the pharynx are thought to be due to this organism. No occupational hazard from HHV-6 has been proved in dentistry, but the virus may well be transmitted in saliva.

HUMAN HERPESVIRUSES 7 AND 8 (KAPOSI SARCOMA–ASSOCIATED HERPESVIRUS)

These viruses have been recently identified: human herpesvirus 7 (HHV-7) is a T-lymphotropic virus and is implicated in rashes; human herpesvirus 8 (HHV-8) is the agent responsible for **Kaposi sarcoma**, a vascular endothelial tumour commonly seen in HIV disease (see Chapter 30); it is also implicated in sarcoidosis.

The relatively recent discovery of these new herpesviruses in individuals with HIV disease suggests that there are more herpesviruses yet to be uncovered. These viruses appear to be evolving in humans and primates. HHV-6 and HHV-7, in particular, are found in 70–90% of the population and hence considered universal herpesviruses.

RNA Viruses

ORTHOMYXOVIRIDAE

These RNA viruses cause worldwide epidemics of **influenza**. They are subdivided into types A, B and C on the basis of the antigenic properties of their major **nucleocapsid protein (NP)** and viral envelope **matrix protein (M protein)**. In addition to these antigenic differences, they are characterized by a unique mechanism of frequent immunological variations within the subtypes. These variations are due to structural changes in the surface spike glycoproteins: **haemagglutinin (H antigen)** and **neuraminidase (N antigen)**. The nomenclature of influenza viruses is based on the H and N antigens. For instance, the first pandemic influenza virus was called H1N1, and the current avian flu virus is H5N1. Influenza epidemics are due to the emergence of a new virus strain containing a haemagglutinin (and sometimes a neuraminidase) that differs from that of previously circulating viruses, so that the population has no (herd) immunity to the new haemagglutinin. Antigenic variation may occur due to:

- **antigenic drift**, as a result of minor changes in the amino acid sequence of the haemagglutinin; these viruses survive because they are less susceptible to the antibodies most common in the population at the time
- **antigenic shift**, which constitutes the appearance of a new antigenic type unrelated or only distantly related to earlier types because of **genetic reassortment**; it occurs infrequently and has only been identified in influenza A (four major antigenic shifts have occurred since 1933).

These antigenic shifts are critically important in the production of vaccines for influenza: the vaccine used in previous years may have little or no effect because of these phenomena.

INFLUENZA

Clinical Features

Symptoms of influenza are sudden and appear 1–2 days after exposure. Major symptoms are high fever, accompanied by myalgia, sore throat, headache, cough and nasal congestion. Pneumonia is the most common serious complication; it is caused by secondary bacterial infection of the respiratory tract with weakened defences.

Epidemiology. Epidemic illness is common in nonimmune or partially immune populations. Transmission occurs by aerosolization and subsequent inhalation of virus-laden respiratory secretions during sneezing and coughing (**droplet spread**). Rapid spread of illness may occur in confined populations (e.g., nursing homes, classrooms).

Treatment and Prevention. Only symptomatic treatment is indicated. **Amantadine** is helpful for relieving symptoms and enhancing the effectiveness of immunization. The low success rate (about 70%) of the vaccination is mainly due to the difficulty of predicting the proper antigenic profile of the influenza strain; this unfortunately cannot be determined until the onset of the particular disease cycle.

AVIAN INFLUENZA OR BIRD FLU (H5N1 VIRUS)

The first known cases of avian influenza caused by H5N1 were discovered in Hong Kong in 1997, and since then sporadic outbreaks have occurred, mainly in Southeast Asia. Usually, such infections are preceded by lethal outbreaks of H5N1 influenza in waterfowl, which are the natural hosts of these viruses and therefore normally have asymptomatic infection. The acquisition by the viruses of characteristics that enhance virulence in humans and their potential for wider distribution by infected migrating birds have caused renewed pandemic concern. The factors that account for the severe symptoms of viral influenza are still not well understood. However, it is believed that the **cytopathic effects of the virus itself and the cytokines** evoked by the infection account for both local and systemic effects that are life-threatening.

Clinical Features

H5N1 infection and its replication in the respiratory tract have been shown to injure directly the nasal and tracheobronchial epithelium, possibly due to virus-induced cellular apoptosis and resulting loss of respiratory epithelial cells. These may account for symptoms such as cough, depressed tracheobronchial clearance and altered pulmonary function.

Incubation is thought to be 7–12 days after exposure. Major symptoms are high fever, sore throat, headache, chest pain and cough, bleeding nose and gums, and diarrhoea. These may lead to pneumonia, encephalitis and organ failure. The predicted death rate of avian flu ranges from 60% to 90%.

Epidemiology. From 2003 to 2014, a total of 407 persons have died due to bird flu worldwide, mainly in Southeast Asia (death rate: 58%).

Treatment and Prevention. Preventive measures include good personal hygiene, thorough adherence to routine hand-washing, respiratory precautions such as wearing masks and avoiding crowded places during an outbreak. The **routine flu vaccine is ineffective against avian flu**. Drugs such as **oseltamivir** (Tamiflu) reduce the severity of infection if taken within 2 days of initial symptoms. Patients may need quicker and larger doses. In dentistry, additional precautions or transmission-based precautions must be implemented during an outbreak situation (see Chapter 36).

PARAMYXOVIRIDAE

The paramyxoviruses are enveloped, RNA viruses with an unsegmented genome. They cause major diseases of infancy and childhood. There are four groups of paramyxoviruses:

- parainfluenza virus
- mumps virus
- measles virus
- respiratory syncytial virus (RSV).

Parainfluenza and mumps viruses are antigenically related.

PARAINFLUENZA VIRUSES

The parainfluenza viruses cause human respiratory infections, especially in autumn and winter.

Clinical Features

The major diseases caused by parainfluenza viruses, particularly in young children and infants, are laryngotracheobronchitis (croup), bronchiolitis and pneumonia. When adults are infected with any parainfluenza type, the **common cold** is the usual result.

Epidemiology. Parainfluenza viruses are spread through respiratory/droplet secretions. Closed populations, including young children, are especially at risk.

MUMPS VIRUS

Mumps, measles, rubella and varicella (chickenpox) are the common **childhood fevers**. Mumps virus typically causes **parotitis** (mumps) of acute onset involving one or both parotid glands. The attenuated form of the mumps virus, incorporated in the combined **measles–mumps–rubella (MMR) vaccine**, leads to the development of antibody in 95% of vaccines (see also Chapter 35).

MEASLES VIRUS

Another agent of common childhood fever, measles virus causes one of the most highly infectious diseases known. Infection results in permanent immunity.

Clinical Features

Measles is an acute febrile illness with a characteristic **exanthematous rash**. The virus enters through the respiratory tract and multiplies in the respiratory epithelium and regional lymphoid tissue for up to 12 days. In the next (viraemic) phase, the virus spreads throughout the lymphoid tissues and skin. This stage is accompanied by prodromal symptoms: **conjunctivitis, nasal discharge, headache, low-grade fever, sore throat** and **Koplik spots**. The Koplik spots are bluish-white, pinpoint spots surrounded by dark-red areolae, which appear on the buccal mucosa opposite the molar teeth and sometimes near the orifice of the parotid duct. The measles rash appears to result from the interaction between virus-infected cells and either sensitized lymphocytes or antibody–complement complexes. The rash consists of fine, sparse, discrete macules. As the rash develops, the Koplik spots disappear.

Complications. The complications of measles virus infection are serious and could be:

- **respiratory** complications (bronchopneumonia): the most serious; seen in 4% of patients, with or without secondary bacterial infection; **otitis media** occurs in a smaller percentage
- **neurological** complications: including **encephalomyelitis** (with a mortality rate of some 10%) and **subacute sclerosing panencephalitis**; the latter is a rare, progressive, degenerative neurological disease of children and adolescents, causing mental and motor deterioration and death within a year
- **gangrenous stomatitis** and **noma**: seen in certain sub-Saharan African countries; a number of cofactors

such as malnutrition, oral ulceration and acute necrotizing ulcerative gingivitis together with concurrent measles infection lead to progressive gangrene and gross destruction of the orofacial tissues, with consequent disfigurement (see Fig. 33.7).

Epidemiology. Measles is readily transmissible, usually via respiratory secretions and urine, especially during the prodromal phase and when the rash appears.

Prevention. The measles component of the **MMR** vaccine is a live attenuated virus that induces immunity for up to 10 years. However, in developing countries such as West Africa, where universal vaccination in childhood is not feasible, measles remains a severe disease and a major cause of death in childhood.

RESPIRATORY SYNCYTIAL VIRUS

A major agent of lower respiratory tract disease, **respiratory syncytial virus (RSV)** causes worldwide epidemics of respiratory tract infection in infants and young children. Adults, although infected, develop only mild or unapparent symptoms. The virus can cause colds, bronchiolitis and pneumonia, especially during the first 6 months of life. Approximately one-third of infants develop antibodies in the first year of life.

PICORNAVIRIDAE

Picornaviridae are nonenveloped **RNA** viruses with an unsegmented genome. Four members of this family cause significant human disease: polioviruses, coxsackieviruses, echoviruses and rhinoviruses. The first three of these are collectively termed **enteroviruses**.

Polioviruses

Polioviruses are agents of **paralytic poliomyelitis**.

Clinical Features

Poliovirus infection is initiated by **ingestion of infectious virions**, after which primary replication occurs in oropharyngeal and intestinal mucosa. The virus drains into the cervical and mesenteric lymph nodes and then into the systemic circulation. Subsequent replication continues in a number of nonneural sites, leading to a persistent viraemia and spread into the central nervous system.

Paralytic poliomyelitis is unusual and depends on host factors that may predispose individuals to **neural infection**. The incidence and severity of paralytic disease increase with age (e.g., teenagers are more likely than younger children to develop crippling disease).

Epidemiology. Polioviruses have a wide geographic distribution and spread rapidly, especially in densely populated areas with poor sewage control, such as some developing countries. Infection occurs mainly in the hot season and is spread in the faeces. Transmission is primarily by person-to-person contact through pharyngeal secretions, although the disease may spread by infected water.

Prevention. Spread of poliovirus disease has been successfully prevented through widespread immunization with either **killed** (Salk vaccine) or **live attenuated** virus (Sabin vaccine). However, poor immunization practices have led to recent resurgence of the disease in some developing countries.

COXSACKIEVIRUSES

Coxsackieviruses are subdivided into two major groups, **A and B**, on the basis of the lesions they induce in suckling mice. Each group also has several serologically distinct subgroups. Most human coxsackievirus infections are mild and frequently asymptomatic. Serious infection, although rare, results in severe disease. Two diseases caused by **group A coxsackieviruses are of particular dental interest:** herpangina and hand, foot and mouth disease.

HERPANGINA

Herpangina, caused by group A coxsackievirus, is common in children but may affect any age group.

Clinical Features

Herpangina is characterized by fever, headache, sore throat, dysphagia, anorexia and, occasionally, a stiff neck. These symptoms are accompanied by herpeslike oropharyngitis, where the ulceration is predominantly on the tonsil, soft palate and uvula. The small, papulovesicular lesions are about 1–2 mm in diameter, with a greyish-white surface surrounded by red areolae. The disease is self-limiting and lasts for 3–4 days (see also Chapter 35).

HAND, FOOT AND MOUTH DISEASE

Hand, foot and mouth disease, also caused by **group A coxsackievirus**, is a relatively common infection in children. It is easily diagnosed because of its classic distribution in the hands, feet and mouth. The incubation period is about 3–5 days and resolution occurs within a week.

Clinical Features

The disease may begin with facial pain, with tenderness along the course of the parotid duct and a few vesicles around the duct orifice. The onset of the oral and skin eruptions is accompanied by headache, malaise and sore throat, but in many individuals there is little systemic upset. The oral lesions are generally bright-red macules, which later form oval or grey vesicles with red areolae (see Chapter 35). The plantar surface of the feet and the palmar surface of the hands and sometimes the buttocks may be affected. These skin lesions are bright-red macules with pale centres, which develop into thin-walled bullae or small ulcers with surrounding erythema. The lesions in the mouth, and on the hands and feet, are not always seen.

All serotypes of coxsackievirus have a worldwide distribution. They are highly infectious within families and closed communities, and the greatest epidemic spread occurs in summer and autumn. Viral transmission is by the faecal–oral route and from nasal and pharyngeal secretions. These viruses enter through the mouth and nose, multiply locally and spread viraemically (compare polioviruses).

RHINOVIRUSES

The aetiological agents of the **'common cold'** and a group of acute, afebrile upper respiratory diseases, rhinoviruses are readily inactivated at low pH conditions and require an incubation temperature of 33°C for maximal replication; hence, they multiply well in the upper respiratory tract where the incoming air provides low temperature conditions suited to the virus.

Antigenicity

There is a vast array (more than 100) of immunologically distinct groups of rhinoviruses based on a single type-specific antigen—hence, the reason for recurrent colds, as the succeeding infective virus is likely to be antigenically different from the virus that caused the previous episode (i.e., immunity is only effective against **homologous challenge**).

Epidemiology. In a family unit, rhinovirus transmission is usually initiated when a child introduces the virus, which spreads rapidly via nasal secretions. The disease is most common in autumn, winter and early spring. Note, however, that rhinoviruses are not the only agents of the common cold, although they are the major culprits.

TOGAVIRIDAE

Rubella

The agent of rubella (**German measles**) is a togavirus. Rubella is a childhood fever resembling measles, except that it has a milder clinical course and shorter duration. If rubella is contracted in early pregnancy, the virus can cause severe congenital abnormalities and may cause the death of the foetus.

Epidemiology. Rubella is a highly contagious disease spread by nasal secretions. Because of its mild clinical symptoms, the infection is often unapparent, and viral dissemination may be widespread before it is recognized. The disease may spread in the dental clinic environment. Females (especially of childbearing age) should be immunized against the virus: the rubella component of the combined **MMR vaccine** contains a **live attenuated virus**, which confers adequate protection.

OTHER RNA VIRUSES

Other RNA virus families that have not been discussed here include Arenaviridae, Bunyaviridae, Coronaviridae, Reoviridae, Rhabdoviridae and Retroviridae. HIV, which is in the Retroviridae family, is discussed in detail in Chapter 30 because of its major relevance to dentistry.

Viruses and Cancer

Viruses that have the ability to cause cancer are called **oncogenic** viruses. A number of DNA viruses are oncogenic, but only one RNA virus is known to have this potential. The virus groups and the cancers they cause are summarized in the following sections.

PAPOVAVIRUSES

HPVs cause benign warts, malignant carcinomas and cervical cancers.

The **polyomavirus** and the **simian virus 40 (SV40)** are oncogenic in laboratory animals.

ADENOVIRUSES

Adenoviruses are oncogenic in newborn hamsters but not in humans.

HERPESVIRUSES

These are implicated in human cancers (also see previous discussion in this chapter):

- **HSV-2** is a likely coagent of certain variants of **cervical cancer.**
- EBV is associated with Burkitt lymphoma and nasopharyngeal carcinoma.
- **HHV-8** is closely associated with the aetiology of Kaposi sarcoma (an endothelial tumour), which is a well-recognized oral manifestation of HIV infection.

HEPADNAVIRUSES

Hepatitis B virus is a well-known agent of human **hepatocellular carcinoma** (Chapter 29).

RETROVIRUSES

Retroviruses include the human T cell leukaemia viruses (HTLVs):

- **HTLV-I** is the agent of **adult T cell leukaemia**, which is endemic in southwestern Japan and the Caribbean region.
- **HTLV-II** is associated with human **lymphomas**.

Key Facts

DNA VIRUSES

- **Human papillomaviruses (HPV)** are one of the major agents of cervical cancer.
- HPV is associated with **benign epithelial tumours** and, infrequently, oral carcinomas.
- An efficacious vaccine for preventing HPV infections is now available.
- **Adenoviruses** cause **acute respiratory disease** and are ubiquitous, and humans are the only known reservoirs.
- Up to eight different types of human herpesviruses are described; they are neurotrophic and epitheliotropic.
- All herpesvirus infections lead to lifelong viral latency.
- **Herpes simplex** and **herpes zoster** viruses cause **primary** and **reactivation** infection (postprimary infection).
- In general, **herpes simplex virus (HSV) types 1 and 2 (HSV-1 and HSV-2**, respectively) cause **infections 'above the belt'** and **'below the belt'**, respectively (i.e., oral and genital infections).
- Herpetic gingivostomatitis is the primary infection, and herpes labialis is the reactivation infection caused by HSV-1.
- Varicella-zoster **(herpes simplex virus type 3, HSV-3)** causes chickenpox (primary) and zoster/shingles (reactivation) affecting well-defined dermatomes ('belt of roses from hell').
- An efficacious vaccine for chickenpox/herpes zoster is now available.
- Epstein-Barr virus (human herpesvirus 4) causes infectious mononucleosis or glandular fever, oral hairy leukoplakia, nasopharyngeal carcinoma, Burkitt lymphoma and post-transplant lymphoproliferative diseases.
- **Cytomegalovirus** (human herpesvirus 5) causes **asymptomatic infection** in adults; if infection occurs during pregnancy, transplacental passage of the virus may cause serious **developmental defects** or abortion.
- **Human herpesvirus 6** causes **'sixth disease'** (or roseola infantum, exanthem subitum), a rash seen in young children.
- Human herpesvirus 7 is isolated from lymphocytes carrying CD4, not yet associated with disease.
- **Human herpesvirus 8** is the agent of **Kaposi sarcoma**, a vascular endothelial tumour common in human immunodeficiency virus (HIV) disease.

RNA VIRUSES

- Orthomyxoviruses cause pandemics of influenza.
- Their success is due to the ability to undergo rapid antigenic changes (**antigenic shifts** and **antigenic drifts**) of haemagglutinin component of the outer surface spikes of the orthomyxovirus.
- Paramyxoviruses include parainfluenza virus, mumps virus, measles virus and respiratory syncytial virus.
- **Mumps** virus is the major agent of **parotitis** (mumps).
- **Measles** is an acute febrile infection with an **exanthematous** rash; prodromal symptoms of measles include **Koplik spots on the buccal mucosa**.
- Complications of measles include bronchopneumonia, neurological complications and gangrenous stomatitis or noma.
- The measles–mumps–rubella (MMR) vaccine prevents measles, mumps and rubella.
- **Group A coxsackieviruses** cause **hand, foot and mouth disease** of children and **herpangina**; oral lesions are papulovesicular, small and greyish-white.
- **Rhinoviruses** are the agents of the **common cold**.
- **Oncogenic viruses**, or **cancer-causing viruses**, include papillomaviruses, polyomavirus, simian virus, Epstein-Barr virus and human herpesvirus 8, human T cell leukaemia viruses (retroviruses) and hepadnaviruses (causing hepatitis B).

Review Questions (Answers on p. 390)

Please indicate which answers are true and which are false.

21.1. Adenoviruses:
  a. are DNA viruses
  b. cause acute upper respiratory infections
  c. primarily cause zoonotic diseases, and humans are accidental hosts
  d. infections have a seasonal incidence
  e. infections are often treated with antiviral agents

21.2. Human herpesviruses include:
  a. rubella virus
  b. cytomegalovirus (CMV)
  c. Epstein-Barr virus (EBV)
  d. varicella-zoster virus
  e. measles virus

21.3. Primary herpesvirus infections may cause:
  a. gingivostomatitis
  b. herpes labialis
  c. herpetic whitlow
  d. chickenpox
  e. herpes zoster

21.4. Which of the following statements on herpes zoster in the maxillofacial region are true?
  a. it is triggered by reactivation of human herpesvirus 3 in the trigeminal ganglion
  b. it can lead to blindness
  c. pain mimics toothache
  d. it is difficult to diagnose without laboratory testing
  e. patient needs to be kept isolated to prevent the disease from spreading

21.5. Epstein-Barr virus (EBV):
  a. is a human herpesvirus
  b. achieves latency in sensory ganglia
  c. infections will produce a blood film with atypical lymphocytosis
  d. is hosted only by humans
  e. diagnosis has to be confirmed by serological methods

21.6. With regard to Epstein-Barr virus (EBV) infection, which of the following are true?
  a. Burkitt lymphoma is highly prevalent in Africa
  b. nasopharyngeal carcinoma is common among Caucasians
  c. EBV DNA is regularly isolated from nasopharyngeal carcinomas
  d. hairy leukoplakia is a malignancy of the oral cavity
  e. EBV is associated with posttransplant lymphoproliferative disorders

21.7. With regard to human herpesvirus infections, which of the following are true?
  a. cytomegalovirus (CMV) can incur foetal damage in pregnant women
  b. disseminated CMV infections are seen in immunocompromised patients
  c. human herpesvirus 6 infection is an occupational hazard to the dentist
  d. human herpesvirus 8 is responsible for Kaposi sarcoma
  e. human herpesvirus 6 causes a facial rash in children

21.8. Cancrum oris:
  a. is a complication of mumps
  b. is more common in African populations
  c. has malnutrition as a contributory factor
  d. may lead to gross disfigurement
  e. is a sequela of fusospirochetal infection

21.9. Papulovesicular oral lesions are seen in:
  a. measles
  b. herpangina
  c. hand, foot and mouth disease
  d. rubella
  e. mumps

Further Reading

Bagg, J. (1994). Virology and the mouth. *Reviews in Medical Microbiology,* 5, 209–216.

Candotto, V., Lauritano, D., Nardone, M., Baggi, L., Arcuri, C., Gatto, R., Gaudio, R. M., Spadari, F., & Carinci, F. (2017, November). HPV infection in the oral cavity: Epidemiology, clinical manifestations and relationship with oral cancer. *Oral & Implantology (Rome), 10*(3), 209–220. doi:10.11138/orl/2017.10.3.209.

Cleator, G. M., & Klapper, P. E. (2009). The *Herpesviridae*. In A. J. Zuckerman, J. E. Banatvala, P. Griffiths, et al. (Eds.), *Principles and practice of clinical virology* (6th ed.). John Wiley.

Greenberg, M. D. (1996). Herpesvirus infections. *Dental Clinics of North America, 40,* 359–368.

Scully, C., & Samaranayake, L. P. (1992). *Clinical virology in oral medicine and dentistry*. Cambridge University Press.

Scully, C., & Samaranayake, L. P. (2015). Emerging and changing viral diseases in the new millennium. *Oral Diseases, 22,* 171–179.

22 Fungi of Relevance to Dentistry

The study of fungi is called **mycology**. Fungi are **eukaryotic** microorganisms, as opposed to Bacteria and Archaea that are **prokaryotic** organisms (Chapter 2). By far the most important fungus of relevance in dentistry is a yeast belonging to the genus *Candida*. It is an oral commensal in about half of the general population. In this chapter, the general characteristics of some medically important fungi are given, but the emphasis is on fungal infections of the oral cavity: the **oral mycoses**, especially those caused by the *Candida* species. Recent NGS analysis has shown that the oral cavity harbours many different fungal genera and species, and the collective term for this is the **oral mycobiome**. The constituent organisms in the oral microbiome are called the **oral microbiota**.

Morphology

Fungi exhibit two basic structural forms: the **yeast** form (Fig. 22.1) and the **mould** form. While some fungi are capable of existing as both forms **(dimorphic)** at different times, others exist in one form only. This morphological switching depends on factors such as the environment and nutrient supply. Generally, dimorphic fungi exist as moulds in the natural environment (and in laboratory culture) and as yeasts in tissue:

- **Yeasts** are unicellular with spherical or ovoid bodies; all yeasts are similar morphologically on light microscopic examination.
- **Moulds** are multicellular with a variety of specialized structures that perform specific functions. The size and nature of these structures vary with different genera.

Hyphae (singular: *hypha* or *hyphum*) are threadlike tubes containing the fungal cytoplasm and its organelles. They can be considered as the structural units of the mould. The hyphae are divided into unit cells by cross-walls called **septa**. The septa have pores that allow the movement of cytoplasm, and even organelles, between cells. The term **mycelium** is given to the mass of hyphae that forms the mould colony.

Reproduction

Both asexual and sexual modes of reproduction are seen in fungi. It is believed that the sexual forms of fungi are not found in clinical material.

Classification

Taxonomy of fungi is a complex subject not dealt with here. Most of the medically important fungi are classified as **fungi imperfecti**, as their sexual forms have not been identified. Fungi of medical importance are classified into:

- yeasts
- filamentous fungi
- dimorphic fungi.

The following methods are used in the classification of fungi:

1. **Yeasts** are identified by biochemical reactions based on the fermentation and assimilation of carbohydrates,

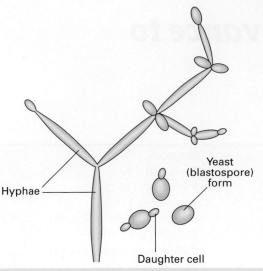

Fig. 22.1   **The yeast (blastospore) and hyphal forms of** *Candida albicans*.

utilization of enzyme substrates and other metabolic activities.

2. **Moulds** are identified by their colour, texture and colonial and microscopic morphology. The specialized asexual reproductive structures of moulds are useful in differentiating various species of moulds.

Cultural Requirements

Medically important fungi require different cultural and growth conditions in comparison to bacteria:

1. The vast majority of medically important fungi grow aerobically.
2. **Sabouraud dextrose agar (SAB)** and variations of it, such as SAB plus antibacterial agents, and **potato dextrose agar (PDA)** are commonly used for laboratory culture of pathogenic fungi.

These mycological media differ from conventional bacteriological media in having a high carbohydrate content (SAB usually contains 3% dextrose or sucrose) and an acidic pH (approximately 4.0). Both these conditions are inhibitory to most bacteria. The SAB medium may also be supplemented with antibiotics to suppress bacterial growth.

Pathogenicity

In general, medically important fungi do not possess the virulent attributes of bacteria such as exotoxins and endotoxins (an exception is the exotoxin **aflatoxin**, produced by *Aspergillus* species); hence they cause **slowly progressive chronic infections** rather than the acute disease commonly seen in bacterial or viral diseases. However, they may cause life-threatening acute infections in immunocompromised patients (e.g., those with acquired immune deficiency syndrome (AIDS)). The oral fungal pathogen *Candida* possesses a number of virulent attributes, including:

- the ability to **adhere** to host tissues and prostheses (e.g., dentures) and form **biofilms**
- the potential to **switch** (e.g., rough to smooth colony formation) and modify the surface antigens, which helps them to evade host recognition
- the ability to develop **hyphae** (filamentous appendages) that helps tissue penetration
- production of extracellular enzymes such as **phospholipase**, **proteinase** and **haemolysin**, which break down physical defence barriers of the host.

Human Mycoses

Human infections caused by fungi can be divided into:

- superficial mycoses
- subcutaneous mycoses
- systemic mycoses.

SUPERFICIAL MYCOSES

Superficial mycoses involve the mucosal surfaces and keratin-containing structures of the body (oral cavity, skin, nails and hair). These infections, relatively common in Western countries, are in general cosmetic problems and are not life-threatening. Superficial mycoses include:

- yeast infections of mucosal surfaces, which lead to **thrush** and similar manifestations (see Chapter 35)
- **dermatophyte** infection of skin, hair and so on, leading to ringworm or similar diseases.

SUBCUTANEOUS MYCOSES

Subcutaneous mycoses involve the subcutaneous tissue and **rarely disseminate**. They are the result of traumatic implantation of environmental fungi leading to chronic progressive disease, tissue destruction and sinus formation. Examples include sporotrichosis and mycetoma (Madura foot), which are common in the tropics and rare in the West.

SYSTEMIC MYCOSES (DEEP MYCOSES)

By far the most serious, and often fatal, systemic mycoses involve the internal organ systems of the body. The organisms are generally acquired through the respiratory tract and spread haematogenously. In the developed world, they are increasingly seen in compromised patients with impaired defence systems and behave as **opportunistic pathogens**, when otherwise they are rather harmless fungi. In the developing world, systemic mycoses (e.g., histoplasmosis, blastomycosis and coccidioidomycosis) can occur even in otherwise healthy individuals.

Opportunistic Fungal Infections

When fungi (such as *Candida albicans*) that are generally innocuous for healthy humans cause disease in compromised patient groups, they are called **opportunistic pathogens**. Such opportunistic mycoses are increasingly common owing to a global rise in compromised individuals such as patients infected with human immunodeficiency

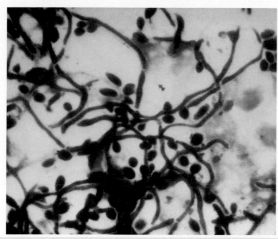

Fig. 22.2 A Gram-stained film of a smear from the fitting surface of the denture of a patient with *Candida*-associated denture stomatitis showing the blastospore (yeast) and hyphal (filamentous) forms of the organism.

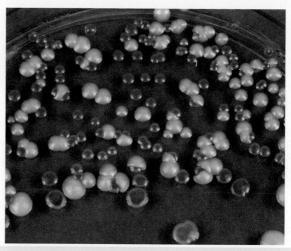

Fig. 22.3 *Candida albicans* and *Candida tropicalis* growing side by side on a special medium (Pagano–Levin agar), which elicits differential colour reactions. Mixed, multi-species oral candidal infections are not uncommon (approx 10–15%).

virus (HIV), recipients of organ transplants on immunosuppressive therapy and patients with cancer on cytotoxic and radiation therapy.

Yeasts

Yeasts are unicellular, oval or spherical organisms, 3–5 μm in diameter (approximately 10 times larger than an average bacterium), and stain positively by the Gram method (Fig. 22.2). They are commonly seen to have lateral projections or buds called **daughter cells**, which gradually enlarge in size until they split off from the parent or mother cell to produce the next generation. Most yeasts develop **pseudohyphae** (chains of elongated budding cells devoid of septa or cross-walls), but only a few develop **true hyphae** (septate hyphae).

Yeasts of the genus *Candida*, the most important fungal pathogen in the oral cavity, also form **pseudohyphae**. This common yeast lives in the oral cavity of about half of the population and is also a resident commensal of the gut. It can cause either **superficial** or **systemic candidiasis** (synonym: **candidosis**). The superficial disease affects:

- the mucosa (mucosal candidiasis)
- the skin (cutaneous candidiasis)
- both the skin and the mucosa (mucocutaneous candidiasis).

The infection is usually **endogenous** in origin. Several species in the genus *Candida* are found in humans, including *Candida albicans*, *Candida glabrata*, *Candida krusei* and *Candida tropicalis* (Fig. 22.3), but *Candida albicans* is responsible for the vast majority of infections (>90%). *Candida auris* is a relatively new emerging *Candida* species, similar to *Candida albicans*. First isolated from the ear (hence the name) of a Japanese patient, it is a multidrug-resistant (so-called 'pandrug resistant') yeast and hence is considered a serious global health threat.

CANDIDA ALBICANS

Habitat and Transmission

Candida albicans is indigenous to the oral cavity, gastrointestinal tract, female genital tract and sometimes the skin; hence infection is usually **endogenous**, although cross-infection may occur—for example, from mother to baby as well as among infant siblings.

Characteristics

Candida albicans typically grows as spherical to oval budding yeast cells 3–5 × 5–10 μm in size. These **yeast-phase** cells are also called **blastospores** (Fig. 22.4), and they should not be confused with bacterial spores. **Pseudohyphae** (elongated filamentous cells joined end to end) are seen especially at lower incubation temperatures and on nutritionally poor media.

Culture and Identification

Cultures grow on Sabouraud medium as **creamy-white colonies**, flat or hemispherical in shape with a beer-like aroma. *Candida albicans* and *Candida dubliniensis* may be differentiated from other *Candida* species by their ability to produce germ tubes and chlamydospores:

- When yeast cells are incubated for 3 h at 37°C in serum, *Candida albicans* and *Candida dubliniensis* form germ tubes (incipient hyphae), whereas other *Candida* species do not (see Fig. 6.15).
- Both *Candida albicans* and *Candida dubliniensis* form round, thick-walled, resting structures called chlamydospores when incubated at 22–25°C with decreased oxygen on a nutritionally poor medium (e.g., cornmeal agar).

However, definitive identification of the species is made on the basis of carbohydrate **assimilation** (aerobic metabolism) and **fermentation** (anaerobic metabolism) reactions and other biochemical tests; **polymerase chain reaction (PCR)** diagnostics should soon replace these methodologies in diagnostic laboratories, especially due to their rapidity.

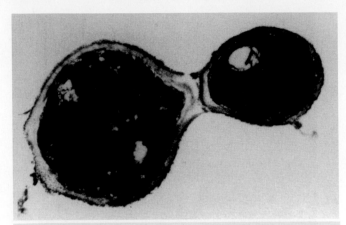

Fig. 22.4   A transmission electron micrograph of a blastospore of *Candida albicans* and a budding daughter cell.

Table 22.1   Factors Predisposing to Oral Candidiasis
Physiological States
▪ Infancy and old age
▪ Pregnancy
Systemic Pathology
▪ Immune defects
▪ Developmental (e.g., chronic mucocutaneous candidiasis syndromes)
▪ Infections (e.g., HIV disease)
▪ Leukaemias/agranulocytosis
▪ Uncontrolled diabetes
▪ Anaemias
▪ Fe and vitamin B_{12} deficiency
▪ Medications
▪ Corticosteroids/antibiotics/cytotoxic drug therapy
Local Host Factors (Oral Milieu)
▪ Unhygienic and or ill-fitting dentures
▪ Xerostomia
▪ Sjögren's syndrome
▪ Old age
▪ Head and neck radiation
▪ High carbohydrate diet
▪ Steroid inhaler use

Pathogenicity

Candida species rarely cause disease in the absence of predisposing factors, a vast number of which have been identified, for both superficial and systemic candidiasis (Table 22.1).

Superficial Candidiasis
1. **Mucosal infection:** The characteristic mucosal lesion of *Candida* is **thrush**. This is classically a white **pseudomembrane** on buccal mucosa and the vagina that can be easily removed by wiping. Other major oral manifestations include **erythematous and hyperplastic variants** (see Chapter 35). Candidal vulvovaginitis is common in women using oral contraceptives and is accompanied by a thick, yeasty-smelling discharge, vaginal itching and discomfort.
2. **Skin infection** is seen particularly on surfaces that are warm and moist. Candidal intertrigo consists of vesicular pustules that enlarge, rupture and cause fissures, and it is especially seen in the obese.
3. **Nappy rash** in children may be caused by *Candida albicans* derived from the lower gastrointestinal tract. Scaly macules or vesicles, associated with intense burning and pruritus, are common in nappy rash.
4. **Candidal paronychia** is a localized inflammation around and under **the nails**, caused by *Candida* when the hands are frequently immersed in water (e.g., in dishwashers and laundry workers).

Mucocutaneous Candidiasis. Mucocutaneous candidiasis involves both the skin and the oral and/or vaginal mucosae. This rare disease is due to heritable or acquired defects in the host immune system or metabolism. Chronic mucocutaneous candidiasis is a rare condition associated with T-cell deficiency (see Chapter 35).

Systemic or Deep Candidiasis. Systemic or deep candidiasis may involve the lower respiratory tract and urinary tract, with resultant **candidaemia** (*Candida* in blood); localization in endocardium, meninges, bone, kidney and eye is common. Untreated **disseminated disease** is fatal. Susceptible settings include organ transplantation, heart surgery, prosthetic implantation and long-term steroid or immunosuppressive therapy. Rarely, a superficial infection is the cause of disseminated disease.

Diagnosis
1. Demonstration of yeasts in Gram-stained smear, followed by culture of specimen on Sabouraud agar.
2. Serology, novel PCR-based molecular methods and blood culture (in suspected candidaemia) are each helpful in the diagnosis of disseminated candidiasis.
3. Histopathological examination of a biopsy of the lesion; demonstration of tissue invasion by fungal hyphae helps establish a causal relationship.

Treatment

In general, *Candida* infections can be treated by four major classes of antifungal drugs: **polyenes**, **azoles**, **allylamines** and **echinocandins** (see Chapter 7). However, the polyenes and the azoles are the most commonly used antifungals in dentistry. The agents used depend upon the type and severity of infection. Superficial infections, such as oral (or vaginal) candidiasis, can usually be treated topically with a polyene (nystatin or amphotericin) or an imidazole (miconazole, clotrimazole).

Systemic infections and disseminated candidiasis require **intravenous amphotericin, or echinocandins** either alone or sometimes in combination with flucytosine. The triazole agent fluconazole, effective for both superficial and systemic mycoses, is the drug of choice in treating *Candida* infections in HIV disease. (However, *Candida krusei* is resistant to fluconazole.) The newer agents, such as **echinocandins** and **terbinafine** (a synthetic allylamine), are very infrequently used in dentistry.

Prevention

Candidiasis is almost always endogenous in origin; therefore, prevention entails correction of predisposing factors. Those who are compromised may require long-term prophylactic antifungal treatment, either continuously or intermittently.

CRYPTOCOCCUS

Cryptococcus neoformans is a pathogenic yeast belonging to the *Cryptococcus* genus. It causes cryptococcosis, especially cryptococcal meningitis.

Habitat and Transmission

This yeast is a ubiquitous saprophyte commonly isolated from soil enriched by pigeon droppings. Infection is initiated by inhalation of airborne yeast cells.

Characteristics

Cryptococcus neoformans is a budding yeast with a thick capsule, 5–15 μm in diameter.

Culture and Identification

Identification is by sputum and spinal fluid culture on Sabouraud agar. Latex agglutination is used to detect the polysaccharide antigen in urine, blood or spinal fluid. Indian ink preparations of spinal fluid are used in the demonstration of the encapsulated yeast (Fig. 22.5).

Pathogenicity

The thick **polysaccharide capsule** of the yeast is highly resistant to host immune defences. Life-threatening infections caused by *Cryptococcus neoformans* have been steadily increasing over the past few decades due to the onset of AIDS and to the expanded use of immunosuppressive drugs. Cryptococci cause an **influenza-like syndrome or pneumonia**. Subsequent fungaemia causes infection of the meninges. Reduced cell-mediated immunity exacerbates the infection; immunocompetent people may occasionally

develop cryptococcal meningitis. Rarely cryptococcal oral ulceration can be seen in compromised patients such as those with HIV infection.

Treatment

Intravenous combination therapy with amphotericin and flucytosine is typical, although the beneficial role of the latter has been questioned. Fluconazole, which penetrates the central nervous system, is also useful.

Filamentous and Dimorphic Fungi and Oral Disease

The foregoing text describes one major group of fungi—yeasts—which are of dental and medical relevance. The other two main groups, **filamentous** and **dimorphic** fungi, usually do not cause oral disease except in immunocompromised groups. During the recent COVID-19 pandemic, oral and maxillofacial infections caused by ***Mucor* species** were reported widely, but mainly from the tropics.

Organisms that are noteworthy and cause **oral ulceration** are *Penicillium marneffei*, *Blastomyces dermatitidis*, *Coccidioides immitis*, *Histoplasma capsulatum* and *Histoplasma duboisii* and various *Mucor* species (Table 22.2).

***Mucor* species** cause mucormycoses that are essentially opportunistic infections caused by fungi belonging to the Mucorales order. After *Candida* and *Aspergillus* species, in general, Mucorales cause the third most common invasive human fungal infection. The advent of COVID-19 has led to a recrudescence of Mucorales infections that were otherwise usually seen in compromised patient groups.

Pathogenicity

In all these cases, infection is usually acquired by inhalation, and the primary lesions are seen in the lungs. In a majority, the initial lesion heals, often asymptomatically, and delayed hypersensitivity develops, with a positive skin test reaction to the appropriate antigen. Progressive disease may affect the lungs, causing cavitation, and/or disseminate widely

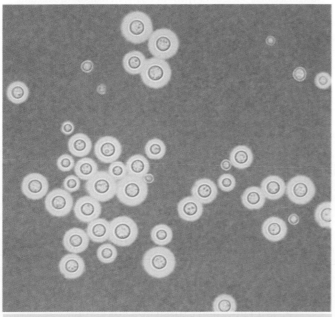

Fig. 22.5 Indian ink preparation of *Cryptococcus neoformans* showing capsules of yeasts, which appear as translucent haloes. (Courtesy Centers for Disease Control and Prevention, Atlanta, USA, and Dr. Leanor Haley.)

Table 22.2 Dimorphic Fungi That May Cause Oral Ulceration, Especially in Immunocompromised Patients

Fungus	Disease	Geographic Distribution
Penicillium marneffei	Penicilliosis	Southeast Asia
Blastomyces dermatitidis	North American blastomycosis	North America, especially Mississippi and Ohio valleys
Coccidioides immitis	Coccidioidomycosis	US from California to Texas; South and Central America
Histoplasma capsulatum	Histoplasmosis	Eastern and central US; occasionally other parts of the world
Histoplasma duboisii	African histoplasmosis	Equatorial Africa
Mucor species	Mucormycosis	Mainly in the dry tropical regions such as the Indian subcontinent

to involve the skin, oral and other mucous membranes and internal organs. Ulceration is the most common presentation in the oral mucosa.

Chronic mucor infections in the maxillary sinuses may spread inferiorly to the palatal area and necrosis and destruction of the palate may ensue, if untreated. On the other hand, superior spread of infection from the palate into the orbital area may cause even blindness in some cases.

Diagnosis

Diagnosis may be by direct demonstration in exudate, sputum or biopsy specimens, isolation in appropriate culture media and/or serology.

Treatment

Amphotericin is the drug of choice; itraconazole is an alternative.

Key Facts

- Fungi are **eukaryotic** microorganisms, as opposed to bacteria, which are **prokaryotes**.
- Fungi exhibit two basic structural forms: the **yeast form** and the **mould form; yeasts** are unicellular with spherical/ovoid bodies, and **moulds** are multicellular with a variety of specialized structures.
- **Hyphae** (singular: hypha or hyphum) are threadlike tubes containing the fungal cytoplasm and its organelles (**mycelium**, a mass of hyphae).
- Fungi of medical importance are classified into **yeasts**, **filamentous fungi** and **dimorphic fungi**.
- The vast majority of medically important fungi grow aerobically on **Sabouraud dextrose agar (SAB)** or its variations.
- *Candida albicans* possesses a number of virulent attributes, including the ability to **adhere** to host tissues/prostheses and form **hyphae**, colonial **switching** and the production of extracellular **phospholipase** and **proteinases**.
- Human infections caused by fungi can be broadly categorized as **superficial**, **subcutaneous or systemic** (deep) mycoses.
- When fungi (such as *Candida albicans*) that are generally innocuous in healthy humans cause disease in compromised patients, the infection is called **opportunistic**.
- *Candida*, a common yeast that lives in the oral cavity of some 50–60% of the population, can cause either **superficial** (mucosal, cutaneous or mucocutaneous) or **systemic** candidiasis.
- Species in the ***Candida*** genus found in humans include *Candida albicans*, *Candida glabrata*, *Candida dubliniensis*, *Candida krusei* and *Candida tropicalis*; *Candida albicans* is responsible for the vast majority of infections (>90%).
- *Candida albicans* is **indigenous to the oral cavity**, gastrointestinal tract, female genital tract and sometimes the skin; hence the infection is usually **endogenous**.

- *Candida albicans* and *Candida dubliniensis* may be differentiated from other *Candida* species by their ability to produce **germ tubes** and **chlamydospores**.
- *Candida* species rarely cause oral disease in the absence of predisposing factors, such as intraoral environmental changes (e.g., unhygienic prostheses, xerostomia) and/or systemic factors such as diabetes and immunodeficiency.
- The three major clinical manifestations of oral candidiasis are **pseudomembranous**, **erythematous** and **hyperplastic variants** (see Chapter 35).
- Demonstration of yeasts in **Gram-stained smear**, positive **culture** on Sabouraud dextrose agar and subsequent confirmation by biochemical or genetic techniques constitute a mycological diagnosis of candidiasis.
- *Candida* infections can be treated by three main groups of agents: the **polyenes**, the **azoles** and the **DNA analogues**, depending on the type and severity of infection.
- The triazole agent **fluconazole** is effective for both superficial and systemic mycoses, and it is the drug of choice in treating *Candida* infections in HIV disease.
- Resistance to azoles is seen in *Candida* species, usually following prolonged treatment, while resistance to polyene group drugs is rare.
- Treatment of candidiasis entails **correction of predisposing factors**, with or without oral or systemic **antifungals**.
- Oral lesions due to fungi other than *Candida* are rare. These fungal lesions, such as **cryptococcosis**, **histoplasmosis** and **penicilliosis**, may be seen in HIV disease and usually respond to intravenous amphotericin therapy.
- **NGS technology** has uncovered the presence of numerous fungal genera and species comprising the **oral mycobiome**; most of these are thought to be innocent commensal organisms, and are rarely pathogenic.

Review Questions (Answers on p. 390)

Please indicate which answers are true and which are false.

22.1. Which of the following statements on fungi are true?
   a. Fungi are eukaryotic organisms.
   b. Fungi are oral commensals in approximately 50% of humans.
   c. The most common fungus in the oral cavity is *Candida glabrata*.
   d. Fungal mycelium contains an abundance of hyphal elements.
   e. Some fungi produce endotoxins.

22.2. Higher frequency of oral candidiasis or oral yeast carriage may be caused by:
   a. leukaemia
   b. diabetes mellitus
   c. frequent eating of sweets by dentulous individuals
   d. smoking
   e. breast cancer

22.3. Cryptococcosis:
   a. is an infection caused by a eukaryote
   b. may present as oral ulceration
   c. is associated with death due to meningitis
   d. can cause cardiac abnormalities
   e. is associated with dog lovers

Further Reading

Calderone, R. A., & Clancy, C. J. (2002). *Candida and candidiasis*. ASM Press.

Kibber, C. C., MacKenzie, D. W. R., & Odds, F. C. (Eds.). (1996). *Principles and practice of clinical mycology*. Wiley.

Reichart, P., Samaranayake, L. P., & Philipsen, H. P. (2000). Pathology and clinical correlates in oral candidiasis and its variants: A review. *Oral Diseases, 6*, 85–91.

Samaranayake, L. P., Cheung, L. K., & Samaranayake, Y. H. (2002). Mycotic infections of the oral cavity. *Dermatologic Therapy, 15*, 252–270.

Samaranayake, L. P., Fakhruddin, K. S., Ngo, H. C., Bandara, H. M. N. M., & Leung, Y. Y. (2022). Orofacial mycoses in coronavirus disease-2019 (COVID-19): A systematic review. *International Dental Journal, 72*(5), 607–620.

Samaranayake, L. P., Leung, W. K., & Jin, L. J. (2009). Oral mucosal infections. *Periodontology 2000, 49*, 39–59.

Samaranayake, L. P., & MacFarlane, T. W. (Eds.). (1990). *Oral candidosis*. Wright.

Seneviratne, C. J., Jin, L. J., & Samaranayake, L. P. (2008). Biofilm lifestyle of *Candida*: A mini review. *Oral Diseases, 14*(7), 582–590.

PART 4

SYSTEMIC INFECTIONS OF RELEVANCE TO DENTISTRY

The aim of this section is to survey the major organ-related, systemic infections that are of particular interest in dentistry. Each infection in general is thematically organized, for the sake of convenience, according to its aetiology, clinical features, pathogenesis, laboratory diagnosis, and treatment and prevention. A new feature of this edition is a concise description of the Coronavirus disease 2019 (COVID-19) incorporated in the chapter on infections of the respiratory tract.

- Infections of the respiratory tract
- Infections of the cardiovascular system
- Infections of the central nervous and locomotor systems
- Infections of the gastrointestinal tract
- Infections of the genitourinary tract
- Skin and wound infections
- Viral hepatitis
- Human immunodeficiency virus infection, AIDS and infections in compromised patients

SYSTEMIC INFECTIONS OF RELEVANCE TO DENTISTRY

23 Infections of the Respiratory Tract

The human respiratory tract is highly susceptible to infectious diseases, and morbidity of this region accounts for the majority of general practitioner consultations and almost a quarter of all absences from work due to illness in the western world. Most respiratory tract infections are mild, associated with cold, damp winter months when coughing and sneezing in enclosed spaces facilitate the spread of disease. Serious infections are seen in the very young and the very old, and in compromised patients, throughout the year.

This said, the pandemic of COVID-19 with millions dying from SARS-CoV-2-associated pneumonias have shed a totally new light on the critical importance of respiratory infections and their spread in the community. In addition, the pandemic has created a new awareness among the public on the value of infection control measures such as mask wearing, respiratory hygiene and the utility of disinfectants and antiseptics, and vaccinations (Chapters 36–38). Although all respiratory infections are important, this chapter highlights the respiratory infections more germane to dental practice. An extended **description of coronavirus infections**, which caused SARS in 2003 and the pandemic of COVID-19 beginning in 2019, is presented in this chapter due to their obvious importance to dentistry.

Respiratory infections can be broadly classified into **upper and lower respiratory tract infections**, although both areas may be simultaneously affected by some agents, notably viruses. The throat, pharynx, middle ear and sinuses are involved in upper respiratory tract infections, whereas lower respiratory tract infections are confined to the trachea, bronchi and lungs.

Normal Flora

In health, the nose and the throat are colonized by commensal bacterial species, while the lower respiratory tract (the lower bronchi and alveoli) contain only a few, if any, organisms. The nose is the habitat of a variety of streptococci and staphylococci, the most significant of which is *Staphylococcus aureus*, especially prevalent in the anterior nares. Other commensal flora of the upper respiratory tract include corynebacteria, *Haemophilus* spp. and neisseriae. In health, these endogenous (and other exogenous) organisms are unable to

Table 23.1 Natural Antimicrobial Defences of the Respiratory Tract

Mucociliary system
Nasal vibrissae
Action of cilia
Mucous glands and goblet cells
Bronchoconstriction
Cough reflex
Nonspecific mucosal defences
Lactoferrin
Lysozyme
α-antitrypsin
Alveolar macrophage system
Mucosal antibody (mainly secretory IgA)
Local cell-mediated immunity

IgA, immunoglobulin A.

gain access to the tissues and cause disease because there is an effective array of defence mechanisms (Table 23.1).

Important Pathogens of the Respiratory Tract

The major causative agents of bacterial and viral respiratory infections of both the upper and lower respiratory tract are illustrated in Fig. 23.1.

Infections of the Upper Respiratory Tract

The following infections of the upper respiratory tract of clinical relevance to dentistry are noteworthy:

- sore throat syndrome
- streptococcal sore throat and scarlet fever
- rheumatic fever
- acute glomerulonephritis
- common cold syndrome
- diphtheria
- Vincent's angina
- infectious mononucleosis (Chapter 21)
- candidiasis (Chapter 22).

SORE THROAT SYNDROME

Clinical Features

Sore throat is a very common symptom that may or may not be accompanied by constitutional changes. A number of agents may cause a sore throat, but the majority, **approximately two-thirds**, of the infections are **caused by viruses**. The major bacterial pathogen involved is **Streptococcus pyogenes (Lancefield group A)**. Sore throat is a frequent precursor of the common cold syndrome (see following).

STREPTOCOCCAL SORE THROAT AND SCARLET FEVER

Clinical Features

Streptococcal sore throat (*syn*. strep throat) is characterized by the redness of the pharynx and tonsils and possible oedema of fauces and soft palate with exudate (acute follicular tonsillitis). Children 5–8 years old are most commonly affected. Spread of infection may cause a peritonsillar abscess (quinsy throat); further spread may cause sinus infection (sinusitis—commonly maxillary sinusitis) or middle-ear infection (otitis media).

Scarlet fever, a childhood disease, is a complication of streptococcal upper respiratory tract infection and is accompanied by an erythematous rash and constitutional upset. It is caused by a **pyrogenic exotoxin-producing streptococcus: *S. pyogenes***. Superantigens (SAgs) secreted by this Group A streptococcus (GAS) usually overstimulate the human immune system, causing an amplified hypersensitivity reaction leading to initial symptoms such as sore throat, high fever and a sandpaper-like scarlet skin rash (hence the name).

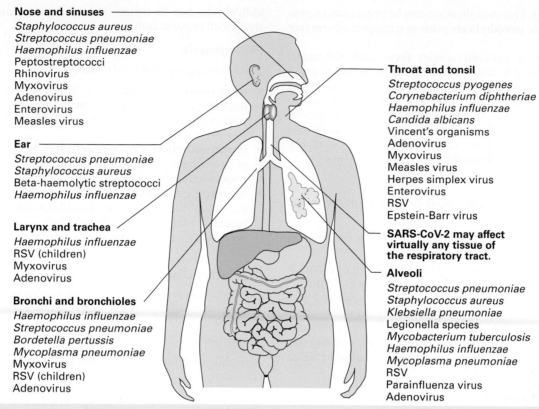

Nose and sinuses
Staphylococcus aureus
Streptococcus pneumoniae
Haemophilus influenzae
Peptostreptococci
Rhinovirus
Myxovirus
Adenovirus
Enterovirus
Measles virus

Ear
Streptococcus pneumoniae
Staphylococcus aureus
Beta-haemolytic streptococci
Haemophilus influenzae

Larynx and trachea
Haemophilus influenzae
RSV (children)
Myxovirus
Adenovirus

Bronchi and bronchioles
Haemophilus influenzae
Streptococcus pneumoniae
Bordetella pertussis
Mycoplasma pneumoniae
Myxovirus
RSV (children)
Adenovirus

Throat and tonsil
Streptococcus pyogenes
Corynebacterium diphtheriae
Haemophilus influenzae
Candida albicans
Vincent's organisms
Adenovirus
Myxovirus
Measles virus
Herpes simplex virus
Enterovirus
RSV
Epstein-Barr virus

SARS-CoV-2 may affect virtually any tissue of the respiratory tract.

Alveoli
Streptococcus pneumoniae
Staphylococcus aureus
Klebsiella pneumoniae
Legionella species
Mycobacterium tuberculosis
Haemophilus influenzae
Mycoplasma pneumoniae
RSV
Parainfluenza virus
Adenovirus

Fig. 23.1   Major causative agents of respiratory tract infections. RSV, respiratory syncytial virus. Note: **SARS-CoV-2 may affect virtually any tissue of the respiratory tract.**

Both extraoral and intraoral manifestations are associated with scarlet fever. A characteristic, virtually pathognomonic facial sign that appears concurrently with the initial skin rash is a **flushed face** with a **circumoral pallor** (i.e., lighter skin around the mouth relative to the other flushed areas of the face).

Intraorally, a yellowish-white coating with red papillae may initially cover the tongue, with the subsequent fading of the coating leaving a residual red tongue termed the '**strawberry tongue**' or '**raspberry tongue**'. The prominence of the filiform and fungiform papillae due to the associated swelling and redness leads to this appearance. As the infection progresses, the dorsum of the tongue becomes swollen and erythematous as a result of the desquamation of the keratinized epithelium of the papillae and the associated inflammation. Fissured lips and **enlarged oedematous tonsils** with exudates are also common oral signs of the infection.

The early diagnosis and treatment of scarlet fever is critical to obviate the development of local and systemic sequelae such as acute rheumatic fever, endocarditis and glomerulonephritis (see below).

Pathogenesis and Epidemiology

The sore throat in particular is common, especially in winter, with the peak incidence in young schoolchildren with inadequate levels and range of antibodies. Transient streptococcal carriage for a few weeks is common after an acute episode.

On the other hand, the incidence of scarlet fever decreased dramatically in the postantibiotic era after the advent of the penicillins. However, there has been a recent recrudescence of scarlet fever, particularly in some parts of Europe, and the reasons for this are as yet unknown.

Late Sequelae of Streptococcal Infection

Immunologically mediated diseases can manifest in susceptible individuals as a late consequence of certain strains of *Streptococcus pyogenes* (group A) infection—namely, rheumatic fever and acute glomerulonephritis.

RHEUMATIC FEVER

Clinical Features

Fever, pain, joint swelling and pancarditis (myocarditis, endocarditis and pericarditis) may occur 2–5 weeks after streptococcal sore throat. **Cardiac manifestations** may lead to permanent **heart damage**. In developed countries, the incidence of rheumatic fever (and related heart disease) has declined markedly, though with sporadic episodes in limited geographic regions. The general reduction in the disease prevalence is possibly owing to changes in the virulence of the bacterium, improved affluence and social conditions, and effective antimicrobial therapy (e.g., penicillins). However, both rheumatic fever and consequent heart disease are still a major problem in the developing world.

The disease clears spontaneously but may lead to chronic valvular diseases of the heart such as stenosis or incompetence of the mitral or aortic valves in about 70% of patients. Affected individuals are **highly susceptible to bacterial endocarditis** later in life, when bacteraemias are created during **dental or surgical procedures** such as scaling. This complication can be prevented by prudent **antibiotic prophylaxis** prior to such procedures (see Chapter 24).

The difference between scarlet fever and rheumatic fever is important to note. *Streptococcus pyogenes* infection first causes either scarlet fever or streptococcal sore throat ('strep throat'). Rheumatic fever is a secondary sequel to streptococcal infection, and it is an immune-mediated event (see also Chapter 11). Scarlet fever need not necessarily lead to rheumatic fever, whereas the latter is always preceded by a streptococcal throat infection.

Pathogenesis

A number of theories have been proposed for rheumatic carditis:

- **rheumatic toxins:** extracellular products of group A streptococci reacting with heart tissue
- **autoimmunity:** induced by the localization of extracellular streptococcal products and antibodies in tissues
- **cross-reactivity:** the group A streptococcus cell wall antigens and glycoproteins of human heart valves share the same antigenic determinants; thus the antibodies produced against the bacterial cell wall may cross-react with the heart valve components, with resultant cardiac complications (Fig. 23.2).

Laboratory Diagnosis

Diagnosis is mainly clinical; **throat swabs** are useful to confirm the presence of *Streptococcus pyogenes*. Swabs cultured on blood agar aerobically and anaerobically yield characteristic **β-haemolytic colonies**, which can subsequently be identified by Lancefield grouping.

Infection can be proved by serological analysis of paired clotted blood samples. Evidence for **antibody to streptolysin O** should be sought (streptolysin O is a haemolysin produced by *Streptococcus pyogenes*). Antibodies to other streptococcal products such as hyaluronidase and DNAase may also be demonstrated immediately after an infection.

Treatment

β-haemolytic streptococci are universally sensitive to penicillin. Erythromycin is an alternative in cases of penicillin hypersensitivity. After eradication of *Streptococcus pyogenes* with penicillin, reinfection must be prevented by long-term prophylaxis.

ACUTE GLOMERULONEPHRITIS

Acute glomerulonephritis is another immunological complication that may follow streptococcal sore throat (and sometimes streptococcal skin infection). The latent period between infection and symptoms is shorter than in rheumatic fever.

Clinical Features

The condition presents 1–3 weeks after the sore throat; characteristically there is haematuria, albuminuria and oedema that manifests as a puffed face, especially on waking, and as the day wears on, ankle oedema often develops. The disease spontaneously clears in the majority of individuals, but in others kidney damage may progressively lead to renal failure.

Pathogenesis

The following are proposed theories:

- **nephrotoxins:** production of toxic substances by nephritogenic streptococci, including streptolysin, cell wall extracts and uncharacterized diffusible substances released by the cells
- **immunological cross-reactivity:** between antigens of protoplasts of nephritogenic streptococci and soluble components of glomerular basement membrane
- **immune complexes:** thought to be formed by combinations of antistreptococcal antibody with either streptococcal antigens already circulating in the blood or deposited on the basement membranes.

Laboratory Diagnosis

A clinical diagnosis is confirmed by past or present streptococcal infection.

Treatment

Penicillin is useful if the organism is still present at the infective focus.

COMMON COLD SYNDROME

A number of viruses, such as coronaviruses, adenoviruses and rhinoviruses, cause the common cold, although rhinoviruses are by far the most common culprit.

Clinical Features

A brief incubation period of 2–4 days and acute illness last up to a week with a nonproductive cough lasting up to 2–3 weeks. The average adult has up to two attacks per year. Symptoms include sneezing, nasal obstruction and discharge, sore throat accompanied possibly by headache, mild cough, malaise and a chilly sensation and fever. Secondary bacterial infection may lead to otitis media, sinusitis and bronchitis or pneumonia in children.

Pathogenesis

Virus enters the upper respiratory tract and multiplies in the surface epithelium of the nasal mucosa, leading to increased nasal secretion and oedema. Virus is essentially transmitted through close contact and through air in confined spaces; self-inoculation by hand contamination is considered a more important route than airborne transmission.

Antibodies develop in most individuals after an acute episode but provide limited protection due to rapid decline in antibody levels and also due to multiple rhinovirus serotypes or other common cold viruses circulating during a single season.

Treatment

Only symptomatic treatment is possible. Many attempts at vaccine preparation have failed, and antiviral drugs are

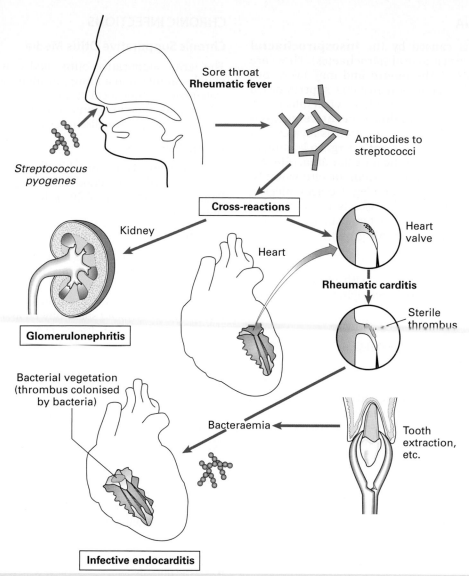

Fig. 23.2 Pathogenesis and sequelae of rheumatic carditis. *Note:* Streptococcal sore throat and/or scarlet fever may lead to rheumatic fever; the former is a direct result of streptococcal infection, whereas rheumatic fever is due to an immunological sequel of the streptococcal sore throat (events leading to infective endocarditis are also illustrated).

equally ineffective. Nasal spray of interferon-α has shown some promise in preventing the spread of rhinoviruses.

DIPHTHERIA

Diphtheria is caused by *Corynebacterium diphtheriae* (three main biotypes: **gravis, intermedius and mitis**). It was a common disease in the young prior to the advent of the DTP vaccine (see below).

Clinical Features

After an incubation period of 2–5 days, a severe, acute inflammation of the upper respiratory tract, usually the throat, sets in. Severity of the disease is related to the infecting strain of the organism and the extent of the grey-white membrane that covers the fauces. The membrane is a product of a serocellular exudate. **Nasal diphtheria** is often milder than **laryngeal diphtheria**, which is serious because of respiratory tract obstruction.

Pathogenesis

Corynebacteria produce a powerful exotoxin that is **cardiotoxic and neurotoxic**. This toxin diffuses throughout the body, affecting the myocardium, adrenal glands and nerve endings.

Epidemiology

Diphtheria is rare in developed countries because of the successful **diphtheria–tetanus–pertussis** (DTP) vaccine immunization programme. Outbreaks occur in nonimmunized populations, especially in the developing world.

Treatment

Antitoxin must be used in addition to penicillin or erythromycin.

VINCENT'S ANGINA

Vincent's angina is caused by the **fusospirochaetal complex** (fusobacteria and oral spirochaetes). These are normal commensals of the mouth and may overgrow, mainly as a result of poor oral hygiene superimposed on nutritional deficiency, leukopenia or viral infections. The outcome may be **necrotizing ulcerative gingivitis** (Vincent's stomatitis) if the infection is localized in the mouth (Chapter 33) or **Vincent's angina** leading to massive tissue involvement in the tonsillar area. (Similar fusospirochaetal infections may occur in bite wounds, lung abscesses, bronchiectasis and leg 'tropical' ulcers.) The primary cause of these diseases is the anaerobic environment, due to local or systemic factors, which precipitate polymicrobial anaerobic growth.

Treatment

Penicillin or metronidazole combined with effective debridement, along with removal of the underlying cause of tissue breakdown.

Infections of the Paranasal Sinuses and the Middle Ear

Infections of the paranasal sinuses and the middle ear can either be acute or chronic, and they are often initiated as a secondary complication of a viral infection of the respiratory tract (e.g., a common cold). Some important examples are:

- acute infections
- otitis media
- sinusitis
- chronic infections
- chronic suppurative otitis media
- chronic sinusitis.

ACUTE INFECTIONS

Otitis Media

Inflammation of the **middle ear** may be caused by infection spreading via the eustachian tube, especially after a common cold. Mainly a childhood disease characterized by earache; recurrences are common.

Sinusitis

Inflammation frequently affecting frontal and/or maxillary sinuses is a familiar symptom of the common cold but resolves spontaneously. However, pain and tenderness with purulent discharge may indicate bacterial infection, in which case antibiotic therapy is indicated. **Maxillary sinusitis may present as toothache** in some individuals.

Aetiology

Both otitis media and sinusitis are due to endogenous infection (from reservoirs in the nasopharynx) by bacteria such as *Haemophilus influenzae*, *Streptococcus pneumoniae* and *Streptococcus pyogenes*.

Treatment

Amoxicillin, ampicillin, erythromycin.

CHRONIC INFECTIONS

Chronic Suppurative Otitis Media

The term 'suppurative otitis media' is given to chronic middle-ear infection and suppuration (pus formation) associated with pathological changes. It can recur at intervals throughout childhood and also in adulthood. The main symptoms are profuse discharge and pain.

Chronic Sinusitis

Chronic sinusitis is associated with headache, painful sinuses, nasal obstruction and mucopurulent discharge. Patients may also complain of toothache if the maxillary sinuses are affected.

Aetiology

The aetiology is the same as in acute infections, with endogenous spread of infection from the indigenous upper respiratory tract flora. In addition, other organisms such as *Staphylococcus aureus* and a range of enterobacteria and anaerobes (*Bacteroides* spp.) may be associated. The role of these organisms in the disease process is not clear.

Treatment

Antibiotic treatment is required, guided by antibiotic sensitivity testing of isolates. Nasal decongestants may be helpful.

Infections of the Trachea and Bronchi

Infection and consequent inflammation of the larynx (laryngitis), trachea (tracheitis) and bronchi (bronchitis) are common after viral infections of the upper respiratory tract. The following important diseases are outlined in this section:

- bronchitis
- cystic fibrosis
- pertussis (whooping cough).

BRONCHITIS

Acute bronchitis in a patient with a healthy respiratory tract is usually a minor complaint possibly due to a viral infection. However, secondary bacterial infection of the damaged respiratory mucosa may result in severe attacks in those with a history of chronic bronchitis, bronchiectasis or asthma. Acute exacerbation of chronic bronchitis is a serious disease.

Aetiology

Two major agents are *Haemophilus.influenzae* and *Streptococcus pneumoniae*. *Moraxella catarrhalis* and *Mycoplasma pneumoniae* may also be involved in some cases.

Clinical Features

A dry cough that later turns productive with expectoration of yellow-green sputum; fever.

Pathogenesis and Epidemiology

Bronchitis is primarily an endogenous infection due to the organisms mentioned above. However, chronic bronchitis is the result of a vast number of additional aetiological factors including previous lung disease, smoking, poor housing, low socioeconomic class, urban dwelling, atmospheric pollution, and damp, cold and wintry weather conditions.

Diagnosis

The diagnosis is mainly clinical; sputum samples are cultured to isolate and to determine the antibiotic sensitivity profile of the aetiological agents.

Treatment

Ampicillin or amoxicillin, tetracycline, co-trimoxazole (combination of sulfamethoxazole and trimethoprim) and erythromycin are all used in the treatment, depending on the culture and sensitivity results. In chronic bronchitic patients, antibiotic treatment should begin early in the infection to reduce severity.

RESPIRATORY INFECTIONS IN CYSTIC FIBROSIS

Respiratory infection is a major problem in patients with cystic fibrosis. This inherited defect leads to production of **abnormally thick mucus** that blocks the respiratory 'tubes' and tubular structures in many different organs. However, the most disabling feature of this condition is **chronic respiratory tract infection** due to compromised natural defence mechanisms of the airways. The aetiological agents are usually *Staphylococcus aureus*, *Streptococcus pneumoniae* and *Pseudomonas aeruginosa*. The biofilms of the latter, in particular, within the thick mucous mass, are not easily penetrated by antibacterials, leading to chronic recalcitrant infections.

PERTUSSIS (WHOOPING COUGH)

Pertussis is caused by *Bordetella pertussis*.

Clinical Features

An acute childhood disease (usually in the first year) with tracheobronchitis, the disease has an insidious onset. First stage is the **catarrhal stage** (about 2 weeks), which leads to a **paroxysmal stage** characterized by a cough and indrawing of breath that creates a 'whoop' (hence the name). There is a very low fatality rate, but morbidity is high, leading to sequelae such as bronchiectasis.

Pathogenesis and Epidemiology

Droplet spread; the attack rate in unprotected siblings may be as high as 90%. Whooping cough occurs in epidemic proportions every few years, especially in unvaccinated populations.

Laboratory Diagnosis

A pernasal swab or cough plate of charcoal-blood or Bordet–Gengou medium confirms the diagnosis. A **pernasal swab** is obtained by passing a swab along the floor of the nose to sample nasopharyngeal secretions; a cough plate is obtained by holding the culture plate in front of the mouth when coughing. The organisms grow as mercury drop colonies on charcoal-blood agar.

Treatment and Prevention

Antibiotics are of little help; DTP vaccine is an effective preventive measure (see Chapter 37).

Lung Infections

The following noteworthy infections are outlined:

- pneumonia (including severe acute respiratory syndrome [SARS] and COVID-19)
- legionnaires' disease
- respiratory tuberculosis (TB)
- empyema

PNEUMONIA

Despite the diverse array of antibiotics available today, pneumonia remains a significant cause of morbidity and mortality in the very young, the very old and the immunocompromised. Pneumonia can be categorized into three main types:

1. **lobar** (or **segmental**) **pneumonia:** consolidation is limited to one lobe or segment of the lung
2. **bronchopneumonia:** usually bilateral, with consolidation scattered throughout the lung fields
3. primary **atypical** or **virus pneumonia:** with patchy consolidation of the lungs.

The aetiological agents of different types of pneumonia are given in Table 23.2.

Lobar Pneumonia and Bronchopneumonia

Clinical Features. These include fever, malaise, rapid arterial pulse and leukocytosis (in bacterial pneumonias); central cyanosis and breathlessness; cough and purulent sputum often laced with blood (in lobar pneumonias); and herpes labialis of the lips. Pleuritic chest pain may occur in pneumococcal pneumonias, and there may be signs of lung consolidation on chest examination.

Pathogenesis and Epidemiology. Lobar pneumonia is mainly caused by exogenous organisms, although the patient's own upper respiratory tract flora may sometimes be an endogenous cause. The major agent of disease is the pneumococcus. However, of some 80 serotypes of pneumococci,

Table 23.2   Aetiological Agents of Pneumonia

Pneumonia Variant	Main Pathogens
Bronchopneumonia and lobar pneumonia	*Streptococcus pneumoniae*
	Streptococcus pneumoniae
	Haemophilus influenzae
	SARS coronavirus (SARS-CoV-1)
	MERS coronavirus (MERS-CoV)
	SARS coronavirus-2 (SARS-CoV-2)
Atypical pneumonias	*Mycoplasma pneumoniae*
	Coxiella burnetii
	Chlamydia psittaci
Legionnaires' disease	*Legionella* spp.

SARS, severe acute respiratory syndrome.

only a few are implicated in the disease process. *Staphylococcus aureus* and *Haemophilus influenzae* are the other organisms involved.

The organisms invade the lung and deprive the alveolar cells of essential nutrients, thereby causing their destruction and death. This process is amplified in pneumococcal pneumonia by the **resistance of the pneumococci to phagocytosis** (due to the capsules) and the production of toxins such as **pneumolysins**.

The causative organisms of **bronchopneumonia** are similar to those of lobar pneumonia: pneumococci, *Staphylococcus aureus* and *Haemophilus influenzae* are common; coliforms are sometimes implicated. Staphylococcal bronchopneumonia frequently follows influenza and bronchitis in the elderly and infirm and may lead to death.

Other notable organisms that cause pneumonia are *Moraxella pneumoniae*, *Coxiella burnetii* and *Chlamydia psittaci*.

Laboratory Diagnosis. A properly taken, **early-morning sample of sputum** (as this is likely to be the most purulent) is essential for culture. Blood culture may be useful for diagnosing lobar pneumonia.

Treatment and Prevention. Antibiotic therapy is dictated by sensitivity tests; penicillins are the first choice. For pneumococcal pneumonia, selective prophylaxis with pneumococcal vaccine is advised for high-risk groups (e.g., debilitated, institutionalized elderly people).

Primary Atypical Pneumonia

A pneumonia is atypical when its causative agent cannot be isolated in ordinary laboratory media and/or when its clinical picture does not resemble that of pneumococcal pneumonia. The major agent of primary atypical pneumonia is the virus-like organism *Moraxella pneumoniae* (see Chapter 20), although others such as *Legionella* may be involved (Table 23.2). Mycoplasmal pneumonia has an incubation period of 1–3 weeks and is endemic in the community.

Severe Acute Respiratory Syndrome (SARS) and Coronavirus Disease 2019 (COVID-19)

Both severe acute respiratory syndrome (SARS) and coronavirus disease 2019 (COVID-19) are caused by coronaviruses; the former is due to SARS-CoV-1, and the latter is due to SARS-CoV-2 (Chapter 4). They are human and animal pathogens of great importance, as shown by the pandemic of COVID-19.

Coronaviruses usually inhabit animals such as bats but may cause human infection when they **cross the so-called 'species barrier'** from animals to humans. One such notable event occurred in 2013 in Guangzhou, China, and led to the SARS epidemic, whereas the second major epochal event occurred 6 years later at the end of 2019, precipitating what is now known as the COVID-19 pandemic. The origin of the SARS-CoV-2 is still shrouded in mystery, although the disease was first described in Wuhan, China.

Another such coronavirus infection of lesser severity and significance called the **Middle East respiratory**

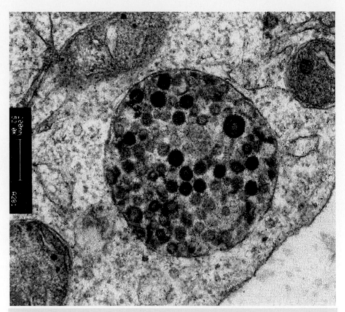

Fig. 23.3   A transmission electronic micrograph of the severe acute respiratory syndrome coronavirus (SARS-CoV-1) particles in the alveolar tissue of a patient.

syndrome coronavirus (MERS-CoV) ensued in 2012 in Saudi Arabia. This virus, like SARS-CoV-2, also originated in bats but later transmitted to dromedary camels. MERS was a relatively well-contained infection with less than 3000 being infected worldwide to date. (MERS is not further discussed here).

SEVERE ACUTE RESPIRATORY SYNDROME (SARS)

Severe acute respiratory syndrome (SARS) was the first, severe, readily transmissible, emerging infection of the 21st century. Caused by the SARS-CoV-1 (Fig. 23.3), it was recognized in 30 countries within a short period of 6 months. Unfortunately, a large number of **health care workers succumbed** to the disease in the early period of infection, prior to the discovery of the virus and its mode of spread. Fortunately, no documented cases of SARS have been described since the first outbreak in 2003.

Clinical Features, Pathogenesis and Epidemiology

Nonspecific early symptoms such as fever, malaise, chills, headache, cough and sore throat are followed by shortness of breath a few days later. Some patients deteriorate rapidly, which leads to **acute respiratory distress** requiring hospitalization and ventilatory support. The disease is difficult to differentiate from other atypical pneumonias, and, if not recognized early and promptly managed, death due to respiratory failure occurs in 10%, particularly in the elderly.

The virus spreads by the **airborne** route through droplets or aerosols. However, no cases of disease transmission through a dental clinic setting have been reported. Infectivity of the virus during the prodrome of about 6 days is low, but it is high during the febrile period. The virus is relatively robust and hence survives in **urine, faeces and in mixed saliva for up to 4 days**, leading to further spread under unhygienic conditions.

Laboratory Diagnosis

The earliest diagnosis methods included serodiagnosis with acute and convalescent sera, enzyme-linked immunosorbent assay (ELISA), haemagglutination and electron microscopy of respiratory secretions or stool samples. Rapid polymerase chain reaction–based diagnostic methods under development appear to be reliable.

Treatment and Prevention

There is no proven treatment or vaccine, as yet. The mainstays of prevention are isolation of patients, quarantine of those exposed, travel restrictions and use of appropriate protective clothing by health care workers during disease outbreaks.

CORONAVIRUS DISEASE 2019 (COVID-19)

There is a vast literature on COVID-19, and the description that follows here is a highly abbreviated account of the virus and the disease. (*Note:* Readers are advised to keep abreast of the current literature on the topic as the disease dynamics are ever changing.)

Epidemiology

In the latter part of 2019, a novel coronavirus was identified as the cause of a cluster of pneumonia cases in Wuhan, China. It rapidly spread, resulting in an epidemic throughout China, and this was followed by a **global pandemic**. In February 2020, the World Health Organization (WHO) designated the disease as COVID-19 (acronym for **co**ro**na**virus **d**isease 20**19**) and its etiological agent as severe acute respiratory syndrome coronavirus 2 (SARS-CoV-2) (Fig. 23.3). Since then, several mutants of varying degrees of infectivity and virulence have emerged from the original wild-type strain, such as Alpha, Beta, Gamma, Delta and Omicron. The latter and its progeny, are the currently circulating major variants.

At the time of this writing (September 2023), COVID-19 has claimed approximately 7 million lives with over 695 million cases reported globally. SARS-CoV-2 is more infectious than SARS or MERS, and elderly and compromised patients with comorbidities are at the greatest risk of fatality. COVID-19 has significantly impacted people worldwide, transforming their social, hygiene and behavioural practices as well as their life style, either directly or indirectly.

Virology

Infectivity. The extremely high infectivity of SARS-CoV-2 is thought to be due to (1) its high reproduction number, so-called R_0 value between 2 and 6 (i.e., the expected number of secondary cases produced in a completely susceptible population), (2) the relatively long prodromal period and (3) the asymptomatic carrier state of 30–40%.

Furthermore, once it reaches human tissues, SARS-CoV-2 has an inherent avidity and an affinity to recognize and bind to the **angiotensin converting enzyme 2 (ACE2)** receptors. These receptors are present in virtually *all eukaryotic cells*, and therefore the viral **spike proteins** (Fig. 4.5) can latch onto any human cell, though it preferentially binds to those of the respiratory epithelium in the first instance (Fig. 23.4).

Transmission modes. Many; respiratory droplets (talking, coughing, sneezing), contact with contaminated surfaces or objects (fomites), short-range aerosol and airborne transmission from suspended (entrained) droplets in air, especially in poorly ventilated and/or crowded indoor settings and hospitals.

Saliva and SARS-CoV-2

SARS-CoV-2 is always present in mixed saliva of COVID-19 patients and is highly likely to be present in asymptomatic carriers as well. Salivary gland cells and cells from mixed saliva exhibit ACE2 receptors for spike antigens of the virus, indicating these could be viral reservoirs. Both acellular and cellular salivary fractions from asymptomatic individuals incubating the infection may transmit SARS-CoV-2 ex vivo. It is also known that the salivary viral burden correlates well with COVID-19 symptoms, including taste loss. Furthermore, upon recovery, asymptomatic individuals exhibit sustained salivary IgG antibodies against SARS-CoV-2.

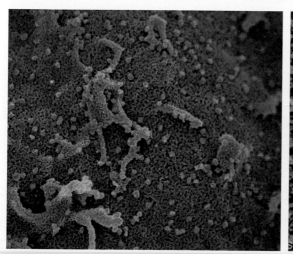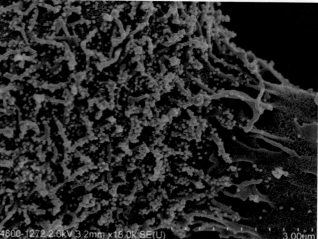

Fig. 23.4   A pseudo-coloured (left) and a black-and-white (right) scanning electron micrographs (SEM) depicting numerous budding, fully developed SARS-CoV-2 particles emerging from laboratory cultured infected cells. (The numerous small spheres are the viral particles on the cell surface (Magnification 18,000×). (Images courtesy of Professor John Nicholls and the University of Hong Kong.)

Hence saliva is both a **potential vehicle of SARS-CoV-2 transmission** and a useful **diagnostic fluid** for COVID-19 infection.

Clinical Features Including Orofacial Manifestations

Incubation period. Ranges from 1–14 days; some, such as the newer Omicron variant, has a relatively shorter incubation period of around 3 days.

Clinical manifestations. A broad clinical spectrum ranging from asymptomatic infection to septic shock and multiorgan dysfunction. Thus COVID-19 exhibits protean manifestations similar to bacterial infections such as syphilis (Chapter 27).

Disease classification. Based on the severity of the presentation classified as **mild, moderate, severe, and critical**.

Most common symptoms: Fever, fatigue, dry cough, and diarrhea.

Mild disease: Presents with symptoms of an upper respiratory tract infection such as dry cough, mild fever, nasal congestion, sore throat, headache, muscle pain, and malaise; radiographic features are absent.

Moderate disease: Typically present with cough, shortness of breath, and tachypnea.

Severe disease leading to critical illness: Presents with severe pneumonia, acute respiratory distress syndrome (ARDS), sepsis or septic shock and radiographic features. Severe disease may lead to critical illness with respiratory arrest and or other multiorgan manifestations, and finally death. Older people and those with comorbidities (e.g., hypertension, heart and lung disease, diabetes, obesity or cancer) are at higher risk of developing severe disease.

Unfortunately, it is estimated that 10%–20% of people may continue to experience mid- and long-term effects of COVID-19, including fatigue, respiratory and neurological symptoms collectively known as 'post–COVID-19 condition' or **'long COVID'**. However, these symptoms usually improve with time.

Orofacial Manifestations

Most common are the afflictions of the **chemosensory system**, which dictates the ability to **taste** (dysgeusia, hypogeusia, ageusia) and **smell** (hyposmia, anosmia); also called – sensorineuronal deficit. **Dysgeusia** or aberrations of taste is considered a hallmark of the disease.

The aetiology of dysgeusia is attributed to:

- direct viral infection and damage to the **taste buds** located in the filiform, fungiform and vallate papillae
- viral infection of the tongue **keratinocytes** and the associated cell death and desquamation blocking the taste buds
- virus infecting the **supporting cells** of the taste buds.

Importantly though, dysgeusia is almost always temporary with normal taste sensation returning by 4–6 weeks after recovery from acute COVID-19 illness.

In addition, a number of other minor orofacial manifestation of COVID-19 have been infrequently reported thus far (Table 23.3). The presentation and frequency of oral manifestations appear to be higher in older, hospitalized cohorts with comorbidities and severe COVID-19.

Laboratory Diagnosis

Tests for the identification of viral RNA or humoural responses are the basis for laboratory diagnosis (Fig. 23.5). The tests are basically divided into three categories:

Table 23.3 Orofacial Manifestations of COVID-19

Relatively more common:

Sensorineuronal deficit (most common)

Loss of taste (dysgeusia, ageusia, hypogeusia)

Loss of smell (hyposmia, anosmia)

Ulcerative lesions (less common)

Aphthous-like lesions (ALL)

Herpetiform/zosteriform lesions

Erosive lesions

Erythema multiforme (EM)-like target lesions

Relatively less common:

White/red plaques/patches

Angina bullosa-like lesions

Necrotizing periodontal disease

Postinflammatory pigmentation

Mucositis

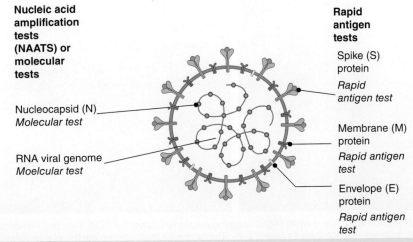

Fig. 23.5 SARS-CoV-2 viral components used in rapid antigen tests (right) and molecular tests (left).

- *Rapid antigen tests (RATs):* Useful for provisional diagnosis; detect protein markers on the outside of the virus (Fig. 23.5); can be self-administered, and most can be used in point-of-care (POC) settings such as dental surgeries; results available within minutes
- *Real-time polymerase chain reactions (RT-PCRs; syn: nucleic acid amplification tests NAATS):* to detect molecular RNA of the pathogen; usually required to confirm a RAT test; **gold standard confirmatory test** usually done in laboratory settings (some could be self-administered)
- *Serology and adaptive immune response tests:* Useful from the second week of symptoms onward after a serological response is mounted; these tests could also monitor **postvaccination antibody** levels
- *Viral specimens:* Nasopharyngeal specimens remain the recommended specimens, whereas nasal mid-turbinate, anterior nasal or oropharyngeal swabs are acceptable alternatives.

Treatment

Mild disease symptoms are managed with over-the-counter medicines, such as acetaminophen (Tylenol) or ibuprofen (Motrin, Advil).

Antiviral drugs: The combination antivirals **nirmatrelvir** and **ritonavir** (trade name Paxlovid), as well as **molnupiravir** and **remdesivir**, are effective in all age groups against COVID-19 and its variants. To be effective, the drugs should be started **within 7 days of symptom onset** and administered for 3 days; they are usually given to high-risk patients.

Prevention

General measures: The risk of COVID-19 transmission can be mitigated by wearing well-fitted masks, covering coughs and sneezes and maintaining a distance of at least 6 feet from others (social distancing), frequent hand hygiene and avoiding crowded venues during outbreaks.

Other preventive measures include quarantine of patients and those exposed, as well as proper use of personal protective clothing by dental care workers during disease outbreaks (Chapter 37).

Vaccines: Vaccination is the most effective way to prevent COVID-19, particularly to prevent serious infection and death. A variety of vaccine types (mRNA, DNA, viral vector, subunit and attenuated) are available (Chapters 10 and 37). The most popular vaccine type appears to be the mRNA vaccines.

LEGIONNAIRES' DISEASE

Legionnaires' disease is caused by *Legionella pneumophila* and other *Legionella* species.

Clinical Features, Pathogenesis and Epidemiology

An increasingly common cause of pneumonia with significant mortality, legionnaires' disease typically affects middle-aged smokers, often in poor general health. The illness **resembles influenza** and may lead to respiratory failure; associated symptoms are mental confusion, renal failure and gastrointestinal upsets.

The organism is a **saprophyte** that often exists in soil and stagnant water. Airborne spread is associated with cooling towers of air-conditioning systems and with

Table 23.4 Groups at Risk of Tuberculosis
Children and young adults
Contacts of patients with active infection
Immunosuppressed individuals (e.g., HIV, drug therapy)
Health care workers in close contact with patients
Socially disadvantaged poor, in crowded urban environments
Individuals with alcoholism, diabetes mellitus or silicosis

HIV, human immunodeficiency virus.

complex modern plumbing systems; person-to-person airborne spread has not been documented. Concern has been expressed in the past that legionellae may multiply in **stagnant water in dental unit water systems**, and patients may be exposed to this health hazard when three-in-one syringes are used. Such fears appear to be unfounded.

Laboratory Diagnosis, Antibiotics and Prevention

See Chapter 19.

RESPIRATORY TUBERCULOSIS

Up to one-third of the global population is thought to be infected by the tubercle bacillus with up to 3 million deaths each year. Respiratory tuberculosis (TB) is the preeminent fatal disease of the middle- and low-income countries. Caused by *Mycobacterium tuberculosis* and other atypical mycobacteria (Chapter 19). TB is reemerging as a result of i) the human immunodeficiency virus (HIV) pandemic and ii) the bacilli that are gradually acquiring resistance to the conventional antituberculous drugs. These diseases are classified as either **multidrug-resistant tuberculosis (MDR-TB) or XDR-TB** depending on the degree of the antibiotic resistance of the bacilli. The latter, severe variant of the disease is virtually untreatable as the bacilli are not killed by any of the currently available anti-tuberculous drugs. Persons at increased risk of TB including dentists and their assistants, who are exposed to infectious droplet particles from their patients. Nevertheless, successfully BCG vaccinated need not have these concerns (Table 23.4).

Clinical Features and Pathogenesis

Respiratory TB is a **chronic granulomatous disease** with **protean manifestations** that mainly affects the lungs, although other organs and tissues are frequently involved. Infection is initiated after inhalation of contaminated aerosol droplets. The disease can be divided into primary infection and postprimary infection.

Primary Infection

The primary focus of pulmonary TB is generally the **apical regions of the lungs**, including the upper part of the lower lobe and the lower part of the upper lobe. This takes the form of a primary complex—the local lesion (**Ghon focus**) with enlargement of the regional hilar lymph nodes. Within 3–6 weeks, the patient's cellular immunity is activated and replication of the bacilli will cease in most patients. The **primary infection is entirely symptomless** or sometimes associated with malaise, anorexia and weight loss. Cough is not a significant finding at this stage.

The primary infection is usually contained, and the active focus may become walled off and fibrotic. Antibiotic treatment at this stage may also resolve the infection. Without such intervention, however, the disease may progress in some, leading to death. The resultant systemic spread of disease may cause:

- tuberculous bronchopneumonia
- miliary TB: haematogenous spread of the bacilli with multiple infective foci throughout the body
- tuberculous meningitis
- bone and joint TB
- renal TB.

Postprimary Infection

There may be a latent period of months or years before the tubercle bacilli initiate active disease after primary infection. Such postprimary infection commonly involves the lungs, leading to **caseous necrosis and fibrosis**. The symptoms of postprimary disease are loss of appetite and weight, tiredness, fever and night sweats, cough, sputum and haemoptysis. Breathlessness due to pleural effusion, pneumothorax and lung collapse may occur if not treated.

Treatment

Treatment of TB is complex and depends on combination drug therapy to suppress the emergence of resistant bacilli. The recommended drugs in the UK are isoniazid, rifampicin, pyrazinamide and ethambutol. Treatment is usually initiated in the hospital, after which **directly observed treatment short-term (DOTS)** is given for up to 8 months.

Prevention

Vaccination with a live, attenuated, bovine *Mycobacterium* strain, **bacille Calmette–Guérin (BCG)**, provides immunity for most but not all. The vaccine is given to those who are Mantoux test negative.

The **Mantoux test** is an intradermal injection in the arm of purified protein derivative (PPD) from *M. tuberculosis* cultures. A hard lesion of 10 mm or more in diameter 48–72 h after injection indicates either active disease or past infection. Mantoux testing is not totally reliable as false negatives may occur.

The BCG vaccine is most effective in children and less so in adults. One disadvantage of the vaccine is that, while it may or may not confer protection, it will yield a positive (Mantoux) skin test, which precludes the usefulness of the latter test as a means of detecting early infection.

Other methods of preventing TB include improving social and living conditions and nutrition.

EMPYEMA

Empyema or **pus in the pleural space** is almost always caused by secondary bacterial spread entering the pleural space as a result of:

- TB, lung abscess or complication of pneumonia
- thoracic surgery or trauma
- hepatic or subphrenic abscess.

The organisms involved are similar to those that cause the primary infection; treatment depends on drainage and removal of the infected fluid and appropriate antibiotic therapy.

Fungal Infections of the Lower Respiratory Tract

Inhalation of pathogenic spores or yeast cells may cause a number of fungal infections of the lower respiratory tract, especially in persons who are immunocompromised. Such infections are becoming increasingly prevalent because of the pandemic HIV infection; they include blastomycosis, coccidioidomycosis, cryptococcosis and histoplasmosis. Pneumonias due to *Pneumocystis jirovecii* (PJP) are particularly common in patients with acquired immune deficiency syndrome (AIDS) and are the leading cause of death in HIV disease; patients are treated with co-trimoxazole (sulfamethoxazole and trimethoprim) and aerosolized pentamidine.

Respiratory Infections and Dentistry

Respiratory infections are of special concern to dentists, as patients will regularly present for treatment during the prodromal period, occasionally in the acute phase or the recovery stage of infections. This is particularly the case with COVID-19, as a significant proportion of viral carriers appear to be asymptomatic and ambulatory. The most common mode of transmission of respiratory infections is the airborne route, although direct or indirect contact with contaminated fomites may spread infections such as COVID-19 (see Chapter 36).

The majority of infections that may spread in the dental clinic are thought to be caused by viruses, and it has been documented that dental personnel tend to suffer more from viral upper respiratory tract infections than the average individual. Such cross-infection may be minimized by wearing a face mask and by appropriate ventilation of the surgical suite. It is noteworthy that the COVID-19 pandemic and the advent of highly transmissible SARS-CoV-2 variants such as Omicron and lineage strains have led to further reinforcement of infection control measures in dentistry and adoption of so called 'transmission-based precautions'.

The transmission of a number of severe bacterial infections such as diphtheria, pertussis and TB as well as viral infections such as hepatitis B and COVID-19 can be mitigated by immunization of the dental team as appropriate (Chapter 37).

General anaesthesia should never be administered to patients with respiratory tract infection, as this may cause reduced respiratory efficiency due to increased secretions and obstruction of the airways. Dental personnel suffering from acute respiratory infection should not attend work, as they may transmit the infection to other staff and to their patients.

Key Facts

- Human **respiratory tract infections** account for **the majority of general practitioner consultations** and for almost a quarter of all absences from work due to illness in the western world.
- The **nose** is the **habitat of a variety of streptococci** and **staphylococci**, the most significant of which is *Staphylococcus aureus*, especially prevalent in the **anterior nares**.
- The major **bacterial pathogen** in the **sore throat syndrome** is *Streptococcus pyogenes* (Lancefield group A).
- *Streptococcus pyogenes* is the agent of childhood scarlet fever.
- Scarlet fever may present extraorally as a facial skin rash and intraorally as a '**strawberry tongue**' or '**raspberry tongue**'.
- **Rheumatic fever**, **rheumatic carditis** and **acute glomerulonephritis** are immunologically mediated diseases that may manifest as a late consequence of *Streptococcus pyogenes* infection such as streptococcal sore throat or scarlet fever.
- **Rheumatic fever** may lead to permanent **endocardial damage**, and infected individuals are highly susceptible to **bacterial endocarditis** later in life, when **bacteraemias** are created during **dental or surgical procedures**.
- Prudent **antibiotic prophylaxis** prior to such procedures in susceptible individuals prevents bacterial endocarditis.
- **Diphtheria**, a severe, acute inflammation of the upper respiratory tract, usually the throat, is due to *Corynebacterium diphtheriae*; **prevention** is by the **diphtheria–tetanus–pertussis (DTP) vaccine**.
- **Corynebacteria** produce a powerful **exotoxin** that is **cardiotoxic** and **neurotoxic**, affecting the myocardium, adrenal glands and nerve endings.
- **Vincent's angina**, caused by the **fusospirochaetal complex** (fusobacteria and oral spirochaetes), can be treated by either **penicillin or metronidazole**.
- Both **otitis media** and **sinusitis** are due to endogenous infection with bacteria such as *Haemophilus influenzae*, *Streptococcus pneumoniae* and *Streptococcus pyogenes*.
- Pneumonia can be categorized into lobar or segmental pneumonia bronchopneumonia and primary atypical or virus pneumonia.
- **Lobar pneumonia** is mainly caused by **exogenous organisms** (major agent: pneumococcus) and sometimes by the patient's own upper respiratory tract flora.
- The major agent of primary atypical pneumonia is *Mycoplasma pneumoniae*.
- **SARS-CoV-2** is the third virus of the coronavirus family to cause epidemics/pandemics in the 21st century, after **SARS-CoV-1** and **MERS** coronavirus.
- **SARS-CoV-2** and its derivative variants (such as Alpha, Beta, Gamma, Delta and Omicron) are the agents of the **COVID-19** pandemic that began in 2019.
- The extremely high infectivity of SARS-CoV-2 is due to the ability of its **spike proteins** to recognize and **bind to ACE2 receptors** on all human (eukaryotic) cells and its ability to survive on inanimate surfaces for a few days; these then act as **fomites**.
- COVID-19 infection is basically classified as **mild, moderate, severe and critical disease**, with the latter eventually leading to death.
- **Dysgeusia** is considered the hallmark oral manifestation of COVID-19 infection; various types of oral ulcerations have also been reported as common, particularly in severe disease.
- COVID-19 could be provisionally diagnosed by **rapid antigen tests (RAT)** and confirmed by **real-time polymerase chain reaction (RT-PCR)** tests; **serology** is useful to detect past infection and the efficacy of vaccines.
- **Prevention** of COVID-19 is essentially through measures that mitigate inhalation of airborne viral particles (e.g., masks, social distancing, respiratory hygiene and personal protective equipment) and, **most importantly, vaccines**.
- A number of vaccines are available to prevent COVID-19, and the most popular type is the **mRNA vaccines**.
- **Legionnaires' disease** is caused by *Legionella pneumophila* and other *Legionella* species that are saprophytic and exist in soil and stagnant water.
- Up to one-third of the global population is infected with *Mycobacterium* species that cause tuberculosis.
- **Tuberculosis is reemerging** as a result of both the **human immunodeficiency virus (HIV) pandemic** and the bacilli that are gradually acquiring **resistance to the conventional antituberculous drugs**—so-called multidrug-resistant tuberculosis (**MDR-TB and XDR-TB**).
- **Treatment of tuberculosis is complex** and depends on combination drug therapy (e.g., directly observed treatment (**DOT**)).
- **Vaccination** with a live, attenuated, bovine *Mycobacterium* strain, **bacille Calmette–Guérin (BCG)**, provides **immunity from tuberculosis** for most but not all. The vaccine is given to those who are Mantoux test-negative.

Review Questions (Answers on p. 390)

Please indicate which answers are true and which are false.

23.1. Which of the following statements on pharyngitis are true?
    a. Gram-positive cocci in chains in a smear from a throat swab are diagnostic of a bacterial cause.
    b. A course of oral penicillin is always advisable to prevent complications.
    c. It may lead to immunological sequelae.
    d. The aetiological agent can be predicted by visual examination of the throat.
    e. When associated with rhinorrhoea, sneezing and conjunctival irritation, it is likely to be of viral aetiology.

23.2. Which of the following statements on the common cold are true?
    a. It may have a seasonal variation in incidence.
    b. It is commonly caused by respiratory syncytial viruses.
    c. It is often self-limiting.
    d. It might lead to exacerbation of asthma in some individuals.
    e. Hand-washing is one of the important preventive methods.

23.3. Pharyngitis caused by *Streptococcus pyogenes*:
   a. is often seen in children
   b. commonly presents as stridor
   c. has peritonsillar abscess formation as a common complication
   d. frequently gives rise to rheumatic fever
   e. has penicillin as the drug of choice

23.4. Rheumatic fever:
   a. may lead to glomerulonephritis
   b. pathogenesis is due to invasion of cardiac tissues by *Streptococcus pyogenes*
   c. is more common in children than in adolescents
   d. may increase the risk of bacterial endocarditis in later life
   e. may lead to permanent heart damage

23.5. Otitis media:
   a. is an infrequent complication of common cold
   b. risk is increased in the presence of congenital oropharyngeal malformations
   c. calls for culturing a swab taken from the external auditory meatus to point to the aetiological agent
   d. has mastoiditis as a known complication
   e. rarely causes brain abscess due to direct extension

23.6. Vincent's angina:
   a. is associated with poor oral hygiene and concomitant viral infections
   b. is a polymicrobial infection with fusobacteria and spirochaetes
   c. may be associated with acute ulcerative gingivitis
   d. can be cured by antibiotics alone
   e. is common in immunodeficient patients

23.7. COVID-19:
   a. is caused by SARS-CoV-1
   b. may lead to loss of taste and smell
   c. can be cured by antivirals in cases of severe disease
   d. can be definitively diagnosed by rapid antigen tests
   e. is relatively common in those with comorbidities

23.8. Which of the following statements on scarlet fever are true?
   a. It is caused by Lancefield Group B beta hemolytic streptococci
   b. Rheumatic fever could be a sequel
   c. It is more common in children than in adolescents
   d. Circumoral pallor is a presenting feature
   e. Maculo-papular lesions may follow the skin rash

Further Reading

Fakhruddin, K. S., Samaranayake, L. P., Buranawat, B., & Ngo, H. (2022). Oro-facial mucocutaneous manifestations of Coronavirus Disease-2019 (COVID-19): A systematic review. *PLOS One, 17*(6), e0265531.

Huang, N., Pérez, P., Kato, T., et al. (2021). SARS-CoV-2 infection of the oral cavity and saliva. *Nature Medicine, 27*, 892–903. https://doi.org10.1038/s41591-021-01296-8.

Matusubara, V., Christoforu, J., & Samaranayake, L. (2023). Recrudescence of scarlet fever and its implications for dental professionals. *International Dental Journal, 73*, 331–336.

Mims, C., Playfair, J., Roitt, I., et al. (1998). Upper respiratory tract infections. In *Medical microbiology* (2nd ed., Ch. 15 and 17). Mosby.

Phelan, J. A., Jimenez, V., & Tompkins, D. C. (1996). Tuberculosis. *Dental Clinics of North America, 40*, 327–341.

Samaranayake, L. P., Fakhruddin, K. S., & Panduwawala, C. (2020). Sudden onset, acute loss of taste and smell in coronavirus disease 2019 (COVID-19): A systematic review. *Acta Odontologica Scandinavica, 78*(6), 467–473.

Samaranayake, L. P., Fakhruddin, K. S., Mohammad, O. E., & Panduwawala, C. (2022). Attributes of dysgeusia and anosmia of coronavirus disease 2019 (COVID-19) in hospitalized patients. *Oral Diseases, 28*, 891–898.

Shanson, D. C. (1999). Infections of the lower respiratory tract. In *Microbiology in clinical practice* (3rd ed., p. 14). Butterworth-Heinemann.

Van-Arsdall, J. A., et al. (1983). The protean manifestations of legionnaires' disease. *Journal of Infection, 7*, 51–62.

24 Infections of the Cardiovascular System

In health, the cardiovascular system is sterile, but a few organisms may enter the blood stream (even in health) during routine procedures such as tooth-brushing, especially in the presence of periodontitis. However, these bacteria have only a transient existence, as the efficient defences of the blood quickly destroy them.

Bacteraemia, Septicaemia and Sepsis Syndrome

DEFINITIONS

Bacteraemia: literally 'bacterial presence in the blood', where the bacterial burden in blood is usually very low and is clinically insignificant (i.e., bacteraemia is **asymptomatic**). Bacteraemia could be produced simply by brushing of teeth or chewing, especially in the presence of periodontitis. Additionally, a number of invasive dental procedures may cause bacteraemia, and this has major clinical significance. Such 'seeding' of bacteria carried through the blood circulation to distant sites (i.e., so-called 'hematogenous seeding') such as heart valves may be the initial event that leads to infective endocarditis.

Septicaemia: literally 'sepsis of the blood', seen when large numbers of organisms **enter** and/or **actively multiply** and persist in the blood stream, producing clinical signs and symptoms such as hypotension, fever and rigors.

Sepsis syndrome: a systemic response to microbial products or constituents circulating in the blood mediated by inflammatory cytokines (see Septicaemia and Sepsis Syndrome below).

SEPTICAEMIA AND SEPSIS SYNDROME

Aetiology

Some common predisposing factors and agents that cause septicaemia are shown in Table 24.1.

Pathogenesis and Clinical Features

Once the blood stream is invaded by microbes, the host responds by activating its defence mechanisms, leading to the production of a cascade of **inflammatory cytokines** (e.g., interleukin-1, tumour necrosis factor; see Chapter 10). The cytokine release is orchestrated by endotoxins of Gram-negative bacteria, peptidoglycan of Gram-positive bacteria and exotoxins from both these groups. Generally, these cytokines are beneficial in eliminating

Table 24.1 Some Common Predisposing Factors and Agents of Septicaemia

Predisposing Factor	Agent
Abdominal sepsis	Enterobacteria
	Bacteroides fragilis
	Enterococcus faecalis
Infected wounds, burns	*Staphylococcus aureus*
	Streptococcus pyogenes
	Enterobacteria
Osteomyelitis	*Staphylococcus aureus*
Pneumonia	*Streptococcus pneumoniae*
Intravascular devices	*Staphylococcus aureus*
	Staphylococcus epidermidis
	Enterobacteria
Food poisoning	*Salmonella* spp.
	Campylobacter spp.
Meningitis	*Streptococcus pneumoniae*
	Neisseria meningitidis
	Haemophilus influenzae
Immunosuppressed patients	Enterobacteria
	Staphylococcus aureus, etc.

the organisms, but excessive production may lead to organ dysfunction and circulatory septic shock: the **sepsis syndrome**.

Some of these patients are said to develop the **systemic inflammatory response syndrome (SIRS)** depending on their clinical signs; these include hypotension, fever, rigors, oliguria and renal failure. Sometimes the infection may trigger a pathological activation of the coagulation system (**disseminated intravascular coagulation (DIC)**) and, due to the resultant consumption of platelets and clotting factors, severe **bleeding disorders**.

Diagnosis

Blood should be cultured for a diagnosis of septicaemia. As the number of organisms circulating in the blood may vary from time to time, depending on the disease condition, more than one blood culture may be required; whenever possible, this should be carried out before antibiotic therapy is instituted. Several positive cultures are required to ensure that the culture result is not due to contamination from the venepuncture site. Cultures from sites suspected to be causing the infection are useful (e.g., pus from an abscess) to establish and localize the infective focus.

Treatment

The principles of therapy are:

- aggressive bactericidal (rather than bacteriostatic) intravenous antimicrobial therapy in adequate dosage
- stabilization of the haemodynamic status (e.g., intravenous fluids, cardiogenic drugs, oxygen)
- identification of the focus of infection and appropriate action (e.g., removal of a foreign body, surgical intervention by draining an abscess).

Infections of the Heart

Important pathogens that cause **pericarditis**, **myocarditis** and **endocarditis** are shown in Fig. 24.1. Of these, infective endocarditis is the most important disease of relevance to dentistry.

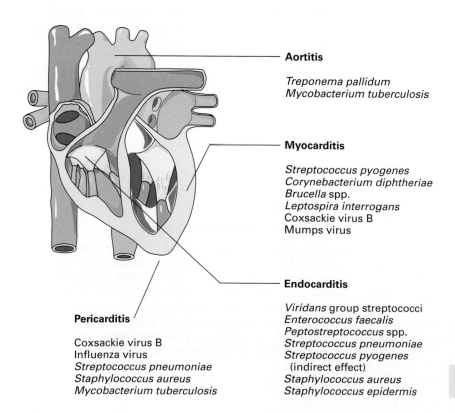

Aortitis

Treponema pallidum
Mycobacterium tuberculosis

Myocarditis

Streptococcus pyogenes
Corynebacterium diphtheriae
Brucella spp.
Leptospira interrogans
Coxsackie virus B
Mumps virus

Endocarditis

Viridans group streptococci
Enterococcus faecalis
Peptostreptococcus spp.
Streptococcus pneumoniae
Streptococcus pyogenes
 (indirect effect)
Staphylococcus aureus
Staphylococcus epidermis

Pericarditis

Coxsackie virus B
Influenza virus
Streptococcus pneumoniae
Staphylococcus aureus
Mycobacterium tuberculosis

Fig. 24.1   Major infectious agents of aortitis, myocarditis, endocarditis and pericarditis.

INFECTIVE ENDOCARDITIS

Definition

Inflammation of the endocardium of the heart valves, and sometimes the endocardium around congenital defects, resulting from an infection.

Microbial Aetiology

Bacteria are predominantly involved, although other organisms, such as fungi, rickettsiae and chlamydiae, may occasionally cause endocarditis (Table 24.2). More than 80% of infective endocarditis is caused by streptococci and staphylococci. The position held by the *viridans* group of organisms in the league table indicates the major role played by the oral commensals in causing this life-threatening disease. It is noteworthy that nearly all patients with *viridans* endocarditis have a previous heart lesion, and about a quarter give a history of a recent dental procedure as a precipitating factor.

Clinical Features

Although two clinical forms of the disease—**acute** and **subacute**—have been identified, the line of demarcation between these forms is not often clear. The acute form is a rapidly progressive condition and is caused by bacteria such as *Streptococcus pneumoniae*, *Staphylococcus aureus* and *Streptococcus pyogenes*. The subacute form is more insidious and chronic, and it progresses rather slowly. The agents of this form of the disease are less virulent bacteria, such as *viridans* streptococci, *Staphylococcus epidermidis* and *Enterococcus faecalis*.

Signs and Symptoms

The classic signs are fever, malaise, loss of weight, anaemia, splinter haemorrhages, petechiae, cardiac murmur, haematuria and splenomegaly.

Diagnosis

Clinical signs supported by positive blood culture are used to make the diagnosis. Repeated culture may be necessary to isolate the causal organism owing to the low-grade bacteraemia. If possible, blood should be collected when the temperature of the patient rises, indicating fever due to bacteraemia. At least 10 mL of blood should be collected prior to antibiotic therapy and cultured under aerobic and anaerobic conditions (see Fig. 6.4). Any agent isolated from two different blood culture sets (on separate occasions) is considered significant. Identification and antibiotic sensitivity tests are then performed on the isolate.

Pathogenesis and Epidemiology

Infective endocarditis normally occurs in patients with some pathological condition of the endocardium, although those with apparently normal heart valves may rarely be affected. The predisposing conditions include valve prostheses, septal defects, atheroma of the valve, congenital valve deformities and pre-existing rheumatic fever (Table 24.3). Infective endocarditis is the end result of the sequential interaction of events shown in Fig. 23.2:

1. A breach of the endocardium, or an abnormality of the endocardial surface per se, is the first event that makes the valvular surface finally succumb to infection. Such a breach may occur because of the acute inflammatory valvulitis of rheumatic fever (consequential to *Streptococcus pyogenes* infection; see Fig. 23.2) or in congenital heart diseases such as aortic valve disease and ventricular septal defect, when alterations of the blood flow patterns (haemodynamic turbulence) may result in the deposition of fibrin and platelets at foci where high-velocity jets of blood hit the valvular surface.
2. The microscopic platelet aggregates that form on the breached endocardium detach and **embolize** harmlessly or stabilize and **consolidate** through fibrin deposition, forming a sterile **thrombus**. The latter is a potential trap for circulating microbes. Such sterile thrombus formation is called **nonbacterial thrombotic endocarditis**. Platelets also have the potential to adhere to other 'foreign' surfaces such as prosthetic valves.
3. The next critical event occurs when organisms circulating in the blood (e.g., after a tooth extraction or scaling) attach to or become trapped in the thrombotic endocardium or the prosthetic device. The resultant

Table 24.2 Causative Microorganisms in Infective Endocarditis

Microorganisms	Cases (%)
Total streptococci	**60**
Viridans group	35
Enterococcus faecalis	13
Microaerophilic streptococci	3
Anaerobic streptococci	2
Others	7
Total staphylococci	**25**
Staphylococcus aureus	20
Staphylococcus epidermidis	5
Miscellaneous	**5**
Culture-negative	**10**

Table 24.3 Cardiac Valvular Disease Predisposing to Infective Endocarditis

Disease	Degree of Risk
Aortic valvular disease	High
Prosthetic valves	
Mitral insufficiency	
Ventricular septal defect	
Patent ductus arteriosus	
Coarctation of aorta	
Previous infective endocarditis	
Mitral valve prolapse and stenosis	Intermediate
Pulmonary and tricuspid valve disease	
Degenerative (calcific) aortic valve disease	
Nonvalvular intracardiac prosthetic implants	
Atrial septal defect	Low/negligible
Coronary artery disease	
Cardiac pacemakers	
Arteriosclerotic plaques	

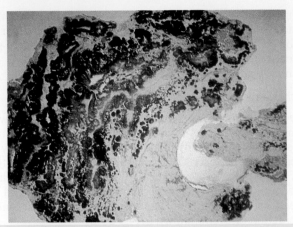

Fig. 24.2 A stained section of an infected heart valve teeming with Gram-positive streptococci (black colonisation). The heart valve was recovered from a rabbit subjected to experimental induction of infective endocarditis.

platelet–fibrin–bacterial mass, now called the **bacterial vegetation**, constitutes the primary pathology of infective endocarditis (Figs. 23.2 and 24.2).

4. Once the organisms are attached to the lesion, they multiply and colonise this niche in an exuberant manner. As a result, further aggregation of platelets and fibrin deposition ensues, protecting the organisms from the body defences. The organisms now reside in a sanctuary inaccessible to phagocytes by virtue of the **fibrin–platelet barrier**. Further, the bacteria may be sheltered from antibiotics and host antibodies, as the vegetation is essentially **avascular** in nature. As a result, it is necessary to use an intensive course of **prolonged, high-dose antibiotic therapy** to eradicate such an infective focus.

5. Even if endocarditis is successfully treated, the healed valve is permanently scarred and thickened, and such residual abnormalities make the patient highly vulnerable to episodes of reinfection.

Treatment

High-dosage single or combination antibiotic therapy, guided by the microbiological findings from the blood culture, is necessary. The antibiotic regimen selected should be:

- **bactericidal** and not bacteriostatic
- **parenterally** delivered
- **prolonged**, of several weeks' duration (usually up to 4 weeks).

The rationale behind management is:

1. to eradicate the organisms totally, without leaving residual pockets or reservoirs
2. to administer high concentrations of antibiotic so that it may penetrate, by diffusion, into the focal aggregates of bacteria in the avascular cardiac vegetations
3. to assess antibiotic levels in blood regularly, by **laboratory monitoring**, throughout the treatment period. Special sensitivity tests such as the **minimum inhibitory concentration (MIC)** and **minimum bactericidal concentration (MBC)** of the antibiotic (see Chapter 6) need to be performed regularly to ascertain the **optimal level** of antibiotics that should be present in the circulation to eradicate the organisms and to avoid the **toxic effects** (e.g., nephrotoxicity, ototoxicity) of aminoglycosides such as gentamicin, which is commonly prescribed in combination with other drugs.

INFECTIVE ENDOCARDITIS AND DENTISTRY

The oral cavity acts as a portal of entry for organisms causing bacteraemia, and dental manipulations may set in motion the disease process leading to infective endocarditis. Bacteraemia can occur during a number of dental procedures, as shown in Table 24.4. These include routine

Table 24.4 Examples of Invasive and Noninvasive Dental Procedures and Their Likelihood of Creating a Bacteraemia (*Note: This not an exhaustive list.*)

Invasive Dental Procedures (likely to create a bacteraemia)	Noninvasive Dental Procedures (unlikely to create a bacteraemia)
■ Placement of matrix bands	■ Infiltration or block local anaesthetic injections in noninfected soft tissues
■ Placement of subgingival rubber dam clamps	■ Supragingival scaling and polishing
■ Subgingival restorations including fixed prosthodontics	■ Supragingival restorations
■ Surgical or nonsurgical endodontics	■ Supragingival orthodontic bands and separators
■ Intraligamentary injections	■ Removal of sutures
■ Preformed metal crowns/stainless-steel crowns (PMCs/SSCs)	■ Taking radiograph
■ Full periodontal examinations (including pocket charting in diseased tissues)	■ Placement or adjustment of orthodontic or removable prosthodontic appliances
■ Root surface instrumentation/subgingival scaling	
■ Incision and drainage of abscess	
■ Dental extractions	
■ Surgery involving elevation of a mucoperiosteal flap or mucogingival area	
■ Placement of dental implants including temporary anchorage devices, mini-implants	
■ Uncovering implant substructures	
■ Reimplantation of teeth	

tooth **extractions, surgical or nonsurgical endodontics, gingivectomy, root-planing, scaling** and **flossing, intraligamentary injections** and **reimplantation** of avulsed teeth. The frequency of bacteraemia is also related to the preoperative **oral sepsis** of the patient and the degree of **trauma** and **tissue injury**; a routine activity such as tooth-brushing may also cause bacteraemia, depending on the degree of oral sepsis.

The real risk of development of infective endocarditis in a patient 'at risk' following dental procedures is difficult to ascertain, and the evidence base is rather contradictory; it has been estimated that bacteraemias vary between 10% and 90%. Clearly, a proportion of infections is associated with random transient bacteraemias that commonly follow mastication, and even tooth brushing, in patients with chronic periodontitis.

INFECTIVE ENDOCARDITIS PROPHYLAXIS

As eventual development of endocarditis may well be the most common potentially fatal complication of dental treatment, all dentists must have a good working knowledge of the problem and the appropriate preventive measures.

Accurate Identification of At-Risk Patients

The main risk conditions are shown in Table 24.3. Dentists usually identify patients at risk from their medical history. It is also important to obtain confirmatory and expert information from the patient's medical practitioner.

Patient Awareness of Risk Status and Dental Involvement in Cardiac Clinics

Warning cards given to patients with cardiac disease increase their awareness of the disease. Additionally, in the US, a **wallet card** containing information on the proper antibiotic dose (Table 24.4), if endocarditis prophylaxis is warranted, may be obtained by patients from the American Heart Association.

Dentists should be part of the medical team involved in the preoperative and postoperative management of patients undergoing cardiac surgery who are at risk.

Preventive Dental Care

Susceptible patients should be exposed to risky operative procedures as rarely as possible; this can be best achieved by careful and intensive oral hygiene instruction, dietary advice and regular dental examinations. The aim should be to reduce the amount of treatment to the absolute minimum necessary for the maintenance of a healthy natural dentition for life. The need to administer prophylactic antibiotics for dental procedures that could produce a bacteraemia capable of initiating infective endocarditis must be weighed carefully, and the *respective guidelines in each jurisdiction should be adhered to strictly.*

Awareness of Postoperative Morbidity

Even when antibiotic cover has been provided, patients at risk should be instructed to **report any unexplained illness** because of the insidious origin of infective endocarditis.

Cardiac Patients Who Need Antibiotic Prophylaxis

There is some controversy as to the need of antibiotic prophylaxis solely to prevent infective endocarditis in people at risk, undergoing either dental or nondental procedures. Hence, the British recommendations (National Institute for Health and Care Excellence (NICE) Guidelines), as opposed to the US recommendations, state that **there is *no* need for routine antibiotic prophylaxis for *any* dental procedure** due to the following reasons:

- There has been no consistent association between having an interventional procedure, dental or nondental, and the development of infective endocarditis.
- Regular tooth brushing presents a greater risk of infective endocarditis than a single dental procedure because of repetitive exposure to bacteraemia with oral flora.
- The clinical effectiveness of antibiotic prophylaxis is not proven.
- Antibiotic prophylaxis against infective endocarditis for dental procedures may lead to a greater number of deaths through fatal anaphylaxis than might a strategy of no antibiotic prophylaxis, and thus such prophylaxis is not cost-effective.
- The likelihood of emergence of antibiotic-resistant organisms.

British and US Guidelines on Prophylaxis Against Infective Endocarditis in Patients Undergoing Interventional Procedures

BRITISH GUIDELINES

Adults and children with the following cardiac conditions should be considered as being at increased risk of developing infective endocarditis:

- acquired valvular heart disease with stenosis or regurgitation
- hypertrophic cardiomyopathy
- previous infective endocarditis
- structural congenital heart disease, including surgically corrected or palliated structural conditions, but excluding isolated atrial septal defect, fully repaired ventricular septal defect or fully repaired patent ductus arteriosus, as well as closure devices that are judged to be endothelialized
- valve replacement.

Any episodes of infection in the aforementioned categories of people at risk of infective endocarditis should be investigated and treated promptly to reduce the risk of endocarditis developing.

Patient Advice

People at increased risk of infective endocarditis should be offered clear and consistent information about prevention, including:

- the benefits and risks of antibiotic prophylaxis, and an explanation of why antibiotic prophylaxis is no longer routinely recommended

- the importance of maintaining good oral health
- symptoms that may indicate infective endocarditis and when to seek expert advice
- the risks of undergoing invasive procedures, including nonmedical procedures such as body piercing or tattooing
- why chlorhexidine mouthwash is not offered as prophylaxis against infective endocarditis as there is no evidence base to substantiate its effectiveness.

US GUIDELINES

Compared with previous American Heart Association (AHA) guideline recommendations, there are currently relatively few patient subpopulations for whom antibiotic prophylaxis may be indicated prior to dental procedures that may create a bacteraemia. These include only those patients with an underlying condition that poses **the highest risk of an adverse outcome** from infective endocarditis such as:

- heart failure
- aortic root abscess
- need for cardiac valve replacement
- need for complex surgical revisions in patients with congenital heart disease
- recurrent streptococcal infective endocarditis.

Dental Procedures That Need Antibiotic Prophylaxis

The aforementioned groups of patients must be given antibiotics for all dental procedures that involve manipulation of gingival tissue or the periapical region of teeth or perforation of the oral mucosa as these procedures may cause bacteraemia.

Presurgical antibiotic regimens for a dental procedure according to the American Heart Association Guidelines can be found at the following Further Reading (Wilson et al., 2021). Similar antibiotic regimens have been declared by European and Australian authorities.

It should be borne in mind that these recommendations are regularly reviewed by the authorities, and practitioners need to keep abreast of such developments.

ANTIBIOTIC PROPHYLAXIS FOR MISCELLANEOUS CONDITIONS

Prosthetic Cardiac Valve

The dental management of patients with a prosthetic cardiac valve can be undertaken by dentists under antibiotic cover if they fall into a category of patients described in AHA guidelines (as described above), provided patients require local anaesthesia and are not hypersensitive to penicillin. If the patient has received penicillin more than once within the past month, oral clindamycin should be given. Furthermore, the antibiotics should be prescribed through consultation with the patients' cardiologist.

Third Molar Surgery

A number of properly controlled trials have conclusively indicated that antimicrobial agents **have no significant effect** on swelling, pain, trismus or postoperative infection in third molar surgery.

Dental Implants

Surgical placement of dental implants is an elective procedure performed under relatively aseptic conditions. Hence, it **does not warrant antibiotics either pre- or postsurgically**, although many surgeons prefer to do so worldwide. A number of reviews have indicated that pre- or postsurgical antibiotics during implant placement are of dubious value.

(Please see Chapter 25 for antibiotic prophylaxis for arthroplasties.)

Key Facts

- In health, the cardiovascular system is sterile, but a few organisms may transiently enter the blood stream during routines such as tooth brushing.
- **Bacteraemia is asymptomatic** and the bacterial burden in blood is very low, whereas in **septicaemia** large numbers of **organisms enter and/or actively multiply** and persist in the blood stream, producing clinical signs and symptoms such as hypotension, fever and rigors.
- Bacteraemias can occur after numerous dental procedures (Table 24.4), but to the extent to which they may cause endocardial infection is uncertain.
- **Sepsis syndrome** is a systemic response to microbial products or constituents circulating in the blood mediated by inflammatory cytokines.
- Infective endocarditis is defined as the inflammation of the endocardium of the heart valves, and sometimes the endocardium around congenital defects, caused by an infection.
- More than 80% of infective endocarditis is caused by streptococci and staphylococci.

- Infective endocarditis is **diagnosed** by positive **blood culture**; repeated culture may be necessary to isolate the causal organism.
- The **predisposing conditions** for infective endocarditis include valve prostheses, septal defects, atheroma of the valve, congenital valve deformities and pre-existing rheumatic fever.
- **High-dose single or combination antibiotic therapy**, guided by the microbiological findings from the blood culture, is necessary to treat infective endocarditis.
- **Infective endocarditis prophylaxis** is based on accurate identification of patients at risk, patient awareness of risk status, dental involvement in cardiac clinics, preventive dental care, antibiotic prophylaxis **according to the local guidelines** and patient awareness of postoperative morbidity.
- Cardiac **patients who may need antibiotic cover** (as dictated by US guidelines) include those with congenital cardiac defects, prosthetic cardiac valves, previous history of endocarditis, and cardiomyopathy after cardiac transplantation.
- Drugs used in antibiotic prophylaxis of infective endocarditis include amoxicillin, clindamycin, cephalexin and clarithromycin.

Review Questions (Answers on p. 390)

Please indicate which answers are true and which are false.

24.1. Bacteraemia:
   a. may be produced by tooth brushing
   b. will occur in healthy individuals
   c. differs from septicaemia in that there is no active multiplication of organisms
   d. might lead to endocarditis in patients with rheumatic carditis
   e. always precedes septicaemia

24.2. Which of the following statements on infective endocarditis are true?
   a. normal oral flora are key agents
   b. it can precipitate cardiogenic shock
   c. it is always managed by parenteral antibiotics
   d. it can always be diagnosed by a single blood culture
   e. congenital cardiac defects significantly increase the risk

24.3. When obtaining blood for bacteriological cultures:
   a. a total of 2 mL blood is sufficient
   b. the procedure should be done before the commencement of antibiotics
   c. the procedure is likely to yield the best result if collected at peaks of temperature
   d. multiple specimens are required
   e. all of the above are true

24.4. Endocarditis:
   a. is always precipitated by a microbial infection
   b. is caused by *Viridans* streptococci that cause rheumatic fever, which leads to it
   c. always requires more than a single antibiotic
   d. can be prevented by education of susceptible groups
   e. due to enterococci is commonly of endogenous origin

24.5. According to the American Heart Association (AHA) guidelines, prophylaxis against endocarditis in patients undergoing dental procedures is necessary if they have:
   a. heart failure
   b. certain congenital heart diseases
   c. recurrent streptococcal endocarditis
   d. third molar surgery
   e. atherosclerosis

Further Reading

Antibiotic prophylaxis prior to dental procedures. https://www.ada.org/en/resources/research/science-and-research-institute/oral-health-topics/antibiotic-prophylaxis.

Lever, A., & Mackenzie, I. (2007). Sepsis: Definition, aetiology and diagnosis. *British Medical Journal, 335*, 879–883.

Martin, M. V., Kanatas, A. N., & Hardy, P. (2005). Antibiotic prophylaxis and third molar surgery. *British Dental Journal, 198*, 327–330.

National Institute for Health and Care Excellence (NICE). (2016, July). NICE Guidelines: Prophylaxis against infective endocarditis. https://www.nice.org.uk/guidance/cg64/chapter/Recommendations#prophylaxis-against-infective-endocarditis.

Oliver, R., Roberts, G. J., & Hooper, L. (2004). Penicillins for the prophylaxis of bacterial endocarditis in dentistry (Cochrane review). *Australian Dental Journal, 49*, 3.

Scottish Dental Clinical Effectiveness Program. (2018). Antibiotic prophylaxis: Implementation advice for National Institute for Health and Care Excellence (NICE) Clinical Guideline 64 Prophylaxis Against Infective Endocarditis. https://www.sdcep.org.uk/published-guidance/antibiotic-prophylaxis.

Wilson, W. R., Gewitz, M., Lockhart, P. B., Bolger, A. F., DeSimone, D. C., Kazi, D. S., & Baddour, L. M. (2021). Prevention of viridans group streptococcal infective endocarditis: a scientific statement from the American Heart Association. *Circulation, 143*(20), e963–e978. Table 5. https://doi.org/10.1161/CIR.0000000000000969.

25 Infections of the Central Nervous and Locomotor Systems

Infections of the Central Nervous System

As the cerebrospinal fluid is devoid of effective antimicrobial defences, generalized infection rapidly sets in when pyogenic organisms enter the subarachnoid space and the cerebrospinal fluid. This may be caused by:

- **direct spread** due to trauma and resultant breach of the integuments of the central nervous system
- **seeding** via blood from a peripheral infective focus.

MENINGITIS

Inflammation of the meninges, the membranes that cover the brain and spinal cord, is classified according to the aetiological agent, as:

- **bacterial meningitis** (also called pyogenic or polymorphonuclear meningitis)
- **viral meningitis** (also called aseptic or lymphocytic meningitis).

Bacterial Meningitis

Bacterial meningitis is more severe than the viral type and remains a serious cause of morbidity and mortality despite antibiotic therapy. Prompt diagnosis is of the essence in preventing disabling sequelae of infection and death.

Clinical Features. Symptoms include severe headache, fever, vomiting, photophobia and convulsions leading to drowsiness and unconsciousness. Signs are mainly those of **meningeal irritation** (i.e., neck and spinal stiffness) and **Kernig's sign** (pain and resistance on extending the knee when the thigh is flexed). These cardinal signs and symptoms may be absent in neonatal meningitis and meningitis in the elderly and the immunocompromised. Sequelae include encephalopathy (altered cerebral function), cranial nerve palsies, cerebral abscess, obstructive hydrocephalus and subdural effusion of sterile or infected fluid.

Aetiology. The common types of bacterial meningitis and the major agents are:

- meningococcal meningitis: *Neisseria meningitidis*
- haemophilus meningitis: *Haemophilus influenzae*, capsulated (Pittman type b)
- pneumococcal meningitis: *Streptococcus pneumoniae*
- tuberculous meningitis: *Mycobacterium tuberculosis* and other mycobacteria.

Table 25.1　Cerebrospinal Fluid in Meningitis

	Normal	Acute Pyogenic	Tuberculous	Aseptic
Appearance	Clear	Turbid	Clear or opalescent	Usually clear
Total protein	Normal	Greatly increased	Increased	Normal
Glucose	Normal	Greatly reduced or absent	Reduced	Normal
Lactate	Normal	Raised	Considerably raised	Normal
Cell count	Lymphocytes 0–3 × 10⁹/l	Greatly increased; polymorphs	Increased; mainly lymphocytes but some polymorphs	Increased lymphocytes

Epidemiology, Treatment and Prevention

MENINGITIS DUE TO NEISSERIA AND HAEMOPHILUS SPECIES. *Neisseria meningitidis* (the meningococcus) is the main agent of meningitis in the UK and US, and most infections are caused by group B strains. The disease is common in children and young adults. Penicillin is the drug of choice: cefotaxime and chloramphenicol are alternatives. Haemophilus meningitis is mostly seen in children between 1 month and 4 years old and is treated with chloramphenicol or cefotaxime. Pneumococcal infection, common in older patients and those without a functioning spleen, is treated with penicillin. Tuberculous infection is managed by 'triple therapy', as described in Chapter 23.

Meningitis may spread quickly in close household contacts. Avoiding overcrowding in living and working conditions is helpful. Chemoprophylaxis with antibiotics (e.g., rifampicin) in meningococcal infection can eliminate the carrier state, which may develop in some.

Meningitis Due to Other Organisms. Rarely, other organisms, such as *Listeria monocytogenes*, *Leptospira interrogans* and *Cryptococcus neoformans* (a fungus), may cause meningitis.

Laboratory Diagnosis. Examination of the cerebrospinal fluid, usually obtained by a **lumbar puncture**, is essential. Changes that occur in the cerebrospinal fluid, depending on whether the aetiology is acute pyogenic, tuberculous or viral, dictate appropriate and timely therapy (Table 25.1). Cerebrospinal fluid should also be centrifuged and the deposit Gram-stained and cultured to isolate and identify the causative agent. Blood cultures are also useful in the diagnosis of bacterial meningitis.

Treatment. Treatment is dictated by the causative organism and its antibiotic sensitivity; because of the serious nature of the illness, empirical therapy with two or three antibiotic drugs is given immediately.

Viral Meningitis

Aetiology. Viral or aseptic meningitis can be caused by many agents, as shown in Table 25.2.

Pathogenesis. The major routes of viral entry into the body are the respiratory and gastrointestinal tracts. From these portals, viruses spread to the central nervous system

Table 25.2　Major Causes of Viral Meningitis and/or Encephalitis

Echovirus
Mumps virus
Coxsackievirus
Herpes simplex virus
Adenovirus
Measles virus
Influenza virus
Varicella-zoster virus

by direct migration via the olfactory nerves or indirectly via blood. Cells involved in viral spread include capillary endothelial cells, epithelial cells of the choroid plexus and infected leukocytes.

Epidemiology. Children and young adults are the most affected.

Treatment. Viral meningitis is a benign, self-limiting condition and requires only symptomatic treatment. No antiviral drugs are indicated as the condition resolves in 1–2 weeks.

ENCEPHALITIS

Infection of the brain substance (as opposed to the meninges) is called encephalitis. This is a somewhat artificial division as patients often show signs and symptoms of meningitis and encephalitis at the same time.

Aetiology

The most frequently involved viruses are herpes simplex virus, mumps virus and arboviruses.

Pathogenesis

Encephalitis occurs after childhood illnesses such as measles, chickenpox and rubella, and rarely after immunization with vaccines such as pertussis. Affected patients often die or have debilitating sequelae.

Treatment

In contrast to viral meningitis, encephalitis is a very serious disease that needs prompt and specific antiviral therapy such as intravenous aciclovir.

POLIOMYELITIS

Aetiology

Poliomyelitis is caused by poliovirus types 1–3, belonging to the Picornaviridae.

Pathogenesis

The portal of infection is the mouth, and the virus multiplies in the lymphoid tissue of the pharynx and the intestine. It then enters the blood stream and causes a viraemia, with resulting spread into the central nervous system, causing neurological disease. The disease is an influenzalike illness, with meningitis and encephalitis. In some, damage to the anterior horn cells of the spinal cord leads to respiratory failure (requiring artificial ventilation) or permanent lower motor neuron weakness and paralytic poliomyelitis.

Epidemiology and Prevention

Although epidemics were common in the past, poliomyelitis is now rare in the West, owing to effective polio vaccine. However, the disease is still prevalent in developing countries, where universal vaccination programmes are difficult to implement, despite the goal of the World Health Organization (WHO) to eradicate the disease by the year 2000. Polio vaccines are of two types: the killed (Salk) vaccine and the live attenuated (Sabin) vaccine (Chapter 37).

CEREBRAL ABSCESS

Aetiology

Many bacteria may cause brain abscesses. These include streptococci (*Streptococcus milleri* and *Streptococcus pneumoniae*) enterococci (*Enterococcus faecalis*), staphylococci, anaerobic cocci and coliforms. The infections are mostly polymicrobial (i.e., mixed infections) in nature.

Pathogenesis

The infective agent may reach the brain through the blood or by direct extension. In the latter case, a brain abscess may result as a direct extension of sinus infection caused by oral bacteria or, rarely, as a complication of acute or chronic dental infection. Infection may also follow traumatic injury to the maxillofacial region.

Treatment

Operative drainage and excision of the abscess (if well encapsulated) is supplemented by antibiotic therapy. β-lactam group antibiotics and gentamicin are very popular; metronidazole is also used because of its good penetration into abscesses and as anaerobes are frequently involved.

TETANUS

Aetiology

Tetanus is caused by infection with *Clostridium tetani* (drumstick bacillus).

Clinical Features

After an incubation period of 5–15 days, the exotoxins produced by the organisms precipitate severe and painful muscle spasms:

- **lockjaw**—spasm of masseter muscles
- **risus sardonicus**—facial grimace due to spasm of facial muscles
- **opisthotonos**—arched body due to spasm of the more powerful extensor muscles of the body (see Fig. 13.4).

Pathogenesis

Contamination of wounds with tetanus spores derived from dust, manured soil or rusty objects results in spore germination and release of the powerful **exotoxins tetanospasmin and tetanolysin** (see Chapters 5 and 13). Although the bacteria remain localized at the site of infection, the exotoxins are absorbed at the motor nerve endings and diffuse centripetally towards the anterior horn cells of the spinal cord, blocking the normal inhibitory impulses that control motor nerve function, with resultant sustained contraction of the muscles. Wounds of the face, neck and upper extremities are more dangerous than those of the lower extremities as they have a shorter incubation period and result in more severe disease.

Epidemiology

The main source of spores is **animal faeces**. The incidence is higher in the developing world because of lack of immunization and poor standards of wound care. Although tetanus is commonly associated with deep penetrating wounds, it can often result from superficial abrasions (e.g., thorn pricks). **Neonatal tetanus** due to infection of the umbilical stump is common in rural areas of developing countries.

Diagnosis

Diagnosis is mainly clinical as bacteriological confirmation frequently fails. Swab or exudate from the wound typically shows 'drumstick bacilli'; biochemical identification and confirmation by mouse pathogenicity are described in Chapter 13.

Treatment

1. **Supportive treatment:** muscle relaxants to control spasms, sedation and artificial ventilation (for respiratory muscle paralysis).
2. **Antitoxin:** given intravenously in large doses to neutralize the toxin; it is of little use in the late stage of disease.
3. **Antibiotics:** penicillin or tetracycline to prevent further toxin production.
4. **Debridement:** excision and cleaning of the wound.

Prevention

Active immunization with adsorbed tetanus vaccine, also called toxoid (a component of diphtheria–tetanus–pertussis vaccine), should be given in childhood (during the first year of life and before school or nursery-school entry).

Prophylaxis of Wounded Patients

- If the patient is **immune**, a booster dose of toxoid or adsorbed tetanus vaccine should be given if the primary course (or booster dose) was given more than 10 years previously, *along with* human antitetanus immunoglobulin if the wound is dirty and more than 24 h old.
- If the patient is **nonimmune**, human antitetanus immunoglobulin should be given, followed by a full course of tetanus toxoid by injection.
- Penicillin may be given as prophylaxis, not only to prevent tetanus but also to avoid pyogenic infection.

Booster doses of toxoid 10 years after the primary course and again 10 years later maintain a satisfactory level of protection. Any adult who has received five doses is likely to have lifelong immunity.

Infections of the Locomotor System

The two major infections associated with the locomotor system (i.e., bones and joints) are acute septic arthritis and osteomyelitis.

Natural defences in the locomotor system include:

- specialized macrophages in the synovial membranes of joints (highly phagocytic)
- a few mononuclear cells, complement and lysozyme of synovial fluid
- a rich vascular plexus traversing the medulla and cortex of bone with integral defences.

Important pathogens are listed in Fig. 25.1.

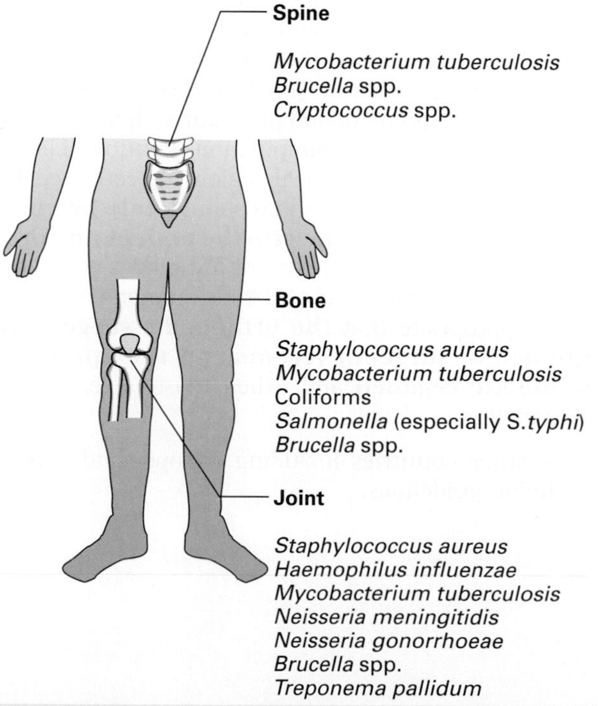

Spine

Mycobacterium tuberculosis
Brucella spp.
Cryptococcus spp.

Bone

Staphylococcus aureus
Mycobacterium tuberculosis
Coliforms
Salmonella (especially S.*typhi*)
Brucella spp.

Joint

Staphylococcus aureus
Haemophilus influenzae
Mycobacterium tuberculosis
Neisseria meningitidis
Neisseria gonorrhoeae
Brucella spp.
Treponema pallidum

Fig. 25.1   Major infectious agents of the locomotor system.

ACUTE SEPTIC ARTHRITIS

Aetiology

Commonly associated bacteria are *Staphylococcus aureus*, *Haemophilus influenzae*, *Streptococcus pneumoniae* and other streptococci, *Neisseria gonorrhoeae* and nonsporing anaerobes such as *Bacteroides* spp. Other infrequent but notable agents are *Mycobacterium tuberculosis*, *Salmonella* spp. and *Brucella* spp.

Clinical Features

Limitation of movement with swelling, redness and severe pain are the cardinal symptoms; usually, only a single joint is involved. Crippling and permanent joint damage may result despite antibiotic therapy.

Pathogenesis

The condition may result from:

- traumatic injury through the joint capsule
- haematogenous spread, usually as a complication of septicaemia
- extension of osteomyelitis or spread of infection from an adjacent septic focus
- complication of rheumatoid arthritis
- infection of joint prosthesis.

Epidemiology

Acute septic arthritis occurs most commonly in children. Sources of infection are many and include sepsis of the skin, nasopharynx, sinuses, lungs, peritoneum and genital tract. The source of infection of artificial joints could be the patient, the operating team or the theatre air.

Laboratory Diagnosis

Diagnosis is by direct film observation and culture of aspirated joint fluid; blood culture; culture of specimens from the suspected primary focus of infection (e.g., throat, genital tract); and serological tests for salmonellosis and brucellosis, if suspected.

Treatment

Initial antibiotic therapy is given on an empirical or 'best-guess' basis. Early administration of antibiotics, immediately after the specimen is taken, is essential to prevent chronic sequelae. Antibiotics may be injected directly into the joint or given systemically.

REACTIVE ARTHRITIS

Reactive arthritis is the term given to acute arthritis affecting one or more joints; it develops 1–4 weeks after infection of the genitals – **postsexual reactive arthritis** or gastrointestinal tract – **postdysenteric reactive arthritis**. The causative agent in postsexual reactive arthritis is *Chlamydia trachomatis*; almost all patients are men. Postdysenteric reactive arthritis may follow infections with *Salmonella*, *Shigella*, *Yersinia* or *Campylobacter*.

Reactive arthritis should be differentiated from septic arthritis as **it is not due to joint infection**. It is thought to be mediated by immunological mechanisms, and there is an apparent genetic predisposition to the disease.

OSTEOMYELITIS

Osteomyelitis can be divided into **acute and chronic** forms. Acute infection usually occurs in children under 10 years old, whereas the chronic variety is more common in adults.

Aetiology

Acute. Mostly *Staphylococcus aureus* (some 75% of cases); other agents include *Haemophilus influenzae* (in preschool children), *Streptococcus pyogenes*, *Streptococcus pneumoniae* and other streptococci; *Salmonella*, *Brucella* and nonsporing anaerobes rarely.

Chronic. *Staphylococcus aureus* is most common; rarely *Mycobacterium tuberculosis*, *Pseudomonas aeruginosa*, Salmonella and Brucella spp.

Pathogenesis

Any septic lesion can be the source of the organism (e.g., a boil or pustule); spread to bone is usually haematogenous. Infection at all ages may be a result of major trauma (e.g., compound fracture) that exposes bone tissue to the environment.

Laboratory Diagnosis

Diagnosis is by **blood culture** (a number of cultures may be required to isolate the infective agent(s), which circulate in the blood in very small numbers); culture of pus from the bony focus—pus may be obtained by needle aspiration or by open surgery; and by specimens from the related infective focus (e.g., 'cold abscess' pus in tuberculosis).

Treatment

Antibiotics alone are helpful if started early in the disease, by the parenteral route first and the oral route later. Penicillinase-resistant penicillin (such as flucloxacillin) should be given first if culture results are not available as *Staphylococcus aureus* is the predominant agent. Drugs that penetrate bone well (such as fusidic acid and clindamycin) are alternatives. Erythromycin is an alternative in patients who are hypersensitive to penicillin.

Surgery may be needed to drain pus and remove sequestra, if any.

Osteomyelitis of the Jaws

Osteomyelitis of the jaws (see also Chapter 34) is uncommon owing to the relatively high vascularity of the jaws, especially the maxilla; therefore, the mandible is more commonly affected than the maxilla. The following predisposing conditions are noteworthy:

- **bone disease**, such as Paget's disease or osteopetrosis, fibrous dysplasia, bone tumours
- **irradiation** of the jaws for cancer therapy (e.g., nasopharyngeal carcinoma)

- **trauma** superimposed on debilitating conditions such as malnutrition as well as immunocompromised states.

Arthroplasties and Antibiotic Prophylaxis for Dental Procedures

More than a million hip replacements are carried out each year worldwide, and the number of other artificial joints inserted is also rising, so that infections associated with arthroplasties have become more common. However, there is a paucity of literature on infections precipitated by hematogenous seeding of oral bacteria during arthroplasties, and whether patients with arthroplasties should be given antibiotic prophylaxis during invasive dental treatment.

GUIDELINES FOR ANTIBIOTIC PROPHYLAXIS FOR PROSTHETIC JOINT IMPLANTS AND HIP JOINT REPLACEMENTS

There is wide consensus that patients with prosthetic joint implants, including total hip replacements, **do not require antibiotic prophylaxis**, because the risks of prophylaxis outweigh the benefits. Nevertheless it is important that the possible need for prophylactic cover should be **discussed with the patient's doctor** before dental treatment starts. Furthermore, there should be liaison between orthopaedic surgeons and dentists to **render patients dentally fit** prior to insertion of replacements or implants.

The current American Heart Association (AHA) guidelines on prosthetic joint replacement are provided below.

According to AHA there are relatively few patient subpopulations for whom antibiotic prophylaxis may be indicated prior to certain dental procedures.

- In general, for patients with prosthetic joint implants, prophylactic antibiotics are not recommended prior to dental procedures to prevent prosthetic joint infection.
- However, for patients with a history of **complications associated with their joint replacement surgery** who are undergoing dental procedures that induce bacteremia (e.g., gingival manipulation or mucosal incision or surgery in the periapical region of teeth; see Table 24.4), prophylactic antibiotics should **only be considered after consultation with the patient and orthopedic surgeon** in cases where antibiotics are deemed necessary. Furthermore, AHA recommends that it is most appropriate that **the orthopedic surgeon (not the dental surgeon) recommend the appropriate antibiotic regimen** and, when reasonable, write the prescription.

Most other countries including Europe, and Australia have similar guidelines.

Key Facts

- The **cerebrospinal fluid is sterile** and devoid of effective antimicrobial defences; it may be infected either directly from a contiguous focus (e.g., due to trauma) or indirectly via blood from a peripheral infective focus.
- **Meningitis**, defined as the inflammation of the meninges, can be broadly categorized as **bacterial meningitis** (also called pyogenic or polymorphonuclear meningitis) or **viral meningitis** (also called aseptic or lymphocytic meningitis).
- The common types (and agents) of bacterial meningitis are meningococcal meningitis (*Neisseria meningitidis*), haemophilus meningitis (*Haemophilus influenzae*), pneumococcal meningitis (*Streptococcus pneumoniae*) and tuberculous meningitis (*Mycobacterium tuberculosis* and others).
- Examination of the **cerebrospinal fluid**, obtained by a **lumbar puncture,** is mandatory for diagnosis of the different types of bacterial meningitis.
- Viral or aseptic meningitis can be caused by many agents, and the major routes of entry are the respiratory and gastro-intestinal tracts.
- Viral meningitis is usually benign and self-limiting, requiring only symptomatic treatment; no antiviral therapy is indicated.
- Polio vaccine is of two types: the **killed (Salk) vaccine** and the **live attenuated (Sabin) vaccine**; the latter given orally is the more popular.
- Contamination of wounds with *Clostridium tetani* spores derived from dust, manured soil or rusty objects results in spore germination and release of the powerful exotoxins **tetanospasmin** and **tetanolysin** to cause tetanus.
- Tetanus is **managed by supportive measures** (e.g., muscle relaxants, sedation and artificial ventilation), **antitoxin, antibiotics** (penicillin or tetracycline) and **wound debridement**.
- Tetanus-preventive measures are active immunization with **formol toxoid** (a component of diphtheria–tetanus–pertussis **(DTP) vaccine** given in childhood) and booster doses of toxoid once every 10 years for risk groups.
- Osteomyelitis can be divided into **acute** (seen in children under 10 years old) and **chronic osteomyelitis** (common in adults).
- The acute form of osteomyelitis is mostly caused by *Staphylococcus aureus* (some 75% of cases); in chronic osteomyelitis, *Staphylococcus aureus* is most common; rarely *M. tuberculosis*, *Salmonella* and *Brucella* spp.
- **Osteomyelitis of the jaws is uncommon** owing to their high vascularity (especially the maxilla).
- Predisposing conditions that result in osteomyelitis of the jaws include bone disease (e.g., Paget's disease, osteopetrosis, fibrous dysplasia, bone tumours), irradiation and trauma superimposed on debilitating conditions such as malnutrition, and immunocompromised states.
- In general, routine antibiotic prophylaxis should not be offered to patients with a history of arthroplasties.

Review Questions (Answers on p. 391)

Please indicate which answers are true and which are false.

25.1. Common causative agents of acute bacterial meningitis include:
   a. *Neisseria meningitidis*
   b. non-typable *Haemophilus influenzae*
   c. *Streptococcus pneumoniae*
   d. *Staphylococcus aureus*
   e. *Leptospira interrogans*

25.2. Signs and symptoms of acute bacterial meningitis include:
   a. headache
   b. nuchal rigidity
   c. photophobia
   d. vomiting
   e. all of the above

25.3. Aseptic meningitis:
   a. commonly has a viral aetiology
   b. can be easily differentiated from pyogenic meningitis at presentation
   c. has a seasonal incidence
   d. cerebrospinal fluid cultures often become positive
   e. cerebrospinal fluid examination usually shows an elevated lymphocyte count

25.4. Poliomyelitis:
   a. is caused by an RNA virus
   b. spreads by the faecal–oral route
   c. leads to flaccid paralysis
   d. causes death due to cardiac failure
   e. can be prevented using a live vaccine

25.5. Cerebral abscesses:
   a. are often due to monomicrobial infections
   b. may follow traumatic injury to the maxillofacial region
   c. can manifest with focal neurological signs
   d. may rarely need surgical drainage
   e. may be caused by oral flora

25.6. Tetanus:
   a. is the result of direct invasion of the anterior horn cells by *Clostridium tetani*
   b. results in painful muscle spasms and spastic paralysis
   c. may be present when a patient presents to the dentist with trismus
   d. treatment of the acute case is with toxoid and penicillin
   e. could be prevented by a single dose of tetanus toxoid

25.7. Osteomyelitis of the jaw:
   a. is relatively uncommon
   b. is more common than those of long bones
   c. has anaerobes as the common causative agents
   d. is a complication of irradiation therapy
   e. may be complicated by pre-existing bone disease

Further Reading

American Academy of Orthopaedic Surgeons/American Dental Association. (2012). Prevention of orthopaedic implant infection in patients undergoing dental procedures: Evidence-based clinical practice guideline. https://www.aaos.org/globalassets/quality-and-practice-resources/dental/pudp_guideline.pdf.

Quinn, R. H., Murray, J. N., Pezold, R., & Sevarino, K. S. (2017). American Academy of Orthopaedic Surgeons appropriate use criteria for the management of patients with orthopaedic implants undergoing dental procedures. *Journal of Bone and Joint Surgery, American Volume, 99*(2), 161–163.

Shanson, D. C. (1999). *Infections of the central nervous system*. In *Microbiology in clinical practice* (3rd ed., Ch. 11). Butterworth-Heinemann.

Shanson, D. C. (1999). Bone and joint infections. In *Microbiology in clinical practice* (3rd ed., Ch. 18). Butterworth-Heinemann.

Thornhill, M. H., Gibson, T. B., Pack, C., Rosario, B. L., Bloemers, S., Lockhart, P. B., Springer, B., & Baddour, L. M. (2023). Quantifying the risk of prosthetic joint infections after invasive dental procedures and the effect of antibiotic prophylaxis. *Journal of the American Dental Association, 154*(1), 43–52.e12. doi:10.1016/j.adaj.2022.10.001.

26 Infections of the Gastrointestinal Tract

Normal Flora

In healthy, fasting individuals, the **stomach is either sterile or may contain only a few organisms**, because of its low pH and the endogenous enzymes. However, the microbiome of both the upper and lower intestines is vast and complex and is considered an essential 'organ' in providing nourishment, regulating epithelial development and instructing innate immunity of the host. As in the oral cavity, the intestinal tract harbours a multitude of uncultivable, and yet to be discovered, microbiota.

The **small intestine** may be colonized with **streptococci, lactobacilli and yeasts** (especially *Candida albicans*); the proportions of these and other organisms vary, depending on dietary habits. In the ileum, a typical Gram-negative flora (e.g., *Bacteroides* spp. and Enterobacteriaceae) is seen, and the **large intestine has a dense population** of varied flora. These include members of the Enterobacteriaceae, *Enterococcus* *faecalis, Bacteroides* spp., *Clostridium* spp., bifidobacteria and anaerobic streptococci. The anaerobes outweigh the aerobes by a lot and comprise the vast majority of the bacteria in the large intestine. Roughly 20% of the **faeces contains** bacteria, approximately 10^{11} **organisms per gram**.

IMPORTANT PATHOGENS

Gastrointestinal infections are a major cause of morbidity and mortality worldwide. For example, recent studies have revealed that, globally, severe diarrhoea and dehydration are responsible each year for the death of over 1.5 million children under the age of 5 years. Most of these diseases are preventable and are caused by poor food quality, low levels of personal hygiene, poor sanitation and lack of quality pipeborne water systems.

A diverse array of infections of the gastrointestinal tract are caused by an equally varied population of microbial agents (Fig. 26.1). The agents of diarrhoeal diseases, including those that are considered common agents of **food poisoning**, are listed in Table 26.1. The common bacterial **diarrhoeal diseases** in the developed world include those caused by:

- *Campylobacter* spp.
- *Shigella* spp.
- *Salmonella* spp.
- *Escherichia coli*
- *Staphylococcus aureus*
- *Clostridium welchii*
- *Vibrio cholerae*.

Less common diarrhoeal diseases include those caused by *Clostridium difficile*, the agent of hospital-acquired (nosocomial) infectious diarrhoea, and *Bacillus cereus*, a common agent of food poisoning.

Common Diarrhoeal Diseases

CAMPYLOBACTER SPP.

Campylobacter coli and *Campylobacter jejuni* are among the most common diarrhoea-inducing agents in the Western world. They are curved, slender, Gram-negative bacilli present in the gut as well as in the oral cavity. Several ***Campylobacter* species are commonly found in the oral cavity**, and a few, such as *Campylobacter rectus*, *Campylobacter gracilis* and *Campylobacter showae*, have been implicated in human periodontal disease.

Pathogenesis and Epidemiology

Symptoms vary from mild to severe, with any part of the small or large intestine affected. Dogs and cats are probable sources of infection, but **mass-produced poultry** is the most common source. Eating contaminated food is a common cause of infection; note that campylobacters do not multiply in food. Patients may become symptomless carriers after recovery.

Diagnosis

A specimen of stool cultured on selective media will indicate the diagnosis.

Treatment

The infection is self-limiting; erythromycin is useful to relieve symptoms, and ciprofloxacin is an alternative.

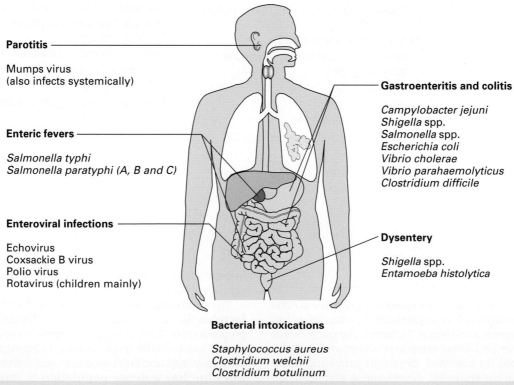

Parotitis

Mumps virus
(also infects systemically)

Enteric fevers

Salmonella typhi
Salmonella paratyphi (A, B and C)

Enteroviral infections

Echovirus
Coxsackie B virus
Polio virus
Rotavirus (children mainly)

Gastroenteritis and colitis

Campylobacter jejuni
Shigella spp.
Salmonella spp.
Escherichia coli
Vibrio cholerae
Vibrio parahaemolyticus
Clostridium difficile

Dysentery

Shigella spp.
Entamoeba histolytica

Bacterial intoxications

Staphylococcus aureus
Clostridium welchii
Clostridium botulinum

Fig. 26.1   Major infectious agents of the gastrointestinal tract.

Table 26.1 Aetiological Agents of Diarrhoeal Diseases

Occurrence	Bacterial	Viral	Protozoal
Common	*Campylobacter* spp.[a]	Rotavirus	*Entamoeba histolytica* (amoebic dysentery)
	Shigella spp.		
	Salmonella spp.[a]		
	Escherichia coli[a]		
	Staphylococcus aureus[a]		
	Clostridium welchii[a]		
Uncommon	*Clostridium difficile*	Adenovirus	*Giardia lamblia* (giardiasis)
	Bacillus cereus[a]	Astrovirus	
		Norwalk virus, calicivirus[c]	
Rare	*Vibrio cholerae*[b]		

[a]Common agents of food poisoning.
[b]Rare in the developed world but very common in developing countries such as Bangladesh and India.
[c]Not discussed in text.

Prevention

Food and personal hygiene.

SHIGELLA SPP.

Shigella causes **bacillary dysentery**, as opposed to amoebic dysentery caused by intestinal amoebae. It is an important cause of morbidity and death in young children, particularly in the developing world.

Aetiology

The genus *Shigella* contains four species: *Shigella dysenteriae*, *Shigella flexneri*, *Shigella boydii* and *Shigella sonnei*.

Pathogenesis and Epidemiology

Infection is by ingestion of organisms. Once ingested, the bacteria attach to the mucosal villus epithelium, then enter and multiply in these cells. The resultant death of the infected cells initiates an inflammatory reaction in the submucosa and lamina propria. Finally, necrosis and ulceration of the villus epithelium ensue, resulting in **blood and mucus in the stool**. This type of severe reaction is usually due to *Shigella dysenteriae*, which is known to produce a potent **enterotoxin** and a **cytotoxin**. This infection may be life-threatening.

Dysentery due to other *Shigellae* spp. is generally milder and varies from asymptomatic excretion to a severe attack of diarrhoea with abdominal pain. *Shigella sonnei* is the usual agent of dysentery in the UK, whereas *Shigella boydii* is common in the Middle East and Southeast Asia.

Spread of the disease is from hand to mouth. It usually occurs in nursery schools where the **index case** (i.e., the person with the disease) contaminates hands at the toilet and further contaminates lavatory handles and hand towels if personal hygiene is deficient. Subsequent handling of these bacteria-laden **fomites** (inanimate surfaces acting as vehicles of disease transfer) by healthy individuals results in hand-to-mouth transmission of the agents, leading to the disease. Thus '**food, flies** and **fomites**' are classical means of spread.

Diagnosis

The diagnosis is made by examination of stool sample and culture on MacConkey agar and selective media such as desoxycholate citrate agar (DCA). Pale, non-lactose-fermenting (NLF) colonies are then isolated and identified by biochemical tests; serological identification is performed subsequently.

Treatment

Antibiotics are of little use except in *Shigella dysenteriae* infection, where trimethoprim (first-line drug), ampicillin or tetracycline may be used.

Prevention

Attention to personal hygiene, good sanitation with safe, pipeborne water and adequate sewage disposal are important. All these measures are difficult to implement in conditions of poverty and poor housing.

SALMONELLA SPP.

A large number of different *Salmonella* species exist, together with an even more bewildering number of serotypes (about 1500). Of these, about 14 are important pathogens. The common diarrhoea-causing organism is *Salmonella typhimurium*. The other major pathogens of this group are *Salmonella typhi* and *Salmonella paratyphi-A*, -*B* and -*C*, which cause enteric fever, a septicaemic illness in which diarrhoea is a late feature of the disease.

Pathogenesis and Epidemiology

The genesis of *Salmonella* food poisoning is poorly understood. Patients have mild gastrointestinal disturbances with an incubation period of about 1–2 days. Abdominal pain, diarrhoea (with or without fever) and vomiting are commonly present. Septicaemia is rare.

The organism is found in **domestic animals and poultry** and is spread via the faecal–oral route. On entering the gastrointestinal tract, the salmonellae may either produce an enterotoxin (similar to toxigenic *Escherichia* *coli*) or invade the mucosa of the small intestine (like *Shigella* spp.).

Diagnosis

Examination of a stool sample and culture on MacConkey (indicator) medium and selective media such as DCA or Wilson–Blair medium; pale, NLF colonies on MacConkey medium and black, shiny colonies on Wilson–Blair medium. Subsequent identification is by biochemical tests and determination of serological status. The major antigens that are useful for the serotyping of salmonellae are the 'O' (somatic or body antigen) and the 'H' (flagellar) antigens.

Treatment

Treatment is rarely necessary. Antibiotics are contraindicated except in septicaemic cases; antibiotic therapy prolongs the carriage of the organism in the convalescent phase.

Prevention

Prevention includes control of animal food quality, good farming and abattoir practices, rigorous kitchen hygiene and good personal hygiene among food handlers, and exclusion of known human carriers (**excretors**) from food handling. However, the best form of prevention is thorough cooking of food and avoidance of consumption of raw or partly cooked eggs and other animal-derived food.

ESCHERICHIA COLI

Escherichia coli is a normal commensal of the gastrointestinal tract, but certain strains, for some unknown reason, can behave as pathogens. As described in Chapter 15, they produce **enterotoxins**, and the enteroinvasive strains have the ability to invade the gut mucosa.

Pathogenesis and Epidemiology

There are two types of *Escherichia coli* diarrhoea:

- infantile gastroenteritis
- traveller's diarrhoea.

Infantile Gastroenteritis. Accompanied by acute and profuse diarrhoea, this infection has an incubation period of 1–3 days. The disease is mainly caused by enteropathogenic *Escherichia coli* (EPEC), but in a minority of cases, enterotoxigenic *Escherichia coli* (ETEC) strains contribute (Chapter 15). It is common in the developing world because of poor sanitation and poverty; infection spreads directly from case to case and via fomites (see above for shigellae), and in some cases the mother may be the source of infection.

Traveller's Diarrhoea. Accompanied by abdominal pain and vomiting, this infection is usually self-limiting, with a short incubation period of 1–2 days. The most frequent cause of diarrhoea in travellers (thus named 'Delhi belly', 'Tokyo two-step', etc.), it is usually spread by contaminated food.

Diagnosis

- **Infantile gastroenteritis:** faecal culture and identification of lactose-fermenting colonies in MacConkey's agar (compare with *Salmonella* and *Shigella*); confirmation by serology. (*Note:* Viruses such as rotavirus may cause similar gastroenteritis and should be included in a differential diagnosis.)
- **Traveller's diarrhoea:** owing to the self-limiting nature of the disease, diagnosis is usually made clinically.

Treatment

In **infantile diarrhoea**, treatment is by rehydration and correction of fluid loss and electrolyte balance. No antibiotics are necessary for either of the *Escherichia coli* diarrhoeas. **Traveller's diarrhoea** is self-limiting.

Prevention

- **Infantile gastroenteritis:** Scrupulous hygiene in neonatal units and personal hygiene of nursing staff are required; patients with diarrhoea should be screened. In the developing world, improved sanitation, housing, pipeborne water supplies and antenatal health education will all help.
- **Traveller's diarrhoea:** public health measures.

Haemorrhagic Syndromes Due to *Escherichia coli*

Though not diarrhoeogenic, two important haemorrhagic syndromes caused by *Escherichia coli* are noteworthy here. **Haemorrhagic colitis** is seen in children and adults, whereas **haemolytic uraemic syndrome** is mainly seen in children. Both produce outbreaks and sporadic infections; death may be the outcome in either. The agent is *Escherichia coli* (mainly of the serotype O157) that produces **cytotoxins** VT1 and VT2 (demonstrated in the laboratory by their cytopathic effect on cultured monkey kidney cells called 'Vero cells'); due to their verotoxigenicity, these *Escherichia coli* strains are known as verotoxigenic *Escherichia coli* (**VTEC**; Chapter 15). These toxins are also called Shiga-like toxins. The main source of infection is beef.

STAPHYLOCOCCUS AUREUS

Staphylococcus aureus is a common cause of **diarrhoea due to food poisoning**. Symptoms ensue very quickly after the food intake, as the *Staphylococcus aureus* enterotoxin is preformed in food.

Pathogenesis and Epidemiology

The *Staphylococcus aureus* **enterotoxin** has a local action on the gut mucosa, with resultant nausea and vomiting (and occasional diarrhoea) within a few hours after the food intake. Cooked food that is not stored at 4°C or frozen immediately but left at room temperature is the usual source of infection. The organism usually reaches the food from a staphylococcal lesion on the skin of a food handler and, if left at ambient or warm temperatures, may multiply in food and liberate the enterotoxin. The toxin is relatively heat-resistant; on heating contaminated food, the *Staphylococcus aureus* cells usually die, leaving the active toxin in the food, which is ingested. Milk or milk products such as cream or custard may also act as sources of toxin.

Diagnosis

Diagnosis is by culture of faecal specimens, suspected food or vomitus (Chapter 11).

Treatment

The disease is self-limiting; hence no treatment is required.

Prevention

Prevention is by good food hygiene, quick refrigeration or freezing of leftover food, and exclusion of food handlers with septic lesions.

CLOSTRIDIUM WELCHII

Clostridium welchii, responsible for gas gangrene (see Chapter 13), also causes food poisoning.

Pathogenesis and Epidemiology

Heat-resistant spores of *Clostridium welchii* survive in contaminated food during the heating procedure, and subsequently multiply in deep, relatively anaerobic parts of the food (e.g., in meat pies). After the food is ingested, **sporulation** (spore formation) occurs in the gastrointestinal tract, and an enterotoxin is produced, which alters the membrane permeability of the small intestine, causing diarrhoea.

Diagnosis

Diagnostic procedures are not usually performed. However, isolation of the same serotype of *Clostridium welchii* from the victim and the food is indicative of the disease source.

Treatment

Treatment is symptomatic; no antibiotics are necessary.

Prevention

Good food hygiene, including adequate cooking of food to kill the organisms, is required.

CHOLERA

Though rare in the West, cholera is a relatively common disease in some parts of the world, especially in Southeast Asia (e.g., Bangladesh). It is mainly caused by *Vibrio cholerae* O1. Approximately 1.3–4 million people around the world get cholera each year, and 21,000–143,000 people die from it.

Pathogenesis and Epidemiology

Vibrio cholerae **infects only humans** and is transmitted via the faecal–oral route. Contaminated food and water are the main reservoirs of infection. **Human carriers are frequently asymptomatic** and may be incubating or convalescing from the disease. Once ingested, the organism colonizes the small intestine and secretes a protein exotoxin (an enterotoxin).

A large number of cholera vibrios (about 1 billion) need to be ingested for them to survive the acids of the stomach. They then adhere to the brush border of the intestine (by secreting a mucinase that dissolves the protective glycoprotein of the intestinal cells), multiply and secrete the enterotoxin (**choleragen**). The toxin stimulates the activity of the enzyme adenyl cyclase of the intestinal cells and increases the flow of water and electrolytes into the bowel lumen, leading to a **massive, watery diarrhoea without inflammatory cells**. Morbidity and death are due to dehydration and electrolyte imbalance. If fluid balance is adjusted promptly, the diarrhoea is self-limiting in about 7 days.

Clinical Features

The hallmark of cholera is nonbloody, frothy and colourless diarrhoea: '**rice-water stools**'. The incubation period varies from 6 h to 5 days. There is no abdominal pain, and symptoms are mainly due to dehydration, which also brings about cardiac and renal failure. The mortality rate is about 40% without treatment.

Diagnosis

Diagnosis is by culture of faeces on selective media (e.g., thiosulphate–citrate–bile salts–sucrose (TCBS) agar).

Treatment

Prompt, adequate replacement of **water and electrolytes** (oral or intravenous). Tetracycline, although not essential, reduces the duration of symptoms and carriage of organisms in the faeces.

Prevention

Clean water supply, adequate sewage disposal and good personal hygiene are all important. A vaccine, made of killed organisms, is of limited use and does not interrupt transmission.

Less Common and Uncommon Diarrhoeal Diseases

CLOSTRIDIUM DIFFICILE

Clostridium difficile is the agent of **antibiotic-associated pseudomembranous colitis**, a mild and self-limiting disease. Rarely, life-threatening fulminant infection may set in.

Pathogenesis and Epidemiology

The organism is a normal commensal of the gut in some 3% of the population. Antibiotics (especially clindamycin, cephalosporins and, less frequently, ampicillin) suppress drug-sensitive normal flora, allowing *Clostridium difficile* to multiply and produce two toxins: an **enterotoxin** and a **cytotoxin**. These initiate the diarrhoea and the resultant **pseudomembranes** (yellow-white plaques) on the colon visualized by sigmoidoscopy.

Outbreaks are commonly reported in long-stay wards and hospitals.

Diagnosis

Clinical diagnosis is by proctosigmoidoscopy to detect the pseudomembranes. The toxin in stool samples can be detected by its toxic effect on cultured cells.

Treatment

Withdraw the offending antibiotic and replace fluids. Oral vancomycin, which is active against anaerobes, should be given.

Prevention

No specific measure is preventive, but prescribe antibiotics only when necessary.

BACILLUS CEREUS

Bacillus cereus is an aerobic, spore-forming Gram-positive bacillus commonly found in soil, air and dust.

Pathogenesis and Epidemiology

The organisms can contaminate rice and soups or can survive cooking by **sporulation**. When the food is stored at room temperature, reheated or fried quickly, the spores germinate into vegetative forms, multiply and liberate an **enterotoxin**. The latter, when ingested with contaminated food, causes diarrhoea either within 1–2 h (short incubation) or within 6–18 h (long incubation). The disease is commonly associated with Chinese restaurants because of their bulk use of rice.

Diagnosis

Laboratory diagnosis is not usually done.

Treatment

Symptomatic treatment only is required as the disease is self-limiting.

Prevention

Prevention is by adequate food hygiene and correct storage of food.

ENTERIC FEVER

The term 'enteric fever' is given to **typhoid** and **paratyphoid** infections caused by *Salmonella typhi* and *Salmonella paratyphi-A*, *-B* and *-C*, respectively; *Salmonella paratyphi-A* and *-C* are common in the tropics, whereas type *B* is common in Europe. Both diseases are due to salmonellae that are significantly more virulent and hence more invasive than those responsible for food poisoning.

Clinical Features

Typhoid Fever. The onset of typhoid fever is slow, with fever and constipation (compare diarrhoea and vomiting of *Salmonella enteritidis*). After the first week (following the 2- to 3-week incubation period), the bacteria enter the blood stream (i.e., bacteraemia), with resultant high fever, delirium and tender abdomen with '**rose spots**' (rose-coloured papules on the abdomen). The disease begins to resolve by the third week, but severe complications such as intestinal haemorrhage or perforations may occur if the disease is not promptly treated. About 3% of typhoid patients become **chronic carriers** of the organism, a favourite reservoir of which is the gall bladder.

Paratyphoid Fever. Paratyphoid fever is a milder febrile illness than typhoid fever. It is of short duration with transient diarrhoea or symptomless infection.

Pathogenesis and Epidemiology

In typhoid fever, the organism takes a complicated route inside the body after entering the alimentary tract (Fig. 26.2). The pathogenicity of salmonellae appears to depend both on their ability to survive and grow inside macrophages and on the potency of their endotoxin (O antigen of the lipopolysaccharide). Further, the typhoid bacilli possess a glycolipid, the virulence (Vi) antigen, that protects the organism from phagocytosis.

The reservoir of infection is the human gut, during both the **acute** and the **carrier** phases of the infection (which may last up to 2 months after the acute illness). Spread occurs via water, food or the faecal–oral route. Small numbers of *Salmonella typhi* can cause typhoid fever, whereas large doses of *Salmonella paratyphi* are required to initiate paratyphoid fever.

Diagnosis

Diagnosis is by isolation of the organisms from blood (first week of disease), stools and urine (second and third weeks) in selective media such as MacConkey's agar, DCA or bismuth sulphite agar or in fluid enrichment media. Identification is by biochemical tests (e.g., **API** test) and **serology** (screening for H and O antigens by appropriate antisera). Further typing with bacteriophages (**phage typing**) can be performed.

Widal Test. When *Salmonella typhi* cannot be isolated, the diagnosis can be made serologically by demonstrating a rise in antibody titre in the patient's serum. This classic test, called the **Widal test**, consists of demonstrating antibodies to flagellar H antigen (using formalized bacteria) and somatic O antigen (using boiled bacteria) of *Salmonella typhi* and *Salmonella paratyphi-A* and *-B*. Interpretation of the test is difficult if the patient has been immunized with typhoid vaccine.

Treatment

Chloramphenicol, co-trimoxazole and ciprofloxacin are useful drugs, both in the treatment of acute typhoid fever and of the carrier state.

Prevention

Good personal hygiene and public health measures (i.e., safe water supplies, adequate sewage disposal and supervision of food processing and handling) are of great importance. Carriers of the organism should not be employed in the food industry. Immunization is useful. Two types of vaccine are available for travellers to—or those living in—endemic areas:

- heat-killed *Salmonella typhi*, given as two doses (4–6 weeks apart), subcutaneously
- live attenuated *Salmonella typhi* (Ty 21a) given orally, in three doses, on alternate days.

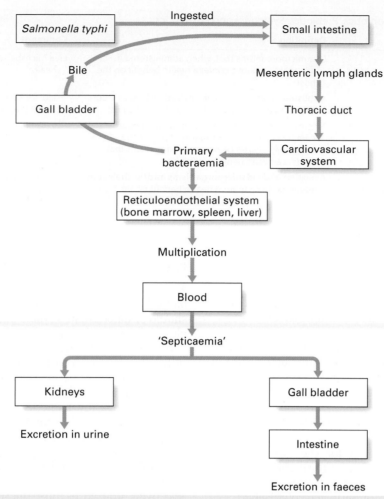

Fig. 26.2 Pathogenesis of typhoid fever.

Nonbacterial Causes of Diarrhoea

The foregoing lists the major causes of bacterial diarrhoea. It is important to realize that there are a number of **viral** and **protozoal** agents that may cause diarrhoea. These major nonbacterial causes of diarrhoea are briefly outlined in the following section (also see Table 26.1).

INFANTILE GASTROENTERITIS DUE TO ROTAVIRUS

Apart from *Escherichia coli* diarrhoea in children, the major cause of infantile gastroenteritis is rotavirus infection. This infection, seen mainly in older children and sometimes in adults, may be accompanied by respiratory illness. Laboratory diagnosis is by electron microscopy of stools for viral particles or enzyme-linked immunosorbent assay (ELISA) for antigen in stools.

PROTOZOAL DIARRHOEAL DISEASES

Amoebiasis (Amoebic Dysentery)

Caused by *Entamoeba histolytica*, the symptoms of amoebic dysentery vary from fulminating colitis to absence of symptoms. The disease is common in the tropics and is usually acquired via food contaminated by the cysts of the organism.

The drug of choice is metronidazole.

Giardiasis

Infection with *Giardia lamblia*, **a flagellate protozoan** with a pear-shaped body, gives rise to symptoms of abdominal discomfort, flatulence and diarrhoea; malabsorption and steatorrhoea may develop in chronic infection. Both children and adults are affected, and it is a common bowel pathogen in countries throughout the world.

The drug of choice is metronidazole.

PROBIOTICS AND GASTROINTESTINAL INFECTIONS

Probiotics are defined as **live microorganisms that, when administered in adequate amounts, confer a health benefit on the host**. The use of probiotics to prevent and treat a variety of diarrhoeal diseases as well as to maintain general gastrointestinal health has gained favour in recent years. However, the overall efficacy of these treatments and the mechanisms by which probiotics ameliorate gastrointestinal infections are yet not fully defined.

Table 26.2   Definitions of Probiotics, Prebiotics, Synbiotics and Postbiotics

Term	Definition	Comment
Probiotics (e.g., *Bifidobacterium animalis* subsp. *lactis Lactobacillus reuteri*)	Live microorganisms that, when administered in adequate amounts, confer a health benefit on the host	Live microbes that are beneficial for the host health
Prebiotics (e.g., inulin)	A substrate that is selectively utilized by host microorganisms conferring a health benefit on the host	'Food' for beneficial microbes such as lactobacilli that provide a health benefit
Synbiotics (e.g., *B. lactis* BB-12 + inulin)	A combination prebiotic and a probiotic mixture comprising live microorganisms and substrate(s) selectively utilized by host microorganisms that confers a health benefit on the host	Also defined as complementary synbiotics
Postbiotics (e.g., heat-killed *Akkermansia mucinophila* ATCC BAA-835)	A mixture of **dead microorganisms and/or their components** that confers a health benefit on the host	Intact nonviable microbes or their cell fragments; purified metabolites are not considered as postbiotics

Probiotic bacteria currently used include:

- *Lactobacillus acidophilus* (most widely used), *Lactobacillus plantarum*, *Lactobacillus brevis*, *Lactobacillus bulgaricus*
- *Bifidobacterium bifidum*, *Bifidobacterium infantis*
- *Streptococcus thermophilus*.

Probiotics may be delivered to the host via capsules, in powder form or laced in food (such as the lactobacilli) in various milk-related manufactured products.

Mechanisms of Action

Postulated mechanisms by which probiotics may help the host include:

- competing against pathogens for the same essential nutrients, leaving less available for the pathogen
- competitive binding to host adhesion sites and reducing the surface area available for pathogen colonization
- evoking signalling pathways in immune cells leading to secretion of cytokines that target the pathogen
- attacking pathogens and killing them directly by releasing bacteriocins or other toxic chemicals.

Probiotics, Prebiotics, Postbiotics and Synbiotics

The terms 'probiotics', 'prebiotics', 'synbiotics' and 'postbiotics' are commonly used in the medical literature and should be differentiated (Table 26.2). Definitions and examples of these are also given below.

Prebiotics. Defined as a substrate that is selectively utilized by host microorganisms conferring a health benefit on the host. These are usually specialized plant fibers, such as inulin, which act like nutrients that stimulate the growth of healthy bacteria ('lunch for good bacteria'). Prebiotics are found in many fruits and vegetables, especially those with complex carbohydrates, such as fiber and resistant starch.

Synbiotics. A **combination prebiotic and probiotic** mixture comprising live microorganisms and substrate(s) selectively utilized by host microorganisms that confer a health benefit on the host.

Postbiotics. A mixture of **dead microorganisms and/or their components** that confers a health benefit on the host.

Key Facts

- The human intestinal microbiome and its constituent endogenous microbiota are vastly complex; the majority of the organisms are 'uncultivable' and yet to be identified.
- The usual method of spread of gastrointestinal pathogens is the **faecal–oral route**.
- The common bacterial causes of diarrhoea are *Campylobacter* spp., *Shigella* spp., *Salmonella* spp., *Escherichia coli*, *Staphylococcus aureus*, *Clostridium welchii* and *Vibrio cholerae*.
- These organisms may **invade** the gut, causing systemic disease (e.g., typhoid) or proliferating to produce locally acting toxins that **focally damage** the gastrointestinal tract (e.g., cholera).
- The genus *Shigella* contains four species: *Shigella dysenteriae*, *Shigella flexneri*, *Shigella boydii* and *Shigella sonnei*.
- A large number of different *Salmonella* species exist (together with about 1500 serotypes), of which about 14 are important pathogens. The common **diarrhoeogenic** organism is *Salmonella typhimurium*.

- The term 'enteric fever' is given to **typhoid** and **paratyphoid** infections caused by *Salmonella typhi* and *Salmonella paratyphi-A*, -B and -C, respectively.
- *Escherichia coli* is a normal commensal of the gastrointestinal tract, but certain strains cause infantile gastroenteritis and traveller's diarrhoea.
- Distinct groups within the *Escherichia coli* species, such as enteropathogenic *Escherichia coli* (EPEC) and enterotoxigenic *Escherichia coli* (ETEC), exhibit different pathogenic mechanisms: some are invasive, others toxigenic.
- Cholera, a relatively common disease, especially in Southeast Asia, is mainly caused by *Vibrio cholerae* O1.
- The hallmark of cholera is non-bloody, frothy and colourless diarrhoea (rice-water stools); morbidity and death are due to dehydration and electrolyte imbalance.
- The terms **probiotics, prebiotics, synbiotics and postbiotics** are commonly used to define various sources of food mainly for healthy gut bacteria (Table 26.2).

Review Questions (Answers on p. 391)

Please indicate which answers are true and which are false.

26.1. Which of the following statements on the microbial flora of the gastrointestinal tract are true?
   a. it is modulated by the dietary intake
   b. aerobic bacteria outnumber the anaerobes in the colon
   c. *Candida albicans* may colonize the small intestine in healthy individuals
   d. the presence of *Escherichia coli* necessarily indicates infection
   e. *Salmonella* spp. are members of the normal flora

26.2. Dysentery:
   a. is often caused by viruses
   b. caused by *Shigella sonnei* is more severe than that caused by *Shigella dysenteriae*
   c. often spreads by faecal contamination of water sources
   d. is also caused by *Vibrio cholerae*
   e. can be prevented by good personal hygiene

26.3. *Salmonella* spp.:
   a. consist of more than 1500 serotypes
   b. cause predominantly foodborne infections
   c. form pink-coloured colonies on MacConkey's agar
   d. possess endotoxins
   e. infections in humans may lead to persistent carriage

26.4. *Escherichia coli*:
   a. could be a transient oral flora
   b. is a known cause of traveller's diarrhoea
   c. forms lactose-fermenting colonies on blood agar
   d. some strains demonstrate cytopathic effects
   e. enterotoxigenic variant (enterotoxigenic *Escherichia coli* (ETEC)) causes dysentery

26.5. Match the organism responsible for each of the clinical situations mentioned below:
   a. antibiotic-associated pseudomembranous colitis
   b. food poisoning associated with reheated fried rice
   c. predominantly nausea and vomiting a few hours after a suspected meal
   d. occurrence of copious amount of diarrhoeal stools resembling 'rice water'
   e. major agent responsible for infantile diarrhoeas
      1. *Bacillus cereus*
      2. *Staphylococcus aureus*
      3. *Clostridium difficile*
      4. *Vibrio cholerae*
      5. rotavirus

Further Reading

Britton, R. A., & Versalovic, J. (2008). Probiotics and gastrointestinal infections. *Interdisciplinary Perspectives on Infectious Diseases*, e1–e10. doi:10.1155/2008/290769.

Mims, C., Playfair, J., Roitt, I., et al. (1998). Gastrointestinal tract infections. In *Medical microbiology* (2nd ed., Ch. 20). Mosby.

Shanson, D. C. (1999). Infections of the gastrointestinal tract. In *Microbiology in clinical practice* (3rd ed., Ch. 15). Butterworth-Heinemann.

27 Infections of the Genitourinary Tract

Normal Flora and the Natural Defences of the Genitourinary Tract

Akin to the oral microbiome, the vaginal microbiome and the constituent microbiota form a mutually beneficial relationship with their host and have a major impact on health and disease.

Our understanding of the vaginal microbiome and its composition, structure and function has significantly broadened over the last decade due to the cultivation-independent methods based on the analysis of 16S ribosomal RNA (rRNA) and next-generation sequencing (NGS) technology.

In asymptomatic, otherwise healthy adult women, a **complex microbial community** exists in the vagina. The predominant species that **keep the vaginal pH low** and appear to prevent the growth of potential pathogens belong to the **genus *Lactobacillus***. For instance, their suppression by antibiotics may lead to overgrowth of the yeast *Candida albicans* found in relatively low numbers in the healthy vagina.

Other common groups of vaginal organisms include diphtheroids, streptococci, coliforms and a diverse array of anaerobes. Approximately 20% of women of child-bearing age carry group B β-haemolytic streptococci in the vagina. These may be acquired by the neonate during passage through the birth canal, resulting in serious infections such as meningitis and sepsis.

Unlike the vagina and vaginal tract, **the bladder, urinary tract and urine are normally sterile**, but the voided urine often becomes contaminated by flora from the distal portions of the urethra, such as *Staphylococcus epidermidis*, coliforms, diphtheroids and streptococci. Additionally, in females the organisms present in the distal part of the urethra may include contaminants from the gut flora, such as enterobacteria and lactobacilli.

The **flushing action of the urine** is arguably the most important defence factor of the urethra in both males and females. Bactericidal mechanisms in the bladder mucosa, including **local antibody response and lysozyme**, play an important role in preventing ascending infection of the urinary tract.

IMPORTANT PATHOGENS

Important genitourinary tract pathogens are listed in Fig. 27.1 and Table 27.1.

Sexually Transmitted Infections

More than 1 million sexually transmitted infections (STIs) are acquired every day worldwide. They are essentially transmitted by sexual intercourse and may affect both heterosexual and homosexual partners. Varying patterns of sexual behaviour can result in such infections manifesting in the oral cavity, oropharynx and rectum; STIs frequently—but not invariably—produce genital lesions; several produce severe systemic disease that may even lead to death, such as human immunodeficiency virus (HIV) infection and hepatitis B.

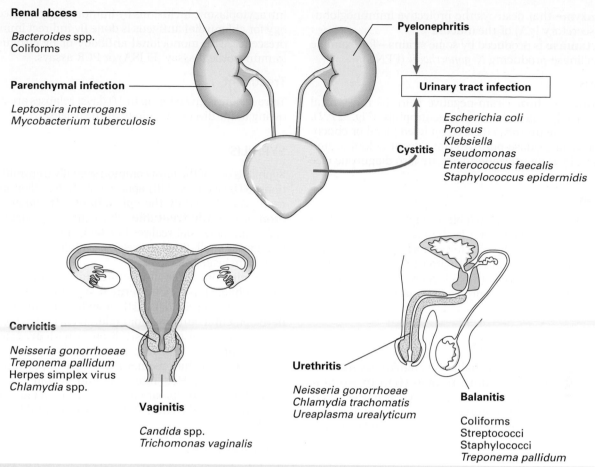

Renal abcess

Bacteroides spp.
Coliforms

Parenchymal infection

Leptospira interrogans
Mycobacterium tuberculosis

Pyelonephritis

Urinary tract infection

Escherichia coli
Proteus
Klebsiella
Pseudomonas
Enterococcus faecalis
Staphylococcus epidermidis

Cystitis

Cervicitis

Neisseria gonorrhoeae
Treponema pallidum
Herpes simplex virus
Chlamydia spp.

Vaginitis

Candida spp.
Trichomonas vaginalis

Urethritis

Neisseria gonorrhoeae
Chlamydia trachomatis
Ureaplasma urealyticum

Balanitis

Coliforms
Streptococci
Staphylococci
Treponema pallidum

Fig. 27.1   Major infectious agents of the genitourinary tract.

GONORRHOEA

Gonorrhoea is caused by *Neisseria gonorrhoeae* (the gonococcus).

Clinical Features

In women: acute **urethritis**, increased vaginal secretions with purulent discharge. In men: acute gonococcal urethritis with severe **dysuria** and purulent discharge. The disease may involve the **rectum** and **oropharynx**. Pharyngitis, sore throat, tonsillitis and gingivitis may occur because of gonococcal infection, especially from orogenital contact in homosexual men. **Asymptomatic infection** is common in both men and women. Complications include prostatitis, salpingitis and occasionally haematogenous spread, causing arthritis, septicaemia and meningitis.

Pathogenesis and Epidemiology

Gonococcal infection has been reported only in humans. The infection is limited to the mucosa of the anterior urethra in men and the cervix of women. In the newborn, **gonococcal conjunctivitis** may occur due to **cross-infection** from the mother's birth canal.

Three virulence factors have been identified:

1. an **endotoxin** that inhibits the ciliary activity of the fallopian tubes and retards the expulsion of the gonococcus

Table 27.1   Sexually Transmitted Diseases

Disease	Agent
BACTERIAL INFECTIONS	
Gonorrhoea	*Neisseria gonorrhoeae* (the gonococcus)
Syphilis	*Treponema pallidum*
Vaginitis	*Gardnerella vaginalis*, anaerobes
Chancroid	*Haemophilus ducreyi*
VIRAL INFECTIONS	
Genital herpes	Herpes simplex virus (type 2 mainly)
Genital warts	Human papillomavirus (see Fig. 21.1)
Hepatitis B[a]	Hepatitis B virus
AIDS	Human immunodeficiency virus (HIV)
Monkeypox (Mpox)[a]	Mpox virus
OTHERS	
Lymphogranuloma venereum	*Chlamydia trachomatis* types L_1–L_3
Granuloma inguinale (donovanosis)	*Calymmatobacterium granulomatis* (a *Klebsiella*-like microorganism)
Pubic lice (crabs)	*Pthirus pubis*
Genital scabies	*Sarcoptes scabiei*
Nonspecific urethritis	*Chlamydia trachomatis* types D–K
Trichomoniasis	*Trichomonas vaginalis*
Vaginal thrush	*Candida albicans*

[a]Not always sexually transmitted.

2. an **enzyme** that destroys the protective immunoglobulins (secretory IgA) of the mucosa
3. **β-lactamase** is produced by some strains—for example penicillinase-producing *N. gonorrhoeae* (PPNG).

Diagnosis

Gram smears show Gram-negative pairs of the typical kidney-shaped gonococci inside neutrophils (Fig. 27.2). **Swabs** from the urethra cultured on lysed blood or chocolate agar yield oxidase-positive, translucent colonies, and rapid carbohydrate utilization tests are also diagnostic (see Chapter 14).

Treatment

A choice of antibiotics is available: a single dose of 500 mg of intramuscular ceftriaxone is the current antibiotic of choice, particularly in the US. However a large, single, curative oral dose of amoxicillin (with probenecid to delay renal excretion), spectinomycin (for β-lactamase-positive gonococci) or erythromycin (children or pregnant women) could be used.

NONSPECIFIC URETHRITIS

One of the most common sexually transmitted diseases, nonspecific urethritis is seen **more in men than in women**. It is caused by more than one agent, but *Chlamydia trachomatis* is the most common cause. A mycoplasmal organism ('bacteria' without a cell wall), *Ureaplasma urealyticum*, may also cause significant morbidity. In females urethritis is usually accompanied by cervicitis.

Clinical Features

In men the acute purulent urethral discharge resembles that of gonorrhoea. Female patients with urethritis may report dysuria, intermittent vaginal bleeding and discharge.

Diagnosis

Smears and swabs of urethral or cervical discharge are diagnostic. Culture is now rarely done. Smears are examined for

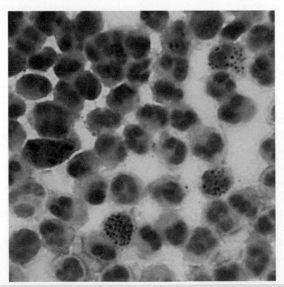

Fig. 27.2 Smear of a urethral pus exudate in gonorrhoea showing polymorphs and intracellular Gram-negative gonococci.

intracytoplasmic inclusions by immunofluorescence. Serology for chlamydial antigens is done by indirect immunofluorescence with monoclonal antibody or by enzyme-linked immunosorbent assay (ELISA) or PCR assays.

Treatment

Tetracycline is given for up to 10 days; relapses are common owing to the diverse aetiology of the disease.

SYPHILIS

Syphilis is one of the most common sexually transmitted infections (STIs) globally, with approximately 6 million infections each year. Caused by the **spirochaete *Treponema pallidum***, it is **easily treatable**, although symptoms may fade before an individual realizes he/she is infected, or they may not appear at all. If left untreated, syphilis can cause serious long-term health problems.

Syphilis contracted during pregnancy can be passed on to the child, causing **congenital syphilis**. This is the second leading cause of stillbirth globally and can have severe developmental outcomes for children carried to term.

It is also one of the classic diseases with **protean manifestations** (i.e., affecting virtually all organ systems of the body), and has reemerged as an important disease associated with HIV infection and sexual promiscuity. Important due to its late and severe sequelae, syphilis is preventable, and treatable with effective and inexpensive antibiotics.

Clinical Features

Syphilis has an incubation period of 10–90 days (average 3 weeks) and is characterized by four main clinical stages: **primary, secondary, tertiary** and **late or quaternary** (Fig. 27.3).

Primary Syphilis. A **painless red papule** develops at the inoculation site of the spirochaete, some 3 weeks (range 9–90 days) after the contact; this may be in the labia, vagina, cervix, penis or oral mucosa. The papule then produces the **chancre** of primary syphilis: a flat, red, indurated, **highly infectious** ulcer with a serous exudate. Enlarged, painless **regional lymphadenopathy** is common at this stage. The chancre disappears spontaneously within 3–8 weeks.

Secondary Syphilis. This stage is reached 6–8 weeks later and lasts for 1–3 months. A generalized **mucocutaneous spread** of the spirochaetes ensues at this stage and the lesions appear as papules on the skin and oral ulcers (see Chapter 35). The ulcers may coalesce to give the characteristic **'snail tracks'** and **mucous patches** in about one-third of those affected (Fig. 27.4). These lesions, like the primary chancre, are **highly infectious**. Other manifestations are generalized lymphadenopathy and **condylomata** (warts) of the anus and vulva; rarely, periostitis, arthritis and glomerulonephritis may be seen.

Tertiary Syphilis. The most destructive phase of the disease occurs 3–10 years after primary syphilis. Lesions appear as characteristic **gummata/gumma** or granulomatous nodules of the skin, mucosa, bone and other internal organs. Gummata commonly break down to produce

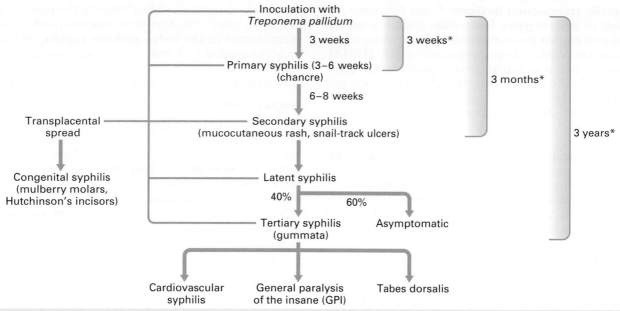

Fig. 27.3 Natural history of untreated syphilis; (*aide-memoire*: approximatelty 3 weeks, 3 months and 3 years for primary, secondary and tertiary syphilis onset, respectively) * Approximate figures.

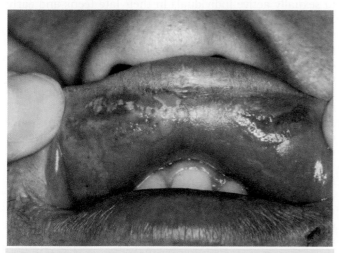

Fig. 27.4 *Mucous patches (on the patient's right)* and a snail-track ulcer (*left*) of the oral mucosa in a patient with secondary syphilis.

shallow, punched-out ulcers. In the oral cavity, gummata may rarely break down to produce **palatal perforations**, leading to **oronasal fistulae**. These lesions are **not infective**, as the tissue damage is due to a delayed type of hypersensitivity reaction.

Late or Quaternary Syphilis. This occurs 10–20 years after primary syphilis. The two main clinical forms of late syphilis are **cardiovascular syphilis** and **neurosyphilis**, with resultant pathology of the aorta and the nervous system, respectively.

Latent Syphilis. This may be seen in some after many years without any symptoms. The disease lies dormant without any clinical signs (except for positive serology) and may manifest as cardiovascular or neurosyphilis.

Congenital Syphilis. *Treponema pallidum* is one of the few microorganisms that has the ability to **cross the placental barrier**; thus the foetus may be infected during the second or third trimester from a syphilitic mother (either in the primary or secondary stage of syphilis). The disease will manifest in the infant as:

- **latent infection:** no symptoms but positive serology
- **early infection:** lesions such as skin rashes, saddle nose, bone lesions and meningitis appear up to the end of the second year of age
- **late infection:** after the second year of age, lesions include **Hutchinson's incisors** (notching of incisor teeth), **mulberry molar teeth** (due to infection of the enamel organ in the foetus), interstitial keratitis, bone sclerosis, arthritis, deafness.

Diagnosis

Direct Microscopy. Spirochaetes in exudate from primary or secondary lesions were identified by dark-ground microscopy, now rarely done. Care should be taken to differentiate *Treponema pallidum* from commensal oral spirochaetes (*Treponema denticola*) when oral lesions are examined. (*Note: Treponema pallidum* cannot be grown in laboratory media but can be propagated in the **testes of rabbits**.)

Serology. Antigens used for syphilis serology are of two types:

1. **Cardiolipin** or **lipoidal antigen:** Although not derived from the spirochaete, it is sensitive for detecting antibody. The most popular test that uses this antibody is the Venereal Diseases Reference Laboratory (**VDRL**) test; it is simple and sensitive, but biological false-positive reactions are common. As the antibody disappears after treatment, it can be used to monitor the efficacy of antimicrobial therapy (Table 27.2).

2. **Specific treponemal antigen:** Using *Treponema pallidum* as antigen gives fewer false-positive reactions and tests remain positive after treatment. The tests are *Treponema pallidum* haemagglutination test **(TPHA)**, fluorescent treponemal antibody absorption test **(FTA-ABS)**, which detects both IgM and IgG antibody, and **ELISA.** The last is increasingly used as a screening test to detect IgG antibody, although some false positives may result.

The interpretation of syphilis serology is complex (because of the many medical conditions that yield false-positive reactions) and is not further discussed here.

Recently, it has been shown that **real-time polymerase chain reaction** (rtPCR) is a fast, efficient and reliable test for the diagnosis of primary syphilis, but has no added value for the diagnosis of secondary syphilis.

Treatment

Penicillin (large doses, for up to 3 weeks) is the drug of choice. Erythromycin or tetracycline can be used if the patient is hypersensitive.

NOTES ON SOME COMMON SEXUALLY TRANSMITTED DISEASES

HIV Infection

This is a pandemic infection commonly transmitted by sexual intercourse and is also a disease of enormous importance for health care personnel (see Chapter 30).

Trichomoniasis

A common protozoal infection in women is caused by *Trichomonas vaginalis*. It is transmitted mainly by sexual intercourse: in men, the infection is often symptomless; in women, it manifests as a chronic vaginal infection ranging from a yellow, offensive discharge with vaginitis to symptomless or low-grade infection.

- **Diagnosis** is by culture of swabs in special media or examination of direct smear for motile, flagellated protozoa.
- **Treatment:** metronidazole.

Candidiasis

Candidiasis is a yeast infection commonly transmitted by sexual intercourse; it is frequently seen in women but rarely in men. *Candida albicans* is the most frequent causative yeast; the disease is characterized by **white membranes in the vulva and the vagina**, which may be accompanied by a watery discharge; many cases are symptomless.

Diagnosis and treatment are as described in Chapter 22.

Herpes Genitalis

Mainly due to **herpes simplex type 2 virus**, but as a result of sexual promiscuity, type 1 viruses (which are more or less confined to oral regions) are frequently implicated. The lesions are **vesicular and painful**, and seen in anogenital regions. The primary lesion, associated with fever and inguinal lymphadenopathy, is more protracted and painful than the secondary recurrences. **Asymptomatic infection is common** in both men and women; hence sexual spread of the disease is common.

Diagnosis and treatment are described in Chapter 21.

Hepatitis B

See Chapter 29.

Human Papillomavirus

Human papillomavirus (HPV) infection is one of the **most common sexually transmitted infections** mainly seen in sexually active individuals in their late teens and early 20s. HPV can exist as harmless commensals on oral mucosal surfaces (see Chapter 21). More than 200 different HPV genotypes have been identified, and some, such as **HPV-16 and HPV-18, are agents of oral cancers and precancers**. The major benign clinical manifestations of HPV infection are **oral papilloma/condyloma and focal epithelial hyperplasia**.

HPV infections can be prevented by **efficacious vaccines**. A number of widely available multivalent vaccines can protect against specific HPV genotypes.

Monkeypox (Mpox) Infection. Monkeypox infection caused by the monkeypox (Mpox) virus (related to the now extinct smallpox virus) is a highly contagious disease first documented in humans in the 1970s. Since then, sporadic outbreaks of Mpox have been reported in many countries, though most cases have been restricted to **endemic areas in Africa**. However, the recent emergence of Mpox in the West and evidence indicating person-to-person transmission, have been a major concern.

The recent cases of Mpox were mainly **sexually transmitted**, particularly among gay, bisexual and other men who had sex with men. The disease in such situations is usually contracted through direct contact with the infectious rash, scabs, crusts or fluids from sores, saliva or infected bodily fluids, including respiratory secretions.

The prodromal symptoms of Mpox include fever, headache, myalgia, backache, chills, fatigue and, in particular, generalised lymphadenopathy, which distinguishes it from chickenpox. **Mucosal lesions in the mouth appear first**—therefore, dentists are well placed to identify the disease at an early stage of infection—followed by skin lesions on the face and extremities, including palms and soles, and sometimes extending to the genital region. The rash will undergo the typical **macular, papular, vesicular and blister stages** (Fig. 27.5). Finally, the blisters break, forming a black scab that eventually falls off.

Table 27.2   Serological Tests for Syphilis

Stage of Disease	VDRL	TPHA	FTA-Abs
Primary	+ or −	−	+
Late primary	+	+ or −	+
Secondary and tertiary	+	+	+
Late (quaternary)	+	+	+
Latent	+ or −	+	+
Treated syphilis	−	+	+
Congenital syphilis	+	+	+

Note: The efficacy of treatment can be monitored by the VDRL test.
FTA-Abs, fluorescent treponemal antibody-absorption test; *TPHA, Treponema pallidum* haemagglutination test; *VDRL,* Venereal Diseases Reference Laboratory.

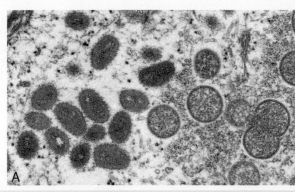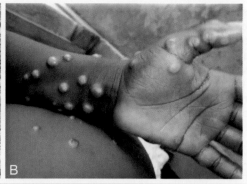

Fig. 27.5 Mpox virus and skin lesions. (Panel A) An electron micrograph showing mature, oval, mulberry-shaped Mpox virus particles (*dark on left*), and spherical immature virions (*light on right*). (Panel B) Papular and vesicular skin lesions of a patient with Mpox. (Sources: A, Cynthia S. Goldsmith, Russell Regnery; Courtesy CDC Image library; B, Photo from WHO homepage. Source: https://www.who.int/health-topics/monkeypox#tab=tab_1).

Mpox is usually a **self-limiting disease** with symptoms lasting between 2 and 4 weeks. In general, the case fatality rates of the current epidemic have been between 3% and 6%, though slightly higher among children.

A vaccine specific for Mpox is under development, although the **smallpox vaccine is effective** in curbing the infection.

CONTROL OF SEXUALLY TRANSMITTED DISEASES

Although control is difficult, **tracing of sexual partners** of infected individuals is essential to prevent spread of disease in the community. Patients are requested to name consorts, and the latter should submit themselves to examination and treatment. In the long term, prevention of sexually transmitted diseases, including HIV infection, is far more important in reducing health care costs of the community.

Urinary Tract Infections

Urinary tract infections are common, especially in women, despite the availability of a spectrum of antibiotics. They are defined as follows:

- **bacteriuria:** multiplication of bacteria in urine within the renal tract (more than 10^5 organisms per millilitre of urine is considered to be significant bacteriuria (i.e., evidence of urinary tract infection))
- **pyuria:** presence of pus cells (polymorphs) in urine
- **cystitis:** infection of the bladder
- **pyelonephritis:** infection of the pelvis and parenchyma of the kidney
- **urethritis:** infection of the urethra.

Cystitis, pyelonephritis or urethritis may occur either singly or in combination.

IMPORTANT PATHOGENS

Causative agents are many and varied (see Fig. 27.1), but ***Escherichia coli* is the most common**, accounting for 60–80% of infections. Some *E. coli* strains are more invasive than others, possibly as a result of the possession of capsular or K antigens, which inhibit phagocytosis, and their superior ability to adhere to the uroepithelium with the aid of the pili on cell surfaces.

Other organisms that commonly cause infection include:

- *Staphylococcus saprophyticus:* commonly seen in sexually active women under 25 years of age
- *Proteus mirabilis:* causes about 10% of infections
- *Klebsiella* spp.: resistant to a number of antibiotics (multiple antibiotic resistant)
- *Staphylococcus aureus* and *Pseudomonas aeruginosa:* seen after instrumentation or catheterization.

Note: **Acute** urinary tract infection is mostly **monomicrobial** in origin, whereas **polymicrobial** infection with more than one organism is common in **chronic** infections.

CLINICAL FEATURES

Urinary tract infection is mainly a disease of women, with a male-to-female ratio of 1:10. Clinical features of cystitis include dysuria, urgency, suprapubic pain, increased frequency and haematuria. Fever, loin pain and tenderness are signs of pyelonephritis.

LABORATORY DIAGNOSIS

- **Microscopy:** wet films and Gram-stained films used for detection of red blood cells, polymorphs, bacteria and epithelial cells.
- **Culture:** usually on nutrient agar and MacConkey's agar. As the number of organisms in the sample indicates the degree of infection, this can be assessed semi-quantitatively by appropriate plating out.

TREATMENT

An array of oral antibiotics excreted in urine in high concentrations is available, including trimethoprim, co-trimoxazole, ciprofloxacin and nitrofurantoin. Therapy depends on the aetiological agent and its antibiotic-sensitivity pattern.

Dentistry and Genitourinary Infections

It is important for the dentist to be aware of sexually transmitted diseases, as many of them manifest frequently in the oral cavity as a result of atypical sexual habits and the escalating sex industry worldwide. Indeed, some consider the oral cavity as a sexual organ. Furthermore, organisms that may cause sexually transmitted diseases (e.g., herpes, HIV infection) may have the propensity to be transmitted in the clinical setting, from the patient to the dentist, by direct contact or indirectly via contaminated instruments if appropriate infection control measures are not implemented.

Urinary tract infections are of no direct relevance to dentistry except insofar as patients are taking antibiotics, which may either affect the oral flora or, rarely, interact with drugs prescribed by the dentist. Indeed, the potential of metronidazole to kill anaerobic bacteria was first detected by an astute dentist who noted the resolution of acute ulcerative gingivitis in a patient under his care who was undergoing treatment for vaginal trichomonal infection with this drug (at that time prescribed solely as an antiprotozoal agent).

Key Facts

- The **predominant vaginal microbiota** in adult women comprises lactobacilli; other microorganisms are diphtheroids, streptococci, anaerobes and coliforms.
- **The urine** in the bladder is **normally sterile**, but the voided urine often becomes contaminated with flora on the distal portions of the urethra.
- The **flushing action** of the urine is the most **important defence factor** of the urethra in both males and females.
- A large group of infections is transmitted by sexual intercourse (both heterosexual and homosexual), and varying patterns of sexual behaviour can result in infections manifesting in the oral cavity, oropharynx and the rectum.
- **Gonorrhoea**, caused by *Neisseria gonorrhoeae* (the gonococcus), causes acute urethritis with purulent discharge.
- Gonorrhoea may involve the rectum and oropharynx with resultant pharyngitis, sore throat, tonsillitis and gingivitis (especially from orogenital contact).
- Virulence factors of *N. gonorrhoeae* include an endotoxin, a protease that destroys secretory immunoglobulin A (IgA), and β-lactamase production in some (penicillinase-producing *N. gonorrhoeae* (PPNG)).
- **Syphilis** caused by *Treponema pallidum* (syphilis spirochaete) is a classic disease with **protean manifestations** and is characterized by four main clinical stages.
- **In primary syphilis, chancre** (a flat, red, indurated, highly infectious ulcer with a serous exudate) is seen both on the oral and on the vaginal mucosae is the hallmark feature.
- **Secondary syphilis** is characterized by a generalized mucocutaneous spread of spirochaetes and lesions that appear as papules on the skin, and infectious oral ulcers **(snail-track ulcers)**.
- In **tertiary syphilis**, noninfective lesions appear as characteristic **gummata/gumma** or granulomatous nodules

of the skin, mucosa, bone and other internal organs. Intraorally, gummata may break down to produce palatal perforations, leading to oronasal fistulae.
- The two main clinical forms of **late or quaternary syphilis** are cardiovascular syphilis and neurosyphilis.
- **Dental lesions** in **congenital syphilis** include **Hutchinson's incisors** (notching of incisor teeth) and **mulberry molar teeth** (due to infection of the enamel organ in the foetus).
- **Syphilis** is mainly **diagnosed by serology** (Venereal Diseases Reference Laboratory (VDRL) test) with either the specific treponemal antigen or cardiolipin or lipoidal antigens.
- Causative agents of **urinary tract infection** are many, but *Escherichia coli* **is the most** common, accounting for 60–80% of infections.
- Most oral human papillomavirus (HPV) lesions are benign papillomas.
- Over 200 different HPV genotypes have been identified, and some, such as **HPV-16 and HPV-18**, are agents of **oral cancers and precancers**.
- Efficacious vaccines are available to prevent HPV transmission.
- **Monkeypox (Mpox)**, previously confined mainly to the African continent, is now seen in the West as a sexually transmitted infection.
- The prodromal symptoms of Mpox include fever, headache, myalgia, chills, fatigue and, in particular, generalised lymphadenopathy, which distinguishes it from chickenpox.
- Oral mucosal lesions are the usually the first to appear in Mpox, followed by skin lesions on the face and extremities; hence, dentists are well placed to identify the disease at an early stage.

Review Questions (Answers on p. 391)

Please indicate which answers are true and which are false.

27.1. Purulent urethral discharge in a sexually active male:
   a. is commonly of gonococcal origin
   b. should warrant investigations for other sexually transmitted diseases
   c. necessitates screening of the sexual partner/s
   d. may not yield any organism in a Gram-stained smear
   e. is often associated with dysuria

27.2. In a healthy individual, which of the following anatomical loci are considered sterile?
   a. urinary bladder
   b. distal urethra
   c. vagina
   d. fallopian tubes
   e. ureters

27.3. The finding of Gram-negative intracellular diplococci in a direct smear from a throat swab:
   a. is indicative of gonococcal infection
   b. should be followed with culture and biochemical tests
   c. may signify a sexually acquired infection
   d. needs empirical treatment with rifampicin
   e. indicates that the patient is at risk of developing meningitis

27.4. Genital ulcerations are seen in:
   a. gonorrhoea
   b. syphilis
   c. candidiasis
   d. genital herpes
   e. trichomoniasis

27.5. Oral manifestations of syphilis include:
   a. Hutchinson's incisors in congenital syphilis
   b. snail-track ulcers in primary syphilis
   c. mulberry molars in tertiary syphilis
   d. chancre in secondary syphilis
   e. palatal perforation in tertiary syphilis

Further Reading

Beale, M. A., Marks, M., et al. (2021). Global phylogeny of *Treponema pallidum* lineages reveals recent expansion and spread of contemporary syphilis. *Nature Microbiology, 6*, 1549–1560. doi:10.1038/s41564-021-01000-z.

Brooks, J. F., Carroll, K. C., Butel, J. S., et al. (Eds.). (2013). Neisseriae. In *Jawetz, Melnick & Adelberg's medical microbiology* (26th ed., pp. 285–293). McGraw Hill.

Brooks, J. F., Carroll, K. C., Butel, J. S., et al. (Eds.). (2013). Spirochetes and other spiral organisms. In *Jawetz, Melnick & Adelberg's medical microbiology* (26th ed., pp. 327–338). McGraw Hill.

Samaranayake, L., & Anil, S. (2022). The monkeypox outbreak and implications for dental practice. *International Dental Journal, 72*(5), 589–596. doi:10.1016/j.identj.2022.07.006.

Sun, C. X., Bennett, N., Tran, P., Tang, K. D., Lim, Y., Frazer, I., Samaranayake, L., & Punyadeera, C. (2017). A pilot study into the association between oral health status and human papillomavirus-16 infection. *Diagnostics (Basel), 7*(1), 11. doi:10.3390/diagnostics7010011.

28 Skin and Wound Infections

Normal Flora

The microbiome of the skin is complex and has a thriving community of bacterial flora with a few commensal fungi. These microbiota comprise 10^3–10^4 organisms per square centimetre of skin and fall into two major categories:

- **normal or resident flora:** a stable population of organisms in terms of numbers and composition
- **transient flora:** essentially 'in transit' but may multiply for a short period; are quickly eliminated because of competition from the normal flora.

The main resident flora of the skin includes staphylococci, principally *Staphylococcus epidermidis* (asymptomatic carriage of *Staphylococcus aureus* is common in specific niches such as the anterior nares and axillae and in hospital personnel), propionibacteria, micrococci and diphtheroids. Most of them are located superficially in the stratum corneum, but some are found in the hair follicles and act as a reservoir, replenishing the superficial flora—for example, after hand-washing. The composition of the normal microbiota in specific anatomical niches of the skin such as the scalp, axillae and pubic area differs considerably because of ecological differences in the pH, temperature and nutrients (e.g., sebum, fatty acids, urea). Continuous **desquamation** of the stratum corneum and the impervious nature of the epithelium are major barriers for invading organisms. Other antimicrobial defences include **lysozyme** (in sweat, sebum and tears), **bacteriocins** produced by commensals and **fatty acids** produced from hydrolysis of sebum triglycerides.

Skin Infections

The major forms of skin infections and the agents involved are shown in Table 28.1.

BACTERIAL SKIN INFECTIONS

Staphylococcal Infections

Boils, styes, carbuncles, sycosis barbae and angular cheilitis are all caused by staphylococci. A **boil** is a common, circumscribed infection of the hair follicle with central suppuration; pus eventually discharges and the boil heals, leaving no scar. **Carbuncles**, now rare, are large abscesses that occur at the back of the neck, especially in people with diabetes. They are associated with constitutional upset and malaise. **Sycosis barbae** is a staphylococcal skin infection involving the shaving area of the face.

Streptococcal Infections

In contrast to staphylococcal infections, which generally remain localized, streptococcal infections of the skin tend to spread subcutaneously and may lead to the following conditions.

Cellulitis. *Streptococcus pyogenes* group A is the most common offender, although *Staphylococcus aureus* may be involved in some cases. Cellulitis is a serious disease as **subcutaneous spread of infection** may carry the pathogen to lymphatic and blood vessels, resulting in marked constitutional upset and septicaemia.

Table 28.1   Agents of Some Important Skin Infections[a]

Aetiological Agent	Skin Infection
Bacteria	
Staphylococcus aureus	Abscesses (boils), impetigo, pustules, carbuncles, toxic epidermal necrolysis (Ritter's disease), omphalitis, angular cheilitis, sycosis barbae
β-haemolytic streptococci	Cellulitis, impetigo, erysipelas
Propionibacterium acnes	Acne
Mycobacterium tuberculosis	Lupus vulgaris
Mycobacterium ulcerans	Swimming pool granuloma
Mycobacterium leprae	Leprosy
Actinomyces israelii	Actinomycosis (cervicofacial)
Treponema pallidum	Syphilis
Haemophilus ducreyi	Chancroid
Viruses	
Herpes simplex virus	Cold sore, herpetic whitlow
Varicella-zoster virus	Chickenpox, shingles
Papovaviruses	Papillomas, warts
Coxsackievirus A	Hand, foot and mouth disease
Fungi	
Candida spp.	Chronic mucocutaneous candidiasis
	Angular cheilitis
Various dermatophytes	Ringworm, etc.

[a]Infections caused by protozoa and insects are not given.

Erysipelas. A distinctive type of cellulitis caused by *Streptococcus pyogenes* is usually seen in **elderly adults**. Lesions are typically on the face and limbs; the lesion distribution on the face is often **butterflylike** with a characteristic **'orange-peel'** texture of the skin and induration; the patient may be acutely ill with high fever and toxaemia.

Impetigo. In this disease of **young children**, vesicles appear on the skin around the mouth and later become purulent, with characteristic honey-coloured crusts; both *Streptococcus pyogenes* and *Staphylococcus aureus* are involved.

Necrotizing Fasciitis

Necrotizing fasciitis is a rapidly progressing infection involving the full thickness of the skin down to the fascial planes, causing extensive necrosis and tissue loss. The skin looks initially normal, but the infection spreads surreptitiously along the fascial planes, destroying the blood supply to the skin, which discolours and becomes necrotic within hours (hence the tabloid term **'flesh-eating bacteria'**). The patient is severely ill with toxaemia and shock, and may die within 24 h. Formerly called 'streptococcal gangrene', it can be caused by mixed flora comprising staphylococci, strict anaerobes and Enterobacteriaceae; the major offending organism is the **Lancefield Group A Streptococcus:** *Streptococcus pyogenes*. Management entails prompt excision of skin, antibiotics and supportive therapy (see Chapter 11).

Angular Cheilitis

Inflammation of one or both angles of the mouth, especially in denture-wearing elderly people, may be related to ***Staphylococcus aureus* and/or *Candida* infection**. However, many other predisposing factors such as malnutrition and iron deficiency anemias are involved, and the **dentist should be aware of the management** of this condition (see Chapter 35: Fig. 28.1). (Synonyms for angular cheilitis include 'perleche' and 'angular stomatitis'.)

Acne

Caused by *Propionibacterium acnes*, acne is a common and disfiguring facial infection of **adolescents**. The disease is a disorder of the **pilosebaceous system** and is precipitated by the

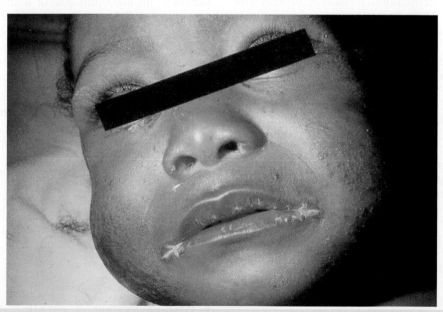

Fig. 28.1   Bilateral angular cheilitis in a malnourished African child. A number of non infective, predisposing cofactors may contribute to this condition (see also Fig 35.9).

excessive production of fatty acids and lipases by the follicular bacteria. This leads to an inflammatory response and blockage of the sebaceous duct that drains the sebum from the gland to the skin surface. Accumulation of sebum and consequent low-grade, propionibacterial (and sometimes staphylococcal) infection is the final outcome. Clearly **hormonal imbalances** also play a role, as the lesions generally resolve during the post-pubertal period. Long-term, low-dose antibiotic therapy may alleviate acne in **chronic, long-term, recalcitrant infection**.

Leprosy

Caused by *Mycobacterium leprae*. The organism lives in human skin and nerves and is transmitted by prolonged contact to cause a chronic granulomatous disease. There are two types: the **lepromatous** and the **tuberculoid** forms (Fig. 28.1; see Chapter 19).

Gram-Negative Infections

Gram-negative infections, less frequent than Gram-positive infections, are mostly associated with the moist areas of the skin such as the groin, axillae and perineum. Organisms involved include *Pseudomonas aeruginosa* and *Bacteroides* spp.

Diagnosis of Bacterial Skin Infections

Swabs and smears of pus and exudate from lesions are adequate; Gram-stained smears will generally indicate whether staphylococci or streptococci are involved. Swabs inoculated on blood agar (both aerobically and anaerobically) demonstrate the nature of haemolysis produced by streptococci (α-, β- or no haemolysis); subsequent confirmation of the identity of isolates is by appropriate tests (e.g., coagulase test, API tests).

VIRAL SKIN INFECTIONS

Herpes simplex viruses (human herpesviruses 1 and 2) cause recurrent **cold sores** and **genital lesions**; **herpetic whitlow** may be an occupational disease of dentists and nursing staff (see Fig. 21.2). Varicella-zoster virus (human herpesvirus 3) may cause **chickenpox** (primary lesion) and **shingles** of the skin (either in the facial or other dermatomes). Human herpesvirus 6 and human parvovirus B19 cause **exanthem subitum** and the **'slapped-cheek' syndrome**, respectively; both are innocuous self-limiting diseases that cause facial rash and redness, mainly in children (see Chapter 21). Papovaviruses cause the common **wart**, and coxsackievirus A16 infection may result in **hand, foot and mouth disease** (Table 28.1).

Note that many infectious diseases such as rubella, chickenpox, measles and glandular fever manifest as macules (spots) or papules (pimples) on the skin.

Diagnosis of Viral Skin Infections

Diagnostic methods include serology for antibody studies; swab or vesicular fluid for tissue culture; and electron microscopy (see Chapter 6).

FUNGAL SKIN INFECTIONS

Fungal skin infections are mainly caused by dermatophytes and the yeast *Candida*. As their name implies, dermatophytes

(which include *Microsporum*, *Epidermophyton* and *Trichophyton*) live in keratinized tissues, especially hair, nails and skin squames. *Candida* species are common opportunistic pathogens that may cause both skin and mucosal infections (see Chapter 35).

Wound Infections

SURGICAL WOUND INFECTION

Surgical wound infection accounts for approximately one-quarter of hospital-acquired **(nosocomial)** infections. It is a significant cause of morbidity, prolonging the hospital stay of surgical patients, and frequently results in death.

Aetiology

Staphylococcus aureus and *Escherichia coli* are the major pathogens, but other coliforms such as *Pseudomonas aeruginosa* and *Klebsiella* spp. may be involved. If the wound is contaminated (e.g., large bowel), anaerobes, *Clostridium* spp. and *Bacteroides* spp. may also be involved. Most wound infections are polymicrobial in nature.

Clinical Features

Wound edges become reddened, with or without pus formation; sometimes a wound abscess may form unnoticed in the deeper layers and eventually discharge through the suture line. Patients may or may not be pyrexial, depending on the degree of infection. Surgical wound infection may result in:

- spread of infection either to adjacent tissues or into the blood, causing **septicaemia** (see below)
- **wound dehiscence** (breakdown of the wound), necessitating **resuture**.

Pathogenesis and Epidemiology

The infection could be either **endogenous** or **exogenous**. The source of an exogenous infection could be an infected person in an adjoining bed, or a carrier, who might be a member of staff. Reservoirs of infection include human skin, environmental dust and inanimate objects **(fomites)** such as bed linens. The mode of cross-infection could be **direct or indirect contact**, or the **airborne** route. Many factors affect the incidence of wound infection; these include:

- type of wound: **clean** (i.e., no incision through respiratory, gastrointestinal or genitourinary tract), **contaminated** (e.g., following surgery in a site with a normal flora) or **infected** (e.g., drainage of an abscess)
- overcrowded wards
- length of stay in the hospital (shorter hospital stay carries a lesser risk of infection)
- length of the operation (longer operation carries a greater infectious risk)
- presence of foreign bodies and drains
- general health of the patient.

Prevention

Infection may be avoided by:

- rigid observation of **aseptic** and **antiseptic techniques** during both patient preparation and the operation itself

- rigid observation and implementation of **infection control theatre protocols**
- appropriate theatre **clothing**, as transmission of infection from humans is the single most important cause of wound infection
- **positive-pressure ventilation** within the operating room to prevent ingress of contaminated air and dust from the external hospital environment
- **isolation** of patients with discharging wounds to prevent the dissemination of pathogens—that is, **source isolation**, where the patient is the source of infection (compare **protective isolation** of susceptible patients—for instance, a bone marrow transplant patient, from infectious agents)
- carefully chosen **preoperative antibiotic prophylaxis** in specific situations (e.g., colonic surgery).

INFECTIONS OF BURNS

Major burns create large, moist, exposed surfaces that are ideal for bacterial growth because the protective skin cover has been lost.

Aetiology

Common organisms that infect burns are *Streptococcus pyogenes*, *Pseudomonas aeruginosa* and *Staphylococcus aureus*; infection is usually polymicrobial.

Pathogenesis and Epidemiology

Bacteria colonize burn wounds within 24 h if appropriate prophylaxis is not given, with eventual cellulitis of adjacent tissues and septicaemia. *Streptococcus pyogenes*, in particular, is a frequent cause of septicaemia; *Pseudomonas aeruginosa* has a special ability for surviving in burnt tissue and in burn wards, but it is not as virulent as *Streptococcus pyogenes*.

DIAGNOSIS OF WOUND INFECTIONS

Swabs of exudate, tissue or pus are cultured on conventional media (blood agar, MacConkey's agar, Robertson's medium); the smears of the tissue or exudate are Gram-stained and examined for organisms.

CLOSTRIDIAL WOUND INFECTIONS

Wound infections (described above), which are suppurative, differ clinically from those caused by clostridia (Gram-positive, anaerobic, spore-forming rods; Chapter 13). These infections are severe but, fortunately, rare. The two major clostridial wound infections are **tetanus**, caused by *Clostridium tetani*, and **gas gangrene**, due to three different but related organisms: *Clostridium welchii*, *Clostridium novyi* and *Clostridium septicum*.

Tetanus

See Chapter 25.

Gas Gangrene

Gas gangrene is caused by *Clostridium welchii* (60–65%), *Clostridium novyi* (20–40%) and *Clostridium septicum* (10–20%).

Clinical Features. Spreading gangrene of the muscles is accompanied by toxaemia and shock. The involved tissues are **black** and **oedematous** with a **foul-smelling serous exudate**; they exhibit the sign of **crepitus** (palpable crackling on pressure due to subcutaneous movement of gas bubbles) as a result of the production of gaseous metabolites by the multiplying clostridia.

Pathogenesis and Epidemiology. A serious disease with a high mortality rate, very often requiring the excision or amputation of the affected area or limb, gas gangrene is a result of the toxins and enzymes produced by clostridia thriving on damaged and devitalized tissues, which provide ideal conditions for anaerobic growth. The organisms produce a variety of toxins, one of which is a **lecithinase** that damages cell membranes; other enzymes produce gaseous by-products within tissue compartments, helping to spread the infection further.

Clostridia can be commonly isolated from faeces, and their spores are ubiquitous in nature.

Laboratory Diagnosis. See Chapter 13.

Treatment. Gas gangrene is treated with:

- **surgical debridement:** including wide excision or even amputation of affected areas
- **antibiotics:** large doses of penicillin, with or without metronidazole
- **hyperbaric oxygen:** may be given, if available, to reduce anaerobiosis of affected tissues.

Prevention. Debridement and amputation should be performed as appropriate. Prophylactic penicillin should be administered for surgical procedures in the area of the thigh, perineum and buttocks (as clostridia are commensals in these regions).

Key Facts

- The skin has a thriving microbiome of **resident** and **transient** flora; there are about 10^3–10^4 organisms per square centimetre of skin.
- The principal resident flora of the skin are *Staphylococcus epidermidis*, propionibacteria, micrococci and diphtheroids.
- **Asymptomatic carriage** of *Staphylococcus aureus* is common in sites such as the **anterior nares** and axillae and in hospital personnel.
- Boils, styes, carbuncles, sycosis barbae and angular cheilitis may all be due to staphylococcal infection, with several predisposing factors playing a role.
- Subcutaneous spread of infection or **cellulitis** is caused by *Streptococcus pyogenes* (group A), sometimes with *Staphylococcus aureus*.
- **Necrotizing fasciitis** is the term given to rapidly progressing infection involving the full thickness of the skin, including the fascial planes, causing **extensive necrosis, tissue loss, toxaemia** and **shock**.
- **Angular cheilitis** or stomatitis is mainly caused by *Staphylococcus aureus* and/or *Candida* infection, but other predisposing factors are involved.
- **Acne**, a common, disfiguring facial infection of adolescents, is caused by *Propionibacterium acnes*.
- *Mycobacterium leprae*, the agent of **leprosy**, lives in human skin and nerves and is transmitted by prolonged contact to cause two types of chronic granulomatous disease: the **lepromatous form** and the **tuberculoid form**.
- **Surgical wound infections** account for approximately one-quarter of hospital-acquired (nosocomial) infections.
- *Staphylococcus aureus* and *Escherichia coli* are the major agents of surgical infection.
- **Factors affecting** the incidence of **wound infection** include the type of wound (clean, contaminated or infected), overcrowded wards, length of stay in hospital, length of the operation, foreign bodies and drains, and the general health of the patient.
- Common organisms that infect **burns** are *Streptococcus pyogenes*, *Pseudomonas aeruginosa* and *Staphylococcus aureus*; infection is usually **polymicrobial**.
- The two major **clostridial wound infections** are **tetanus**, caused by *Clostridium tetani*, and **gas gangrene**, due to *Clostridium welchii*, *Clostridium novyi* or *Clostridium septicum*.

Review Questions (Answers on p. 391)

Please indicate which answers are true and which are false.

28.1. Which of the following statements about human skin are true?
a. a stable population of microorganisms is found
b. hair follicles act as reservoirs of pathogenic bacteria
c. bacteriocins act as a major inhibitory factor for invading organisms
d. sebum has antibacterial properties as it contains lysozyme
e. Gram-negative infections are more common than Gram-positive infections

28.2. With regard to skin infections, which of the following statements are true?
a. staphylococcal skin infections usually remain localized
b. cellulitis is predominantly caused by *Staphylococcus aureus*
c. necrotizing fasciitis may have a polymicrobial aetiology
d. angular cheilitis could present as a mixed bacterial and fungal infection
e. infections by dermatophytes can affect hair and nails

28.3. Which of the following statements on postoperative wound infections are true?
a. they are a major cause of nosocomial infections
b. coliforms are thought to be major pathogens
c. they can lead to wound dehiscence and septicaemia
d. prolonged operation time is not considered a risk factor
e. incidence may be reduced by preoperative antibiotic prophylaxis

28.4. Gas gangrene:
a. is exclusively caused by *Clostridium welchii*
b. often affects the lower limbs
c. classically exhibits crepitus in affected tissues
d. often necessitates amputation of the affected limb
e. hyperbaric oxygen has a place in treatment

28.5. Identify and match the major aetiological agent responsible for the skin conditions given below:
a. acne
b. folliculitis
c. cellulitis
d. impetigo
e. slapped-cheek syndrome
1. *Propionibacterium acnes*
2. *Staphylococcus aureus*
3. *Streptococcus pyogenes*
4. *Staphylococcus epidermidis*
5. parvovirus B19

Further Reading

Mims, C., Playfair, J., Roitt, I., et al. (1998). Infections of the skin, muscle, joints, bone and hemopoietic system. In *Medical microbiology* (2nd ed., Ch. 3). Mosby.

Murray, P. R., Rosenthal, K. S., Kobayashi, G. S., et al. (1998). Superficial, cutaneous and subcutaneous mycoses. In *Medical microbiology* (3rd ed., Ch. 69). Mosby.

Shanson, D. C. (1999). Skin infections and infestations. In *Microbiology in clinical practice* (3rd ed., Ch. 17). Butterworth-Heinemann.

29 Viral Hepatitis

Viral hepatitis is a devastating chronic disease that affects millions worldwide, particularly those in developing countries. Relatively recent data from the World Health Organization (WHO) indicate that hepatitis B infection alone accounts for more than 1 million deaths worldwide while there are around 296 million individuals living with hepatitis B, and over 58 million living with hepatitis C.

A clear understanding of viral hepatitis is, therefore, essential for all dental practitioners, particularly in view of the **blood-borne nature** of the disease, its serious sequelae and the potential of transmitting the infection in the dental clinic.

Hepatitis can be due to a number of **other noninfective causes**, such as **alcohol abuse, trauma or drug-induced toxicity**. However, in global terms viral infections are by far the single most important cause of hepatitis. These include infections with herpes simplex virus, cytomegalovirus and Epstein–Barr virus, but the vast majority of viral liver diseases are one of the following:

- hepatitis A (infectious hepatitis, short-incubation hepatitis)
- hepatitis B (serum hepatitis)
- hepatitis C
- hepatitis D (delta hepatitis)
- hepatitis E (enterically transmitted hepatitis)
- hepatitis G.

These may be classified into two groups based on the viral transmission route:

1. **Faecal–oral route:** hepatitis A and hepatitis E (highly unlikely to be transmitted in dentistry)
2. **Parenteral route:** hepatitis B, hepatitis C, hepatitis D and possibly hepatitis G (could be transmitted in dentistry).

The various types of viral hepatitis differ in severity of infection, morbidity, mortality rate, presence or absence of a carrier state and frequency of long-term sequelae such as cirrhosis and cancer. The main differences between the hepatitides caused by these viruses are shown in Table 29.1.

Signs and Symptoms of Hepatitis

The common symptoms and signs of hepatitis include **malaise, jaundice, dark urine and pale, fatty stools**. These, together with results of serum and urine biochemistry and specific serology tests, facilitate the diagnosis of viral hepatitis. Investigation typically reveals abnormal liver function with raised levels of serum transaminases and bilirubin, as well as bilirubinuria. Specific serological tests are now available to detect hepatitis A, B, C, D and E antibodies.

Table 29.1 Epidemiological and Clinical Features of Hepatitis Viruses

	Hepatitis A	Hepatitis B	Hepatitis C	Hepatitis D	Hepatitis E	Hepatitis G
Synonym	Infectious hepatitis	Serum hepatitis	Hepatitis C	Delta hepatitis	Hepatitis E	Hepatitis G
Genus	*Hepatovirus*	*Orthohepadnavirus*	*Hepacivirus*	*Deltavirus*	*Hepevirus*	*Flavivirus*
Type of virus	ssRNA	dsDNA	ssRNA	ssRNA	ssRNA	RNA
Incubation period	2–7 weeks	1–6 months	2–26 weeks	2–12 weeks	6–8 weeks	?
Transmission	Predominantly faecal–oral	Predominantly parenteral	Predominantly parenteral	Parenteral	Predominantly faecal–oral	Parenteral
Carrier state	No	Yes	Yes	Yes	No	Yes
Oncogenic	No	Yes	Yes	?	No	No
Severity of hepatitis	±	++	+	+	±	±
IMMUNITY						
Passive immunization	Hyperimmune globulin	Hyperimmune globulin	None	Hyperimmune globulin	None	?
Active immunization	Vaccine (hepatitis A)	Vaccine (hepatitis B)	None	Vaccine (hepatitis B)	None	None

ds, double-stranded; *ss*, single-stranded.

Hepatitis A

The hepatitis A virus (HAV) is a small (27 nm) **RNA virus** belonging to the picornavirus group (which also includes poliovirus and coxsackieviruses). The virus is inactivated by ultraviolet light, by exposure to water at 100°C for 5 min and by exposure to 2% glutaraldehyde for 15 min.

EPIDEMIOLOGY

Hepatitis A commonly occurs in **developing parts of the world** where sewage disposal measures and food hygiene are unsatisfactory. Only 10–13% of the population in developed countries has been exposed to the virus by the age of 20. It is usually contracted by the **faecal–oral route** from **contaminated food and water**. Children and young people are most often infected, and for this reason a history of hepatitis in childhood would, in most instances, be indicative of a hepatitis A infection.

CLINICAL FEATURES

The mean incubation period is 30 days (range 2–7 weeks). Patients are infectious before the onset of symptoms during the prodromal phase and just before the onset of clinical disease.

Jaundice is common in adults and rare in young children. There are **no chronic sequelae**. Some patients continue to excrete HAV in faeces during weeks 1–3 of the illness, and HAV may also be present in saliva (100 particles per mL) throughout this period.

DIAGNOSIS

Diagnosis is by demonstration of HAV antigen in faeces. Serological tests demonstrate immunoglobulin M (IgM)-class anti-HAV antibodies in serum during the acute or early convalescent phase (**IgG-class antibodies** appear later in the disease and **confer enduring protection** against the disease). Additional test may include rtPCR to detect hepatitis A virus RNA.

Unlike hepatitis B, **no carrier state** is associated with the disease. This, together with its faecal–oral transmission, implies that hepatitis A transmission in the dental clinic is highly unlikely.

PROPHYLAXIS

Passive immunization by **hyperimmune globulin** is effective against clinical illness, particularly when administered in the early incubation period. However, the main use of short-term, preexposure prophylaxis is for travellers to hepatitis A–endemic areas, such as some parts of the developing world. Several **vaccines** of inactivated HAV produced in human cell culture are available. Immunization (two doses: an initial and a booster 6–12 months after) is safe and effective and recommended for dental and other professionals working with institutionalized patients. A **combined vaccine for hepatitis A and B** is now available.

HEPATITIS A AND DENTISTRY

HAV is not a significant infection risk in dentistry as the route of transmission is faecal–oral. **Close contact with saliva** may transmit infection as saliva can contain some HAV. Rarely, infection has been transmitted by needle-stick injury, and there is a single reported episode of transmission from a surgeon to a patient. **Standard infection control measures** are adequate to prevent transmission in dental practice.

Hepatitis B

The hepatitis B virus (HBV) is a **DNA hepadnavirus** (*hepa*: liver + DNA), which is structurally and immunologically complex. Electron microscopy of HBV reveals three distinct particles (Fig. 29.1):

- **Dane particle** (42 nm): the complete infective virus
- **spherical** forms (22 nm): noninfective
- **tubular** forms (22 × 100 nm): noninfective.

Being a **hepatotropic** virus, HBV will reside and multiply in hepatocytes after entering the body and will cause hepatic injury and inflammation (hepatitis) to varying degrees. During the viral multiplication process within the hepatocytes, different components of the virus (surface antigen proteins and the DNA, etc.) are produced in disproportionate amounts ('surplus to need'). Due to the overproduction of such noninfectious surface proteins of the virus (termed hepatitis B surface antigens [HBsAgs]), they circulate freely in the serum for prolonged periods after the acute hepatitis episode. HBsAg appear as tubular and spherical bodies in the serum of infected individuals (Fig. 29.1).

The central **core** of the HBV consists of a single-stranded DNA, an enzyme (DNA polymerase) and a core antigen (HBcAg). Although this antigen is rarely found in the serum, a breakdown product of HBcAg, termed hepatitis B 'e' antigen (HBeAg), may be found in the serum and is a marker of active infection.

EPIDEMIOLOGY

The prevalence of hepatitis B varies greatly in different parts of the world: it is higher in African and Asian countries than in the Americas, Australia and western Europe (Fig. 29.2); in urban than in rural areas; and in men than in women. In developed countries, the risk of exposure to hepatitis B is high in certain categories of people, as shown in Table 29.2. Several variants of HBV are now known, and when these involve rearrangement of the surface antigens, existing vaccines may not be protective. This has come to light as a few individuals who had been successfully immunized against HBV but who were at high risk of infection nevertheless contracted hepatitis B. A variant HBV, HBV-2, has been described in West Africa, the Middle East, Spain, France, Taiwan, New Zealand and the US, and another has been reported from Italy, Greece and the UK. Both variants are able to infect persons immunized against the original genotype of HBV.

CARRIER STATE AND IDENTIFICATION OF CARRIERS

Most patients who contract hepatitis B **recover within a few weeks without any sequelae** (Fig. 29.3). However, serological markers of previous HBV infection are invariably present in these patients for prolonged periods. Such markers take the form of antibodies to various components of the

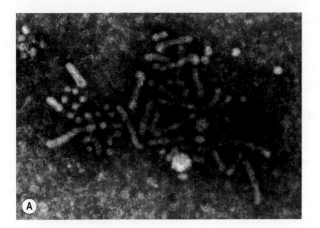

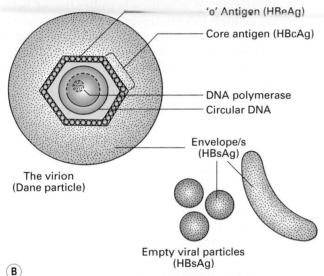

'o' Antigen (HBeAg)

Core antigen (HBcAg)

DNA polymerase
Circular DNA

Envelope/s
(HBsAg)

The virion
(Dane particle)

Empty viral particles
(HBsAg)

Fig. 29.1 Hepatitis B virus: (A) scanning electron micrograph; Note the banana shaped, tubular HBsAg particles (B) a diagrammatic rendering of hepatitis B virus and particles. *HBsAg*, hepatitis B surface antigen.

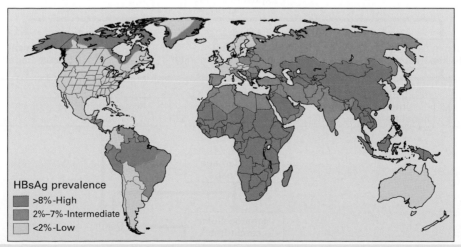

HBsAg prevalence
>8%-High
2%–7%-Intermediate
<2%-Low

Fig. 29.2 Geographic distribution of chronic hepatitis B virus infection. HBsAg, hepatitis B surface antigen. (Courtesy the Centers for Disease Control and Prevention, US.)

HBV. A minority (2%–5%) fail to clear HBV by 6–9 months and consequently develop a **chronic carrier state**. This state more frequently follows **anicteric** HBV infection (i.e., infection without jaundice). The converse of this is that a majority of infections that lead to jaundice resolve without a carrier state. Hence a history of jaundice in a patient in most instances indicates little or no risk in terms of hepatitis B transmission.

The chronic carriers of hepatitis B infection fall into two main groups: those with **chronic persistent hepatitis** (the so-called 'healthy carrier state') and those with **chronic active hepatitis** (Fig. 29.3). In chronic persistent hepatitis, the patient does not develop liver damage and is generally in good health, although the liver cells persistently produce viral antigen (HBsAg) because of the integration of the viral genome into the DNA of the hepatocytes. The second group of chronic carriers (i.e., chronic active hepatitis) are extremely infectious as they harbour the infective Dane particles in their blood. In addition, they are very susceptible to **cirrhosis and hepatocellular carcinoma**. Nonetheless, the chronic active hepatitis group represents a small minority of hepatitis B patients. In general, infection with HBV leads to complete recovery in most individuals, whereas only about 2–5% develop a carrier state. These two disease states elicit characteristic serological profiles in the affected individual during various phases of the disease, as shown in Figs. 29.4 and 29.5.

DIAGNOSIS AND SEROLOGICAL MARKERS

Diagnosis of HBV is complicated by the variety of serological markers and the complex sequelae of the disease itself. Table 29.3 summarizes the significance of the serological markers described below:

1. **HBsAg:** This indicates that the person is a carrier and potentially infective. This state can persist for months until recovery, or for years in chronic carrier states.
2. **anti-HBs:** Antibody to HBsAgs appears in serum during the recovery phase and is long-lived; its presence indicates recovery and immunity to further HBV infection; also seen in high titre after successful vaccination for HBV, as the active ingredient of the hepatitis B vaccine is HBsAg.
3. **HBeAg:** Hepatitis B 'e' antigen **is indicative of active disease or high infectivity**. Infectivity of this particle is so high that even 0.0001 mL of serum containing the particle may transmit the disease; its prolonged persistence in serum indicates the possibility of chronic liver damage.
4. **anti-HBe:** Antibody to hepatitis B 'e' antigen appears in the serum soon after the appearance of HBeAg and indicates partial recovery from infection and a low level of infectivity; its absence, in the presence of HBeAg, indicates high infectivity and possible chronic carrier state.
5. **anti-HBc:** Antibody to hepatitis B core antigens appears at the onset of symptoms in acute hepatitis B, and is a measure of *both IgM and IgG, and persists for life.* The presence of total anti-HBc indicates previous or ongoing infection with hepatitis B virus in an undefined time frame. This antibody outlasts all the other aforementioned antibodies.

Clinical interpretation of the presence or absence of various serological markers of hepatitis B infection is complex, and should be left to clinicians conversant with the subject.

Table 29.2	Hepatitis B High-Risk Population Groups

SELECTED PATIENT GROUPS

Patients requiring frequent large-volume transfusions of unscreened blood/blood products (e.g., in haemophilia)

Institutionalized patients with learning difficulties

Patients with a recent history of jaundice

Patients in renal dialysis units

Immunosuppressed/immunodeficient patients

POPULATION GROUPS

Injecting drug abusers

Promiscuous homosexual men

Female prostitutes

Migrants from developing countries

Health care and laboratory personnel (especially surgeons)

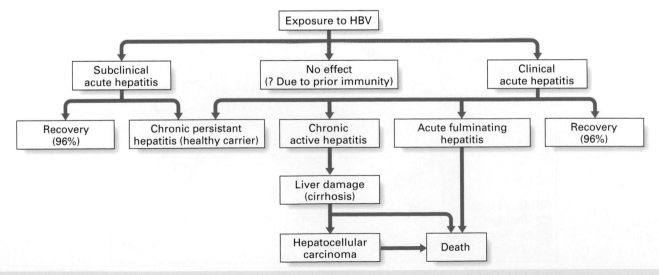

Fig. 29.3 Possible sequelae of exposure to hepatitis B virus (HBV). Values in parentheses indicate percentage recovery.

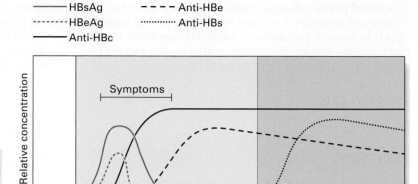

Fig. 29.4 Typical profile of hepatitis B serological markers after recovery from infection. *Anti-HBc*, antibody to hepatitis B core antigen; *anti-HBe*, antibody to hepatitis B 'e' antigen; *anti-HBs*, antibody to hepatitis B surface antigen; *HBeAg*, hepatitis B 'e' antigen; *HBsAg*, hepatitis B surface antigen.

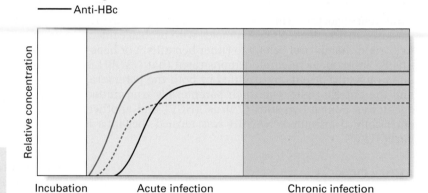

Fig. 29.5 Hepatitis B chronic carrier state: no seroconversion. *Anti-HBc*, antibody to hepatitis B core antigen; *HBeAg*, hepatitis B 'e' antigen; *HBsAg*, hepatitis B surface antigen.

Table 29.3 Serological Markers of Hepatitis B Infection and Their Interpretation

Risk status	HBsAg	HBeAg	Anti-HBe	Anti-HBsAg	Total Anti HBC
High/low risk	Positive	Unknown	Unknown	Negative	Positive
High risk	Positive	Positive	Negative	Negative	Positive
Low risk	Positive	Negative	Positive	Negative	Positive
Immune due to previous infection	Negative	Negative	Positive or negative	Positive	Positive
Immune due to vaccination	Negative	Negative	Negative	Positive	Negative
Not infected or vaccinated	Negative	Negative	Negative	Negative	Negative

anti-HBe, antibody to hepatitis B 'e' antigen; *anti-HBs*, antibody to hepatitis B surface antigen; *HBeAg*, hepatitis B 'e' antigen; *HBsAg*, hepatitis B surface antigen.

HEPATITIS B AND DENTISTRY

To date over 400 health care workers, including dental surgeons, have been infected with hepatitis B in clinical settings. Most were surgeons; in dentistry, the risk of infection is greater among oral surgeons and periodontists than among general dental practitioners. Standard infection control procedures were often lacking when such transmission occurred.

This said, the number of health care workers, including dentists, contracting infection reported since the introduction of the hepatitis B vaccine programme in 1987 has been small. However, there is an ever-present danger of hepatitis B transmission in dentistry if dental personnel are not vaccinated, or are vaccinated but with inadequate seroconversion (see below).

Although the usual mode of transmission of hepatitis B is from the patient to the dentist, there are at least eight recorded outbreaks where dentists have transmitted the disease to patients.

Intraorally, the **greatest concentration of HBV is at the gingival sulcus** as a result of the continuous serum exudate, which is small in healthy people but greatly increased in diseased states—for example, periodontitis; the virus is present in mixed saliva but not in parotid or submandibular saliva (Table 29.4).

Special precautions are not necessary when treating carriers of hepatitis B (or any other disease), as standard infection control precautions, routinely employed in dentistry irrespective of the clinical status of the patient (see Chapter 36), should prevent disease transmission.

PROPHYLAXIS

See Chapters 10 and 37.

TREATMENT

In chronic carriers of the virus, oral nucleoside analogs, which have potent activity against HBV and fewer side effects than previously prescribed interferon therapy, appear to be the preferred option.

Hepatitis C

Some years ago, the term 'non-A non-B hepatitis' (NANBH) was used to describe a disease complex with probable infective origin that did not belong to either hepatitis A or hepatitis B. Subsequent research demonstrated that NANBH is due to infective agents transmitted by both the parenteral and the enteric route. One such parenterally transmitted agent was named 'hepatitis C virus' (HCV) and another, enterically transmitted, NANBH was termed 'hepatitis E virus' (HEV).

AETIOLOGY

Hepatitis C is caused by an **enveloped RNA virus** related to the **flaviviruses**. The virus has yet to be grown in

culture or visualized ultrastructurally. It may exist as one of at least six different genotypes. Some patients may be infected with more than one genotype. The viral RNA can remain intact for at least 7 days at room temperature. Thus, although the infectivity of HCV is still unclear, it is essential that adherence to standard infection control is observed at all times.

EPIDEMIOLOGY

Hepatitis C is globally prevalent. According to the WHO, about **3% of the world population** has been infected with hepatitis C, and there are more than 170 million chronic carriers at risk of developing liver cirrhosis or cancer. There may, however, be considerable regional and ethnic group variation (Fig. 29.6).

Blood, blood products, intravenous immunoglobulins and donated organs have transmitted HCV, although newer methods of HCV detection have reduced, but not entirely eradicated, such risk. Injecting drug abusers, transfusion recipients and patients with haemophilia receiving blood products are other groups who are at risk. The disease occurs in 5%–10% of transfusion recipients, leading to chronic hepatitis in about half of them.

DIAGNOSIS

The diagnosis of HCV infection is serological. Assays using the enzyme-linked immunosorbent assay (ELISA) technique can detect **antibodies to HCV envelope or core proteins.** Polymerase chain reaction (PCR) assays are also very sensitive and specific and can detect early infection. Most HCV-infected persons are HCV seropositive within 6 months of infection. Because of this delay in antibody response, donated blood may not be screened effectively.

CLINICAL FEATURES

- The incubation period varies from 2–26 weeks (average 6–7 weeks).
- The initial infection is often asymptomatic, especially in children and young adults, whereas some 40% of adults

Table 29.4	Concentration of Hepatitis B in Body Fluids	
High	**Moderate**	**Low/Undetectable**
Blood	Mixed saliva	Urine
Wound exudates	Semen	Sweat, tears
	Vaginal fluid	Breast milk
		Parotid/submandibular saliva

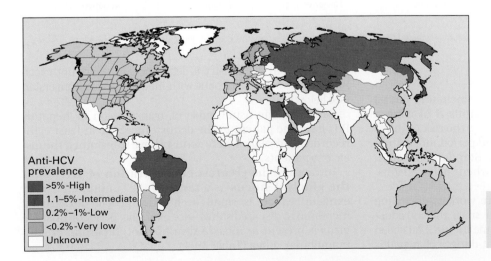

Anti-HCV prevalence
- >5%-High
- 1.1–5%-Intermediate
- 0.2%–1%-Low
- <0.2%-Very low
- Unknown

Fig. 29.6 Prevalence of hepatitis C virus (HCV) infection among blood donors. (Courtesy the Centers for Disease Control and Prevention, US.)

may have acute symptoms. Hence, many are unaware of their infection or the eventual outcome.

- A minority can have persistent viraemia without serological or clinical evidence of hepatic disease. Infection with HCV rarely gives rise to fulminant hepatic failure.
- HCV **can be secreted in the saliva** and has been detected in the salivary glands.
- About 25% of infected patients develop jaundice, and up to 60% can have histological evidence of chronic liver disease. Cirrhosis may eventually develop in up to 80% of chronically HCV-infected persons.
- Interestingly, the link between HCV and hepatocellular carcinoma appears to be even stronger than that for HBV.
- Factors thought to influence the extent of liver disease include HCV genotype, gender, age at infection and the extent of immunodeficiency.

SEQUELAE OF CHRONIC HCV INFECTION

Persistent chronic infection develops in approximately 80% of infected persons, and the course of infection may run for 20 or more years. Approximately 70% of those with chronic HCV will develop chronic liver disease. The virus may also cause mixed cryoglobulinaemia, thyroid disorders, diabetes mellitus and thrombocytopenia.

TREATMENT

A new infection with HCV does not always require treatment, as the immune response in some people will clear the infection. However, when HCV infection becomes chronic, treatment is necessary and must be managed with antivirals. Currently several antiviral medications are available, including entecavir, tenofovir and lamivudine. These can clear the viraemia and reduce the risk or slow down the development of liver sequelae.

PREVENTION

At present, there is **no passive or active immunization programme for HCV** infection. All immunization methods appear to be unsatisfactory as reexposure of HCV-infected patients to different strains of HCV still results in reinfection. This reflects the possible different subtypes of HCV and their rapid rate of mutation. By the same token, prophylaxis with immunoglobulins confers little, if any, immunity.

HEPATITIS C AND DENTISTRY

- *Possible* oral manifestations of HCV infection include **lichen planus**, **oral malignancy** and **salivary gland disease**; the underlying pathogenic mechanisms of these HCV-related lesions are not clear but may reflect immunogenetic factors or the presence of antiepithelial antibodies.
- There is no unequivocal evidence of transmission of HCV as a consequence of dental treatment.
- Saliva of up to 50% of patients with acute and chronic hepatitis C infection may contain HCV RNA; other studies have failed to detect HCV in saliva.

- Needle-stick injuries are the most common way in which HCV is transmitted in clinical settings, although health care workers are not at especial risk of infection. The risk of HCV infection after a needle-stick injury with HCV-contaminated blood may be 3%–10% (approximately 10 times greater than for human immunodeficiency virus (HIV)).
- There are a number of studies indicating a significant positive association between oral lichen planus and HCV seropositivity. This association may have geographic variations.
- Studies of dental staff in the UK and Taiwan have shown no raised incidence of HCV infection, but their counterparts in the US (particularly oral surgeons) may be susceptible to HCV carriage.
- Immunoglobulin therapy or interferon therapy has been suggested as a possible management procedure for a needle-stick injury involving blood from an HCV-infected patient. The efficacy of either approach remains to be determined.

Hepatitis D (Delta Hepatitis)

Delta hepatitis is caused by **a 'defective' RNA virus**, which coexists with HBV (Fig. 29.7). Hepatitis D virus (HDV) is the smallest animal virus known and contains a nucleoprotein, a delta antigen and an outer surface protein. The outer coat of the delta virus is 'borrowed' HBsAg, and hence the virus cannot survive independently without the hepatitis B viral particles. Consequently, delta infection is only seen as a:

- **co-infection** in a patient with hepatitis B
- **superinfection** in a carrier of hepatitis B.

Both usually cause an episode of acute hepatitis. Co-infection usually resolves, whereas superinfection frequently causes chronic delta infection, leading to chronic active hepatitis (Fig. 29.8).

EPIDEMIOLOGY

It has been estimated that about 15 million persons are infected with HDV worldwide, as about **5% of HBV**

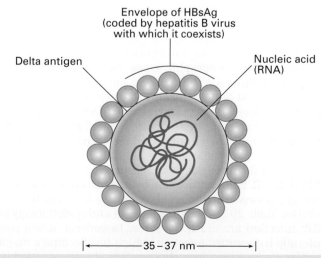

Envelope of HBsAg
(coded by hepatitis B virus
with which it coexists)

Delta antigen

Nucleic acid
(RNA)

|←——— 35 – 37 nm ———→|

Fig. 29.7 Hepatitis D (delta) virus. HBsAg, hepatitis B surface antigen.

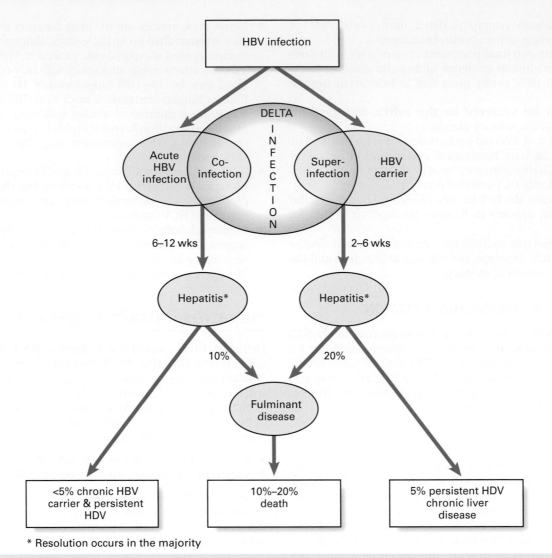

Fig. 29.8   Sequelae of hepatitis delta virus (HDV) infection. *HBV,* hepatitis B virus. * Resolution occurs in the majority.

carriers are HDV-positive. In nonendemic areas such as the US and northern Europe, HDV is mainly confined to persons frequently exposed to blood and blood products, particularly drug addicts. Up to 4% of US blood donors have evidence of previous HDV infection. It is noteworthy that HDV infection is not common in most groups in Southeast Asia. Geographic areas with a high incidence of delta hepatitis are the Amazon basin, parts of Africa, the Middle East and Arab countries, where 30%–90% of HBsAg carriers with liver disease are infected. Delta infection occurs rarely in the susceptible population of northern Europe and is virtually confined to parenteral drug abusers.

Routes of delta transmission appear to be similar to those of hepatitis B, with the infection being most commonly seen among persons at high risk of acquiring hepatitis B infection (see Table 29.2). The transmission and epidemiology of HDV infection are much the same. In general, it is a parenterally transmitted infection, which has become a major problem in injecting drug abusers. It is also transmitted by sexual or close contact with HDV-infected persons. However, sexual transmission of HDV appears to be less common than for HBV, and HDV infection is uncommon in men who have sex with men.

CLINICAL FEATURES AND DIAGNOSIS

The incubation period of HDV infection ranges from 2–12 weeks, and most infections lead to jaundice. The virus produces acute hepatitis, which usually resolves, but may precipitate fulminant liver disease. The latter is 10 times more frequent in HDV infection than in HBV infection alone. Chronic hepatitis is a common sequela of HDV infection, and 70% of those affected develop cirrhosis. The role, if any, of HDV in hepatic carcinogenesis is unclear.

Diagnosis is by detection of delta antigen (using ELISA) in serum and/or by the appearance of delta antibody. Delta infection does not respond well to interferon therapy.

PROPHYLAXIS

As the delta virus is dependent on HBV for replication, successful immunization with the hepatitis B vaccine will prevent delta infection.

HEPATITIS D AND DENTISTRY

The main route of HDV transmission is parenteral, in either blood or blood products. Sexual transmission may occur sometimes within households, and perinatally if mothers are positive for HDV and HBeAg. It is unclear whether saliva is a vehicle.

There is at least one report of HDV transmission in dentistry in the US, where up to 700 cases were recorded. At least four dentists were infected; one oral surgeon became an HBV carrier and was thought to have infected several patients.

Hepatitis E

HEV is a relatively newly described **RNA virus** that bears some similarities to the Caliciviridae. Transmission is via the **faecal–oral route**, by ingesting contaminated drinking water. Hepatitis E outbreaks are common in Africa, Asia and Latin America, especially in countries with poor sewage disposal facilities. In these geographic regions, different HEV viruses are responsible for the infection. Intrafamilial and parenteral spread is rare. In most instances the disease follows a benign pattern like that of hepatitis A, with a low mortality rate of 1%–2%. The infection is infrequently associated with fulminant hepatitis. The disease can be diagnosed by Western blot, ELISA and PCR assay.

Because of its mode of transmission, the virus does not pose a major risk of cross-infection in dentistry.

Hepatitis Viruses of Unclear Pathogenicity

These include hepatitis G virus (HGV), transfusion transmitted virus (TTV), SEN virus and possibly hepatitis F virus.

HEPATITIS G

It has become increasingly evident that there are patients with acute or chronic hepatitis who are not infected by the hepatitis viruses A–E described earlier (hence the designation non-A–E hepatitis). Thus another hepatitis agent isolated from a surgeon (whose initials were GB) with acute hepatitis is now called the hepatitis G virus (HGV).

HGV is an RNA virus of the Flaviviridae family and a distant relative of HCV. It is estimated that approximately 0.3% of patients with acute viral hepatitis may be attributed solely to HGV.

Infections with HGV appear more common among injecting drug abusers and people with haemophilia (i.e., frequent blood product recipients). HGV does not seem to elicit a strong immune response, and indeed no cases have symptoms like the other hepatitis viruses. Carrier rate (in the US) is between 2% and 5% in the general population.

Hepatitis G and Dentistry

HGV RNA is present in whole saliva of infected individuals, but transmission through this route has not been determined. No data are available on the transmission of hepatitis G or the rate of HGV carriage among dental personnel.

No vaccine is available; implementation of standard infection control measures should be adequate to prevent transmission of this virus in dentistry.

TRANSFUSION-TRANSMITTED VIRUS (TTV)

Both hepatitis G virus and TTV may produce posttransfusion hepatitis. Described in 1997, transfusion-transmitted virus (TTV) is a **nonenveloped, single-stranded DNA virus** possibly belonging to the Parvoviridae family. It has been isolated from persons in the UK, Japan and Brazil, especially older blood donors. The most remarkable feature of TTV is the extraordinarily high prevalence of chronic viraemia in apparently healthy people (up to nearly 100% in some countries). It may be transmitted parenterally, but this route has not been confirmed.

SEN VIRUS

SEN viruses (SEN D and SEN H), so called after the initials of the patient from whom the virus was isolated, are single-stranded, circular DNA viruses. They are strongly associated with transfusion-related non-A–E hepatitis. The vast majority of SEN virus–infected recipients did not develop hepatitis.

No information on either TTV or SEN virus salivary carriage or transmission in dental settings is available.

A NOTE ON HEPATITIS F VIRUS

Hepatitis F is a poorly defined hepatitis virus of uncertain significance. Viral particles were found in the stool of posttransfusion, non-A, non-B, non-C, non-E hepatitis cases. Injection of these particles into Indian rhesus monkeys caused hepatitis, which was then named 'hepatitis F'. However, these initial findings have not been confirmed and the original observation is now thought to be incidental.

Key Facts

- Viruses are by far the most important agents of hepatitis and include hepatitis A, B, C, D, E and G (the existence of hepatitis F has been queried).
- These **hepatotropic viruses** are classified into two groups depending on the transmission route. The **faecal–oral route**: hepatitis A and hepatitis E (highly unlikely to be transmitted in dentistry), and the **parenteral route**: hepatitis B, C and D and possibly hepatitis G (could be transmitted in dentistry).
- The various types of viral hepatitis differ in severity of infection, morbidity, mortality rate, presence or absence of a carrier state and frequency of long-term sequelae such as cirrhosis and cancer.
- **Hepatitis A virus (HAV):** 27 nm, RNA virus, belongs to the picornavirus group; clinical disease mild; no chronic carrier state.
- **Hepatitis A vaccine** is safe and effective and recommended for professionals working with institutionalized patients. A combined vaccine for hepatitis A and B is available.
- **Hepatitis B virus (HBV)** is a double-shelled DNA virus; on electron microscopy, three distinct particles are seen: the infective Dane particle and the noninfective, spherical and tubular forms.
- The central **core** of the HBV consists of single-stranded DNA, an enzyme (DNA polymerase) and a core antigen (HBcAg). Although this antigen is rarely found in serum, a breakdown product of HBcAg, termed 'hepatitis B 'e' antigen (HBeAg)', may be found in serum and is a marker of active infection.
- **HBV** is transmitted by **body fluids:** blood-to-blood contact, and perinatal and sexual transmissions are the major routes.
- The **diagnosis** of HBV is serological with initial **screening for hepatitis B surface antigen (HBsAg).**
- Appearance of antibody to HBsAgs (anti-HBs) heralds recovery and immunity to further HBV infection; high titres of anti-HBs are seen as successful vaccination for HBV (as the active ingredient of the hepatitis B vaccine is HBsAg).
- **HBV vaccine** is safe, effective and relatively long-lasting, and also protects against hepatitis D infection.
- The number of dental care workers contracting hepatitis B since the introduction of the vaccine programme has been small, but there is an ever-present danger of HBV transmission if personnel are not vaccinated, or vaccines do not

seroconvert (up to 5%). Hence antibody levels should be ascertained after a vaccine course.
- **Intraorally**, the greatest concentration of **HBV is at the gingival sulcus** as a result of the continuous serum exudate, which is small in health but greatly increased in diseased state.
- Hepatitis C is due to an **enveloped RNA virus** that may have up to six different genotypes. Some patients may be infected with more than one genotype.
- Persistent chronic hepatitis C virus (HCV) infection may develop in some 85% of those infected, and the course of infection may run up to 20 years.
- Possible oral manifestations of HCV infection include **lichen planus**, **oral malignancy** and **salivary gland disease**.
- Saliva of up to 50% of patients with acute and chronic hepatitis C infection may contain HCV RNA; some studies have failed to detect HCV in saliva.
- The risk of infection after a needle-stick injury with HCV-contaminated blood may be 3%–10% (compare 0.4% for human immunodeficiency virus (HIV) and 0.007% for HBV).
- **Delta hepatitis** is caused by a '**defective' RNA virus** (hepatitis D virus (HDV)), which coexists with HBV and hence is seen as a **co-infection** in a hepatitis B patient or a **superinfection** in a hepatitis B carrier.
- The transmission and epidemiology of HDV infection are similar to HBV, and the virus is a major problem, especially in injecting drug abusers.
- **Hepatitis E virus** is an RNA virus that resembles the Caliciviridae, transmitted via the faecal–oral route mainly by ingesting contaminated drinking water.
- **Hepatitis viruses of unclear pathogenicity** include hepatitis G virus (HGV), transfusion transmitted virus (TTV), SEN virus, and hepatitis F virus.
- **Hepatitis G virus** is a flavivirus, present in **whole saliva** of infected individuals, common among injecting drug abusers and haemophiliac patients; disease associations have yet to be defined.
- **Transfusion-transmitted virus (TTV)** is a recently described, hepatotrophic, non-enveloped, single-stranded DNA virus; it causes post-transfusion hepatitis and may be transmitted parenterally. No information on TTV salivary carriage or transmission in dental settings is available.

Review Questions (Answers on p. 391)

Please indicate which answers are true and which are false.

29.1. Of the viruses causing hepatitis, which of the following are likely to be transmitted in the dental clinic/office?
   a. hepatitis A virus (HAV)
   b. hepatitis B virus (HBV)
   c. hepatitis C virus (HCV)
   d. hepatitis E virus (HEV)
   e. hepatitis G virus (HGV)

29.2. In a patient with a history of jaundice, which of the following serological pictures (in the left column) is congruent with the clinical status (in the right column)?

a. hepatitis B surface antigen (HBsAg) positivity	1. chronic carrier state
b. hepatitis Be antigen (HBeAg) positivity.	2. high infectivity
c. antibody to hepatitis B core antigen (anti-HBc) positivity	3. past hepatitis B infection
d. antibody to hepatitis B surface antigen (anti-HBs) positivity	4. acute hepatitis B infection
e. immunoglobulin M (IgM) anti-HBc	5. recent infection with hepatitis B virus

29.3. Delta hepatitis virus infection:
 a. is always associated with HBV infection
 b. is common among intravenous drug abusers
 c. increases the risk of fulminant hepatitis in patients who are chronic hepatitis B carriers
 d. responds well to interferon treatment
 e. can lead to a persistent carrier state

29.4. Which of the following scenarios may pose an arguable risk of hepatitis transmission?
 a. a paediatric dentist sustains a (blood) contaminated needle-stick injury when treating a child with hepatitis A infection
 b. a child shares the same eating utensils with a mother with hepatitis B infection
 c. a dental surgery assistant sustains a (blood) contaminated needle-stick injury when managing a patient with asymptomatic HBV infection
 d. while cleaning the toilet in a clinic, the attendant's intact skin comes into contact with faecal matter
 e. a dental technician sustains a cut from a partial denture clasp from an HBeAg-positive patient

29.5. A dentist who has not been immunized for hepatitis B is found to be both HBsAg-positive and HBeAg-positive. The dentist may:
 a. be infected with both HBV and HEV
 b. transmit hepatitis B to patients
 c. transmit hepatitis E to patients
 d. develop hepatocellular carcinoma later in life
 e. attend clinic as standard infection control procedures have been instituted

Further Reading

Brooks, J. F., Carroll, K. C., & Butel, J. S. et al. (Eds.) (2013). Hepatitis viruses. In *Jawetz, Melnick & Adelberg's medical microbiology* (26th ed., pp. 507–526). McGraw Hill.

Karaylannis, P., & Thomas, H. (1997). Hepatitis G virus: Identification, prevalence and unanswered questions. *Gut, 40,* 294–296.

Klein, R. S., Freeman, K., Taylor, P. E., et al. (1999). Occupational risk of hepatitis C virus infection among New York City dentists. *Lancet, 338,* 1539–1542.

Scully, C., & Samaranayake, L. P. (1992). *Clinical virology in oral medicine and dentistry.* Cambridge University Press.

Zuckerman, A. J., & Harrison, T. J. (1994). Hepatitis viruses. In Zuckerman, A. J., Banatvala, J. E., & Pattison, J. R. (Eds.), *Principles and practice of clinical virology* (3rd ed., Ch. 2). John Wiley.

30 *Human Immunodeficiency Virus Infection, AIDS and Infections in Compromised Patients*

Human Immunodeficiency Virus Infection and Acquired Immune Deficiency Syndrome

Statistics on the human immunodeficiency virus (HIV) are startling. Since the beginning of the epidemic over four decades ago, some 84.2 million people have been infected with the HIV, and as of 2021 about 40.1 million had succumbed to the infection or related complications. Globally, 38.4 million people were living with HIV at the end of 2021. Although the burden of the epidemic varies considerably among countries and regions, sub-Saharan Africa is the current epicentre of the disease, with a staggering 9% affected, compared with 1.2% prevalence worldwide (Fig. 30.1). Worldwide, less than one person in five at risk of HIV has access to basic HIV prevention services.

Although HIV infection is now a global pandemic, acquired immune deficiency syndrome (AIDS) was only described in 1981, in young homosexual men in the US. The disease appears to have **originated in Africa,** where cases have been revealed from as long ago as 1959. The virus causes depletion of CD4+ T-helper lymphocytes over many years; as a consequence, patients succumb to opportunistic infections, particularly ***Pneumocystis jirovecii* pneumonia and oral candidiasis**, as well as neoplasms, especially Kaposi's sarcoma.

After infection with HIV, there is a **prolonged asymptomatic period** that may last up to 10 years, but the risk of developing severe immunodeficiency and AIDS increases with time. Thus, the clinical spectrum of HIV infection is broad, ranging from asymptomatic or mild infection to severe clinical illness and profound immunodeficiency. The variety of clinical manifestations seen in AIDS has spawned a number of definitions of the disease. However, the US

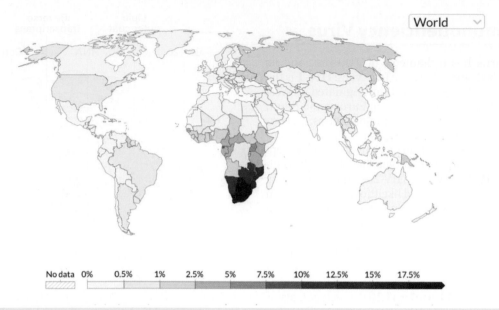

Fig. 30.1   Global data on the share of people 15–49 years old who are infected with HIV as of 2019. (Courtesy the World Health Organization).

Table 30.1   Centers for Disease Control and Prevention Classification of HIV Infection

HIV INFECTION STAGE, BASED ON AGE-SPECIFIC CD4+ T-LYMPHOCYTE COUNT OR CD4+ T-LYMPHOCYTE PERCENTAGE OF TOTAL LYMPHOCYTES

	Age on Date of CD4 T-Lymphocyte Test					
	<1 Year		1–5 Years		6 Years Through Adult	
Stage[a]	Cells/μL	%	Cells/μL	%	Cells/μL	%
1	≥1500	≥34	≥1000	≥30	≥500	≥26
2	750–1499	26–33	500–999	22–29	200–499	14–25
3	<750	<26	<500	<22	<200	<14

[a]The stage is based primarily on the CD4+ T-lymphocyte count; the CD4+ T-lymphocyte count takes precedence over the CD4 T-lymphocyte percentage, and the percentage is considered only if the count is missing.
Note: If none of the above apply (e.g., because of missing information on CD4 test results), the stage is U (unknown).

Centers for Disease Control and Prevention (CDC) has rationalized and revised these definitions to include all patients with **CD4⁺ cell counts of less than 200 per mL**.

The battle to conquer HIV infection and AIDS is fought on many fronts, consuming millions of dollars, and thus far all efforts at producing a preventive vaccine have failed. However the introduction of antiviral regimens such as **highly active antiretroviral therapy (HAART)** has increased life expectancy in those with HIV infection and has dramatically reduced complications, while suppressing viral replication to undetectable levels.

The impact of HIV and AIDS on the practice of clinical dentistry has been enormous: first, because of the regimentation in infection control it has spawned throughout the profession and, second, because of the many oral manifestations and their management, of which the practising dentist has to be aware.

DEFINITIONS

- **HIV infection:** infection with HIV, an RNA retrovirus.
- **HIV disease:** the resulting immunodeficiency and the appearance of attendant diseases (i.e., not all HIV-infected persons will have symptomatic disease).

- **AIDS:** a term given to a group of disorders characterized by a profound cell-mediated immunodeficiency consequential to irreversible suppression of T lymphocytes by the HIV. These disorders are called **AIDS-defining illnesses** and include parameters such as CD4 lymphocyte count below $200 \times 10^6/l$, oropharyngeal candidiasis, hairy leukoplakia, and so on.
- Additionally, confirmed cases can be classified in one of five HIV infection stages (0, 1, 2, 3 or unknown) based on **age-specific lymphocyte counts** (Table 30.1).

RETROVIRIDAE

HIV is a lymphotropic virus that belongs to the family **Retroviridae**. Viruses in this family are **RNA viruses** and comprise three subfamilies:

- **Lentiviruses** cause slowly progressive disease and are cytopathic in nature; they include HIV-1 and HIV-2.
- **Oncoviruses** include those that cause tumours: human T cell leukaemia virus type I (HTLV-I), which causes adult T cell leukaemia–lymphoma (ATLL); and HTLV-II, associated with hairy cell leukaemia.
- **Spumaviruses** are not recognized human pathogens.

Human Immunodeficiency Virus

This lentivirus virus has a diameter of 100 nm, and its structure is described later. There are two types: **HIV-1** is the most prevalent; **HIV-2** is a variant that originated in West Africa and has spread to Central Africa, Europe and South America. Type 1 is classified into two major groups: M, containing 10 genetically distinct subtypes (A–J), and O, containing a heterogeneous collection of viruses. HIV-2, except for its antigenic and nucleic acid profile, has similar biological properties to HIV-1. However HIV-2 is characterized by lower transmissibility and reduced likelihood of progression to AIDS. It may also escape detection when commercial test kits essentially developed for HIV-1 are used. The following discussion relates to the widely prevalent HIV-1.

The structure of HIV is shown in Fig. 30.2. It consists of:

1. an envelope containing virus-specific **'coat' proteins** (e.g., glycoproteins **gp41 and gp120**), which can act as antigens. Glycoprotein gp120 has a 'rugger-ball' configuration and plays an important role in the initial events leading to infection. These coat proteins undergo almost continual structural changes, which hamper the development of effective vaccines
2. a pyramid-shaped **central core** with three major **core proteins**, of which **p24** is especially antigenic; antibodies to this form the basis of most serological testing (the HIV test)
3. a **genome of RNA** within the core, comprising two identical molecules of **single-stranded RNA** (ssRNA)
4. two molecules of an enzyme, **reverse transcriptase** (an RNA-dependent DNA polymerase), essential for transcribing the RNA code of the virus to a DNA code during viral multiplication (so that it may integrate into the host cell DNA).

STABILITY OF HIV

The survival of HIV under varying conditions has been investigated.

- HIV is relatively easily destroyed by heat (autoclave and hot-air oven); the virus is inactivated by a factor of 100-fold each hour at a temperature over 60°C.
- The virus may survive up to 15 days at room temperature and at body temperature (37°C).
- HIV is totally inactivated (>10^5 units of infectivity) by exposure for 10 min at room temperature to the following disinfectants: 2% glutaraldehyde, sodium hypochlorite (10,000 ppm available chlorine, equivalent to 1:10 dilution of domestic bleach), 50% ethanol, 35% isopropanol or 0.3% hydrogen peroxide.
- When HIV is present in clotted blood in a syringe or other material, exposure to undiluted bleach for at least 30 s is necessary for its inactivation.

Important: The preceding figures indicate the limits of survival at very high starting concentrations of HIV (up to 1000 times more than the levels found in the blood of patients) under experimental conditions. Also, the efficacy of the mentioned disinfectants is affected by a variety of factors

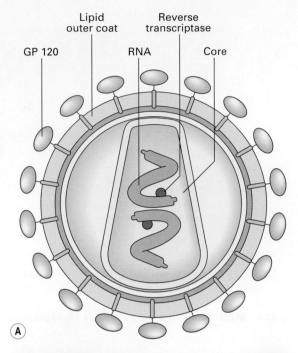

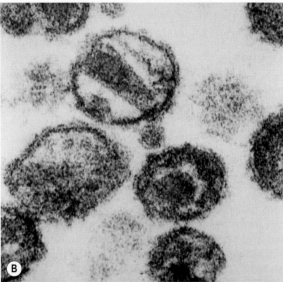

Fig. 30.2   Human immunodeficiency virus. (A) Structure. (B) Scanning electron micrograph of virions showing the pyramid-shaped central core.

such as the associated organic bioburden. Hence, care and strict adherence to protocols are essential when dealing with HIV-contaminated material.

VIRAL REPLICATION

See Chapter 10.

TRANSMISSION OF HIV

The virus is most commonly acquired through **sexual activity** with an infected partner. The virus can enter the body through the lining of the vagina, vulva, penis, rectum or mouth during sex. The infection can also be transmitted by exchange of **infected blood,** or other body fluids such as breast milk, and is not transmitted by social contact or casual, nonsexual contact. Currently, **heterosexual sex** is the major mode of transmission worldwide. Other notable transmission modes include sharing of needles, vertical transmission in utero, breast-feeding and transfusion of infected blood or blood products (factor VIII concentrate). Occasional cases of HIV infection result from needle-stick injuries in health care settings. The question of HIV transmission among health care workers, including dentists, is addressed at the end of this chapter.

Saliva and HIV Transmission

There is only a very slim possibility that HIV may be transmitted by saliva, for the following reasons:

1. Only a small minority of HIV-infected individuals harbour the virus in whole saliva (e.g., in one study HIV was detected in mixed saliva of 5% of infected individuals and in only 1 of 15 parotid saliva samples). In any case, HIV virions cannot exist in a cell-free state in saliva, and rough estimates indicate that there is less than one infectious particle of HIV per mL of mixed saliva.
2. Saliva contains **immunoglobulin A (IgA) group antibodies** to HIV proteins (p24, gp120, gp160), which may neutralize the infectivity of the virus and are the basis of salivary kits used for HIV testing in epidemiological studies.
3. Other HIV-inhibitory factors in saliva include high-molecular-weight **mucins** thought to entrap the virus, **proline-rich proteins** and a serine protease inhibitor termed **salivary leukocyte protease inhibitor (SLPI).** SLPI possibly blocks cell surface receptors needed for entry of HIV into cells.
4. The virus loses its infectivity when exposed to mixed saliva for 30 min.
5. Animal studies have shown that it is not possible to transmit HIV by surface application of the virus on the oral mucosa, although it was transmitted in this manner through vaginal mucosa.
6. The dose of HIV required for infection is far higher than that for hepatitis B virus (the risk of acquiring hepatitis B infection from a contaminated needlestick injury is 6%–30%, compared with a 0.4% risk of contracting HIV infection).

Epidemiology

The main groups of individuals affected are:

- **promiscuous individuals**, both **homosexuals** and **heterosexuals:** 75% of all infection has been acquired through sexual intercourse; the current male-to-female ratio is 3:2 (infections in homosexuals were levelling off due to increased awareness of the disease and safe-sex practices, but a recent increase has been reported)
- **injecting drug abusers:** some 10% of infection globally; 26% in the US
- **persons receiving blood** or **blood products:** about 1% globally (mainly a problem of the developed world)
- **offspring of infected mothers:** varying transmission rates reported, 10%–50%; most infections are acquired at birth, a few are acquired in utero and the rest are acquired through breast-feeding.

THE GLOBAL PANDEMIC

As mentioned, by the end of 2022 an estimated 39 million people worldwide were living with HIV, and some 40 million have died of the infection or related illnesses between the beginning of the pandemic and 2021. Of those succumbing to AIDS, 90% are living in developing countries, especially in Asia and Africa.

The estimated annual increase in new cases of HIV disease worldwide is about 20%, but this varies widely in different geographic locales. For instance, the annual increase is about 11% in the Americas, 26% in Africa and 167% in Asia, indicating the staggering explosion of the disease in the latter region. In those countries, AIDS is overwhelmingly a heterosexually transmitted disease, and there are about equal numbers of male and female cases.

It is surmised that the rapid dissemination of HIV globally, especially in the latter part of the 20th century, was promoted by mass migration of rural inhabitants to urban centres together with international movement of infected refugees as a consequence of civil disturbances, tourism and business travels.

Globally, a silver lining in the deadly HIV story was the introduction of **highly active antiretroviral therapy (HAART)** that has increased life expectancy in HIV infection and dramatically reduced complications, suppressing viral replication to undetectable levels.

Although millions of dollars have been spent to develop a vaccine for HIV, it is still not a reality. **Preexposure prophylaxis (PrEP)** and **monoclonal antibody therapies** may provide a bridge until a vaccine is developed (see later in this chapter).

Acquired Immune Deficiency Syndrome

NATURAL HISTORY OF THE DISEASE

AIDS is an insidious disease, characterized by **opportunistic infections** (fungal, viral and mycobacterial), **malignancies** (especially Kaposi's sarcoma and lymphomas that may be virally induced) and **autoimmune disorders** (Fig. 30.3).

The average **time to development of AIDS is 8–11 years** in most adults in the developed world, and much less in the developing world due to aggravating cofactors such as malnutrition and intercurrent infection (e.g., malaria). A few individuals (some 2%) have not developed AIDS despite antibody positivity. Overall, almost half of those diagnosed with AIDS will die. Untreated, the median survival is about 1 year from the time of diagnosis, and 95% will die within 5 years.

Mean time for seroconversion after exposure to HIV is 3–4 weeks, with the onset of an acute **seroconversion illness** similar to glandular fever. Most will have antibodies within 6–12 weeks after infection, and virtually all will be positive within 6 months. Symptoms of such seroconversion

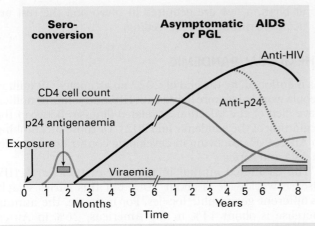

Fig. 30.3 Key events in HIV infection. *PGL*, persistent generalized lymphadenopathy.

Table 30.2 Opportunistic Infections, Neoplasms and Miscellaneous Complications of HIV Disease

Opportunistic Infections	
Mucocutaneous	Human herpesviruses 1, 2, 3, 4, 5, 8
	Human papillomaviruses
	Molluscum contagiosum
	Nontuberculous mycobacteria
	Candida albicans
	Staphylococcus aureus
	Histoplasmosis
Gastrointestinal	Cryptosporidiosis
	Microsporidiosis
	Isosporiasis
	Giardiasis
Respiratory	*Pneumocystis jirovecii*
	Aspergillosis
	Candidosis
	Cryptococcosis
	Histoplasmosis
	Zygomycosis (mucormycosis)
	Strongyloidiasis
	Mycobacteria, including tuberculosis
	Staphylococcus aureus
	Streptococcus pneumoniae
	Haemophilus influenzae
	Toxoplasmosis
	Cytomegalovirus (CMV)
Meningitis	Creutzfeldt–Jakob agent
Encephalitis	Papovaviruses
	Cryptococcus neoformans
	Toxoplasma gondii
Neoplasms	
	Kaposi's sarcoma
	Lymphoma
	Squamous cell carcinoma
	Leukaemia
Miscellaneous	
	Encephalopathy
	Thrombocytopenic purpura
	Lupus erythematosus
	Seborrhoeic dermatitis

include fever, malaise, rash, oral ulceration and, occasionally, encephalitis and meningitis. In some, the disease may then become quiescent and asymptomatic for several years (range 1–15 years or more) for reasons yet unknown. Some of them may have **persistent generalized lymphadenopathy (PGL)**, where the enlarged lymph nodes are painless and asymmetrical in distribution and involve submandibular and neck nodes. In HIV disease classification, patients with these symptoms are categorized as **group A** (see Table 30.1).

Progressive disease leads to other features, including fatigue, fever, weight loss, candidiasis, diarrhoea, hairy leukoplakia, herpes zoster and perianal herpes, and these illnesses are sometimes referred to as the **AIDS-defining complex**. Patients with these symptoms and signs of progressive illness are categorized as **group B**.

Finally, a percentage of HIV-infected individuals develop **full-blown AIDS** (50–70%, depending on drug therapy and other associated cofactors; median life expectancy is 18 months). These individuals are in **group C**. The AIDS-defining conditions are subdivided into opportunistic infections and secondary neoplasms, and include Kaposi's sarcoma, pneumocystis pneumonia (PCP) and many other exotic infections (Table 30.2).

The CDC disease classification also incorporates **blood CD4 lymphocyte count**, as a decrease in the latter is associated with adverse prognosis (see Table 30.1).

OPPORTUNISTIC INFECTIONS AND NEOPLASMS IN AIDS

The opportunistic infections, neoplasms and other features of AIDS and its prodrome are listed in Table 30.2.

Pneumocystis jirovecii Pneumonia

This pneumonia is caused by a fungus, *Pneumocystis jirovecii*, previously thought to be a protozoan (*Pneumocystis carinii*). The fungus grows within the lung alveoli. Seen in 80% of patients, it is the immediate cause of death in 20% of those dying with AIDS. The condition is treated with aerosolized pentamidine.

Toxoplasmosis

Protozoal infection with *Toxoplasma gondii* is seen in 15% of AIDS patients, affecting especially the central nervous system.

Atypical Mycobacteriosis

Atypical mycobacteriosis is present in about 40% of patients in the West; caused by **Mycobacterium avium complex (MAC)** infections due to mycobacteria such as *Mycobacterium avium* and *Mycobacterium intracellulare*. In some countries, up to one-quarter of people who are HIV-positive are infected with *Mycobacterium tuberculosis*, which may be increasingly drug resistant (multidrug-resistant tuberculosis (MDR-TB); see Chapter 19).

Table 30.3 Oral Manifestations of HIV Disease

Strongly Associated	Less Common Associates	Sometimes Seen
Candidiasis	Herpes simplex or zoster infection	Exotic fungal infections (ulcers)
Erythematous	Human papillomavirus infections	Cryptococcosis
Pseudomembranous	Mycobacterial infections	Histoplasmosis
Linear gingival erythema		Penicilliosis
Hairy leukoplakia		
Kaposi's sarcoma (not in Asia)	Unilateral/bilateral swelling of salivary glands	Drug reactions
Necrotizing (ulcerative) gingivitis	Dry mouth	Cranial neuropathies
Necrotizing (ulcerative) periodontitis	Ulceration (nonspecific)	Facial palsies
	Melanotic hyperpigmentation	Trigeminal neuralgia
Non-Hodgkin's lymphoma		Recurrent aphthous stomatitis

Candidiasis and Herpesvirus Infections

(See later in this chapter.)

OROFACIAL MANIFESTATIONS OF HIV INFECTION

The **earliest indicators** of HIV infection may manifest **in the oral cavity,** and some 50 disease entities that may affect the orofacial region of HIV-infected patients have been described. However, with the advent of HAART therapy (see later in this chapter), the prevalence of oral manifestations has been dramatically reduced. The more common orofacial manifestations of HIV infection are (Table 30.3):

- **fungal infections:** oral candidiasis (erythematous and pseudomembranous variants mainly); linear gingival erythema and angular cheilitis (both are possibly due to mixed bacterial and fungal infections)
- **viral infections:** hairy leukoplakia, Kaposi's sarcoma, herpes infections, papillomas
- **bacterial infections:** gingivitis and periodontitis
- **cervical lymphadenopathy** and **lymphomas** such as non-Hodgkin's lymphomas (not discussed further).

Oral Candidiasis

Oral candidiasis (usually **erythematous or pseudomembranous variants** of candidiasis) is very common in HIV infection, especially at the early stage of the disease; it is a reliable and ominous prognostic indicator of the disease progression to AIDS (the earlier the appearance of oral candidiasis, the worse the prognosis). **Oesophageal candidiasis** frequently accompanies oral candidiasis and is usually managed by azole drugs, commonly fluconazole. However, azole resistance is increasingly common.

Linear gingival erythema and angular cheilitis are possibly due to mixed fungal and bacterial infections (see Chapter 35).

Viral Infections

Viral infections include herpetic stomatitis, herpes zoster, Kaposi's sarcoma and others such as hairy leukoplakia and papillomas of viral origin.

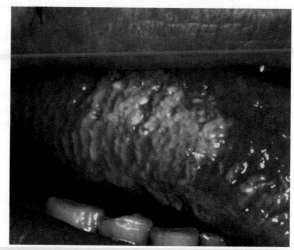

Fig. 30.4   Hairy leukoplakia of the lateral border of the tongue in a patient with AIDS.

Herpetic Stomatitis. A 10% prevalence of herpetic stomatitis in HIV-infected persons has been reported. Herpes simplex infections are mainly intraoral, sometimes extensive and persistent, but **rarely disseminate**. A minority suffer from herpes zoster and papillomavirus infections. The latter manifests as oral papillomas, warts or condylomata.

Kaposi's Sarcoma. Caused by human herpesvirus 8, this is a **multifocal systemic tumour** due to proliferating microvascular and fibroblastic processes, seen mostly in sexually transmitted HIV infection.

Hairy Leukoplakia. This classically appears as an asymptomatic, greyish-white to white, corrugated lesion on the tongue, either unilaterally or bilaterally (Fig. 30.4). The aetiological agent is the **Epstein–Barr virus**. (*Note:* It is also seen in patients belonging to other risk groups, and uncommonly in healthy individuals.) As more than three-quarters of HIV-infected patients with hairy leukoplakia develop AIDS within 3 years, it is considered to indicate a poor prognosis.

Necrotizing (Ulcerative) Gingivitis and Necrotizing (Ulcerative) Periodontitis

An unusual type of recalcitrant, aggressive periodontal disease has been identified in those who are infected with HIV. The disease begins as a form of gingivitis that mimics acute ulcerative gingivitis. However, it differs from the latter as the disease progresses unceasingly despite routine management protocols such as metronidazole therapy, debridement and scrupulous oral hygiene. The anterior gingiva is most commonly affected. In some patients, HIV gingivitis has a very destructive course, leading to periodontitis with loss of soft tissue and bone, sequestrum formation and, in extreme cases, tooth exfoliation.

DIAGNOSIS

History and clinical criteria are of utmost importance in the provisional diagnosis of HIV infection, but laboratory investigations, **after appropriate professional counselling**, are required for confirmation of the disease.

The first step in **serodiagnosis** is the **enzyme-linked immunosorbent assay** (ELISA) or agglutination screening tests for serum antibodies. Up to about 2% of the ELISA tests are either false positive or false negative: hence a positive ELISA must be retested in duplicate samples. If two or more of the latter ELISA results are positive, confirmatory testing has to be done by a **Western blot assay**. Thus, these are the principles and ethics of diagnosis:

1. Apply a minimum of two methodologically different assays.
2. Repeat the test 2–3 months later, as there is a 'window' period between acquisition of infection and the development of antibodies (see Fig. 30.2).
3. Do not divulge positive results until confirmed using the strictest criteria. Maintain confidentiality of the results at all times.

The following are other laboratory diagnostic methods:

- **Virus isolation** mainly from lymphocytes in peripheral blood: essentially limited to research laboratories due to the lengthy and laborious procedures involved
- **Detection of viral nucleic acids or antigens** by various polymerase chain reaction techniques (very useful for detecting HIV in newborns as their plasma is contaminated with HIV antibodies from the mother). A high viral load in the plasma of infected individuals predicts a more rapid progression to AIDS than a low viral load.

MANAGEMENT

A number of antimicrobial agents are used in the management of HIV and its related infections. The two main groups of drugs used to suppress HIV proliferation are these:

1. **Reverse transcriptase inhibitors:** These drugs inhibit the reverse transcriptase enzyme of HIV, and are subdivided into:
   - **nucleoside (analogue)** reverse transcriptase inhibitors, including zidovudine (azidothymidine (AZT)), the first drug introduced in this category; didanosine (ddI); lamivudine (3TC); stavudine (d4T); and zalcitabine (ddC)
   - **non-nucleoside** reverse transcriptase inhibitors (e.g., nevirapine).
2. **Protease (proteinase) inhibitors**, including saquinavir, ritonavir, indinavir and nelfinavir, which inhibit proteins essential for viral reproduction, such as reverse transcriptase and integrase.

Other relatively new drugs include *fusion inhibitors* (approved in 2003), which block the HIV envelope from merging with the host CD4 cell membrane; *entry inhibitors* (2007), which block virus entry into cells; and *integrase inhibitors* (2007), which interfere with the viral enzyme required for HIV replication.

Combination 'cocktail' therapy with nucleoside analogues and protease inhibitors is far more effective than monotherapy with individual drugs. However, the side effects and the cost of treatment are both barriers to such 'cocktail' therapy. HAART consists of two nucleoside inhibitors and one protease inhibitor. There is significant clinical improvement in HAART therapy, yet the virus persists intracellularly as a provirus, only to reemerge if or when therapy is reduced.

Preexposure prophylaxis (PrEP) for prevention of contracting infection, before exposure, in a combination oral pill Emtricitabine/tenofovir is recommended; this does not cure the disease.

A large number of antimicrobial drugs are also used prophylactically to prevent emergence of fungal, bacterial and viral infections, and as therapeutic supportive measures to prolong the quality of life in these patients.

Prevention of HIV Infection

- Public education programmes aiming at changing sexual behaviour and promoting 'safe sex', especially the use of **barrier contraceptives**, will continue to be the mainstay of HIV prevention into the foreseeable future.
- Introduction of **preexposure prophylaxis (PrEP)** with oral antivirals has been a leap forward in prevention. When pills are taken as prescribed, PrEP reduces the risk of getting HIV from sex by about 99% and the risk from injection drug use by at least 74%.
- Free distribution of **sterile needles** to injecting drug abusers has proved useful.
- **Antiretroviral drugs** to HIV-infected mothers and their newborns have been extremely effective with some 50% reduction in infection transmission to **the neonates**.
- Transmission in health care settings can be prevented by appropriate **personal protective equipment** (see Chapter 37).
- The likelihood of an HIV vaccine becoming available within the next 5 years is low, as the virus (1) mutates rapidly from one generation to another, thus evading host immune cells, (2) is not expressed in all cells that are infected, and (3) is not cleared by the host immune cells after primary infection. However, a number of **candidate vaccines** are undergoing trials, and the approach to vaccine development is shown in Fig. 30.5. A major obstacle for vaccine development is the lack of

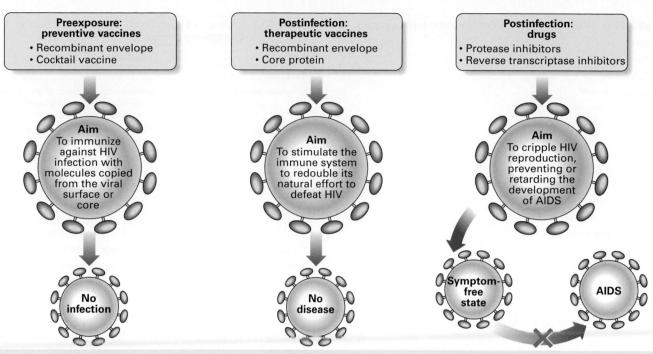

Fig. 30.5   Current approaches to HIV vaccine production and post-infection drug therapy.

an appropriate animal model. Chimpanzees are the only HIV-susceptible animals with a viraemia and antibody response, yet they do not develop immune deficiency.

HIV TRANSMISSION AND DENTAL HEALTH CARE WORKERS

The Risk to Dental Professionals

A number of prospective surveillance studies indicate that there is no risk of HIV transmission by either saliva or blood in routine dental care. However, accidental injuries via contaminated needles are associated with a very low risk of infection (0.3%). In view of the hundreds of thousands of infected patients treated since the advent of the AIDS pandemic, it is highly unlikely that the occupational hazard of dentists contracting HIV infection is greater than that for other health care workers. Additionally, the susceptibility of HIV to many disinfectants, the hygienic environment in most dental surgeries and the use of disposable instruments reduce the risk still further. After close scrutiny of the small number of *alleged* HIV transmission episodes in dentistry, the CDC has stated that there has been **no HIV transmission in dental settings** thus far.

The HIV-Infected Dental Health Care Worker

The disclosure of possible HIV transmission to five patients by an infected dentist (in Florida, US) has raised important ethical, moral and legal issues pertaining to continued delivery of dental care by infected dental personnel. (However, the dental transmission route has now been ruled out as it is believed that the patients acquired the infection from high-risk activities.)

The consensus of professional opinion is that it is the ethical and moral responsibility of dentists who believe that they may be infected with HIV to obtain medical advice and, if found to be infected, to act upon the medical advice, if necessary by modifying the practice of dentistry in some way or by ceasing practice altogether.

Infections in Compromised Patients

A **compromised patient** is a person whose **normal defence mechanisms are impaired**, making the individual more susceptible to infection (e.g., individuals with damaged heart valves, diabetes and immunodeficiency states, including AIDS).

Although the majority of compromised patients are hospitalized, a significant proportion are ambulant community dwellers and likely to seek routine dental care. It is important to note that the drugs and dental treatment provided may interfere with the compromised state and the medications prescribed.

MECHANISMS LEADING TO IMMUNOCOMPROMISED STATES

Immunodeficiency disease can be either **primary** (developmental or genetically determined), which is rare, or **secondary**, due to procedures such as irradiation and cytotoxic drug therapy.

Primary Immunodeficiency

Rarely are children born with congenital deficiency of the immune system. These include deficiencies in B cells, with depressed immunoglobulin production, T-cell deficiency (e.g., thymic aplasia), combined B-cell and T-cell deficiency, and neutrophil dysfunction.

Table 30.4   Main Causes of Secondary Immunodeficiency

Drugs
    Methotrexate
    Cytarabine
Malignant disease
    Acute leukaemia
    Hodgkin's disease
Infections
    AIDS
    Severe viral infections
Deficiency states
    Iron deficiency
Autoimmune disease
    Rheumatoid arthritis
Others
    Diabetes mellitus
    Irradiation

Secondary Immunodeficiency

Secondary immunodeficiency can be due to disease or therapy (Table 30.4).

Disease. Diseases include **neoplasms** of the **lymphoid system** leading to lymphomas (Hodgkin's disease), leukaemia, multiple myeloma and—of special interest—**AIDS** due to HIV infection (see earlier in this chapter). Other diseases such as **diabetes**, **renal failure**, **rheumatoid arthritis** and **autoimmune disease** (e.g., systemic lupus erythematosus) diminish immunity by often complex and incompletely understood mechanisms.

Therapy. Modern medical treatment, especially drugs, radiotherapy and surgical removal of the spleen, may diminish or abolish immune function:

- **drugs:** immunosuppressives, cytotoxic drugs and steroid therapy
- **radiotherapy:** widely used in cancer treatment and a popular regimen for therapy of head and neck cancer. Its adverse effects, in addition to the general suppressive effect of radiotherapy on immune cells, include localized effects on salivary glands and oral mucosa, leading to **xerostomia** and **mucositis** of the oral mucosa, respectively; the latter results in secondary oral infections
- **splenectomy:** This is effective in some but may lead to increased susceptibility to infection with encapsulated bacteria such as *Streptococcus pneumoniae*.

ORAL INFECTIONS IN COMPROMISED PATIENTS

Due to the poor immune functionality associated with the specific underlying conditions decribed above or the management procedures related to the disease, the oral cavity is perhaps the first site where focal infection may be noted in compromised individuals. Such infections may be caused by **endogenous commensal flora** of low pathogenicity (e.g., oral candidiasis) or **exogenous organisms** acquired from the environment (e.g., drug-resistant hospital staphylococci, methicillin-resistant *Staphylococcus*

Table 30.5   Examples of Common Organisms That Cause Infections in Compromised Patients

Agent	Infection
Bacteria	
Enterobacteriaceae	Urinary tract infection, pneumonia, septicaemia, meningitis, oral mucositis, osteoradionecrosis
Mycobacterium tuberculosis and other mycobacteria	Tuberculosis, disseminated disease, IRIS
Staphylococcus aureus	Septicaemia, pneumonia, mucositis, osteoradionecrosis
Streptococcus pneumoniae	Septicaemia
Fungi	
Candida spp.	Thrush, systemic candidiasis, chronic mucocutaneous disease
Cryptococcus neoformans	Meningoencephalitis
Aspergillus and *Mucor* spp.	Disseminated disease
Pneumocystis jirovecii	Interstitial pneumonia (in AIDS)
Viruses	
Herpes simplex virus	Severe cold sores
Cytomegalovirus	Pneumonia, IRIS
Protozoa	
Toxoplasma gondii	Severe toxoplasmosis

IRIS, immune reconstitution inflammatory syndrome.

aureus, coliforms). Virulent organisms and even the most harmless commensals may cause life-threatening disease in these cases (Table 30.5).

Some examples of specific orofacial infections in compromised patients are as follows:

- **Osteoradionecrosis:** Oral cancer is often treated by radiotherapy, and this may lead to tissue necrosis, including bone, due to a decreased number of cells (**hypocellularity**) and a reduction in the number of blood vessels (**hypovascularity**). Resultant death of bony tissue due to a combination of the foregoing effects, or precipitated by trauma (e.g., tooth extraction), may lead to spontaneous bony necrosis, termed **osteoradionecrosis**. Such necrotic tissue may be **secondarily infected** by *Staphylococcus aureus* and/or anaerobes such as *Porphyromonas* and *Prevotella* species. Management of the condition, which is rather difficult, is by **bone-penetrating antibiotics** such as clindamycin and/or metronidazole in combination with surgical debridement, or chlorhexidine irrigation if the site is accessible.
- **Bisphosphonate-associated osteonecrosis:** Osteoporosis is a common condition that leads to calcium loss from the bone. Bisphosphonates are used to **prevent osteoclastic activity** and bone loss. A common adverse side effect of bisphosphonates is failure of bone healing, especially after tooth extraction. Such sockets may be secondarily infected by anaerobes, and irrigation of the tooth socket with chlorhexidine and metronidazole may be helpful.
- **Postirradiation mucositis:** Another complication of irradiation is its effect on the oral mucosa, which reacts in the form of nonspecific inflammation, termed **mucositis**. Microflora associated with mucositis are rather nonspecific and may include Gram-negative aerobes and

Table 30.6   Oral Diseases of Infective Origin Seen in Various Compromised Patient Groups

Condition	Cytotoxic Therapy	Radiotherapy	AIDS	Acute Leukaemia
Mucositis	+	+	−	+
Ulceration	+	+	+	+
Xerostomia	+	+	+	−
Sialadenitis	−	+	±	−
Osteomyelitis	+	+	−	−
Candidiasis	+	+	+	+
Herpes infection	+	−	+	+
Periodontal diseases	−	+	+	+
Dental caries	−	+	−	−

facultative anaerobes such as *Escherichia coli*, *Klebsiella* species and pseudomonads. The condition spontaneously remits after radiotherapy but may be ameliorated by topical application of nonabsorbable antimicrobials.

- **Necrotizing fasciitis:** This is a rapidly progressive, serious infection that may even lead to death and is not uncommon in immunocompromised individuals. Necrotizing fasciitis may be **precipitated by dentoalveolar infection**, and the implicated aetiological agents include the *anginosus* group of streptococci and anaerobes such as *Prevotella* species. Management is by intravenous antibiotics, surgical debridement and hyperbaric oxygen in severe cases.

- **Immune reconstitution inflammatory syndrome:** (Synonyms: **IRIS**, immune recovery syndrome) This condition is seen in some cases of AIDS or immunosuppression, in which the immune system begins to recover—for instance, after antiretroviral therapy—but then responds to a previously acquired opportunistic infection with an overwhelming inflammatory response that paradoxically makes the symptoms of infection worse. IRIS is thought to be precipitated by reconstitution of antigen-specific T-cell–mediated immunity and activation of the immune system against a persisting antigen. The latter may present as intact organisms, dead organisms or debris. Infections most commonly associated with IRIS include cytomegalovirus, herpes zoster, *Mycobacterium avium* complex (MAC), pneumocystis pneumonia and *M. tuberculosis*. Management is by antibiotic or antiviral drugs against the infectious organism, sometimes with corticosteroids to suppress inflammation.

- **Cancrum oris or noma**: See Chapter 33.

Important Cofactors for Oral Infection in Immunocompromised Patients

Cofactors important in oral infection include:

- the **duration** and depth of immunosuppression
- previous or current **antimicrobial therapy** (e.g., broad-spectrum antibiotics promote fungal infection)
- the degree of **oral hygiene** and quality of oral care provided
- the nature of the cytotoxic or immunosuppressive **drug used** (e.g., methotrexate, in particular, causes oral ulceration, which may become secondarily infected).

Clinical Presentation

The presentation of oral infections varies widely, depending on the cofactors previously mentioned. Some conditions are more commonly associated with a particular category of compromised patient than others. For instance, in acute leukaemia, the response to dental plaque is exaggerated, leading to gross gingival swelling, but periodontal disease is not a significant problem during cytotoxic therapy. Oral problems encountered in immunocompromised patients are listed in Table 30.6.

PREVENTION OF INFECTION

General Guidelines

Surveillance. Careful monitoring of the susceptible individual for signs of infection is required; if these occur, treatment should be instituted without delay.

Antibiotics. Avoid the abuse of antibiotics (particularly broad-spectrum antimicrobials) to minimize emergence of resistant flora.

Isolation. Severely ill patients (e.g., those with neutropenia) should be either isolated in a single room with only nursing staff admitted or completely isolated (in a laminar airflow bed or room) and provided with sterilized food.

Specific Guidelines

Pretreatment Management. Pretreatment management includes:

- a careful assessment of the patient's dental health before radiotherapy or immunosuppressive drugs are used
- appropriate restorative or surgical treatment (e.g., extraction of nonrestorable teeth before radiotherapy to prevent osteomyelitis of the mandible)
- oral hygiene instruction and dietary advice (e.g., low-sugar diet, regular fluoride applications).

Management During Treatment.

- Diagnosis and management should be carried out with the assistance of laboratory tests and reports.
- Oral management of patients must be closely linked with the medical treatment, and it is essential that the dentist is regarded as part of the medical team.

Xerostomia and Infection

Xerostomia or dry mouth may be the result of:

- ageing
- drugs (e.g., cytotoxic therapy)

- radiotherapy
- Sjögren's syndrome (primary and secondary).

The resulting chronic dryness of the mucosa and the inadequate salivary cleansing mechanism increase the susceptibility of oral tissues to incidence of:

- caries
- periodontal diseases
- oral candidiasis
- ascending (bacterial) sialadenitis.

Other noninfective sequelae are difficulty in eating and swallowing dry food and in wearing complete dentures; burning sensation of the oral mucosa; and changes in the sense of taste **(dysgeusia)**.

A reduction or absence of salivary secretion has a profound effect on the composition of the normal oral flora. Reduced moisture levels tend to favour growth of bacteria resistant to drying, such as *Staphylococcus aureus*, and inhibit oral commensals adapted to high moisture levels. In addition, the pH of salivary secretions in these patients is low and the oxygen tension (E_h) is high, which may be unfavourable to the growth of bacteria such as *Veillonella*, commensal *Neisseria* and *Micrococcus* spp. Moreover, this environment favours the growth of *Candida* spp.

SEQUELAE OF CHRONIC XEROSTOMIA

Extensive Dental Caries

Dental caries may occur, especially in the **cervical and incisal surfaces** of the teeth and at the margins of dental restorations, sometimes subgingivally.

Prevention. Prevention includes daily fluoride mouth-rinsing; discontinuation of high-sucrose snacks between meals; careful removal of dental plaque by proper, frequent brushing; and regular dental supervision. Severe caries may be controlled by fluoride application.

Periodontal Disease

Periodontal disease, especially gingivitis, is common because of the lack of moisture.

Prevention. Mouthwashes containing 2% chlorhexidine will help control gingivitis and other oral infections.

Candidal Infections

Candida-associated denture stomatitis, angular cheilitis and papillary atrophy of the tongue are frequent.

Prevention. See Chapter 35.

Ascending Parotitis

Ascending parotitis is the result of the absence or reduced natural flushing action of the salivary flow in Stensen's duct.

Prevention. Treat with antibiotics: empirical therapy with penicillinase-resistant penicillins. Pus should be sent for culture and antibiotic sensitivities. Stimulate salivary secretion with sialagogues; if adequate amounts of saliva cannot be stimulated, use a proprietary saliva substitute.

Key Facts

- The **human immunodeficiency virus (HIV)**, an enveloped RNA retrovirus containing the enzyme reverse transcriptase, is the agent of **HIV disease**.
- Not all HIV-infected persons have symptomatic disease; some live a healthy symptom-free life for years.
- **Acquired immune deficiency syndrome (AIDS)** is a group of disorders characterized by a profound cell-mediated immunodeficiency consequential to **irreversible suppression of T lymphocytes** by HIV and associated with opportunistic infection, malignancies and autoimmune disorders.
- AIDS-defining illnesses are characterized by a **CD4 lymphocyte count below 200 × 10⁶/l**, oropharyngeal candidiasis and hairy leukoplakia.
- Two major subtypes of HIV are known: **HIV-1** is more prevalent than **HIV-2**; both subtypes have similar biological properties.
- HIV is characterized by an envelope containing virus-specific **'coat' proteins** (e.g., glycoproteins, gp120); three **core proteins** (e.g., p24); a **genome of RNA**; and two molecules of an enzyme, reverse **transcriptase**.
- HIV is relatively easily destroyed by heat (autoclave and hot-air oven) and disinfectants (e.g., 2% glutaraldehyde and hypochlorite).
- HIV is transmitted by **blood-to-blood, sexual, and perinatal contact**.
- HIV is unlikely to be transmitted by saliva as it is infrequently present and in very low titres in saliva, and salivary **immunoglobulin A (IgA)** and **serine protease inhibitors**

(salivary leukocyte protease inhibitor (SLPI)) neutralize the virus.
- Noteworthy opportunistic infections and neoplasms in AIDS include pneumocystis pneumonia (PCP), toxoplasmosis, atypical mycobacteriosis, candidiasis, herpesvirus infections and Kaposi's sarcoma.
- The earliest indicators of HIV infection may manifest in the oral cavity, and the more common of these are **oral candidiasis**, **hairy leukoplakia**, **Kaposi's sarcoma**, **recurrent ulcers** and **cervical lymphadenopathy**.
- Diagnosis of HIV is performed by screening with **enzyme-linked immunosorbent assay (ELISA) tests** (agglutination test for serum antibodies) and subsequent confirmation by **Western blot assay**.
- The two main groups of drugs used to suppress HIV proliferation are the **reverse transcriptase inhibitors** (nucleoside and nonnucleoside) and **protease inhibitors**.
- **Barrier contraceptives** are the mainstay of HIV prevention for the foreseeable future.
- A **compromised host** is a person whose normal defence mechanisms are impaired, making the individual more susceptible to infection.
- **Immunodeficiency** disease can be either **primary** (developmental or genetically determined), which is rare, or **secondary**, due to procedures such as irradiation and cytotoxic drug therapy.
- The chronic dryness of the mucosa in **xerostomia** leads to caries, periodontal diseases, candidiasis and ascending (bacterial) sialadenitis.

Review Questions (Answers on p. 391)

Please indicate which answers are true and which are false.

30.1. In human immunodeficiency virus (HIV):
 a. the genome consists of two identical single-stranded RNA molecules
 b. envelope proteins undergo continuous structural changes
 c. p24 is an important coat protein
 d. reverse transcriptase activity takes place
 e. the virus can survive in the saliva of HIV-infected individuals

30.2. HIV is likely to be transmitted when:
 a. kissing the cheek of an AIDS patient
 b. having unprotected sex with a prostitute
 c. an HIV-infected dentist does an amalgam filling on a patient
 d. a nurse sustains an injury with a needle-stick, disinfected in 5% ethanol for 5 min and previously used for venepuncture of an AIDS patient
 e. sharing cutlery with an HIV-infected individual

30.3. Which of the following statements on compromised patient groups are true?
 a. mucositis is commonly seen in patients on radiotherapy
 b. oral candidiasis is one of the commonest manifestations in compromised persons
 c. chronic periodontal disease is seen in leukaemic states
 d. appropriate restorative dental procedures must be conducted prior to radiotherapy for oral diseases
 e. dysgeusia is a side effect of xerostomia

30.4. A 65-year-old male receives radiotherapy for his nasopharyngeal carcinoma. Indicate which of the following scenario/s is/are likely to be due to this management mode:
 a. he loses his sense of smell
 b. he has difficulty in wearing his lower full denture
 c. his salivary lactobacillus count is likely to rise
 d. he has reduced gingival bleeding during tooth-brushing
 e. he has swelling of his parotid gland/s

30.5. Which of the following statements on the management of HIV disease are true?
 a. the enzyme-linked immunosorbent assay (ELISA) test is more specific for HIV infection than the Western blot
 b. highly active antiretroviral therapy (HAART) suppresses the oral manifestations of HIV
 c. fluconazole is the antifungal of choice in managing oral candidiasis in HIV disease
 d. hairy leukoplakia, due to a herpes group virus, needs to be managed by excision of the lesion
 e. combination therapy with reverse transcriptase inhibitors and nucleoside analogues is more effective than monotherapy for treating HIV disease

Further Reading

Classification and diagnostic criteria for oral lesions in HIV infection. (1993). EC-Clearinghouse on Oral Problems Related to HIV Infection and WHO Collaborating Centre on Oral Manifestations of Immunodeficiency Virus. *Journal of Oral Pathology and Medicine, 22*(7), 289–291.

Davies, A. N., & Epstein, J. B. (2010). *Oral complications of cancer and its management.* Oxford University Press.

Lewis, M. A. O., & Jordan, R. C. K. (2004). *A colour handbook of oral medicine.* Manson Publishing.

Pillay, D., Geretti, A. M., & Weiss, R. A. (2009). Human immunodeficiency viruses. In A. J. Zuckerman, J. E. Banatvala, P. Griffith, et al. (Eds.), *Principles and practice of clinical virology* (6th ed., Ch. 38). John Wiley.

Samaranayake, L. P. (1992). Oral mycoses in human immunodeficiency virus infection: A review. *Oral Surgery, Oral Medicine, Oral Pathology, 73,* 171–180.

Samaranayake, L. P., & Pindborg, J. J. (1989). Hairy leukoplakia. *British Medical Journal, 298,* 270–271.

Samaranayake, L. P., & Scully, C. (1989). Oral candidosis in HIV infection. *Lancet, 2,* 1491–1492.

Scully, C. (2015). *Scully`s medical problems in dentistry* (7th ed.). Churchill Livingstone.

Tsang, C., & Samaranayake, L. P. (2010). Immune reconstitution inflammatory syndrome (IRIS) after highly active antiretroviral therapy: A review. *Oral Diseases, 16,* 248–256.

PART 5

ORAL MICROBIOTA AND ORAL INFECTIONS

Although all the contents of this book are essential learning for dental professionals, the elements in Part 5 could be considered critical for understanding the basis of oral and maxillofacial infections and their management.

The section begins with a description of the oral microbiota and their interactions with the dynamic oral ecosystem, the oralome. Although a bewildering array of bacterial genera are described in this section, the students are not expected to memorize all of the genera described. However, a basic comprehension of at least the main genera that contribute to oral and systemic diseases is important.

Subsequent chapters are devoted to concise descriptions of oral infections and their management, beginning with the two most common human diseases, dental caries and periodontal disease. There is a vast literature on these subjects, and so only the bare essentials are provided here. Most importantly, this section will demonstrate to the students the relevance of microbiology and infection management to the practice of dentistry.

- Oral microbiota and the oralome
- Microbiology of dental caries
- Microbiology of periodontal disease
- Dentoalveolar and endodontic infections
- Oral mucosal and salivary gland infections

Oral Microbiota and the Oralome

This chapter describes in detail the oral **microbiota** and its living habitat: the oral **microbiome**. Particular emphasis is placed on the all-encompassing oral ecosystem and the dynamic interactions between the hosts and the oral microbes, called the **oralome**, that modulate the life and times of the microbial populations residing in our mouth.

Oral Microbiome and the Oral Microbiota

Humans are not colonized at random, and the microbial residents we harbor and provide shelter for have **coevolved** with us over millions of years. This has led to the realization that the host and its residents together contribute to health and disease as a **holobiont**. According to the latest data from the *Human Cell Atlas*, the adult human body is composed of 37.2 trillion cells. However, when we include the colossal numbers of resident microflora residing in the human body to this eukaryotic cell mass, the cumulative total is thought to exceed several hundred trillion cells. Of the latter total, an overwhelming percentage, some 90%, is thought to comprise the resident microflora, and only 10% are mammalian.

Focusing on the oral ecosystem, bacteria are by far the predominant group of organisms in the oral cavity, and there are probably some 700 common oral species or **phylotypes** of which only 50–60% are cultivable in the laboratory. Of these, approximately 54% are officially named, 14% are unnamed (but cultivated) and 32% are known only as uncultivated phylotypes or **uncultivable flora**. The latter are currently identified using molecular techniques, especially those based on **16S ribosomal RNA (rRNA) sequencing, pyrosequencing, next-generation sequencing (NGS) technology** and **second-generation sequencing technology**. These new genomic technologies together with **bioinformatics** tools provide a powerful means of understanding the role of the oral microbes in health and disease.

A perplexing array of organisms can be found in the oral cavity, which is one of the most heavily colonized parts of the human body. This is due to its unique anatomical structures found nowhere else in the body, such as the nonshedding surfaces of the teeth, epithelial-lined surfaces such as the oral mucosae, gingivae and gingival crevices. Under normal circumstances, this vast array of organisms including bacteria, archaea, fungi, mycoplasmas, protozoa and also the viral flora usually live in harmony in a state of **eubiosis**. However, this state of eubiosis may be perturbed by a variety of extrinsic or intrinsic causes leading to overgrowth of the commensal organisms and/or putative resident pathogens. If such a chaotic state, called **dysbiosis**, is not resolved and the ecobalance between the microbial community and its ecosystem is not restored, various disease states such as caries and periodontal disease may quickly supervene.

DEFINITIONS

Oral microbiota: The totality of all the oral microbes residing in the oral cavity. These include fungi, bacteria, viruses, archaea and protozoa.

Oral microbiome: The totality of the oral microbes, their genetic information and the oral environment within which they interact.

Oralome: The sum total of the dynamic interactions between the ecological community of oral microorganisms in the oral cavity and the host (i.e., microbe-microbe interactions and microbe-host interactions).

The oral microbiome in turn could be divided into six major subcompartments (Fig. 31.1):

- **oral bacteriome** (bacterial component)
- **oral mycobiome** (fungal component; Greek: *mykes* fungus)
- **oral virome/virobiome** (viral component)
- **oral phageome** (phage component)
- **oral archaeome** (archaeal component)
- **oral protozome** (*synonym:* oral protozoome; protozoal component)

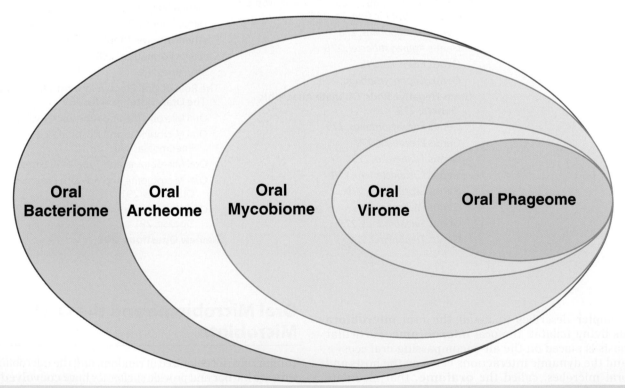

Fig. 31.1 Major compartments of the oral microbiome. Oral bacteriome is by far the biggest component, and oral virobiome and pahgeome (synonym: oral virome) are the smallest. Note the difference between mycobiome and microbiome (Greek: *Mykes* fungus). *Note:* Oral protozome is not shown. Myocplasma species are also infrequently isolated from the oral cavity.

Each of these subcompartments of the oral mcrobiome is described in detail in the account below.

Apart from the aforementioned distinct subcompartments of the oral microbiome, recent reports indicate the existence of a multitude of yet-to-be cultured (or uncultivable) ultra-small bacteria that may fall within the bacteriome group, and these have been classified into a subsector called the **candidate phyla radiation (CPR)** group. Organisms in the CPR group are ultra-small (nanometre range, compared with micron-scale bacteria) and highly abundant (>15% of bacteriome). They are characterized by reduced genomes and unusual ribosomes and appear to be obligate symbionts, living attached to either host bacteria or fungi. The CPR group is also called **microbial dark matter** due to their elusive nature and the dearth of information on their functionality and role in either health or disease.

In recent studies of the structure, function and diversity of the human oral microbiome, evaluated using NGS technology, it has been clearly shown that the oral microbiome is unique to each individual, akin to a '**microbial fingerprint**'. Even healthy individuals differ remarkably in the composition of the resident oral microbiota. Although much of this diversity remains unexplained, diet, environment, host genetics and early microbial exposure have all been implicated in the constituent flora of the climax community.

The oral microbiota exists either suspended in saliva as **planktonic phase** organisms or attached to oral surfaces, in the **biofilm phase** (also called the **sessile phase**—i.e., the **plaque biofilm**). In general, despite the high diversity in the salivary microbiome within and between individuals, little geographic variation can be noticed. Individuals from different parts of the world harbour similar **salivary microbiota**, indicating that host species (i.e., *Homo sapiens*) is the primary determinant of the oral microbiome.

Some oral microbes are more closely associated with disease than others (e.g., *Porphyromonas gingivalis*, a periodontal pathogen), although they commonly lurk within the normal oral flora without harming oral health. This **symbiosis** between beneficial and pathogenic organisms is the key factor that contributes to the maintenance of oral health. In other words, when this **homeostasis** and the symbiotic equilibrium break down—for example, on taking broad-spectrum antibiotics—a state called **dysbiosis** sets in, leading to disease such as caries, periodontal disease and candidal infections. Essentially, in a dysbiotic microbiome, the diversity and relative proportions of species or taxa of the constituent microbiota are disturbed.

On some occasions, specific microbes (mainly lactobacilli) could be administered to help restore a natural healthy microbiome in a given habitat (i.e., to convert a dysbiotic state to a symbiotic state). Such organisms are known as **probiotics** (see Chapter 26).

Oral bacteria can be classified primarily as **Gram-positive** and **Gram-negative** organisms, and secondarily as either **anaerobic** or **facultatively anaerobic** according to their oxygen requirements. Some oral microbes are more closely associated with disease than others, although a vast proportion of these appear to be uncultivable. The following is a synopsis of the major bacterial genera isolated from the oral cavity. Students should refer to the appropriate chapters in Part 3 for detailed information on these organisms.

A NOTE ON THE NOMENCLATURE OF ORAL FLORA

Because of continuing advances in molecular technology, especially those based on 16S rRNA sequences and NGS technology, microbial taxonomy is always in a state of flux. This poses a challenge to both the student and the scientist alike. Despite these changes, some prefer using the traditional nomenclature, whereas others use the new terminology, leading to further confusion. Hence, in the following text both the old and the recent taxonomic changes of oral bacteria are highlighted.

Those who wish to pursue the subject of the oral microbiota and the oral microbiome in further detail need to visit the **H**uman **O**ral **M**icrobiome **D**atabase (HOMD; http://www.homd.org). The HOMD presents a provisional naming scheme for the currently unnamed species so that strain, clone and probe data from any laboratory can be directly linked to a stably named reference scheme.

Oral Microbiota

Oral microbiota is the collective group name for six of its constituents i) oral bacteriome ii) oral archaeome iii) oral mycobiome iv) oral virome v) oral phageome and vi) oral prtozome (Fig. 31.1). These are described in some detail below.

ORAL BACTERIOME

A bewildering array, **approximately 700 species**, of bacteria is found in the oral cavity, making the oral cavity the second-largest bacterial community in the human body, after the gut. However, the most common species belong to four genera:

- Streptococcus
- Gemella
- Granulicatella
- Veillonella.

Of these, Streptococcus and Gemella species are by far the most prevalent.

The following account is a brief description of a notable genera that comprise the oral microbiome, *classified according to their Gram-staining characteristics*.

(*Note:* Clearly, students are not expected to memorize all of the genera described, but a basic comprehension of at least the main genera that contribute to oral and systemic diseases is important.)

GRAM-POSITIVE COCCI

Genus *Streptococcus*

Gram-positive cocci in chains, nonmotile, usually possessing surface fibrils, occasionally capsulate; facultative anaerobes; variable haemolysis but α-haemolysis most common; selective medium: mitis salivarius agar (MSA).

Mutans Group

- **Main species:** *Streptococcus mutans* serotypes c, e, f, k; *Streptococcus sobrinus* serotypes d, g; *Streptococcus criceti* (previously *Streptococcus cricetus*) serotype a; *Streptococcus ratti* (previously *Streptococcus rattus*) serotype b. Oral isolates from monkeys: *Streptococcus ferus*; *Streptococcus macacae*; *Streptococcus downei* serotype h.
- **Cultural characteristics:** high, convex, opaque colonies; produce profuse extracellular polysaccharide in sucrose-containing media (Fig. 11.3); selective medium: MSA + bacitracin agar.
- Main intraoral sites and infections: tooth surface, dental caries.

Salivarius Group

- **Main species:** *Streptococcus salivarius*; *Streptococcus vestibularis*.
- **Cultural characteristics:** large, mucoid colonies on MSA due to the production of extracellular fructans (polymer of fructose with a levan structure). *Streptococcus vestibularis* do not produce extracellular polysaccharide from sucrose; they produce urease and hydrogen peroxide, which lowers the pH and contributes to the salivary peroxidase system, respectively.
- **Main intraoral sites and infections:** dorsum of the tongue and saliva; *Streptococcus vestibularis* mainly reside in the vestibular mucosa (hence the name); not a major oral pathogen.

Anginosus Group

- **Main species:** *Streptococcus constellatus*; *Streptococcus intermedius*; *Streptococcus anginosus*.
- **Cultural characteristics:** carbon dioxide dependent; form small, nonadherent colonies on MSA.
- **Main intraoral sites and infections:** gingival crevice; dentoalveolar and endodontic infections.

Mitis Group

- **Main species:** *Streptococcus mitis*, *Streptococcus sanguinis* (previously *Streptococcus sanguinis*); *Streptococcus gordonii*, *Streptococcus oralis*, *Streptococcus cristatus* (previously *Streptococcus crista*), *Streptococcus parasanguinis*, *Streptococcus oligofermentans*, *Streptococcus sinensis*, *Streptococcus australis*, *Streptococcus peroris*, *Streptococcus infantis*.
- **Cultural characteristics:** small, rubbery (*Streptococcus sanguinis*) or nonadherent (*Streptococcus oralis* and *Streptococcus mitis*) colonies on MSA.
- **Main intraoral sites and infections:** mainly dental plaque biofilms, tongue and cheek, possibly dental caries, infective endocarditis (except *Streptococcus mitis*).

Anaerobic Streptococci

- **Main species:** *Peptostreptococcus anaerobius*, *Micromonas micros* (previously *Peptostreptococcus micros*), *Finegoldia magna* (previously *Peptostreptococcus magnus*) and *Peptoniphilus asaccharolyticus* (previously *Peptostreptococcus asaccharolyticus*); group acronym **GPAC** (Gram-positive anaerobic cocci).
- **Cultural characteristics:** strict anaerobes, slow-growing, usually nonhaemolytic.

- **Main intraoral sites and infections:** teeth, especially carious dentine, periodontal and dentoalveolar abscesses in mixed culture.

Genus *Stomatococcus*

- **Main species:** *Stomatococcus* (formerly *Micrococcus*) *mucilaginous*.
- **Cultural characteristics:** coagulase negative; forms large colonies adherent to blood agar surface, facultative anaerobes.
- **Main intraoral sites and infections:** tongue mainly, gingival crevice; not a major opportunistic pathogen.

Genus *Granulicatella*

- **Genus *Granulicatella*** (previously termed 'nutritionally variant streptococci')
- **Main species:** *Granulicatella adiacens*, *Granulicatella elegans*, *Granulicatella balaenopterae*.
- **Cultural characteristics:** Gram-positive cocci, nonmotile, catalase- and oxidase-negative, non-spore-forming, facultatively anaerobic requiring pyridoxal or L-cysteine for growth (Fig. 31.2). When grown on media without these components, their cell morphology and Gram stainability changes.
- **Main intraoral sites and infections:** A component of normal oral flora and inhabits plaque biofilms, periodontal pockets, and root canals. Increased prevalence in caries, periodontitis and endodontic infections has been noted. Importantly, they cause serious infections such as infective endocarditis.

Genera *Staphylococcus* and *Micrococcus*

See Chapter 11.

GRAM-POSITIVE RODS AND FILAMENTS

These organisms are common isolates from dental plaque biofilms and include actinomycetes, lactobacilli, eubacteria and propionibacteria.

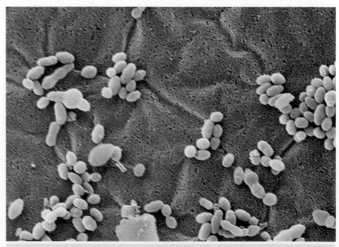

Fig. 31.2   Scanning electron micrograph of *Granulicatella* spp. showing non-spore-forming coccal forms. (Picture courtesy Dr. M. Karched.)

Genus *Actinomyces*

Short, Gram-positive pleomorphic rods:

- **Main species:** *Actinomyces israelii, Actinomyces gerencseriae, Actinomyces odontolyticus, Actinomyces naeslundii* (genospecies 1 and 2), *Actinomyces meyeri, Actinomyces georgiae.* The most important human pathogen is *Actinomyces israelii.*
- **Cultural characteristics:** ferments glucose to give characteristic patterns of short-chain carboxylic acids useful for speciating; strict or facultative anaerobes.
- **Main intraoral sites and infections:** *Actinomyces odontolyticus,* earliest stages of enamel demineralization, and the progression of small caries lesions appear related; *Actinomyces naeslundii* implicated in root surface caries and gingivitis; *Actinomyces israelii* is an opportunistic pathogen causing **cervicofacial and ileocaecal actinomycosis** (Chapter 13). *Actinomyces gerencseriae* and *Actinomyces georgiae* are minor components of healthy gingival flora.

Genus *Lactobacillus*

Gram-positive bacilli:

- **Main species:** *Lactobacillus casei, Lactobacillus fermentum, Lactobacillus acidophilus* (others include *Lactobacillus salivarius, Lactobacillus rhamnosus*).
- **Cultural characteristics:** catalase-negative, microaerophilic; complex nutritional requirements; aciduric, optimal pH 5.5–5.8. Selective medium: Rogosa agar.

- **Main intraoral sites and infections:** common oral inhabitants, but comprise less than 1% of the oral flora. Dental plaque biofilms, usually in small numbers; **advancing front of dentinal caries**. As levels of salivary lactobacilli correlate well with intake of dietary carbohydrates, they may be used to detect the cariogenic potential of the diet. *Lactobacillus* species including some oral species are used as probiotics.

Genus *Eubacterium*

Pleomorphic, Gram-variable rods or filaments:

- **Main species:** *Eubacterium brachy, Eubacterium nodatum, Eubacterium saphenum.* (*Note: Eubacterium timidum* and *Eubacterium lenta,* previously in this group, have now been reclassified as *Mogibacterium timidum* and *Eggerthella lenta,* respectively).
- **Cultural characteristics:** obligatory anaerobes, characterization ill-defined.
- **Main intraoral sites and infections:** plaque biofilms and calculus; implicated in caries and periodontal disease but role unclear; comprise over 50% of the anaerobes of periodontal pockets; *Eubacterium yurii* is involved in '**corn-cob**' formation in dental plaque (see Fig. 31.3).

Genus *Propionibacterium*

Gram-positive bacilli:

- **Main species:** *Propionibacterium acnes* (includes *Propionibacterium propionicus,* formerly *Arachnia propionica*).

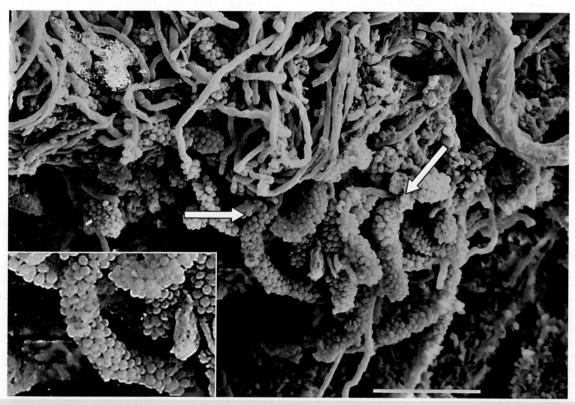

Fig. 31.3 Scanning electron micrograph of a supragingival plaque biofilm showing clearly corn-cob arrangements of cocci aggregated around axial filamentous organisms (arrows), together with other filamentous and coccal forms. *Inset:* a high-power picture of corn-cob arrangement (magnification × 2000; bar 10 μm).

- **Cultural characteristics:** strict anaerobe; morphologically indistinguishable from *Actinomyces israelii* but produces propionic acid from glucose, unlike *Actinomyces israelii*.
- **Main intraoral sites and infections:** root surface caries, plaque biofilms. Possible involvement in dentoalveolar infections.

OTHER NOTABLE GRAM-POSITIVE ORGANISMS

Rothia dentocariosa, a Gram-positive branching filament, is a strict aerobe, found in plaque and occasionally isolated from infective endocarditis.

Bifidobacterium dentium is a Gram-positive strict anaerobe regularly isolated from plaque biofilms; its role in disease is unclear.

GRAM-NEGATIVE COCCI

Genus *Gemella* (previously described as *Neisseria*)

Gram-negative diplococci:

- **Main species:** *Gemella asaccharolyticus*, *Gemella haemolysans*.
- **Cultural characteristics:** asaccharolytic and nonpolysaccharide-producing, facultative anaerobes; oxidase and catalase positive.
- **Main intraoral sites and infections:** isolated in very high numbers from the tongue, saliva, oral mucosa and early plaque biofilm as commensals; may consume oxygen in early stages of plaque formation and provide conditions conducive for the growth of anaerobes; *Gemella haemolysans* has been found to be involved in pulmonary exacerbations of cystic fibrosis patients.

Genus *Neisseria*

Gram-negative diplococci:

- **Main species:** *Neisseria subflava*, *Neisseria mucosa*, *Neisseria sicca*.
- **Cultural characteristics:** asaccharolytic and nonpolysaccharide-producing, facultative anaerobes.
- **Main intraoral sites and infections:** isolated in low numbers from the tongue, saliva, oral mucosa and early plaque biofilm; may consume oxygen in early stages of plaque formation and provide conditions conducive for the growth of anaerobes; rarely associated with disease.

Genus *Veillonella*

Small, Gram-negative cocci:

- **Main species:** *Veillonella parvula*, *Veillonella dispar*, *Veillonella atypica*.
- **Cultural characteristics:** strict anaerobes; selective medium: Rogosa vancomycin agar. Lack glucokinase and fructokinase and hence unable to metabolize carbohydrates; they therefore use lactate produced by other bacteria and raise the pH of the plaque biofilm, and they are considered to be beneficial in relation to dental caries.
- **Main intraoral sites and infections:** isolated from most surfaces, including the tongue, saliva and plaque biofilms. No association with disease.

GRAM-NEGATIVE RODS: FACULTATIVE ANAEROBIC AND CAPNOPHILIC GENERA

Genus *Haemophilus*

Gram-negative coccobacilli:

- **Main species:** *Haemophilus parainfluenzae*, *Haemophilus segnis*, *Haemophilus aphrophilus*, *Haemophilus haemolyticus*, *Haemophilus parahaemolyticus*.
- **Cultural characteristics:** all isolates are facultative anaerobes; growth is enhanced on heated blood agar (chocolate), requires haemin (X factor) and nicotinamide adenine dinucleotide (V factor) for growth.
- **Main intraoral sites and infections:** plaque biofilms, saliva and mucosae; dentoalveolar infections, acute sialadenitis, infective endocarditis.

Genus *Aggregatibacter*

Gram-negative coccobacilli, microaerophilic or capnophilic (carbon dioxide dependent).

- **Main species:** *Aggregatibacter actinomycetemcomitans* (serotypes a–e).
- **Cultural characteristics:** freshly isolated strains contain fimbriae that are lost on subculture. Produces many virulence factors: leukotoxin, epitheliotoxin, collagenase, protease that cleaves immunoglobulin G (IgG).
- **Main intraoral sites and infections:** periodontal pockets; implicated in aggressive forms of periodontal disease (e.g., localized and generalized aggressive periodontitis); some consider as one of the three major 'red complex' or 'keystone' periodontopathogens (Chapter 33). Often isolated from cervicofacial *Actinomyces* infections as co-pathogens.

Genus *Eikenella*

Gram-negative coccobacilli:

- **Main species:** *Eikenella corrodens*.
- **Cultural characteristics:** factor X dependent and microaerophilic; produces corroding colonies on blood agar.
- **Main intraoral sites and infections:** plaque biofilms; dentoalveolar abscesses, infective endocarditis; possibly implicated in some forms of chronic periodontitis.

Genus *Capnocytophaga*

Carbon dioxide dependent, Gram-negative fusiform rods with 'gliding' motility:

- **Main species:** *Capnocytophaga gingivalis*, *Capnocytophaga sputigena*, *Capnocytophaga ochracea*, *Capnocytophaga granulose*, *Capnocytophaga haemolytica*.
- **Cultural characteristics:** capnophilic, medium-sized colonies with an irregular spreading edge.

■ **Main intraoral sites and infections:** plaque, mucosal surfaces, saliva; infections in immunocompromised, possibly destructive periodontal disease. Some strains produce IgA1 protease.

GRAM-NEGATIVE RODS: OBLIGATE ANAEROBIC GENERA

These comprise a large proportion of the plaque biofilms. The classification of this group of organisms is fraught with difficulties, but the advent of new tests such as lipid analysis and molecular approaches have eased the problem to some extent. Most of the oral anaerobes were previously classified under the genus *Bacteroides*. However, advances in taxonomic methods have shown that they belong to two major genera, now termed *Porphyromonas* and *Prevotella*, which differ in their ability to metabolize sugar. Some of these organisms produce characteristic brown-black pigments on blood agar and are referred to collectively as **'black-pigmented anaerobes'** (see Fig. 17.1).

Genus *Porphyromonas*

Gram-negative pleomorphic rods, nonmotile; six serotypes based on capsular polysaccharides (K antigen); asaccharolytic:

■ **Main species:** *Porphyromonas gingivalis, Porphyromonas endodontalis, Porphyromonas catoniae.*
■ **Cultural characteristics:** strict anaerobes, require vitamin K and haemin for growth.
■ **Main intraoral sites and infections:** gingival crevice and subgingival plaque biofilm in small numbers. Associated with chronic periodontitis and dentoalveolar abscess. *Porphyromonas gingivalis* is highly virulent in experimental infections, producing proteases, a haemolysin, collagen-degrading enzymes and cytotoxic metabolites; its capsule is an important virulent attribute; fimbriae helps adhesion. *Porphyromonas endodontalis* is mainly recovered from an infected root canal; it is one of the three major so-called 'red complex' or 'keystone' periodontopathogens (Chapter 33). **Gingipain**, a member of a family of proteases secreted by *Porphyromonas gingivalis* that degrades cytokines (thereby downregulating the host response), have been recovered in **amyloid plaque in neuronal tissue** of persons with **Alzheimer's disease**.

Genus *Prevotella*

Gram-negative pleomorphic rods, nonmotile; moderately asaccharolytic, producing acetic, succinic and other acids from glucose:

■ **Main species:** pigmented species include *Prevotella intermedia, Prevotella nigrescens, Prevotella loescheii, Prevotella corporis, Prevotella melaninogenica*; nonpigmented species include *Prevotella buccae, Prevotella oralis, Prevotella oris, Prevotella oulora, Prevotella veroralis, Prevotella dentalis* (*Bacteroides forsythus*, another nonpigmented species considered an important periodontal pathogen, has now been reclassified as *Tannerella forsythia*).
■ **Cultural characteristics:** strict anaerobes, usually require vitamin K and haemin for growth.

■ **Main intraoral sites and infections:** periodontal pockets, dental plaque biofilm; chronic periodontitis and dentoalveolar abscess.

Genus *Tannerella*

Gram-negative pleomorphic rods, nonmotile; moderately asaccharolytic, producing acetic, succinic and other acids from glucose:

■ **Main species:** *Tannerella forsythia* (previously *Prevotella dentalis*; *Bacteroides forsythus*, forsythia).
■ **Cultural characteristics:** strict anaerobes, usually require vitamin K and haemin for growth.
■ **Main intraoral sites and infections:** periodontal pockets, dental plaque biofilm; chronic periodontitis and dentoalveolar abscess; it is one of the three major so-called 'red complex' or 'keystone' periodontopathogens (Chapter 33).

Genus *Fusobacterium*

Slender, cigar-shaped Gram-negative rods with rounded ends (see Fig. 18.1):

■ **Main species:** *Fusobacterium nucleatum, Fusobacterium alocis, Fusobacterium sulci, Fusobacterium periodonticum.*
■ **Cultural characteristics:** require rich media for growth and are often asaccharolytic, strict anaerobes, usually nonhaemolytic; *Fusobacterium nucleatum* can produce ammonia and hydrogen sulphide from cysteine and methionine and is implicated as an odorigenic organism in halitosis.
■ **Main intraoral sites and infections:** most common isolate is *Fusobacterium nucleatum*; normal gingival crevice, tonsils (*Fusobacterium alocis* and *Fusobacterium sulci*) or periodontal infections (*Fusobacterium periodonticum*); acute ulcerative gingivitis, dentoalveolar abscess.

Genus *Leptotrichia*

Gram-negative filaments with at least one pointed end:

■ **Main species:** *Leptotrichia buccalis.*
■ **Cultural characteristics:** strict anaerobes, with colonies resembling fusobacteria.
■ **Main intraoral sites and infections:** dental plaque biofilm. No known disease association.

Genus *Wolinella*

Gram-negative curved bacilli, motile by polar flagella:

■ **Main species:** *Wolinella succinogenes* (*Wolinella recta* and *Wolinella curva* are now assigned to the Campylobacter genus).
■ Cultural characteristics: strict anaerobe.
■ **Main intraoral sites and infections:** gingival crevice; possible involvement in destructive periodontal disease.

Genus *Selenomonas*

Gram-negative curved cells with tufts of flagella:

■ **Main species:** *Selenomonas sputigena, Selenomonas noxia, Selenomonas flueggei, Selenomonas infelix, Selenomonas diane.*

- **Cultural characteristics:** strict anaerobe.
- **Main intraoral sites and infections:** gingival crevice. No known disease association.

Genus *Treponema*

Motile Gram-negative helical cells, in three main sizes (large, medium and small):

- **Main species:** *Treponema denticola, Treponema macrodentium, Treponema skoliodontium, Treponema socranskii, Treponema maltophilum, Treponema amylovarum, Treponema vincentii.*
- **Cultural characteristics:** all treponemes are strict anaerobes and difficult to culture. Require enriched media with serum. Characterization poor; *Treponema denticola* is asaccharolytic; *Treponema socranskii* ferments carbohydrates to acetic, lactic and succinic acids.
- **Main intraoral sites and infections:** *Treponema denticola* is more proteolytic than others and possesses proline aminopeptidase and arginine-specific protease; it also degrades collagen and gelatin. Found in the gingival crevice; closely associated with acute ulcerative gingivitis, a destructive periodontal disease; one of the so-called 'red complex' or 'keystone' periodontopathogens (Chapter 33).

A NOTE ON UNCULTIVABLE BACTERIA

As stated, it is now estimated that only about 50% of the oral bacteria that can be visualized by microscopy can be cultivated through traditional laboratory culture techniques. The identity and the role of these so-called **uncultivable bacteria (syn; unculturable bacteria)** are mostly an enigma. There are two major reasons why these bacteria cannot be cultured: first, their nutritional requirements are unknown and, second, they coexist in a supportive ecosystem in tandem with neighbouring organisms that sustain them nutritionally as well as physically (through an intricate architectural hierarchy; Figs. 31.3 and 31.4). Some examples of novel species and clones of bacteria detected from subgingival plaque biofilm using 16S rRNA and other techniques such as pyrosequencing are given in Table 31.1.

ORAL MYCOBIOME

For many generations, it was generally thought that fungi belonging to the *Candida* species were the only organisms that could survive within the oralome (Chapter 22), and if other fungi were isolated from oral samples, they were considered transient oral colonizers. Numerous studies using conventional culture techniques have clearly shown that approximately one-half of the population, irrespective of their origin, carries commensal *Candida* species in the oral cavity. In the **'very young, the very old and the very sick'**, these yeasts may proliferate, leading to various forms of opportunistic oral candidal infections due to a dysbiotic mycobiome. (see Chapter 35).

The notion that *Candida* is the supreme fungal inhabitant of the oral microbiome has been overturned by recent NGS studies. It is now clear that, apart from *Candida*,

there is a so-called **basal oral fungal microbiome**, a '**mycobiome**' (Greek: *Mykes*, fungus), comprising many different fungal genera. Some studies have identified up to 101 cultivable and noncultivable fungal species in the oral cavity! The current thinking is that the basal oral mycobiome ranges from relatively common *Candida* species to others such as *Aspergillus, Fusarium, Penicillium* and *Cryptococcus* species. Some of the latter are agents of invasive infections, especially in debilitated and compromised populations.

It is, however, important to note that in terms of the population size, *Candida* species are yet the predominant fungal residents of the oral mycobiome. The most abundant species in this genus is *C. albicans*, followed by *C. glabrata, C. parapsilosis, C. tropicalis, C. krusei* and *C. kefyr.*

ORAL VIROME

It is now thought that viruses and bacteriophages (that usually 'hitch a ride' within viruses) may be indigenous to the oralome, constituting the oral virobiome or oral virome. The viruses may be dormant and silently reside within the lining epithelium or, when appropriate conditions supervene, arrive via the nerve trunks of the trigeminal nerve from time to time to cause disease. The oral virome is highly variable between individuals but remarkably stable over time within each individual. **Herpesviridae** and **Papillomaviridae** are the most common virus families present in healthy oral cavities.

Herpes group of viruses are the predominant constituents of the oral virome as described in Chapter 21. Herpes simplex, for example, causes gingivostomatitis or a subclinical infection, and the virus can subsequently enter a dormant state in the trigeminal ganglion. It may be reactivated in response to external stimuli such as stress and cold weather, and recrudescent infection may manifest as herpes labialis (cold sores). The human papilloma virus, by contrast, resides in some 10% of the human population and may cause papillomas, condylomas and focal epithelial hyperplasia for reasons that are yet unclear. The role of human papilloma and related viruses in oral cancer is currently a hot topic of research.

Viruses with a short, transient oral presence include organisms associated with systemic disease, and these include the mumps and rabies viruses that infest the salivary glands and are secreted in the saliva of affected individuals. Further, viruses causing respiratory tract infections are commonly present in the mouth during the acute phase of these diseases. Noteworthy is the coronaviruses such as SARS-CoV-2, agent of COVID-19, residing in the oral epithelium and salivary gland tissue, particularly during the acute phase of the disease, and sometimes during convalescence. A small proportion of the population can also be asymptomatic oral carriers of SARS-CoV-2 as well.

Similarly, blood-borne viruses such as the hepatitis viruses (hepatitis B, C, D and F) and human immunodeficiency virus (HIV) can enter the mouth via gingival crevicular fluid in affected individuals and shed through mixed saliva. Hence, it is of critical importance to implement standard infection control measures in clinical dentistry (see Chapter 37).

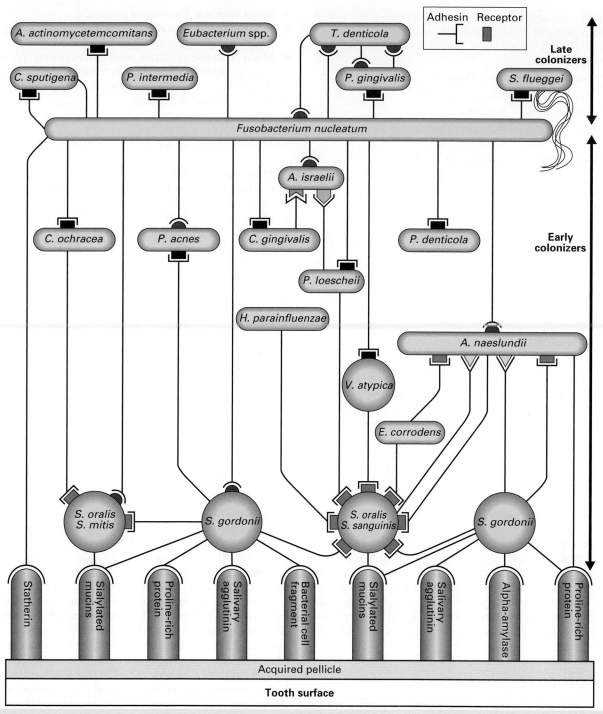

Fig. 31.4 A schematic picture illustrating the various interactions of oral microbial species that lead to plaque biofilm formation. See text for the generic name of the species listed.

ORAL PHAGEOME

Bacteriophage (*syn.* phage) is a virus that has the ability to infect and replicate within bacteria as well as archaea (Chapter 3) Indeed, the vast majority of viruses in the oral cavity are essentially bacteriophages, and they could be considered as a subcomponent of the oral virome. The main bacteriophage families of the healthy oral cavity appear to be **Siphoviridae**, **Myoviridae**, and **Podoviridae**, all belonging to the **Caudovirales** order.

Phages are thought to play a major role in modulating the oral microbiome through mechanisms such as **bacteriolysis and/orlysogeny** (destroying the bacterial host or incorporating its nucleic acid into the host genome) and **spreading antibiotic-resistance genes** from one organism to the other.

These bacteriophages play a decisive role in maintaining a healthy microbiome as their lytic process has the potential to exterminate bacterial species in the community and thereby modify or subvert the communal functions on the

Table 31.1 Examples of Novel Species and Clones of Bacteria Detected in Subgingival Plaque Using 16S Ribosomal RNA (rRNA) and Other Techniques Such as Pyrosequencing

Named Species	Novel Phylotype
Atopobium parvulum	Selenomonas clone
Catonella morbi	Megasphaera clone
Slackia exigua	Eubacterium clone
Filifactor alocis	TM7 (clone 1025)
Dialister pneumosintes	Deferribacteres clone

Note: The significance of these isolates and their role in oral disease is still speculative.

neighboring bacteria. Phages are thought to account for **20–80% of total bacterial death** in the oralome, thus representing a major bacterial-growth limiting factor. For example, phage infestation of two common bacterial species, *Veillonella* spp. and *Streptococcus* spp., may profoundly affect the overall biofilm composition.

ORAL ARCHAEOME

Bacteria and Archaea are morphologically similar organisms and comprise the third domain of life (Chapter 2). Archaea are given the term **extremophiles**, as they are found in extreme environments, such as thermal vents in the deep sea. Some **Archaea produce methane from carbon dioxide** as an energy source for growth A total of five different methanogenic Archaea genera have been isolated from the healthy oral cavity. These are *Methanobrevibacter*, *Methanosphaera*, *Methanosarcina*, *Thermoplasmata* and *Methanobacterium*. The predominant oral Archaea species isolated in most studies is *Methanobrevibacter oralis* and *Methanosarcina mazei*.

The specific role of the archaeome in either health or disease is still unclear. A number of studies have identified increased numbers of *Methanobrevibacter oralis* in periodontitis, periimplantitis and necrotic root canals. As they coexist with periodontal pathogens, such as *Treponema denticola*, *Tannerella forsythia* and *Porphyromonas gingivalis*, they may be associated with this all-too-common infection.

ORAL PROTOZOME

Some consider oral virome and phageome as a single entity as phages are bacterial viruses. Oral protozoans were first noted in very early microscopic studies of plaque samples of patients with very **poor oral hygiene** and **periodontal disease**. Hence, they were thought to be agents of periodontal disease, a notion that has not been proven. They are currently considered **harmless saprophytes** and mere passengers lurking within unhealthy mouths with an abundant provision of **food debris and bacteria** for their sustenance.

Two main protozoon species of the normal microbiome are *Entamoeba gingivalis* and *Trichomonas tenax*.

Genus *Entamoeba*

Large, motile amoebae about 12 μm in diameter:

- **Main species:** *Entamoeba gingivalis*.
- **Cultural characteristics:** strict anaerobe; complex medium; cannot be easily cultured.
- **Main intraoral sites and infections:** periodontal tissues, especially in patients who have received radiotherapy and are on metronidazole. Its role, if any, in periodontal disease is unclear.

Genus *Trichomonas*

Flagellated protozoa, about 7.5 μm in diameter:

- **Main species:** *Trichomonas tenax*.
- **Cultural characteristics:** strict anaerobe; complex medium; difficult to grow in pure culture.
- **Main intraoral sites and infections:** gingival crevice of unhygienic mouths; its role in disease is unclear.

Finally, it is noteworthy that a number of **oral Mycoplasma species** (*Mycoplasma buccale*, *Mycoplasma orale* and *Mycoplasma salivarium*) has been isolated from saliva. There pathogenicity, if any, is yet unknown. (Chapter 20).

The Oral Ecosystem

Ecology is the study of the relationships between living organisms and their environment. An understanding of oral ecology is essential to comprehend the pathogenesis of diseases, such as caries and periodontal disease, caused by oral bacteria.

THE ORAL ENVIRONMENT

The human mouth is lined by **stratified squamous epithelium**. This is modified in areas according to function (e.g., the tongue) and interrupted by other structures such as teeth and salivary ducts. The gingival tissues form a cuff around each tooth, and there is a continuous exudate of **crevicular fluid** from the gingival crevice. A thin layer of saliva bathes the surface of the oral mucosa.

The mouth, being an extension of an external body site, has a natural microflora. This **commensal** (or indigenous, or resident) flora exists in harmony with the host, but disease conditions supervene when this relationship is broken. The predominant dental diseases in humans (caries and periodontal disease) are caused in this manner. In addition to the commensal flora, others (such as coliforms) survive in the mouth only for short periods (**transient flora**). These transient species cannot get a foothold in the oral environment due to the ecological pressure—that is, the **colonization resistance** exerted by the resident flora. Indeed, these residents are considered critical in defending the key portal of entry into the digestive system.

The oral ecosystem comprises the oral flora, the different sites of the oral cavity where they grow (i.e., **habitats**) and the associated surroundings.

Oral Habitats

The major oral habitats are:

- buccal mucosa
- dorsum of the tongue

- tooth surfaces (both supragingival and subgingival)
- crevicular epithelium
- prosthodontic and orthodontic appliances and dental fillings, if present.

Buccal Mucosa and Dorsum of the Tongue. Special features and niches of the oral mucosa contribute to the diversity of the flora—for instance, the cheek mucosa is relatively sparsely colonized, whereas the papillary surface of the tongue is highly colonized because of the safe refuge provided by the papillae. The papillary surface of the tongue has a low redox potential (E_h), promoting the growth of anaerobic flora, and thus may serve as a reservoir for some of the Gram-negative anaerobes implicated in periodontal disease. Further, the keratinized and nonkeratinized mucosae may offer refuge to variants of oral flora.

Some have described various organizational arrangements of the bacteriome of the tongue dorsum, with the tissue surface characterized by a layer of *Actinomyces* spp., followed by a layer of *Streptococcus* spp. taxa, such as *Rothia*, *Gemella* and *Veillonella* spp., present in clusters and stripes in the interior of the biofilm, suggesting that the biofilm grew outwardly from the basal layer.

Teeth. The surfaces of the teeth are the **only nonshedding area of the body** that harbours a microbial population. Masses of bacteria and their products constantly accumulate on tooth surfaces to produce plaque biofilms, in both healthy and disease states. Plaque is a classic example of a **natural biofilm** and is the major agent initiating caries and periodontal disease. In the disease state, there is a shift in the composition of the plaque flora from a symbiotic equilibrium (also called ebiosis) that predominates in the healthy state to a dysbiotic disease state (see Chapters 32 and 33).

A range of habitats are associated with the tooth surface (Fig. 31.5). The nature of the bacterial community varies depending on the anatomical profile of the tooth concerned and the degree of exposure to the environment. For instance, smooth surfaces are colonized by a smaller number of species than pits and fissures while subgingival surfaces are more anaerobic than supragingival surfaces.

Crevicular Epithelium and Gingival Crevice. Although this habitat is only a minor region of the oral environment, bacteria that colonize the crevicular area play a critical role in the initiation and development of gingival and periodontal disease.

Four different layers have been identified in subgingival crevicular biofilms: a **basal layer** (close to the tooth surface) is formed mainly by *Actinomyces* spp., followed by a *second layer* of spindlelike bacteria, such as *F. nucleatum* and *Tannarella* spp.; the *third layer* is formed by filamentous, rod-shaped and coccoid-shaped cells belonging to the *Bacteroides* and other species cluster; the *fourth and final layer* is a 'palisade-like', top, lining layer, which is in close contact with the gingival surface.

Prosthodontic and Orthodontic Appliances and Dental Fillings. If present and not kept scrupulously clean, dental appliances may act as **inanimate reservoirs** of bacteria and yeasts. Yeasts on the fitting surface of full dentures can initiate *Candida*-associated denture stomatitis due to poor denture hygiene.

If not properly cleaned, plaque biofilms may grow to varying extents on amalgam or composite dental fillings depending on their size, shape, location and quality. These may cause **secondary caries** at the margins of fillings, or gingivitis if located near gingivae. Secondary caries lesions should be distinguished from **recurrent caries** lesions which are located underneath dental restorations.

FACTORS MODULATING MICROBIAL GROWTH

Different microenvironments in the mouth support their own microflora, which differ both qualitatively and quantitatively. The reasons for such variations are complex and include anatomical, salivary, crevicular fluid and microbial factors, among others.

Anatomical Factors

Bacterial stagnation areas are created as a result of:

- shape of the teeth
- topography of the teeth (e.g., occlusal fissures)
- malalignment of teeth
- poor quality of restorations (e.g., fillings and bridges)
- nonkeratinized sulcular epithelium.

These areas are difficult to clean, either by the natural flushing action of saliva or by tooth-brushing.

Saliva

Whole (mixed) saliva bathing oral surfaces is derived from the **major** (parotid, submandibular and sublingual) and **minor** (labial, lingual, buccal and palatal) salivary glands. It is a complex mixture of inorganic ions, including sodium, potassium, calcium, chloride, bicarbonate and phosphate; the concentrations of these ions vary diurnally and in stimulated and resting saliva. The major organic constituents of saliva are proteins and glycoproteins (such as mucin), which modulate bacterial growth (Table 31.2) in the following ways:

- adsorption on the tooth surfaces forms a **salivary pellicle**, a conditioning film that facilitates bacterial adhesion
- acting as a readily available, primary source of **food** (carbohydrates and proteins)

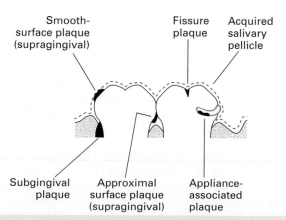

Smooth-surface plaque (supragingival)

Fissure plaque

Acquired salivary pellicle

Subgingival plaque

Approximal surface plaque (supragingival)

Appliance-associated plaque

Fig. 31.5 Habitats associated with tooth surfaces and the nomenclature of plaque biofilm derived from these habitats.

Table 31.2   Specific and Nonspecific Host Defence Factors of the Mouth

Defence Factors	Main Function
NONSPECIFIC	
Epithelial desquamation	Physical removal of microbes
Saliva flow	Physical removal of microbes
Mucin/agglutinins	Physical removal of microbes
Lysozyme-protease-anion	Cell lysis (bactericidal, fungicidal)
Lactoferrin	Iron sequestration (bactericidal, fungicidal)
Apolactoferrin	Iron sequestration (bactericidal, fungicidal)
Sialoperoxidase system	Hypothiocyanite production (neutral pH), hypocyanous acid production (low pH)
Histidine-rich peptides	Antibacterial and antifungal activity
Secretory leukocyte protease inhibitor (SLPI)	Blocks cell surface receptors needed for entry of human immunodeficiency virus (HIV)
Calprotectin	Antimicrobial
Cathelicidin	Antimicrobial
Chitinase and chromogranin	Antifungal
SPECIFIC	
Intraepithelial lymphocytes and Langerhans cells	Cellular barrier to penetrating bacteria and/or antigens
Secretory immunoglobulin A (IgA)	Prevents microbial adhesion and metabolism
IgG, IgA, IgM	Prevent microbial adhesion, opsonins, complement activators
Complement	Activates neutrophils
Neutrophils/macrophages	Phagocytosis

Note: See also Tables 8.1, 8.2 and 8.3.

- **aggregation of bacteria**, thereby facilitating their clearance from the mouth, or deposition on surfaces, contributing to plaque biofilm formation
- **growth inhibition** of exogenous organisms by nonspecific defence factors (e.g., lysozyme, lactoferrin and histatins, which are bactericidal and fungicidal) and specific defence factors (e.g., Igs, mainly IgA and salivary leukocyte protease inhibitor (SLPI), which destroys HIV)
- **maintenance of pH** with its excellent buffering capacity (acidic saliva promotes growth of cariogenic bacteria).

Gingival Crevicular Fluid

There is a continuous but slow flow of gingival crevicular fluid in the healthy state, and this increases during inflammation (e.g., gingivitis). The composition of crevicular fluid is similar to that of serum, and thus the crevice is protected by these 'surrogate'-specific and nonspecific defence factors of serum. Crevicular fluid can influence the ecology of the crevice by:

- **flushing** microbes out of the crevice
- acting as a primary source of **nutrients**: proteolytic and saccharolytic bacteria in the crevice can utilize the crevicular fluid to provide peptides, amino acids and carbohydrates for growth; essential cofactors (e.g., haemin)

can be obtained by degrading haem-containing molecules such as haemoglobin
- maintaining pH
- providing specific and nonspecific **defence** factors: IgG predominates (IgM and IgA are both present to a lesser extent)
- **phagocytosis:** 95% of leukocytes in the crevicular fluid are neutrophils.

Microbial Factors

Microbes in the oral environment can interact with each other both in promoting and suppressing the neighbouring bacteria. Mechanisms that accomplish this include:

- **competition for receptors** for adhesion by prior occupation of colonizing sites and prevention of attachment of 'late-comers'
- **production of toxins**, such as **bacteriocins**, that kill cells of the same or other bacterial species—for example *Streptococcus salivarius* produces an inhibitor (enocin) that inhibits *Streptococcus pyogenes*
- production of **metabolic end-products** such as short-chain carboxylic acids, which **lower the pH** and also act as noxious, antagonistic agents
- use of **metabolic end-products** of other bacteria for **nutritional** purposes (e.g., *Veillonella* spp. use acids produced by *Streptococcus mutans*)
- **coaggregation** with the same species (homotypic) or different species (heterotypic) of bacteria—for example corn-cob formation (Fig. 31.3)
- production of specific messenger chemicals called **quorum-sensing molecules** (such as homoserine lactone) that helps the resident bacteria to communicate (i.e., cross-talk) with each other within a biofilm community and maintain homeostasis of the biofilm. Such microbial cross talk through quorum-sensing molecules may be between bacteria and bacteria (intra-kingdom) or between bacteria and fungi (inter-kingdom).

The foregoing phenomena, which enable the commensal oral flora to suppress or inhibit the growth of exogenous, nonoral organisms and thereby exclude them from their communal neighbourhood habitats, are called **colonization resistance** mechanisms.

Miscellaneous Factors

Local Environmental pH. Many microbes require a neutral pH for growth. The acidity of most oral surfaces is regulated by saliva (mean pH approx. 6.7). Depending on the frequency of intake of dietary carbohydrates, the pH of plaque biofilm can fall to as low as 5.0 as a result of bacterial sugar metabolism. Under these conditions, acidophilic organisms can grow well (e.g., *mutans* group streptococci, lactobacilli, yeast), whereas others are eliminated by competitive inhibition.

Oxidation–Reduction Potential. The oxidation–reduction potential of the environment (E_h) varies in different locations of the mouth. For instance, redox potential falls during plaque biofilm development from an initial E_h of over +200 mV (highly oxidized) to −141 mV (highly reduced) after 7 days. Such fluctuations favour the growth of different groups of bacteria.

Antimicrobial Therapy. Systemic or topical antibiotics and antiseptics affect the oral flora—for instance, broad-spectrum antibiotics such as tetracycline can wipe out most of the endogenous flora and favour the emergence of yeast species.

Diet. Fermentable carbohydrates are the main class of compounds that alter the oral ecology. They act as a major source of nutrients, promoting the growth of acidogenic flora. The production of extracellular polysaccharides facilitates adherence of organisms to surfaces, whereas the intracellular polysaccharides serve as a food resource.

Iatrogenic Factors. Procedures such as dental scaling can radically alter the composition of the periodontal pocket flora of diseased sites and shift the balance in favour of colonization of such sites by flora that are associated with health.

Nutrition of Oral Bacteria

Oral bacteria obtain their food from a number of sources. These include **host resources**:

- remnants of the host diet always present in the oral cavity (e.g., sucrose, starch)
- salivary constituents (e.g., glycoproteins, minerals, vitamins)
- crevicular exudate (e.g., proteins)
- gaseous environment (although most require only a very low level of oxygen) and microbial resources
- extracellular microbial products of the neighbouring bacteria, especially in dense communities such as the plaque biofilm
- intracellular food storage (glycogen) granules.

ACQUISITION OF THE NORMAL ORAL FLORA

1. The infant mouth is **sterile at birth**, except perhaps for a few organisms acquired from the mother's birth canal.
2. A few hours later, the organisms from the mother's (or the nurse's) mouth and possibly a few from the environment are established in the mouth.
3. These **pioneer species** are usually streptococci, which bind to mucosal epithelium (e.g., *Streptococcus salivarius*).
4. The metabolic activity of the pioneer community then alters the oral environment to facilitate colonization by other bacterial genera and species. For instance, *Streptococcus salivarius* produces extracellular polymers from sucrose, to which other bacteria such as *Actinomyces* spp. can attach (Figs. 31.3 and 31.4).
5. When the composition of this complex ecosystem (comprising several genera and species in varying numbers) reaches equilibrium, a **climax community** is said to exist. (*Note:* This is a highly dynamic system.)
6. Oral flora on the child's first birthday usually consists of streptococci, staphylococci, neisseriae and lactobacilli, together with some anaerobes such as *Veillonella* and fusobacteria. Less frequently isolated are *Lactobacillus*, *Actinomyces*, *Prevotella* and *Fusobacterium* species.
7. The next evolutionary change in this community occurs during and *after tooth eruption* when two further niches

are provided for bacterial colonization: the hard-tissue surface of enamel and the gingival crevice. Organisms that prefer hard-tissue colonization, such as *Streptococcus mutans*, *Streptococcus sanguinis* and *Actinomyces* spp., then selectively colonize enamel surfaces, and those preferring anaerobic environments, such as *Prevotella* spp., *Porphyromonas* spp. and spirochaetes, colonize the crevicular tissues. However, the anaerobes do not appear in significant numbers until adolescence. For instance, only 18–40% of 5-year-olds have spirochaetes and black-pigmented anaerobes compared with 90% of 13- to 16-year-olds.

8. A second childhood (in terms of oral bacterial colonization) is reached if all teeth are surgically extracted. Bacteria that colonize the mouth at this stage are very similar to those in a child prior to tooth eruption.
9. Introduction of a prosthetic appliance at any stage changes the microbial composition once again. Growth of *Candida* species is particularly increased after the introduction of acrylic dentures, while it is now recognized that the prevalence of *Staphylococcus aureus* and lactobacilli is high in those age 70 and over. The denture plaque biofilm is somewhat similar to plaque biofilm on the enamel surface; it may also harbour significant quantities of yeast.

The Plaque Biofilm

The plaque biofilm is a tenacious microbial community embedded in an extracellular polysaccharide matrix, attached to either the soft- or hard-tissue surfaces of the mouth, and comprising living and dead bacteria and their extracellular products, together with host compounds, mainly derived from the saliva.

COMPOSITION

The organisms in plaque biofilm are embedded in an organic matrix, which comprises about 30% of the total volume. The matrix is derived from the products of both the host and biofilm constituents. In the gingival area, proteins from the crevicular exudate become incorporated into the plaque biofilm. This matrix acts as a food reserve and as a cement, binding organisms both to each other and to various surfaces.

The microbial composition of dental plaque biofilm can vary widely among individuals; some people are so-called 'rapid plaque formers' and others 'slow plaque formers'. Further, there are large variations in plaque composition within an individual, for example:

- at different sites on the same tooth
- at the same site on different teeth
- at different times on the same tooth site.

DISTRIBUTION

Plaque biofilm is found on dental surfaces and appliances especially in the absence of oral hygiene. In general, it is found in anatomical areas protected from the host defences—for example, occlusal fissures, interproximally or around the gingival crevice. Plaque samples are described in relation to their site of origin and are categorized as: **supragingival**

- fissure plaque: mainly in molar fissures
- approximal plaque: at contact points of teeth
- smooth surface: for example, buccal and palatal surfaces

subgingival, or appliance associated

- full and partial dentures (denture plaque)
- orthodontic appliance-related plaque.

MICROBIAL ADHERENCE AND PLAQUE BIOFILM FORMATION

Adherence of a microbe to an oral surface is an **essential prerequisite for colonization and biofilm formation**. It is also the initial step in the path leading to subsequent infection and invasion of tissues. A number of intrinsic host factors prevent microbial colonization on oral surfaces, and these include (Fig. 31.6):

- the mucosal barrier with constant **desquamation** of the epithelium that dislodges the attached organisms from soft-tissue surfaces
- the dynamic **salivary flow** patterns in different oral niches
- the **muscular movements** of the tongue and cheeks that physically dislodge the biofilms
- the nonspecific and specific defence factors (such as IgA) in saliva
- the **resident community of microbiota** that offers 'colonization resistance' to invading extraneous organisms.

Plaque Biofilm Formation

Plaque biofilm formation is a complex process comprising a number of different stages:

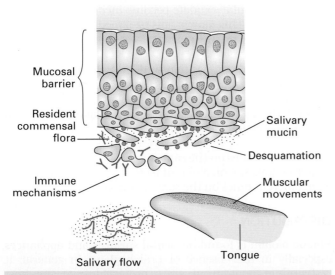

Fig. 31.6   Factors affecting microbial colonization of the oral mucosa.

1. **Pellicle formation.** Adsorption of host and bacterial molecules to the tooth surface forms the acquired salivary pellicle. A thin **layer of salivary glycoproteins** is deposited on the surface of a tooth within minutes of exposure to the oral environment. Oral bacteria initially attach to the pellicle and not directly to enamel (i.e., hydroxyapatite).
2. **Transport.** Bacteria approach the vicinity of the tooth surface prior to attachment, by means of natural salivary flow, Brownian motion or chemotaxis.
3. **Long-range interactions** involve physicochemical interactions between the microbial cell surface and the pellicle-coated tooth. Interplay of van der Waals forces and electrostatic repulsion produces a primary **reversible phase** of net adhesion.
4. **Short-range interactions** consist of stereochemical reactions between **adhesins** on the microbial cell surface and **receptors** on the acquired pellicle. This is an **irreversible phase** in which polymer bridging between organisms and the surface helps to anchor the organisms, after which they multiply on the virgin surface. Doubling times of plaque biofilm bacteria can vary considerably (from minutes to hours), both between different bacterial species and between members of the same species, depending on the environmental conditions.
5. **Coaggregation or coadhesion.** Fresh bacteria now attach onto the already attached first generation of cells (also called pioneer or initial colonizers); these may be bacteria of the same genus or different but compatible genera (Fig. 31.4).
6. **Biofilm formation.** The attached organisms now grow horizontally on the surface and form micro-colonies at first while the aforementioned process continues with a resultant confluent growth and the formation of a biofilm, which matures in complexity as time progresses. Simply defined, biofilm is a complex functional community of one or more species of microbes encased in an extracellular polysaccharide matrix and attached to one another or to a solid surface. The latter could be an inert surface such as tooth enamel, denture acrylic or a plastic catheter or alternatively an organic/living surface such as a heart valve. Architecturally, the biofilm is *not* a flat compact structure resembling an inert piece of concrete. The aggregates of organisms are arranged in columns or mushroom-shaped structures interspersed with water channels that carry metabolites and bring in nutrients (Figs. 5.2 and 5.3).

Thus biofilm formation is a complex, competitive, sequential and dynamic colonization process, and in plaque biofilms, this complexity is further compounded due to the participation of different categories of oral bacteria. Specifically, the **pioneer group** of organisms called '**early or initial colonizers**' that selectively colonize the salivary pellicle during plaque biofilm formation are Gram-positive saccharolytic aerobes and facultative anaerobes that primarily feed on oral glycoproteins and salivary mucins with 80% of the early colonizers being represented by *Streptococcus* species.

After the initial colonization, these early colonizers change their metabolic and gene expression profiles to produce and secrete **extracellular polysaccharides** (EPS), proteins, lipids and extracellular DNA (eDNA). Production

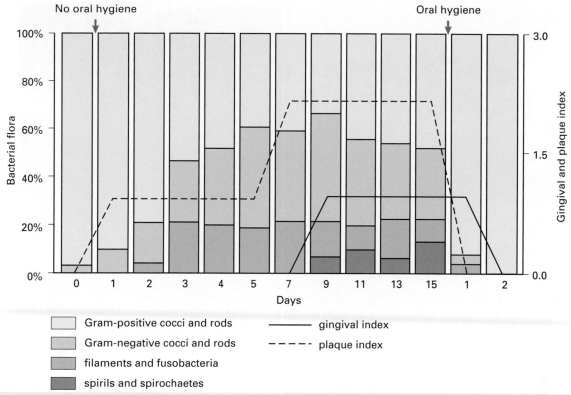

Fig. 31.7 Results from an experimental study showing the predominant groups of organisms comprising the pioneer and the climax community of plaque. Note the relationship between the plaque index and the gingival index. Note the dramatic reduction of the plaque biofilm, as well as the gingival and plaque index, immediately after oral hygeine is initiated (on the 16th day, i.e., depicted here as days 1 and 2 on the right (bottom axis)).

and secretion of EPS confer several advantages to the young biofilm, such as retention of nutrients in the vicinity due and protection from environmental stresses, such as antibiotics and antiseptics diffusing through saliva (e.g., cells embedded in biofilm matrices are up to 1000-fold more tolerant to antibiotics compared to their planktonic counterparts).

The metabolic products of the early plaque biofilm colonizers also radically alter the immediate environment (e.g., create a low redox potential suitable for anaerobes), leading to new colonizers inhabiting the biofilm, with a resultant gradual increase in microbial complexity, biomass and thickness.

Early colonizers are then followed by Gram-negative cocci and rods, and finally by filaments, fusobacteria and spirochaetes. Such an example of a natural succession of plaque flora has been elegantly demonstrated in **'experimental gingivitis' studies**, where groups of individuals, initially subjected to meticulous oral hygiene, were then followed up during a phase of no oral hygiene, and the freshly developing plaque flora was monitored closely. Results of such a study are shown in Fig. 31.7.

As a result of this dynamic process, the plaque biofilm mass reaches a critical size at which a balance between the deposition and loss of plaque bacteria is established; this community is termed the **climax community** (Fig. 31.8).

The **molecular biology** of biofilm formation is complex. Biofilm bacteria appear to maintain their complex structure through continuous secretion of low levels of molecules called **quorum-sensing molecules** (e.g., homoserine lactone, autoinducer-2) that coordinate gene expression. As the number of organisms in the biofilm increases, there is a simultaneous, proportionate increase in the quorum-sensing signals. These activate genes that may be related to additional extracellular polysaccharide production, or reduction of metabolism (for bacteria at the bottom of the matrix) or production of virulent factors, including drug-destroying genes.

Detachment

The bacteria that colonize this climax community may detach and enter the **planktonic** phase (i.e., suspended in saliva) and be transported to new colonization sites, thus restarting the whole cycle.

FURTHER NOTES ON BIOFILMS

The realization of the fact that up to 65% of human infections are caused by organisms encased in biofilms (i.e., **sessile** organisms) as opposed to **planktonic** or free-living forms has resulted in much research and a vast literature on the behaviour of these two rather divergent lifestyles of microbes. There is also a preponderance of biofilms in nature—for instance, as slimy coats that grow in stagnant water or water pipes (see Chapter 38 for biofilms in dental unit water lines). In clinical terms, it is recognized that biofilm organisms are more resistant to antibiotics and chemotherapeutic agents than their planktonic counterparts (see Chapter 5). The problem of drug resistance, however, is not a major concern in dental plaque biofilms due to their ready accessibility to mechanical cleansing measures. However, drug

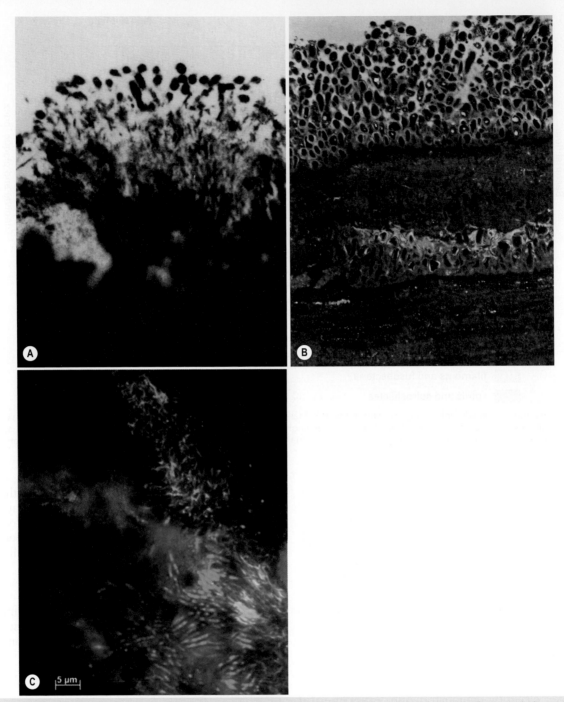

Fig. 31.8 Micrographs of (A) smooth-surface plaque showing the many relationships between different bacterial forms, including palisading and corn-cob formation and (B) mature plaque with compact bacteria and calcification at the base (approximately × 5000). (C) Mature subgingival plaque biofilms stained by fluorescent in situ hybridization (FISH) technique showing nonspecific bacteria (green), group 1 treponemes (orange) and *Fusobacterium* species (magenta) colonizing distinct parts of the biofilm. Some gingival host cell nuclei are stained blue with a nucleic acid stain. (Image courtesy Dr. Annette Motte.)

resistance due to biofilms in other diseased states (e.g., airways infection by *Pseudomonas aeruginosa* in cystic fibrosis) is a major therapeutic problem.

CALCULUS FORMATION

Calcium and phosphate ions derived from saliva may become deposited within deeper layers of dental plaque biofilm (as saliva is supersaturated with respect to these ions). If the plaque biofilm is allowed to grow undisturbed, then the degenerating bacteria in a climax community may act as seeding agents of mineralization. The process is accelerated by bacterial phosphatases and proteases that degrade some of the calcification inhibitors in saliva (statherin and proline-rich proteins). These processes lead to the formation of **insoluble calcium phosphate** crystals that coalesce to form a calcified mass of plaque, termed **calculus**.

Many toothpastes now contain pyrophosphate compounds that adsorb excess calcium ions, thus reducing intraplaque mineral deposition. In general, mature calculus is composed of 80% (dry weight) mineralized material, mostly hydroxyapatite while the remainder (20%) is non-mineralized organic compounds.

Structure

The structure of calculus is shown in Fig. 31.8. Predominant flora are cocci, bacilli and filaments (especially in the outer layers), and occasionally spiral organisms. The bacteria near the enamel surface tend to have a reduced cytoplasm-to-cell wall ratio, suggesting that they are metabolically inactive. Supragingival calculus contains more Gram-positive organisms, whereas subgingival calculus tends to contain more Gram-negative species.

In some areas (especially the outer surface), cocci attach and grow on the surface of filamentous microorganisms, giving a **'corn-cob'** arrangement (Fig. 31.3). The filamentous bacteria tend to orient themselves at right angles to the enamel surface, producing a palisade effect (like books on a shelf). The cytoplasm of some bacteria (mainly cocci) may contain glycogenlike food-storage granules, available as a ready source of nutrition during periods of adversity.

Calculus has a rough surface and is porous, thus serving as an ideal reservoir for bacterial toxins that are harmful to the periodontium (e.g., lipopolysaccharides (LPSs)). Hence, removal of calculus is essential to maintain good periodontal health.

The role of dental plaque biofilm in caries and periodontal disease is discussed in Chapters 32 and 33, respectively.

THE ROLE OF ORAL FLORA IN SYSTEMIC INFECTION: THE ORAL–SYSTEMIC AXIS

Over the last two decades or so, it has been recognized that plaque biofilm–related oral diseases, especially periodontitis, *may* alter the course and pathogenesis of a number of systemic diseases. This is a resurgence of a common belief called **'focal infection theory'** popular in the late 19th and early 20th century, where clinicians believed that oral foci of infection may lead to systemic diseases including heart disease and diabetes. However, it is important to note that definitive evidence for such outcomes are not available as yet, for most of these postulated oral–systemic links. They seem to be mere associations, and *associations do not necessarily prove causality*.

Numerous research groups have now studied the oral–systemic connectivity, and up to some 100 diseases ranging from dementia and Alzheimer's disease to erectile dysfunction have been explored for possible linking pathways! A convincing body of data indicate that the following diseases have a *stronger association* than others with a dysbiotic oral microbiome, particularly periodontal inflammation:

- cardiovascular disease
  - infective endocarditis (see Chapter 24)
  - coronary heart disease: atherosclerosis and myocardial infection
  - stroke
- hospital-acquired (i.e., nosocomial) bacterial pneumonia
- diabetes mellitus

- adverse pregnancy outcomes (e.g., low-birth-weight babies)
- Alzheimer's disease.

At least three major mechanisms linking oral infections to secondary systemic disease have been postulated (Fig. 31.9):

1. **Metastatic infection by physical translocation of organisms**
   i. Microbes gaining entry into the circulatory system through breaches in the oral vascular barrier, as in the case of **bacteraemias** produced during tooth extractions (see Chapter 24), or indeed in the case of periodontitis, through the sites of gingival ulcerations. Periodontal bacteria, such as *Fusobacterium nucleatum*, may also translocate across the foeto-placental barrier, causing adverse pregnancy outcomes.
   ii. In hospital-acquired pneumonias, the oral microbes gain **direct entry** into the respiratory tract and the lungs through the trachea-bronchial tract or through the inserted plastic ventilator shafts.
   iii. **Direct entry** of oral microbes via the saliva into the gut may cause alterations to the gut microbiota, thereby leading to increased gut epithelial permeability and endotoxaemia, which in turn cause systemic inflammation.

2. **Metastatic injury via bacterial by-products**
   Microbial cytolytic enzymes, exotoxins and endotoxin (i.e., LPSs), gaining access to the cardiovascular system in individuals suffering from periodontitis and causing disease at distant sites.

3. **Metastatic inflammation due to immunological injury**
   i. **Proinflammatory cytokines** TNF-α and IL-1β, γ-interferon and prostaglandin E_2 reach high concentrations in periodontitis. Spillover of these mediators into the circulation may induce or aggravate systemic effects. In periodontitis, in particular, locally produced proinflammatory cytokines can enter the systemic circulation and induce an acute-phase response in the liver characterized by increased levels of **C-reactive proteins** (CRP fibrinogen and serum amyloid A), which in turn could contribute to atherosclerosis or intrauterine inflammation.
   ii. Additionally, **soluble antigens** may enter the blood stream from the oral route, react with circulating specific antibodies and form macromolecular complexes, leading to immune-mediated diseases such as Behçet's syndrome.

Of these, the mechanisms linking systemic infection and periodontal disease have been studied the most and the following are now known:

- Factors that place individuals at high risk for periodontitis may also place them at high risk for systemic disease such as atherosclerotic vascular disease. These include tobacco smoking, stress, ageing, race or ethnicity, and male gender.
- Subgingival biofilms are vast reservoirs of especially Gram-negative bacteria, and they are a continuous source of LPSs (i.e., endotoxins), which induce major vascular responses (so-called atherogenic responses). Further, LPSs

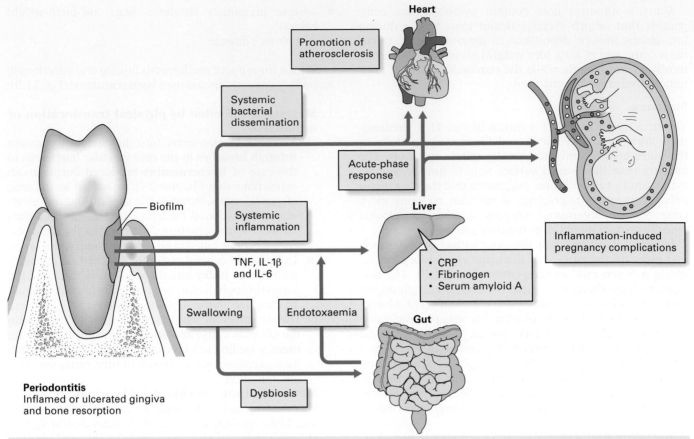

Fig. 31.9 A schematic diagram depicting postulated linking pathways between periodontal inflammation and systemic disease. In particular, the links between periodontitis and atherosclerotic heart disease and adverse pregnancy outcomes are shown (please see text for details). (Adapted, with permission from Macmillan Publishers Ltd., from Hajishengallis, G. (2015). Periodontitis: From microbial immune subversion to systemic inflammation. *Nature Reviews Immunology, 15*, 30–44.). *CRP*, C-reactive protein; *IL*, interleukin; *TNF*, tumour necrosis factor.

upregulate endothelial cell adhesion molecules and secretion of IL-1 and TNF-α.

■ Periodontium is a reservoir of cytokines.

A summary of the postulated mechanisms by which the oral microbiome may cause systemic pathology follows.

Oral Microbiome and Atherosclerosis

The possible link between oral disease and atherosclerotic vascular diseases was first postulated over four decades ago. Since then, a vast number of studies have been conducted and an extensive literature on the subject is available.

The following five mechanisms acting in combination are now thought of as the pathogenic pathways of oral dysbiosis and atherosclerotic plaque formation:

i. **Bacteraemia** from the dysbiotic periodontal/oral microbiome directly invades the arterial wall and promotes atheromatous plaque formation. There are data to show that oral bacteria can invade endothelial cells and phagocytic cells in the atheroma, leading to pathogenic changes and progression of the atheromatous lesions.

ii. Chronically inflamed oral lesions release **inflammatory mediators** such as cytokines (see above) into the blood stream, which promote plaque formation.

iii. **Autoimmunity** to host proteins caused by the host immune response to specific components of oral pathogens that promote plaque formation.

iv. Oral pathogens release specific **bacterial toxins** with pro-atherogenic effects.

v. **Promoting dyslipidemias:** It is known that patients with chronic or aggressive periodontitis have elevated serum levels of low-density lipoprotein (LDL) and triglycerides, as well as decreased levels of high-density lipoprotein (HDL).

Oral Microbiome and Hospital-Acquired Pneumonia

Hospital-acquired pneumonia (HAP) accounts for 25% of all health-care-associated infections and is classified as either **ventilator-associated** or **non-ventilator-associated pneumonia**.

HAP most frequently results from aspiration of oropharyngeal secretions into the lungs through the tubing of ventilators in ventilated patients and from microaspiration episodes of oral microbes into the lungs in nonventilated patients. Oropharyngeal secretions clearly contain a multitude of oral microbes derived either form salivary secretions or biofilm plaque.

By virtue of the fact that hospitalized patients are debilitated and routine oral hygiene measures are restricted, the oral microbiome may harbor a transient population of extraneous organisms that are not usually seen in health. These include coliform organisms (Chapter 5) such as *Escherichia coli*, *Klebsiella pneumoniae*, and *Pseudomonas aeruginosa*, as well as drug-resistant organisms such as methicillin-resistant *Staphylococcus aureus* (MRSA), *Staphylococcus aureus*, and *Streptococcus pneumoniae*. Collectively, oral colonization with these organisms poses a grave risk of both ventilator-associated and nonventilator-associated pneumonia. It is also known that ventilator-associated pneumonias have greater colonization with Gram-negative bacteria as the ventilator tubing may act as reservoirs of coliforms in such situations, especially when they are not regularly replaced.

Oral Microbiome and Type 2 Diabetes

Diabetes and periodontal disease have a so-called '*two-way relationship*' (i.e., uncontrolled diabetes exacerbates periodontal disease while chronic periodontal disease may exacerbate diabetes). Evidence for this includes:

- individuals in some communities, with a high prevalence of severe periodontitis are, in general, at an increased risk of poor glycemic control
- increased frequency of red complex periodontopathogens in plaque of individuals with type 2 diabetes
- treatment of periodontal disease-influenced glycemic control in individuals with both type 1 and type 2 diabetes
- shifts in the overall composition of oral microbiota of patients with diabetes compared to healthy controls have also been reported
- mechanical periodontal therapy is associated with a significant reduction in the hematologic indicators of diabetes (HbA1C) levels

However, more studies are needed to identify the specific oral microbes that contribute to diabetes pathogenesis and to determine the underlying mechanisms by which both an oral and gastrointestinal microbial dysbiosis relate to diabetes.

Oral Microbiome and Adverse Pregnancy Outcomes

The placenta is usually considered to be sterile. However, recent studies point to the existence of a possible pathological **placental microbiome**, which might be involved in pregnancy complications such as miscarriage, intrauterine death, neonatal death, preterm delivery and premature rupture of membranes. These reports indicate that preterm birth rates are significantly higher when bacterial invasion and an IL-6 immune response is present. Some have noted placental and amniotic fluid microbes found in preterm births (e.g., *Fusobacterium nucleatum*, *Actinomyces* spp., *Peptostreptococcus* spp. *and Candida* spp.) were similar to the oral microbiome, suggesting a possible bacteraemia from the oral cavity to the uterus during pregnancy and thereby creating the adverse outcomes.

The mechanisms by which these organisms cause such outcomes are unknown. It has been surmised that direct bacteraemia and subsequent transplacental translocation of oral microbes and/or their by-products, as well as the associated immune mechanisms described above, may play a role.

Oral Microbiome and Alzheimer's Disease

A possible link between oral pathogens and Alzheimer's disease was shown two decades ago, when oral spirochaetes were found in the blood as well as the cerebrospinal fluid of Alzheimer's disease cases but not in healthy controls. Subsequently it was noted that the prevalence of spirochaetal DNA in brain cortex was higher among Alzheimer's disease samples than in controls.

More recently, however, *Porphyromonas gingivalis* DNA was found in the sera of a predominant proportion of Alzheimer's patients, and a protease of the organism, called **gingipain**, was co-localized in amyloid plaque (Tau proteins) of patients' brain tissues. Animal experiments have also confirmed some of these findings, suggesting that a bacteraemia might have driven these pathogens form the oralome into the brain.

Other oral flora apart from *Treponemes* and *Porphyromonas gingivalis* implicated in the aetiology of Alzheimer's disease include the fungal species *Fusarium*, *Alternaria*, *Botrytis*, *Candida*, and *Malassezia*.

To conclude, apart from the well-established link between endocarditis and dental bacteraemia, and hospital-acquired pneumonias and poor oral hygiene, there is no conclusive evidence to indicate that the other postulated diseases mentioned above are either initiated or perpetuated by oral flora and their by-products. The evidence available is circumstantial at best, with a multitude of confounding factors. Therefore, further research is necessary to confirm or refute these observations. Nonetheless, it is beyond doubt that good oral health is important not only to prevent oral disease but also to maintain good systemic health.

Key Facts

- The oral microbiota comprises a diverse group of organisms and includes bacteria, fungi, archaea, protozoa and viruses and phages.
- The six key subdivisions of the oral microbiome are the bacteriome, the mycobiome and the archaeome, the virome, the phageome and the protozome.
- There are probably some 350 different **cultivable species** and a vast proportion of **unculturable flora**, currently identified using molecular techniques. Estimates are that overall, more than 700 species of bacteria inhabit the oralome.
- Streptococci are the predominant supragingival bacteria; they belong to four main **species groups**: *mutans*, *salivarius*, *anginosus* and *mitis*.
- The predominant cultivable species in subgingival plaque biofilm are ***Actinomyces***, ***Prevotella***, ***Porphyromonas***, ***Fusobacterium*** and ***Veillonella*** spp.
- The **oral ecosystem** comprises the oral **flora**, the different **sites** of the oral cavity where they grow (i.e., habitats) and the associated **surroundings**.
- The major oral habitats are the keratinized and unkeratinized buccal mucosa, including the dorsum of the tongue, tooth surfaces, crevicular epithelium and prosthodontic and orthodontic appliances, if present.
- **Adherence** of a microbe to an oral surface is a prerequisite for colonization and is the initial step in the path leading to subsequent infection or invasion of tissues.
- Saliva modulates bacterial growth by (1) providing a **pellicle** for bacterial adhesion, (2) acting as a **nutrient source**, (3) **coaggregating** bacteria, (4) providing nonspecific (e.g., lysozyme, lactoferrin and histatins) and specific (e.g., mainly immunoglobulin A (IgA)) **defence factors** and (5) maintaining **pH**.
- Microbes interact with each other by **competition** for receptors for adhesion, by production of **bacteriocins** plus **antagonistic metabolic end-products** and by **coaggregation**.
- Large masses of bacteria and their products accumulate on tooth surfaces to produce plaque biofilms, present in both healthy and disease states; plaque is an example of a natural **biofilm**.
- Stages in the plaque biofilm formation are **transport** and **adhesion/coadhesion** of bacteria leading to **irreversible attachment** with concomitant extracellular polysaccharide matrix formation.
- **Dental plaque biofilm** can be defined as a tenacious, complex microbial community, found on tooth surfaces, comprising living, dead and dying bacteria and their products, embedded in a matrix of polymers mainly derived from the saliva.
- **Sessile** organisms in biofilms are generally more resistant to antimicrobials than their **planktonic** counterparts due to properties conferred by the thick biofilm matrix and the differentials in the genetic and phenotypic makeup of the sessile forms.
- Recently, it has been recognized that oral plaque biofilm, especially in periodontitis, may alter the course and pathogenesis of a number of systemic diseases. These include atherosclerotic vascular disease, hospital-acquired bacterial pneumonias, type 2 diabetes and adverse pregnancy outcomes.
- However, apart from the well-established link between endocarditis and dental bacteraemia, there is no firm evidence to indicate that the other postulated diseases mentioned above are either initiated or perpetuated by oral flora and their byproducts. It is important to note that **associations need not necessarily prove causality**.

Review Questions (Answers on p. 391)

Please indicate which answers are true and which are false.

31.1. Streptococci comprise a considerable proportion of the normal oral flora. The predominant streptococci found in supragingival sites include:
   a. *Streptococcus pneumoniae*
   b. *Streptococcus mutans*
   c. *Streptococcus salivarius*
   d. *Streptococcus pyogenes*
   e. *Streptococcus mitis*

31.2. Which of the following statements on saliva are true?
   a. a salivary pellicle is always found on the surfaces of the healthy oral cavity
   b. saliva provides nutrition for bacteria
   c. salivary lactoferrin is an antimicrobial agent
   d. coaggregation of bacteria is facilitated by saliva
   e. salivary leukocyte protease inhibitor (SLPI) is antibacterial in nature

31.3. Which of the following are true of plaque biofilms?
   a. organic matrix comprises more than 70% of the mass
   b. the matrix facilitates development of antimicrobial resistance
   c. biofilms on the molar fissures are called supragingival plaque
   d. more than 80% of the mature calculus consists of mineralized material
   e. natural salivary flow is the only mechanism used by organisms to access tooth surfaces

31.4. Which of the following are true with respect to intraoral plaque biofilms?
   a. the initial colonizers are often Gram-negative rods
   b. plaque E_h fluctuations are critical for caries development
   c. early plaque biofilm colonizers reduce the redox potential so that the growth of anaerobes is promoted
   d. planktonic cells comprise the majority of the climax community flora
   e. the degenerating plaque biofilm bacteria may act as nuclei for calculus formation

Further Reading

Aarabi, G., Heydecke, G., & Seedorf, U. (2018). Roles of oral infections in the pathomechanism of atherosclerosis. *International Journal of Molecular Sciences, 19*(7), 1978. doi:10.3390/ijms19071978.

Baker, J. L., Bor, B., Agnello, M., et al. (2017). Ecology of the oral microbiome: Beyond bacteria. *Trends in Microbiology, 25*, 362–374.

Bandara, H. M. H. N., Panduwawala, C. P., & Samaranayake, L. P. (2019). Biodiversity of the human oral mycobiome in health and disease. *Oral Diseases, 25*, 363–371. https://doi.org/10.1111/odi.12899.

Chen, T., Yu, W. H., Izard, J., et al. (2010). The Human Oral Microbiome Database: A Web accessible resource for investigating oral microbe taxonomic and genomic information. *Database (Oxford).* doi:10.1093/database/baq013.

Edgar, W. M., & O'Mullane, D. M. (Eds.). (1996). *Saliva and oral health* (2nd ed.). British Dental Association.

Ghannoum, M. A., Jurevic, R. J., Mukherjee, P. K., et al. (2010). Characterization of the oral fungal microbiome (mycobiome) in healthy individuals. *PLoS Pathogens, 6*, e1000713.

Graves, D. T., Corrêa, J. D., & Silva, T. A. (2019). The oral microbiota is modified by systemic diseases. *Journal of Dental Research, 98*, 148–156.

Hajishengallis, G. (2015). Periodontitis: From microbial immune subversion to systemic inflammation. *Nature Reviews in Immunology, 15*, 30–44.

HOMD. Human Oral Microbiome Database. http://www.homd.org.

Kilian, M., Chapple, I. L., Hannig, M., et al. (2016). The oral microbiome: An update for oral healthcare professionals. *British Dental Journal, 221*, 657–666.

Li, X., Kolltveit, K. M., Tronstad, L., et al. (2000). Systemic disease caused by oral infection. *Clinical Microbiology Reviews, 13*, 547–558.

Marsh, P. D., & Martin, M. V. (2009). *Oral microbiology* (5th ed.). Butterworth-Heinemann.

Parahitiyawa, N. B., Jin, L. J., Leung, W. K., & Samaranayake, L. P. (2009). Microbiology of odontogenic bacteraemia: Beyond endocarditis. *Clinical Microbiology Reviews, 22*, 46–64.

Samaranayake, L. P., & Matsubara, V. H. (2017). Normal oral flora and the oral ecosystem. *Dental Clinics of North America, 61*, 199–215.

32 | *Microbiology of Dental Caries*

Microbiology of Dental Caries

Dental caries is a **chronic, noncommunicable, endogenous infection** caused by the **dysbiosis** of the resident commensal oral microbiome on tooth surfaces. The carious lesion, by contrast, is the result of demineralization of enamel—and later of dentine—by acids produced by dysbiotic plaque microbiota as they metabolize dietary carbohydrates. However, the initial process of enamel **demineralization** is usually followed by **remineralization**, and cavitation occurs when the former process overtakes the latter. Once the surface layer of enamel has been lost, the infection invariably progresses to dentine, with the pulp first becoming inflamed and then necrotic.

DEFINITION

Caries is defined as localized destruction of the tissues of the tooth by bacterial fermentation of dietary carbohydrates.

Epidemiology

Dental caries and periodontal disease could be considered as the two most common diseases affecting humans. Although caries was not uncommon in the developing world, the recent affluence in these regions has resulted in a remarkable upsurge in caries due to the ready and cheap availability of fermentable carbohydrates. By contrast, caries prevalence is falling overall in the developed world due to the increasing awareness of cariogenic food sources and the general improvement in oral hygiene and dental care delivery systems. Caries of enamel surfaces is particularly common up to the age of 20, after which it tends to stabilize. However, in later life, root surface caries becomes increasingly prevalent, due to gingival recession, exposing the vulnerable cementum to cariogenic bacteria.

Classifications

Caries lesions can be classified in many different ways, as per caries activity (active or inactive), adult or childhood, anatomical, International Caries Detection and Assessment System (ICDAS), etc. Details of these are not described here, and only the main features of some newer classifications are given below.

More important, the microbiological basis of caries is virtually similar irrespective of the type of caries, apart from the fact that there are fundamental differences between coronal caries and root caries, by virtue of their ecosystems. Additionally, recent data indicate that early childhood caries (ECC) is associated with a bacterial as well as a fungal flora, mainly comprising *Candida* species.

ANATOMICAL

Dental caries can be classified anatomically with respect to the site of the lesion (Fig. 32.1):

- **pit or fissure caries:** seen in molars, premolars and the lingual surface of maxillary incisors
- **smooth-surface caries:** seen mainly on approximal tooth surfaces just below the contact point
- **root surface caries:** seen on cementum or dentine when the root is exposed to the oral environment
- **enamel or dentinal or cemental caries:** seen in any of these specific anatomical locales
- **recurrent caries:** in any of the above locations but associated with an existing restoration.

AGE-RELATED–CHRONOLOGICAL

- **early childhood caries** (ECC): the presence of one or more decayed (noncavitated or cavitated lesions); missing (due to caries); or filled tooth surfaces in any primary tooth in a child 71 months of age or younger
- **severe early childhood caries** (S-ECC): any sign of smooth-surface caries in a child younger than 3 years of age, and from ages 3–5 years one or more cavitated or missing (due to caries) or filled smooth surfaces in primary maxillary anterior teeth (Fig 32.2). Previously this condition was known as nursing bottle caries and baby bottle tooth decay.

CLINICAL PRESENTATION

The primary lesion of caries is a well-demarcated, chalky-white lesion (Fig. 32.3) in which the surface continuity of enamel has not been breached. This **'white-spot'** lesion **can heal or remineralize**, and this stage of the disease is therefore reversible. However, as the lesion develops, the surface becomes roughened and cavitation occurs. If the lesion is not treated, the cavitation spreads into dentine and eventually may destroy the dental pulp, finally leading to the development of a periapical abscess and purulent infection (see Chapter 34).

Diagnosis

Diagnosis of caries is usually determined by a combination of:

1. **Direct observation.**
2. **Probing.** Probing using a periodontal probe is advised instead of a sharp explorer. Some do not advocate probing, as this may create an incipient breach of the enamel and spread the infection from one tooth surface to another.
3. **Radiographs.** Early white-spot lesions may easily be missed because they cannot be detected by the eye or by radiography. Similarly, it is possible for large carious lesions to develop in pits and fissures with very little clinical evidence of disease.
4. **Experimental methods.** Methods of potential practical value include laser fluorescence for diagnosis of buccal and lingual caries, and electrical impedance (resistance) to detect occlusal caries.
5. **Microbiological tests.** These may be helpful in the assessment of caries (see below).

Aetiology

The major factors involved in the aetiology of caries (Fig. 32.4) are:

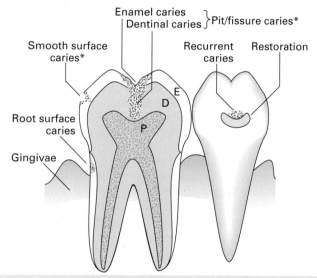

Fig. 32.1 Nomenclature of dental caries. D, dentine; E, enamel; P, pulp. *Also termed occlusal caries.

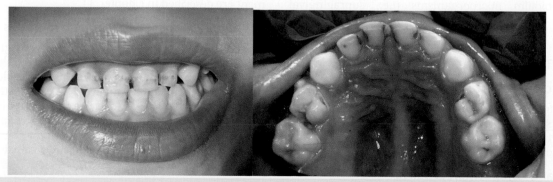

Fig. 32.2 Severe early childhood caries (S-ECC) of the primary dentition (left): anterior view (right), buccal view (left). (Courtesy: Dr. Kausar Fakhruddin.)

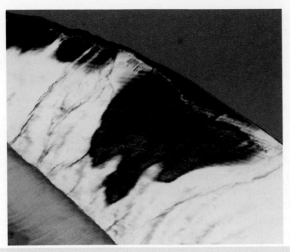

Fig. 32.3   Polarized light microscopic appearance of early enamel caries (ground section). The cone-shaped body of demineralization is evident.

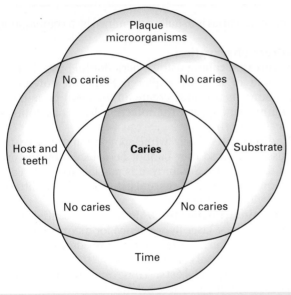

Fig. 32.4   Interplay of major aetiological factors in dental caries (all four factors must act simultaneously for caries to occur).

- host factors (tooth, saliva)
- diet (mainly the intake of fermentable carbohydrates)
- plaque biofilm microorganisms (i.e., supragingival plaque).

HOST FACTORS

Tooth Structure

The structure of enamel, and of dentine in root caries, is important: some areas of the same tooth are much more susceptible to carious attack than others, possibly because of differences in mineral content (especially fluoride).

Flow Rate and Composition of Saliva

The **mechanical washing action** of saliva is a very effective mechanism in the removal of food debris and unattached oral microorganisms. It has a high **buffering capacity**, which tends to neutralize acids produced by plaque biofilm bacteria on tooth surfaces, and it is supersaturated with **calcium** and **phosphorus ions**, which are important in the **remineralization of white-spot lesions**. Saliva also acts as a delivery vehicle for fluoride.

DIET

There is a direct relationship between dental caries and the intake of carbohydrates. The most cariogenic sugar is **sucrose**, and the evidence for its central role in the initiation of dental caries includes:

- increases in the caries prevalence of isolated populations with the introduction of sucrose-rich diets
- clinical association studies
- short-term experiments in human volunteers using sucrose rinses
- experimental animal studies.

Sucrose is highly soluble and diffuses easily into dental plaque biofilm, acting as a substrate for the production of extracellular polysaccharides and acids. Cariogenic streptococci produce water-insoluble **glucan** from sucrose, which, in addition to facilitating **initial adhesion** of the organisms to the tooth surface, serves as a **nutritional source** and a **matrix** for further plaque development. The relationship between sucrose and dental caries is complex and cannot be simply explained by the total amount of sugar consumed. The **frequency of sugar intake** rather than the total amount of sugar consumed appears to be of decisive importance. Also relevant are the **stickiness**, **frequency**, and **concentration** of the sucrose consumed, both factors influencing the period for which sugar is retained in close contact with the enamel surface.

Carbohydrates other than sucrose (e.g., glucose and fructose) are also cariogenic, but less so than sucrose. Polyol carbohydrates, '**sugar alcohols**' (e.g., xylitol), with low cariogenicity have been produced and are sought after as sugar substitutes in products such as chewing gum and baby foods.

MICROBIOLOGY

Microorganisms in the form of dental plaque biofilm are a prerequisite for the development of dental caries. The different types of plaque and the factors involved in their development are described in Chapter 31.

Specific and Nonspecific Plaque Hypothesis

Although *mutans* streptococci have been recognized as the major group of organisms involved in caries, there is some controversy as to whether one or more specific groups of bacteria are principally involved in caries—the **specific plaque hypothesis**—or whether the disease is caused by a heterogeneous mixture of nonspecific bacteria—the **nonspecific plaque hypothesis**.

There is conflicting opinion for and against the specific plaque hypothesis:

- *mutans* streptococci are involved in the initiation of almost all carious lesions in enamel

- *mutans* streptococci are important, but not essential
- the association of *mutans* streptococci and caries is weak and no greater than for other bacteria.

Given the extreme variation in the composition of supra-gingival plaque biofilm from the same site in the same mouth at different times, it is unlikely that the initiation and progression of all carious lesions are associated with specific organisms such as *Streptococcus mutans*. Further, other plaque biofilm bacteria also possess some of the biochemical characteristics thought to be important in cariogenicity. Therefore, it seems likely that combinations of bacteria other than *mutans* streptococci and lactobacilli may be able to initiate carious lesions, and the **plaque flora may be nonspecific** in nature. The current evidence implies that some bacteria (*mutans* streptococci, *Lactobacillus* spp. and *Actinomyces* spp.) may be more important than others in the initial as well as subsequent events leading to both enamel and root surface caries.

The Role of *Mutans* Streptococci

There is a vast literature on the role of the *mutans* streptococci in caries. '**Streptococcus mutans**' is a loosely applied group name for a collection of **seven different species** (*Streptococcus mutans, Streptococcus sobrinus, Streptococcus criceti, Streptococcus ferus, Streptococcus ratti, Streptococcus macacae* and *Streptococcus downei*) and eight serotypes (a–h). They are collectively known as *mutans* streptococci. *Streptococcus mutans* serotypes c, e, and f and *Streptococcus sobrinus* serotypes d and g are the species most commonly found in humans, with serotype c strains being the most prevalent, followed by d and e. The others are rarely encountered. The evidence for the aetiological role of *mutans* streptococci in dental caries includes the following:

- correlations of *mutans* streptococci counts in saliva and plaque with the prevalence and incidence of caries
- *mutans* streptococci can often be isolated from the tooth surface immediately before the development of caries
- positive correlation between the progression of carious lesions and '*Streptococcus mutans*' counts
- production of extracellular polysaccharides from sucrose (which help to reinforce the plaque biofilm and attach the biomass onto the tooth surface, thus permitting a sustained and concentrated assault of the specific enamel, dentinal or cemental surface)
- most effective streptococcus in caries studies in animals (rodents and nonhuman primates)
- ability to initiate and maintain microbial growth and to continue acid production at low pH values
- rapid metabolism of sugars to lactic and other organic acids
- ability to attain the critical pH for enamel demineralization more rapidly than other common plaque biofilm organisms
- ability to produce intracellular polysaccharides (IPSs) as glycogen, which may act as a food store for use when dietary carbohydrates are low
- immunization of animals with specific *Streptococcus mutans* serotypes significantly reduces the incidence of caries.

Note: Not all strains of *mutans* streptococci possess all of the aforementioned properties; thus some strains

are more cariogenic than others. Caries may therefore be an infectious disease in a minority, with a highly pathogenic strain being transmitted from one individual to another. Despite this apparently strong relationship between *mutans* streptococci and caries, a number of longitudinal studies in children have failed to find such a strong correlation.

The Role of Lactobacilli

Lactobacilli were previously believed to be the major causative agents of dental caries. They were considered to be candidate organisms for caries because of:

- their high numbers in most carious lesions affecting enamel (many studies have now shown its high prevalence also in root surface caries)
- the positive correlation between their numbers in plaque biofilm and saliva and caries activity
- their ability to grow in low-pH environments (below pH 5) and to produce lactic acid
- their ability to synthesize both extracellular and IPSs from sucrose
- the ability of some strains to produce caries in gnotobiotic (germ-free) rats
- the fact that their numbers in dental plaque biofilms derived from healthy sites are usually low.

On the negative side, however, lactobacilli are rarely isolated from plaque biofilm prior to the development of caries, and they are often absent from incipient lesions.

Although the role of lactobacilli in the carious process is not well defined, it is believed that:

- they are involved more in the **progression of the deep enamel lesion** (rather than the initiation)
- they are the **pioneer organisms** in the **advancing front** of the carious process, especially in dentine.

The Role of *Actinomyces* spp.

Actinomyces spp. are associated with the development of root surface caries (root lesions differ from enamel caries in that the calcified tissues are softened without obvious cavitation). The evidence for the involvement of *Actinomyces viscosus* in root surface caries is based on:

- association studies *in vivo*
- *in vitro* experimental work with pure cultures
- experimental work in gnotobiotic rodents.

Despite the fact that *Actinomyces* spp. (especially *Actinomyces viscosus*) predominate in the majority of plaque biofilm samples from root surface lesions, some studies have reported both *mutans* streptococci and *Lactobacillus* spp. in these lesions. Furthermore, the sites from which these organisms were isolated appeared to have a higher risk of developing root surface caries than other sites. The role of *Actinomyces* spp. in caries is therefore not clear.

The Role of *Veillonella*

Veillonella is a Gram-negative anaerobic coccus that is present in significant numbers in most supragingival plaque biofilm samples. As *Veillonella* spp. require lactate for growth but are unable to metabolize normal dietary carbohydrates, they use lactate produced by other microorganisms and convert it into a range of weaker and probably less cariogenic organic acids (e.g., propionic acid). Hence this organism may have a **beneficial effect** on dental caries. This protective effect has been demonstrated in vitro and in animal experiments but not in humans.

The Role of *Candida*

The role of fungal flora such as *Candida* spp. in the pathogenesis of caries has been a subject of controversy. The virulence attributes of *Candida* spp.—such as their acidogenicity and aciduric nature, the ability to develop profuse biofilms, ferment and assimilate dietary sugars, and produce collagenolytic proteinases—are all indicative of their latent cariogenic potential. Very recent data indicate the profuse diversity and acidogenicity of the candida-biome of **deep carious lesions of S-ECC**.

Indeed, oral candidal counts have been used by some as a caries risk indicator, akin to lactobacillus or *Streptococcus mutans* counts. The weight of available data tends to imply that *Candida* spp. may play a pivotal role as a **secondary agent**, colonizing an acidic milieu, thus perpetuating the carious process, particularly dentinal caries. On the contrary, others opine that *Candida* is merely a passenger proliferating in an acidic cariogenic milieu, and not a true cariogen.

BIG DATA AND CARIES MICROBIOLOGY

Recent data from next-generation sequencing (NGS) studies have shed new light on the microbiota associated with dental caries. These indicate that many other **noncultivable bacteria are** associated with this complex process. The list of caries-associated bacteria, apart from the traditional organisms such as *mutans* streptococci *Lactobacillus* and *Actinomyces* spp. include species of the following genera: *Atopobium*, *Dialister*, *Eubacterium*, *Olsenella* and *Scardovir* to name a few. The role of these organisms in the caries process is yet to be defined.

PLAQUE BIOFILM METABOLISM AND DENTAL CARIES

The metabolism of plaque biofilm is a complex subject, and the following is a very simplified account.

The main source of nutrition for oral bacteria is saliva. Although the carbohydrate content of saliva is generally low, increased levels (up to 1000-fold) are seen after a meal. To make use of these transient increases in food levels, oral bacteria have developed a number of regulatory mechanisms, which act at three levels:

- transport of sugar into the organisms
- the glycolytic pathway
- conversion of pyruvate into metabolic end-products.

The bacterial metabolism of carbohydrate is critical in the aetiology of caries as the **acidic end-products** are responsible for enamel **demineralization**. The process begins when dietary sucrose is broken down by bacterial extracellular enzymes such as **glucosyl** and **fructosyl transferases**, with the release of **glucose** and **fructose**, respectively. These monosaccharides are then converted into polysaccharides that are either water-soluble or water-insoluble: **glucans** and **fructans**, respectively. **Glucans** are mostly used as a major bacterial **food source**; the **insoluble fructans** contribute to the plaque biofilm matrix while facilitating the adhesion and aggregation of the resident bacteria and serving as a ready, extracellular food source. Some of the sucrose is transported directly into bacteria as the disaccharide or disaccharide phosphate, which is metabolized intracellularly by invertase or sucrose phosphate hydrolase into glucose and fructose. During glycolysis, glucose is degraded immediately by bacteria via the *Embden–Meyerhof pathway*, with the production of two pyruvate molecules from each molecule of glucose. The pyruvate can be degraded further:

- under low sugar conditions, pyruvate is converted into **ethanol, acetate and formate** (mainly by *mutans* streptococci).
- in sugar excess, pyruvate is converted into **lactate** molecules.

Different species produce acids at different rates and vary in their ability to survive under such conditions. The *mutans* streptococci group, being the most **acidogenic** and **aciduric** (acid tolerant), are the worst offenders and reduce the pH of plaque biofilm to low levels, creating hostile conditions for other neighbouring resident biofilm flora. The resultant overall fall in pH to levels below 5.5 initiates the process of enamel demineralization. This characteristic fall in plaque biofilm pH, followed by a slow return to the original value in about an hour, produces a curve that is termed the **'Stephan curve'**.

ECOLOGICAL PLAQUE HYPOTHESIS

A key feature of a number of caries studies is the absence of *mutans* streptococci at caries sites, suggesting that bacteria other than the latter can contribute to the disease process. Conversely, in some studies where *mutans* streptococci were found in high numbers, there was apparently no demineralization of the underlying enamel. This may be due to the presence of lactate-consuming species such as *Veillonella*, or to the production of alkali at low pH by organisms such as *Streptococcus salivarius* and *Streptococcus sanguinis*. These and other related findings have led to the development of the **'ecological plaque hypothesis'** of caries (Fig. 32.5). According to this hypothesis, cariogenic flora found in natural plaque biofilm are weakly competitive and comprise only a minority of the total community. With a conventional diet, levels of such potential cariogenic bacteria are clinically insignificant, and the processes of remineralization and demineralization are in equilibrium. If, however, the frequency of intake of fermentable carbohydrates increases, then the plaque biofilm pH level falls and remains low for prolonged periods, promoting the growth of acid-tolerant (**aciduric**) bacteria while gradually eliminating the communal bacteria that are acid labile. Prolonged low pH conditions also initiate demineralization. This process would turn the balance in the plaque biofilm community in favour of *mutans* streptococci and lactobacilli. The hypothesis also explains, to some extent, the dynamic relationship between the bacteria and the host, so that alterations in major host factors such as salivary flow on plaque biofilm development can be taken into account.

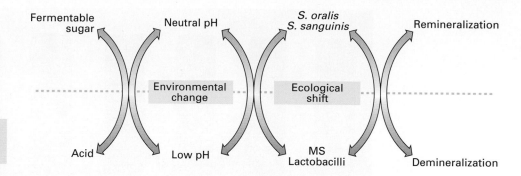

Fig. 32.5 Ecological plaque hypothesis. MS, *mutans* streptococci; S., *Streptococcus*.

Management of Dental Caries

The conventional approach to the treatment of dental caries was to remove and replace diseased tissue with an inert restoration. This approach made no attempt to cure the disease, and the patient often returned some months later requiring further fillings due to new or recurrent caries. By contrast, the modern philosophy in caries management highlights:

- early detection
- the importance of accurate diagnosis
- minimal cavity preparation techniques
- active prevention.

The result of such measures should be less, rather than more, demand for restorative treatment by individual patients.

PATIENT EVALUATION

In patients with a low incidence of caries, a case history and clinical and radiographic examination are probably adequate for treatment planning. However, for patients with **rampant or recurrent caries**, or where expensive crown and bridge work are planned, additional investigations are necessary. These include:

- assessment of dietary habits
- determination of salivary flow rate and buffering capacity
- microbiological analysis (discussed below).

Microbiological Tests in Caries Assessment

Saliva samples can be used to establish the numbers of *mutans* streptococci and *Lactobacillus* spp. in the oral cavity as follows:

1. A paraffin wax-stimulated sample of mixed saliva is collected.
2. In the laboratory, the saliva is appropriately diluted and cultured on selective media (mitis salivarius bacitracin agar for *mutans* streptococci; Rogosa SL agar for *Lactobacillus* spp.
3. The number of typical colonies, i.e., **colony-forming units** (CFUs), is then quantified and extrapolated to obtain the count per mL of saliva:
   - **high caries activity:** >10^6/ml *Streptococcus mutans* and/or >100,000/ml *Lactobacillus* spp.
   - **low caries activity:** <100,000/ml *Streptococcus mutans* and <10,000/ml *Lactobacillus* spp.

Simplified detection kits for estimation of both lactobacilli and *Streptococcus mutans* in saliva are available. The results correlate well with laboratory plate counts, and the tests can be performed in the dental clinic without special facilities (Fig. 32.6).

The presence of high salivary levels of *Streptococcus mutans* or lactobacilli does not necessarily mean that the patient has an increased risk of developing dental caries, as it is a disease of multifactorial aetiology. Other factors, such as **diet, buffering capacity, fluoride content of enamel and degree of oral hygiene**, should also be considered. Further, the presence of large numbers of cariogenic organisms in saliva does not imply that all teeth are caries prone, as the salivary organisms may have originated from a few foci with high caries activity. Therefore, these tests **at best give a generalized approximation of the caries risk**. It should be noted that the microbiological tests used in caries assessment differ from conventional tests used in medical microbiology, where the presence of a pathogen indicates a positive diagnosis (e.g., syphilis). The main uses of microbiology tests in caries assessment are:

- to identify patients who have unusually high numbers of potential pathogens, so that these data can be taken into account when integrating all the factors that may contribute to the carious process in an individual patient
- to monitor the efficacy of caries prevention techniques, such as dietary and oral hygiene advice and the use of antimicrobial agents such as chlorhexidine.

Microbiology of Root Surface Caries

Approximately 60% of individuals in the West age 60 or older now have root caries. This has arisen mainly because of the reduction in enamel caries and the consequential **retention of teeth** later into life, accompanied by **gingival recession**. The soft cemental surfaces thus exposed are highly susceptible to microbial colonization by virtue of their irregular and rough surfaces.

Early studies showed a high prevalence of *Actinomyces naeslundii*, *Actinomyces odontolyticus* and *Rothia dentocariosa* from human root surface caries. However, more recent data suggest a stronger association between lactobacilli, *mutans* streptococci and root caries. Indeed, the presence of lactobacilli is considered to be predictive of subsequent development

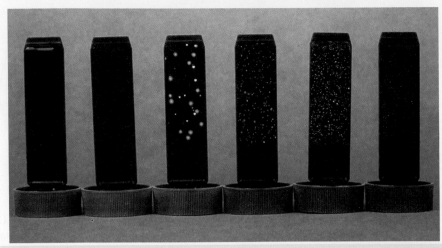

Fig. 32.6 *Dip slide test* **to detect** *mutans* **streptococci in saliva: a high density of white colonies indicates a higher caries risk.** The results shown were derived using saliva from five different individuals. Accordingly, the saliva of the indivdual number three (from left) has a high count of *mutans* streptococci and may have a higher caries risk than the other individuals (a blank control is on the extreme left).

of such lesions. The latter organisms, together with pleo-morphic Gram-positive rods, are also frequent in the deeper dentinal parts of the lesion. Recent molecular analyses of deep dentinal surfaces of root caries lesions, to some extent, confirm previous findings and indicate *mutans* streptococi lactobacilli and *Rothia dentocariosa* to be the predominant species. However, these organisms were associated with a vast number (>40) of new taxa most of them being uncultivable flora!

The current information available therefore suggests:

- a **polymicrobial aetiology** for caries initiation and progression on root surfaces (as in coronal caries)
- **bacterial succession** during the progression of the lesion with deeper lesions having flora different from those of the superficial lesions.

PREVENTION OF DENTAL CARIES

The major approaches to prevention of caries are:

1. **sugar substitutes:** stopping or reducing between-meal consumption of carbohydrates, or substituting noncario-genic artificial sweeteners (e.g., sorbitol, xylitol or Lycasin)
2. **fluorides:** making the tooth structure less soluble to acid attack by using **fluorides**
3. **sealants:** to protect susceptible areas of the tooth (e.g., pits and fissures) that cannot easily be kept plaque free by routine oral hygiene measures
4. **reducing cariogenic flora:** so that even in the presence of sucrose, acid production will be minimal (e.g., oral hygiene aids, antimicrobial agents and possibly immunization)
5. **probiotics** replacement of cariogenic bacteria by organisms with low or no cariogenic potential.

The rationale for these procedures is outlined below.

Sugar Substitutes

Artificial sweeteners or sugar substitutes cannot be absorbed and metabolized to produce acids by the vast majority of plaque biofilm bacteria. Two types of sugar substitute are available:

- **nutritive sweeteners** with a calorific value—for example, sorbitol and xylitol (the sugar alcohols) and Lycasin (prepared from cornstarch syrup)
- **nonnutritive sweeteners**—for example, saccharin and aspartame.

Fluoridation

Fluoride can be delivered to the tooth tissue in many ways. When administered systemically during childhood, it is incorporated during amelogenesis. The best delivery vehicle is the domestic water supply (at a concentration of 1 ppm); failing this, tablets, topical applications of fluoridated gel or fluoridated toothpaste may be used.

Fluoride ions exert their anticariogenic effect by:

1. **substitution** of the hydroxyl groups in hydroxyapatite and formation of fluoroapatite, which is less soluble in acid during amelogenesis
2. promotion of **remineralization** of early carious lesions in enamel and dentine
3. modulation of plaque metabolism by:
   - interference with bacterial membrane permeability
   - reduced glycolysis
   - inactivation of key metabolic enzymes by acidifying the cell interior
   - inhibition of the synthesis of IPSs, especially glycogen.

Fissure Sealants

Sealants prevent caries in pits and fissures by eliminating stagnation areas and blocking potential routes of infection. Early lesions that are well sealed can be effectively arrested by this technique, whereas more extensive lesions may extend into pulp, as the trapped cariogenic bacteria are able to use the carious dentinal matrix as a source of nutrition.

Control of Cariogenic Plaque Biofilm Flora

Control may be achieved by mechanical cleansing, antimicrobial therapy, immunization and replacement therapy.

Mechanical Cleansing Techniques. Conventional tooth-brushing with a fluoridated toothpaste is not very successful in reducing the caries incidence, as it is entirely dependent on the motivation and skill of the patient. Further, it is unlikely that mechanical cleansing even with flossing, interdental brushes and wood sticks will affect pit and fissure caries.

Antimicrobial Agents

CHLORHEXIDINE GLUCONATE. Chlorhexidine gluconate as a 0.2% mouthwash is by far the most effective antimicrobial for plaque control:

- Chlorhexidine disrupts the cell membrane and the cell wall permeability of many Gram-positive and Gram-negative bacteria.
- It is able to bind tenaciously to oral surfaces and is slowly released into the saliva.
- It interferes with the adherence of plaque-forming bacteria, thus reducing the rate of plaque accumulation.
- Compared with other bacteria involved in plaque biofilm formation, *mutans* streptococci are exquisitely sensitive to chlorhexidine and are therefore preferentially destroyed.

Unfortunately, because of the problems of tooth staining and unpleasant taste, chlorhexidine is normally only used for short-term therapy. These mouthwashes may be indicated for special groups such as those who are physically or mentally challenged with poor brushing skills.

SILVER DIAMINE FLUORIDE (SDF). Various formulations of silver diamine fluoride (SDF) have been approved for arresting active caries in children. It is also useful in arresting caries in adult geriatric patients, medically compromised patients and patients with special needs.

POVIDONE IODINE (BETADINE; IDODOPOVIDONE). Povidone iodine is also a less popular alternative used for plaque control.

Active Immunization Against Dental Caries. Using either **cell wall-associated antigens** (antigen I/II) or **glucosyl transferases** (extracellular enzymes) from *mutans* streptococci is effective in reducing experimental dental caries in rats and monkeys. The vaccine may produce its protective effect by:

- inhibition of the microbial colonization of enamel by secretory immunoglobulin A (IgA)
- interference with bacterial metabolism

- enhancement of phagocytic activity in the gingival crevice area due to the opsonization of *mutans* streptococci with IgA or IgG antibodies.

However, convincing proof that any of these mechanisms prevents the development of dental caries *in vivo* is lacking. Vaccination trials on humans have been unsuccessful because of fears of possible side effects, which would be unacceptable as caries is not a life-threatening disease. (The antibodies that develop after immunization with most **antigens** of *mutans* streptococci tend to **cross-react with heart tissue**, and the possibility that heart damage could result has made human vaccine trials very difficult.) Furthermore, the incidence of dental caries is falling in the West, and the disease can be adequately controlled using other techniques.

A caries vaccine could, however, be useful for developing countries with limited dental services and increasing prevalence of caries, and also for prevention of disease in high-risk groups—for instance, children who are mentally or physically challenged.

Passive Immunization. Experimental studies indicate that when the natural levels of oral *mutans* streptococci are suppressed by chlorhexidine, topical application of monoclonal antibodies against antigen I/II of *mutans* streptococci prevents recolonization by the organisms. **Transgenic plants** could be used to produce dimeric antibodies with specificity to antigen I/II of streptococci that are stable in the mouth and persist for longer periods than the monomeric antibody. These new developments have heightened the hopes of an alternative caries-preventive strategy for the future.

Replacement Therapy

Experimental studies indicate that genetically engineered, **low-virulence mutants of *mutans* streptococci** that are deficient in glucosyl transferase or deficient in lactate dehydrogenase activity can be 'seeded' into the oral environment. These organisms can replace their more virulent counterparts and prevent their reemergence. The term **probiotic therapy** (or 'probiotics') is now used for approaches where the offending pathogen is replaced artificially by innocuous commensals that are allowed to obtain a permanent foothold in the locale (e.g., oral cavity, intestines, vagina). It is feasible that replacement therapy of this nature may be exploited to control cariogenic flora in the future. However, assurances of the safety of these replacement strains are needed by both the public and the authorities before these methods are realized.

Key Facts

- **Caries** is defined as localized destruction of the tissues of the tooth by bacterial fermentation of dietary carbohydrates.
- Dental caries is a multifactorial, plaque biofilm-related chronic, noncommunicable infection of the enamel, cementum or dentine.
- **Key factors** in the development of tooth caries are the **host** (susceptible tooth surface and saliva), plaque biofilm **bacteria** and **diet** (mainly fermentable carbohydrates).
- The **initial caries lesion** is the **'white spot'** created by the demineralization of enamel; this is reversible and can be remineralized; cavitation represents irreversible disease.
- The **specific plaque hypothesis** postulates that *mutans* streptococci are important in caries initiation, whereas heterogeneous groups of bacteria are implicated in the nonspecific plaque hypothesis.
- **Lactobacilli** are implicated in the **progression of caries**, especially in the advancing front of the carious lesions (dentinal interface).

- The properties of cariogenic flora that correlate with their pathogenicity are the ability to metabolize sugars to acids rapidly (**acidogenicity**), to survive and grow under low pH conditions (**aciduricity**) and to synthesize extracellular and intracellular polysaccharides.
- **Strategies to control or prevent caries include** sugar substitutes, fluoridation (to increase enamel hardness mainly), fissure sealants and control of cariogenic flora (by antimicrobials, vaccination or passive immunization, or replacement therapy).
- **Microbiological tests** should be undertaken to identify **caries risk** factors in patients with extensive (rampant) or recurrent caries, prior to delivering dental care (e.g., extensive crown and bridge treatment).
- High **salivary or plaque counts of *mutans* streptococci** ($>10^6$/ml) and lactobacilli ($>10,000$/ml) indicate high risk of disease.

Review Questions (Answers on p. 392)

Please indicate which answers are true and which are false.

32.1. Which of the following statements on dental caries are true?
   a. signs of fissure caries can be first detected in dentine
   b. fissure caries is commonly seen in the lingual surface of the incisors
   c. approximately 90% of people over age 60 in the West have root surface caries
   d. smooth-surface caries is mainly seen on adjacent tooth surfaces
   e. recurrent caries is commonly associated with an existing restoration

32.2. The *mutans* group of streptococci are key cariogenic pathogens. Which of the following belongs to the *mutans* group?
   a. *Streptococcus mutans*
   b. *Streptococcus pyogenes*
   c. *Streptococcus sobrinus*
   d. *Streptococcus ratti*
   e. *Streptococcus pneumoniae*

32.3. Which of the following statements supports the role of *mutans* streptococci as cariogenic?
   a. positive correlation of the salivary *mutans* streptococci count and the prevalence of caries
   b. their aciduric and acidogenic characteristics
   c. their isolation from supragingival plaque biofilm samples
   d. production of extracellular polysaccharides
   e. their association with *Veillonella* spp. in root surface caries

32.4. With regard to microbiological evaluation of cariogenic activity, which of the following statements are true?
   a. it can be accomplished by saliva culture on blood agar to isolate *mutans* streptococci
   b. a salivary count of $>100,000$/ml lactobacilli indicate high caries activity
   c. the procedure is more helpful to monitor the response to treatment than making the initial diagnosis
   d. isolation of cariogenic organisms signifies that all teeth are at equal risk of developing caries
   e. it is particularly useful for caries risk diagnosis in high-risk groups

32.5. With regard to prevention of dental caries, which of the following statements are true?
   a. probiotic therapy with 'noncariogenic' bacteria is the most promising approach
   b. caries vaccine may be useful for disease prevention in high caries–risk groups
   c. chlorhexidine mouthwash is by far the most effective approach for plaque reduction
   d. water fluoridation, though effective, leads to other major systemic illnesses
   e. remineralization of early lesions can be accomplished by fluoridated toothpaste

Further Reading

Fakhruddin, K. S., Samaranayake, L. P., Egusa, H., Ngo, H. C., & Pesee, S. (2021). Profuse diversity and acidogenicity of the candida-biome of deep carious lesions of Severe Early Childhood Caries (S-ECC). *Journal of Oral Microbiology, 13*(1), 1964277. doi:10.1080/20002297.2021.1964277.

Kilian, M., Chapple, I. L., Hannig, M., et al. (2016). The oral microbiome: An update for oral healthcare professionals. *British Dental Journal, 221*, 657–666.

Marsh, P. D., Lewis, M. A. O., Marin, M. V., & Williams, D. (2009). *Oral microbiology* (5th ed.). Churchill Livingstone.

Pereira, D., Seneviratne, C. J., Koga-Ito, C. Y., & Samaranayake, L. P. (2018). Is the oral fungal pathogen *Candida albicans* a cariogen? *Oral Diseases, 24*(4), 518–526. doi:10.1111/odi.12691.

Russell, M. W., Chiders, N. K., Michalek, S. M., et al. (2004). A caries vaccine? The state of the science of immunization against dental caries. *Caries Research, 38*, 230–235.

Shen, S., Samaranayake, L. P., Yip, H. K., et al. (2002). Bacterial and yeast flora of root surface caries in elderly, ethnic Chinese. *Oral Diseases, 8*, 207–217.

Zheng, F. M., Yan, I. G., Duangthip, D., Gao, S. S., Lo, E. C. M., & Chu, C. H. (2022). Silver diamine fluoride therapy for dental care. *Japanese Dental Science Review, 58*, 249–257.

33 Microbiology of Periodontal Disease

Periodontal diseases can be defined as **disorders of supporting structures of the teeth**, including the gingivae, periodontal ligament and supporting alveolar bone. Everyone suffers from various degrees of periodontal disease at some point, and it is **one of the major non communicable diseases (NCDs) afflicting humankind**. However, in most people, the common chronic inflammatory diseases involving the periodontal tissues can be controlled using mechanical cleansing techniques and good oral hygiene. A minority experience rapid progressive disease that requires assessment and management by **periodontists**.

The introduction of implants a few decades ago has further expanded the spectrum of periodontal diseases to incorporate **implant-associated periodontal diseases**. To date, millions of implants are in use worldwide, and the supporting alveolar structures of these implants also undergo pathological changes mainly due to a dysbiotic microbiome, and these too have to be managed by dentists as long as the implants are in place, long after their insertion.

This chapter addresses only the microbiological features of periodontal diseases, with a concluding section on infections related to dental implants.

It should also be realised that there are a number of key etiopathologies of periodontal disease, including the **specific and nonspecific host defence mechanisms** (i.e, the host immunity), that play crucial modulating roles (i.e., **modifying factors**); however they are only very briefly addressed here. Furthermore, a vast, growing literature exists on periodontal microbiology, and students should

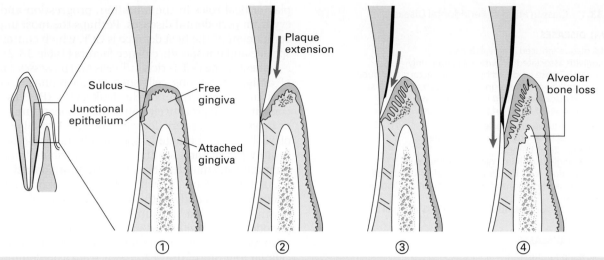

Fig. 33.1 The progression of a marginal periodontium from health to disease. (1) A healthy gingival sulcus with minimal supragingival plaque. (2) Established chronic gingivitis with minor inflammatory enlargement. (3) Long-standing chronic gingivitis with subgingival plaque extension into the pocket. (4) Chronic periodontitis with destruction of the periodontal membrane, alveolar bone loss and apical migration of the epithelial attachment.

refer to the contemporaneous literature to keep abreast of this knowledge base.

The Periodontium

The **periodontium** comprises the **gingivae, periodontal ligament, cementum and alveolar bone** (Fig. 33.1). Although the dentogingival junction is perhaps the most vulnerable site for microbial attack, it is not breached as long as oral hygiene is satisfactory. However, when plaque accumulates close to the gingival margin, the host defences are overcome, and gingival inflammation (gingivitis) and subsequent periodontal inflammation with loss of attachment ensue (periodontitis).

The healthy gingival crevice is a unique environment created by a mineralized structure – the tooth, which is partly embedded in the connective tissue and partly exposed to the oral environment. The gingival crevice is more anaerobic than most locales of the mouth and is constantly bathed by the gingival crevicular fluid (GCF) and its humoral and cellular defence factors as described above. However, dramatic changes occur during the **transition of the crevice into a periodontal pocket**. The **oxygen tension or E_h falls** further and becomes highly anaerobic, and the **flow of GCF increases**. The mostly proteolytic bacteria living in the periodontal pocket **raise the pH to alkaline levels** (pH 7.4–7.8; compared with neutral values in health), which in turn promotes the growth of bacteria such as *Porphyromonas gingivalis*.

The exposed cemental surface of the tooth is first colonized mainly by **pioneer dwellers**, including streptococci and *Actinomyces* spp. **Secondary colonizers** such as *Prevotella* and *Porphyromonas* spp. can adhere to this layer of cells by **coaggregation**. Others, such as *Peptostreptococcus micros*, can adhere to the crevicular epithelium. Thus, the inhabitants and the ecology of a deep periodontal pocket are markedly different from those of the gingival crevice.

Classification of Periodontal Disease

Periodontal disease can be broadly categorized into **gingivitis** and **periodontitis**. These are yet again subdivided into numerous categories. The latest classification of periodontal diseases promulgated in 2017 and currently in force is provided in Table 33.1; an older classification declared in 1999 is given in Table 33.2 for purposes of comparison. The new classification has two key components identifying **a stage and a grade of periodontal disease**. It also provides a structure for treatment planning and for monitoring a patient's response to therapy, and it defines clinical health and distinguishes an intact and a reduced periodontium throughout.

Additionally, the term 'aggressive periodontitis' in the older classification has been expunged, creating a staging and grading system for periodontitis that is based primarily upon attachment and bone loss and classifies the disease into **four stages based on severity** (I, II, III or IV) and **three grades based on disease susceptibility** (A, B or C). However for the sake of simplicity, the term 'aggressive' has been retained in the following sections on the microbiome of periodontal diseases. Moreover, the specific microbial profiles of each of these stages and grades are yet ill defined.

The Progression From Gingivitis to Periodontitis

In gingivitis, the inflammatory process of the superficial gingivae is restricted to the gingival epithelium and the connective tissue without affecting the deeper compartments of the periodontium. In pathological terms, the process is intimately associated with the metabolic activities of the subgingival plaque biofilm microbial communities and the immunoinflammatory infiltrate emanating from the gingival crevice. If this process is not arrested, periodontitis then sets in within

Table 33.1   Classification of Periodontal Diseases

GINGIVAL DISEASES

A. Dental plaque-induced gingival diseases
  1. Gingivitis associated with dental plaque only
  2. Gingival disease modified by systemic factors (e.g., puberty-associated gingivitis, pregnancy-associated gingivitis)
  3. Gingival disease modified by medications
  4. Gingival disease modified by malnutrition

B. Nonplaque-induced gingival lesions
  1. Specific bacterial origin (e.g., gonorrhoea)
  2. Viral origin (e.g., herpes)
  3. Fungal origin (e.g., linear gingival erythema)
  4. Genetic origin (e.g., hereditary gingival fibromatosis)
  5. Gingival manifestations of systemic conditions (e.g., allergic reactions)
  6. Traumatic lesions (factitious, iatrogenic, accidental; e.g., chemical injury)

PERIODONTAL DISEASES

A. Chronic periodontitis
  1. Localized
  2. Generalized

B. Aggressive periodontitis
  1. Localized
  2. Generalized

C. Periodontitis as a manifestation of systemic disease
  1. Associated with haematological disorders
    (i) Acquired neutropenia
    (ii) Leukaemias
    (iii) Others
  2. Associated with genetic disorders
    (i) Familial and cyclic neutropenia
    (ii) Down syndrome
    (iii) Many other rare conditions
  3. Associated with metabolic disorders
    (i) Diabetes mellitus
    (ii) Others

D. Necrotizing periodontal diseases
  1. Necrotizing ulcerative gingivitis (NUG)
  2. Necrotizing ulcerative periodontitis (NUP)

E. Abscesses of the periodontium
  1. Periodontal abscess
  2. Pericoronal abscess
  3. Gingival abscess

F. Periodontitis associated with endodontic lesions combined periodontic–endodontic lesions

G. Developmental or acquired deformities and conditions

the deeper tissues of the periodontium, which may eventually lead to tooth loss (Fig. 33.1). While gingivitis is a major risk factor and a necessary prerequisite for periodontitis, **not all gingivitis cases progress into periodontitis**.

Four types of histopathologic lesions are identified in periodontal disease:

- **the initial lesion**
- **the early lesion**
- **the established lesion**
- **the advanced lesion**, featuring bone loss and clinically manifested as periodontitis.
  (See later for detailed microbiology.)

GINGIVAL CREVICULAR FLUID IMMUNOLOGY

The **specific and nonspecific immune responses** of the host to the subgingival biofilm plaque are considered to play critical roles in the initiation, progression and recovery from periodontal diseases. Perhaps the most important component of the host defence is GCF, which contains both specific and nonspecific defence factors (Table 33.2).

In health, the GCF is rich in T cells and possesses a network of antigen-presenting cells such as macrophages, dendritic cells and polymorphonuclear leukocytes (PMNLs). These constantly and proactively patrol the periodontium and repel or ingest invading periodontopathogens. A small population of $\gamma\delta$ T cells and innate lymphoid cells may also be seen in healthy gingiva and are thought to contribute to protective immunity and maintenance of **tissue homeostasis**.

At the onset of gingivitis, the composition of the GCF changes significantly with increasing influx of B cells and plasma cells with a low number of PMNLs in comparison to periodontitis. As gingivitis progresses from the initial to the advanced stages, a concomitant increased complexity of the cellular infiltrate of the GCF is seen, from a predominant neutrophil infiltrate in the initial lesion, to one containing elevated numbers of macrophages and T cells in the early lesion and, finally, B cells and plasma cells predominating in the established and advanced lesions. Such a host immune response to the subgingival plaque biofilm is protective in nature, as it maintains tissue homeostasis with a balanced host-microbe relationship (eubiosis) and a healthy periodontium.

ROLE OF POLYMORPHONUCLEAR LEUKOCYTES

As mentioned, the small numbers of PMNLs in GCF increase markedly during the onset of gingivitis and periodontitis. The PMNLs migrate from venules and enter the gingival sulcus through the junctional epithelial cells. When PMNLs encounter bacteria, phagocytosis ensues, and the ingested organisms are then killed with a combination of proteolytic and hydrolytic enzymes and other cell-derived killing agents such as hydrogen peroxide and lactic acid. Although phagocytosis can occur in the absence of antibody, the presence of immunoglobulins and complement augments the process. The battle between PMNLs and plaque bacteria may result in:

- death of the pathogen
- death of PMNLs
- mutual extermination of the pathogen and PMNLs
- resultant PMNL autolysis and release of lysosomal enzymes (e.g., hyaluronidase, collagenase, elastase, acid hydrolase).

Thus, PMNLs may have both a protective and a damaging effect on host tissues. Phagocytosis, which may occur within the host tissues and possibly at the interface with subgingival plaque, is important in preventing the microbial ingress into the tissues.

ROLE OF ANTIBODY

Locally derived specific antibodies (IgM, IgG and IgA) to subgingival plaque organisms are found in the GCF. An elevated titre of specific antibody to a periodontopathogen may be:

- protective
- involved in damaging hypersensitivity reactions to the host tissues
- nonspecific and unrelated (i.e., an epiphenomenon).

Table 33.2 Basic Classification of Periodontal Diseases and Conditions

STAGING OF PERIODONTITIS

	Stage I (early/mild)	Stage II (moderate)	Stage III (severe)	Stage IV (very severe)
Interproximal bone loss*	<15% or <2 mm**	Coronal third of root	Mid third of root	Apical third of root
Extent	Described as:			
	Localised (up to 30% of teeth), Generalised (more than 30% of teeth)			
	Molar/incisor pattern			

GRADING OF PERIODONTITIS

	Grade A (slow)	Grade B (moderate)	Grade C (rapid)
% bone loss/age	<0.5	0.5–1.0	>1.0

PERIODONTAL HEALTH, GINGIVAL DISEASES AND CONDITIONS

Periodontal health

Intact periodontium

Reduced periodontium***

Gingivitis: dental biofilm-induced

Intact periodontium

Gingival diseases and conditions: nondental biofilm-induced

PERIODONTITIS

Necrotising periodontal diseases

Periodontitis****

Periodontitis as a manifestation of systemic disease

OTHER CONDITIONS AFFECTING THE PERIODONTIUM

Systemic diseases or conditions affecting the periodontal supporting tissues

Periodontal abscesses and endodontic-periodontal lesions

Mucogingival deformities and conditions

Traumatic occlusal forces

Tooth- and prosthesis-related factors

*Maximum bone loss in percentage of root length.
**Measurement in mm from cemento-enamel junction (CEJ) if only bitewing radiograph available (bone loss) or no radiographs clinically justified (CAL).
***Reduced periodontium due to causes other than periodontitis (e.g., crown-lengthening surgery).
****All patients with evidence of historical or current periodontitis should be staged/graded at initial consultation.

The presence of antibody implies that the T-cell (helper and suppressor) and B-cell interactions occur in periodontal tissues. Cells required for a wide range of immune reactions, present in gingival tissues of periodontitis patients, possess antigen specificity for plaque bacteria. When stimulated, either antibodies (from B lymphocytes) or lymphokines (from T lymphocytes) are produced.

Antibodies and complement present in the periodontal tissues interact to produce hypersensitivity reactions, which may damage host tissues and also contribute to periodontal disease. There is evidence that all four types of hypersensitivity may be involved in the pathogenesis of periodontal disease (Chapter 8).

TIPPING FACTORS LEADING TO PERIODONTITIS

As mentioned, all gingivitis lesions do not lead to periodontitis, and most periodontal lesions resolve without major consequences. However, in a significant proportion of individuals the host response is ineffective, dysregulated and destructive. A multiplicity of factors has been identified as playing a role in either the resistance or susceptibility to periodontitis, and these include:

- **genetic** (some individuals are not susceptible to periodontal disease irrespective of their oral hygiene)
- **epigenetic**
- **environmental** (e.g., smoking, stress, and diet)
- **aging**
- **systemic diseases** (e.g., diabetes).

The next section describes in detail the microbiological features of periodontal disease.

MICROORGANISMS IN SUBGINGIVAL PLAQUE BIOFILM

That the dental plaque biofilm is the essential aetiological agent of the common forms of chronic gingivitis and periodontitis is shown by the following:

1. Epidemiological data indicate a strong positive association between plaque levels and the prevalence and severity of periodontal diseases.
2. Clinical studies in healthy individuals have shown that discontinuation of oral hygiene results in plaque accumulation and subsequent onset of gingivitis (see Fig. 31.4). If plaque is then removed and oral hygiene recommended, the tissues are restored to health.
3. The topical application of certain antimicrobial compounds (e.g., chlorhexidine gluconate) both inhibits plaque formation and prevents the development of gingivitis.

4. Periodontal disease can be initiated in gnotobiotic (germ-free) animals by specific periodontopathic bacteria isolated from human dental plaque (e.g., *Fusobacterium nucleatum*, *Porphyromonas gingivalis*), and the disease can be arrested by administering antibiotics active against that particular organism.

MICROBIOLOGICAL STUDIES OF PERIODONTAL PLAQUE BIOFILM FLORA

As most of the periodontal plaque biofilm flora is anaerobic, special care must be taken to preserve the viability of these organisms during sampling, dispersion and cultivation of plaque samples. Ideally, the sample should be taken from the advancing front of the lesion at the base of the pocket, although in practice this is difficult because of contaminants from the superficial plaque at the top of the pocket. The techniques involved in microbiological studies of pocket flora include:

- **dark-field microscopy** to estimate the different morphological bacterial types **(morphotypes)** present, especially spirochaetes, which are not easily cultivable; the motility of spirochaetes can also be observed
- **cultural studies** using screening methods for the presence of a few, selected periodontopathic microorganisms or in-depth studies using conventional culture techniques to isolate, identify and enumerate all cultivable flora
- **immunological techniques** such as conventional enzyme-linked immunosorbent assay **(ELISA)** and fluorescent antibody techniques
- **molecular biology** techniques using specific DNA probes, and determination of full or partial 16S ribosomal RNA (rRNA) sequences by polymerase chain reaction (PCR) and the newer next-generation sequencing (NGS) technology to identify **uncultivable bacteria** as well as the conventional pathogens; these techniques have revealed the presence of hitherto undescribed bacteria in periodontal pockets. These comprise almost 50% of the flora.

SPECIFIC AND NONSPECIFIC PLAQUE HYPOTHESIS

Although bacteria are definitive agents of periodontal diseases, there are conflicting views as to whether a single or a limited number of species are involved in the disease process—the **specific plaque hypothesis**—or disease is caused by any combination of a wider range of nonspecific bacteria—the **nonspecific plaque hypothesis**.

The Specific Plaque Hypothesis

In certain disease states, such as necrotizing ulcerative gingivitis, the key aetiological agents are fusobacteria and spirochaetes. Furthermore, this disease can be resolved by administering appropriate antibiotics active against anaerobes (e.g., metronidazole). Other studies have convincingly shown the direct involvement of *Aggregatibacter actinomycetemcomitans* in aggressive (juvenile) periodontitis, and disease resolution after therapy with tetracycline, which is active against this organism. These observations led to the theory of specific plaque hypothesis.

The Nonspecific Plaque Hypothesis

This hypothesis proposes that **collective groups or consortia** of different bacteria have the total complement of virulence factors required for periodontal tissue destruction and that some bacteria can substitute for others absent from the **pathogenic consortium**. This hypothesis implies that plaque biofilm will cause disease irrespective of its composition, and it is supported by the clinical findings of numerous bacterial species in diseased periodontal pockets.

It is likely that the two theories represent the extremes of a complex series of host–parasite interactions.

The Ecological Plaque Hypothesis

The ecological plaque hypothesis has also been proposed for the aetiology of periodontal disease. This postulates the following causative process:

1. The reaction of the host to natural **plaque accumulation** in the crevice is an **inflammatory response**.
2. The ensuing **increased GCF flow** provides complex host molecules that can be catabolized by the proteolytic Gram-negative anaerobes that already exist in small numbers in normal plaque flora.
3. The latter organisms **suppress the growth of species** common in the healthy crevice (i.e., facultative anaerobic Gram-positive bacteria mostly), and a **population shift** occurs in the resident flora.
4. These **periodontopathic flora** then produce virulence factors that overwhelm host defences for a time, resulting in **episodic tissue destruction** and disease activity.

This simple yet elegant hypothesis implies that periodontal disease is an **endogenous or an opportunistic infection**, caused by an imbalance in the composition of the resident microflora at a site, owing to an alteration in the ecology of the local habitat (Fig. 33.2).

CLINICAL IMPLICATIONS

The nonspecific plaque hypothesis and the ecology hypothesis imply that periodontal disease may be treated by reducing the plaque to an acceptable level and the maintenance of healthy plaque, or by achievement of total **plaque control**. By contrast, the specific plaque hypothesis implies that therapy should be directed at elimination of specific pathogens—for instance, by appropriate **antibiotic therapy**.

PERIODONTAL HEALTH AND DISEASE

Healthy gingival sulcus has a scant flora dominated by almost equal proportions of **Gram-positive** and **facultative anaerobic** organisms; spirochaetes and motile rods make up less than 5% of the organisms (Table 33.3). With increasing severity of disease, the proportions of **strict anaerobic, Gram-negative** and **motile** organisms increase significantly (Fig. 33.3).

A wide range of microbial products potentially toxic to host tissues have been identified in plaque bacteria; these **virulence determinants** are shown in Table 33.4. If these

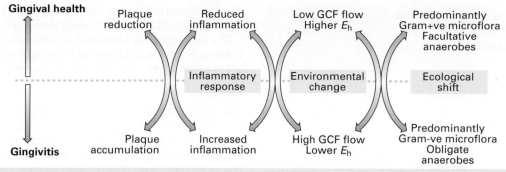

Fig. 33.2   The ecological plaque hypothesis. E_h, redox potential; *GCF*, gingival crevicular fluid.

Table 33.3   Specific and Nonspecific Defence Factors in Gingival Crevicular Fluid

Specific	Nonspecific
B and T lymphocytes	Polymorphs
	Macrophages
Antibodies: IgG, IgA, IgM	Complement system
	Proteases
	Lysozyme
	Lactoferrin

IgG, immunoglobulin G.

toxic products are released into the periodontal tissues, then rapid destructive inflammatory disease could be expected. However, tissue destruction is usually **slow, sporadic** and **episodic**, suggesting the existence of powerful host defence mechanisms, of which little is known. However, the nature of the periodontal disease and its elusive progression or regression could be explicable by the following:

- All clones or clonal types of the pathogen are not equally virulent (e.g., some isolates of *Porphyromonas gingivalis* express virulence and others may not).
- Some pathogens inhabiting the crevice may not possess the requisite genetic elements for virulence expression but may acquire these from other species via phage, plasmids or transposons.
- The pathogen has to be in the right location in a site (e.g., pocket apex adjacent to the epithelium) in adequate numbers to initiate disease.

- Other bacteria in the microbial commune may nullify the expressed virulence factors (e.g., hydrogen peroxide produced by neighbouring *Streptococcus sanguinis* in the commune, either directly or via a host peroxidase system, may inhibit *Aggregatibacter actinomycetemcomitans*).
- Local subgingival environment, such as the temperature, osmotic pressure or the concentration of calcium, magnesium or iron controlled by a global **'regulon'** that in turn affects virulence expression.
- Host susceptibility factors that include defects in PMNL levels or function, smoking, diet, poorly regulated immunological responses, systemic disease such as diabetes and infections (e.g., human immunodeficiency virus (HIV) infection).

Relationship Between Chronic Marginal Gingivitis and Periodontitis

Both chronic marginal gingivitis and periodontitis are **inflammatory diseases**: the lesions of the former are confined to the gingivae; the latter involves destruction of both the connective tissue attachment of the tooth and the alveolar bone. Gingivitis is common in both adults and children, although **early periodontitis is rarely seen before late adolescence**. It is considered that chronic periodontitis is preceded by chronic gingivitis; however, in some cases gingivitis may exist for prolonged periods without progressing to periodontitis. The main stages in

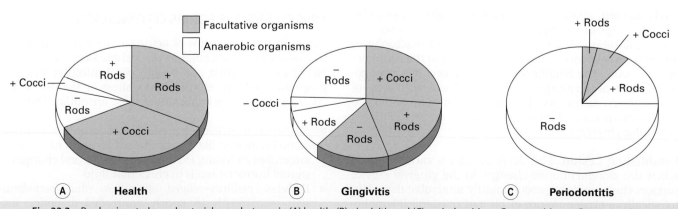

Fig. 33.3   Predominant plaque bacterial morphotypes in (A) health, (B) gingivitis and (C) periodontitis. +, Gram-positive; –, Gram-negative.

Table 33.4 Some Microbial Virulence Determinants in Periodontal Disease

Adhesion, colonization and biofilm formation
Fimbriae
Capsules
Microbial antagonism and synergism
'Corn-cob' formation
Biofilm 'survival mechanisms'
Tissue destruction
Hyaluronidase
Collagenase
Acid phosphatase
Epithelial cell toxin
Evasion of host immunity
Leukocidins
Proteases
Cytotoxins
Siderophores

the development of chronic gingivitis and periodontitis are shown in Fig. 33.1.

CHRONIC MARGINAL GINGIVITIS

Clinical Presentation

The gingivae are red and swollen, with rounded edges; bleeding gums and halitosis are common. However, pain, discomfort and unpleasant taste are uncommon.

Pathogenesis

Plaque-associated gingivitis is divided into three separate but contiguous phases:

1. **initial lesion**: developing within 4 days of plaque accumulation
2. **early lesion**: seen after 7 days
3. **established lesion**: for a variable period afterward.

Initial Lesion. Early histological examination shows an acute inflammatory reaction associated with vasculitis, perivascular collagen destruction, increase in crevicular fluid and polymorphonuclear leukocytosis in the junctional epithelium and crevice. At this stage, no clinical change is evident.

Early Lesion. After about 7 days, clinically recognizable chronic gingivitis with gingival inflammation is seen. A dense infiltration of lymphocytes (75%) with macrophages and plasma cells can be observed, especially at the periphery of the lesion. The lymphocytic infiltrate occupies approximately 15% of the marginal connective tissue with areas of local collagen destruction. Polymorph infiltration of the gingival sulcus peaks 7–12 days following the onset of clinically detectable gingivitis.

Established Lesion. This develops after a variable period when the aforementioned changes in the gingival crevice support the growth of predominantly anaerobic flora. Histologically, a predominance of plasma cells and B lymphocytes is seen, together with a heavy neutrophil infiltrate in the junctional and the newly developed pocket epithelium. It is during this stage that periodontal pocket formation begins.

If oral hygiene is improved at this juncture without the removal of subgingival plaque, then the lesion may persist for years without extending into the deeper periodontal tissues.

Microbiology

Gingivitis is related to the prolonged exposure of host tissues to a nonspecific mixture of gingival plaque biofilm organisms. The microbiological features of the gingival pocket necessarily change during the transition from the initial lesion to the established lesion. In the initial stage, Gram-positive and facultative organisms predominate, including streptococci (see Table 33.3). In the early lesion, *Actinomyces* spp. increase together with proportions of capnophilic species such as *Capnocytophaga* spp. and obligately anaerobic Gram-negative bacteria. For example, in the initial stage of one study (of nonbleeding gingivitis), proportions of *Actinomyces israelii* and *Actinomyces naeslundii* almost doubled. When the disease progresses to the established lesion, where bleeding is seen, the flora further changes, and levels of black-pigmented anaerobes such as *Porphyromonas gingivalis* and *Prevotella intermedia. Tannerella forsythia* increase quantitatively (e.g., 0.1–0.2% of total plaque flora), together with spirochaetes. This consortium of organisms comprises the so-called **red complex, periodontopathogens** (see below).

Management

Treatment is by thorough removal of plaque and calculus deposits, all plaque-retentive factors, and the introduction of good oral hygiene.

THE TRANSITION FROM GINGIVITIS TO PERIODONTITIS

Chronic marginal gingivitis may be present for up to 10 years in some individuals before progressing to periodontitis. This transition may be due to one or a combination of the following:

- selective overgrowth of one or more plaque species due to impairment of the host defences
- infection and proliferation of a newly arrived pathogen (so-called 'periodontopathogens' or 'periodontopathic organisms') in the gingival area
- activation of tissue-destructive immune processes.

MISCELLANEOUS FORMS OF GINGIVITIS

Generally transient forms of acute gingivitis may ensue due to systemic hormonal changes or viral diseases. These include HIV disease, herpetic and streptococcal infection, diabetes, pregnancy, puberty, menstruation, stress or the use of oral contraceptives. More important of these are outlined below:

- *Pregnancy gingivitis:* hormone related; usually seen in the second semester; likely to be due to increased numbers of anaerobes including *Prevotella intermedia* and changes in steroid hormone levels in crevicular fluid
- *Diabetes mellitus–related gingivitis (and periodontitis):* seen mostly in poorly controlled diabetics; diseased sites have more *Capnocytophaga*, and other

periodontopathogens including *Porphyromonas gingivalis* and *Treponema denticola*

- *Acute streptococcal gingivitis:* due to *Streptococcus pyogenes* (Lancefield Group A); usually a sequela of streptococcal sore throat; severe disease with fever, and inflamed erythematous and oedematous gingivae
- HIV disease associated gingivitis (and periodontitis): see Chapter 30
- Acute herpetic gingivostomatitis: see Chapters 21 and 35.

CHRONIC PERIODONTITIS (FORMERLY ADULT PERIODONTITIS)

Periodontitis can be classified into various groups (Table 33.1), but chronic periodontitis is by far the most prevalent disease globally.

Morbidity

About 70–80% of all adults suffer from this universal disease, and chronic periodontitis comprises 95% of all periodontal diseases. Prevalence and severity increase with age.

Clinical Presentation

All the features of the established lesion are present in addition to the following:

- gross gingival inflammation, fibrosis and some shrinkage (Fig. 33.4)
- bleeding pockets of more than 3 mm
- tooth mobility and migration
- irregular alveolar bone loss around the teeth
- gingival recession
- halitosis and offensive taste
- usually little or no pain
- may or may not be associated with systemic disease.

Pathogenesis

The main processes that produce loss of attachment and pocket formation are (Fig. 33.1):

1. The apical spread of subgingival plaque causes the junctional epithelium to separate from the tooth surface (i.e., a **new 'pocket' epithelium** is created).

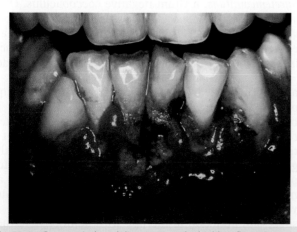

Fig. 33.4 Gross periodontal disease. Note the highly inflamed gingivae and calculus deposits.

2. Inflammatory tissue reactions below the pocket epithelium result in **destruction of the gingival connective tissue, periodontal membrane and alveolar bone**.
3. Apical proliferation of the junctional epithelium results in **migration of the epithelial attachment**.
4. The rate of tissue destruction is not constant but episodic, with periods of quiescence alternating with bouts of bone resorption. A number of patterns of disease activity can occur, ranging from **slowly progressive destruction** to **brief bursts of episodic activity**, which may vary in intensity and duration in different sites in the same mouth. This makes microbiological sampling for disease activity extremely difficult.
5. While the entire dentition may be equally affected, more often the disease distribution is localized, with more severe destruction in molar areas and in anterior segments.

Microbiology

Microorganisms implicated in chronic periodontitis are listed in Table 33.3.

The depth of the periodontal pocket creates a highly anaerobic locale with a shift from neutral to alkaline pH (7.4–7.8). The protein-rich fluid in the pocket encourages the growth of anaerobes, which possess many proteolytic enzymes.

One of the seminal studies widely quoted in the literature has categorized periodontal microbiota into various groups and aggregates, some more associated with periodontal pathology than others These indicate that subgingival plaque has two distinct zones: a zone of Gram-positive cocci and bacilli close to the tooth surface, and a zone of Gram-negative organisms next to the gingival crevice.

The progression from gram-positive bacteria in the superficial regions to gram-negative bacteria active in the apical disease front has been colour coded from yellow to red (corresponding to traffic light colors). Accordingly a total of five closely associated bacterial complexes have been recognized (Fig. 33.5).

Early colonizers – the yellow, green and purple complexes/clusters

- a **yellow complex** consisting of mainly the members of the genus Streptococcus
- a **green complex** of mainly *Capnocytophaga, Campylobacter* and *Eikenella* spp. and *Aggregatibacter actinomycetemcomitans* (Serotype a)
- a **purple complex** mainly consisting of *Veillonella parvula, Actinomyces spp. and Aggregatibacter actinomycetemcomitans (Serotype b)*

The foregoing three groups of species are early colonizers of the tooth surface whose growth usually precedes the multiplication of the predominantly gram-negative orange and red complexes

Late colonizers – the orange and red complexes/clusters

- an **orange complex** consists of *Campylobacter species, Eikenella nodatum, Fusobacterium species, Peptostreptococcus micros,* and *Streptococcus constellatus*
- a **red complex** consists of *Tannerella forsythia, Porphyromonas gingivalis,* and *Treponema denticola*.

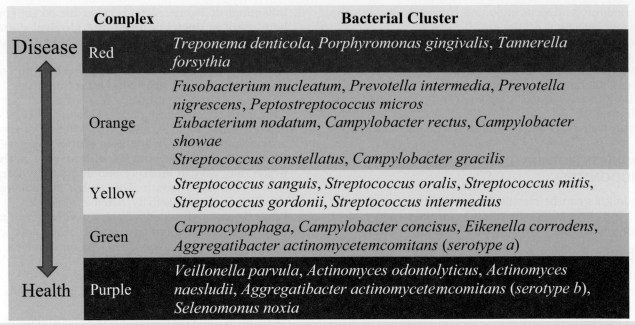

	Complex	Bacterial Cluster
Disease	Red	*Treponema denticola, Porphyromonas gingivalis, Tannerella forsythia*
	Orange	*Fusobacterium nucleatum, Prevotella intermedia, Prevotella nigrescens, Peptostreptococcus micros* *Eubacterium nodatum, Campylobacter rectus, Campylobacter showae* *Streptococcus constellatus, Campylobacter gracilis*
	Yellow	*Streptococcus sanguis, Streptococcus oralis, Streptococcus mitis, Streptococcus gordonii, Streptococcus intermedius*
	Green	*Carpnocytophaga, Campylobacter concisus, Eikenella corrodens, Aggregatibacter actinomycetemcomitans (serotype a)*
Health	Purple	*Veillonella parvula, Actinomyces odontolyticus, Actinomyces naesludii, Aggregatibacter actinomycetemcomitans (serotype b), Selenomonus noxia*

Fig 33.5 Bacterial clusters and major species associated with periodontal health and disease. (Modified from Socransky et al., 1998.)

The orange and **red complex species** are thought to be the major etiologic agents and protagonists at the active front of the periodontal infection and are also termed **keystone periodontopathogens** and represent the climax community of the plaque biofilm in chronic progressive periodontitis. Members of the red complex are rarely found in the absence of members of the orange complex. The evidence for the specificity of these periodontopathogens in active periodontal lesions is derived from:

■ clinical association studies
■ the production of a wide range of factors *in vitro* that can impair the host defences and damage components of the periodontium; these include proteases, collagenases, hyaluronidases and cytotoxins (Table 33.5)
■ infections in experimental animals that have produced both soft tissue destruction and bone resorption.

AGGRESSIVE PERIODONTITIS

Periodontal diseases entities previously classified as juvenile periodontitis (localized and generalized), rapidly progressive periodontitis, early-onset periodontitis and prepubertal periodontitis are now categorized under the common heading of aggressive periodontitis. However, as mentioned above, the new classifiicaiton based on grading and staging of periodontal diseases discourages the use of the term 'aggressive periodontitis'.

Localized and Generalized Aggressive Periodontitis (Formerly Localized/Generalized Juvenile Periodontitis)

Morbidity. The condition is relatively rare—0.1% in young whites—but is more common in West Africans and Asians. It appears around puberty and is relatively common in girls; case clusters are usually seen in families.

Initiation and Course. Approximately around 13 years, with onset of puberty; rather rapid progress with active and quiescent periods.

Clinical Features. In the localized variant, the incisors and/or first permanent molars in both jaws are affected for unknown reasons. Later, other teeth may be involved, producing the appearance of generalized alveolar bone loss (Fig. 33.6). Alternatively, in the generalized variant of the disease, many areas may be involved in a similar manner. The disease is insidious in nature, and lesions are discovered incidentally on radiographs. In some generalized cases, about 50% of the supporting alveolar bone is affected, and teeth may be lost. The condition **may or may not manifest with gingivitis**, and patients can present with various levels of oral hygiene. In contrast to chronic periodontitis, **little plaque or calculus** is present in periodontal pockets. The disease **may be inherited** (autosomal recessive).

Microbiology and Immunology. A majority of patients with aggressive periodontitis have peripheral blood lymphocytes with impaired ability to react to chemotactic stimuli. This deficiency may be associated with, or is a direct cause of, the presence of large numbers of *Aggregatibacter actinomycetemcomitans*, a Gram-negative coccobacillus. Other organisms, such as *Capnocytophaga* spp. and *Porphyromonas gingivalis*, may be synergistically associated with the disease. The evidence for the specific involvement of *Aggregatibacter actinomycetemcomitans* in aggressive periodontitis includes:

■ a high incidence of the organism in subgingival plaque obtained from lesional sites
■ high levels of antibody to *Aggregatibacter actinomycetemcomitans*, which tend to fall after successful treatment
■ the possession of a wide range of potentially pathogenic products, such as leukotoxins, ideally suited to a periodontopathic organism. However, all strains are not equally leukotoxic (compare *Escherichia coli* strains, which are toxigenic and nontoxigenic)
■ successful periodontal therapy with adjunctive tetracycline is associated with disease regression and elimination of the organism from diseased sites.

Table 33.5   Microorganisms Associated With Various Types of Periodontal Disease

Condition	Predominant Microorganisms	Comments
Health	*Streptococcus sanguinis* (previously *Streptococcus sanguis*) *Streptococcus oralis* *Actinomyces naeslundii* *Actinomyces viscosus* *Veillonella* spp.	Mainly Gram-positive cocci with few spirochaetes or motile rods
Chronic marginal gingivitis	*Streptococcus sanguinis* *Streptococcus milleri* *Actinomyces israelii* *Actinomyces naeslundii* *Prevotella intermedia* *Capnocytophaga* spp. *Fusobacterium nucleatum* *Veillonella* spp.	About 55% of cells are Gram-positive with occasional spirochaetes and motile rods
Chronic periodontitis	*Porphyromonas gingivalis* *Prevotella intermedia* *Fusobacterium nucleatum* *Tannerella forsythia* (formerly *Bacteroides forsythus*) *Aggregatibacter actinomycetemcomitans* *Selenomonas* spp. *Capnocytophaga* spp. *Spirochaetes*	About 75% of cells are Gram-negative (90% being strict anaerobes). Motile rods and spirochaetes are prominent.
'Aggressive periodontitis'*	*Aggregatibacter actinomycetemcomitans* *Capnocytophaga* spp. *Porphyromonas gingivalis* *Prevotella intermedia*	About 65–75% of bacteria are Gram-negative bacilli. Few spirochaetes or motile rods are present. These diseases may be associated with cellular immune or genetic defects.

Note: Also see Fig. 33.5. *The term 'aggressive periodontitis' is not used in the most recent classification of periodontal diseases.

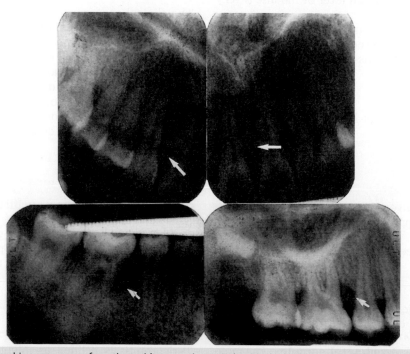

Fig. 33.6   Radiographic appearance of a patient with aggressive periodontitis showing localized periodontal bone loss (*arrows*).

Aggregatibacter actinomycetemcomitans is a rare but recognized pathogen in medical microbiology and has been implicated in actinomycosis (Chapter 13), abdominal and brain abscesses, septicaemia and infective endocarditis.

Management. Mechanical periodontal therapy and attention to oral hygiene are the mainstays of treatment. In many, adjunct therapy with tetracycline (250 mg three times a day for 4 weeks) produces resolution and may reduce the risk of reactivation.

Acute Necrotizing Ulcerative Gingivitis (ANUG)

Necrotizing ulcerative gingivitis, also known as acute necrotizing ulcerative gingivitis (ANUG), is rare in the West but may be seen in developing countries; it is commonly associated with poor and neglected oral hygiene, malnutrition and possibly systemic diseases.

CLINICAL FEATURES

The condition is characterized by actually inflamed, red, shiny and bleeding gingivae with irregularly shaped ulcers, which initially appear on the tips of the interdental papillae. If untreated, the ulcers enlarge and spread to involve the marginal and, rarely, the attached gingivae (Fig. 33.7). The lesions are **extremely painful** and are covered by a **pseudomembrane** (or slough), which can be wiped from the surface. The slough consists of leukocytes, erythrocytes, fibrin, necrotic tissue debris and microorganisms. Characteristically, the patient's breath is malodorous. The patient may complain of an unpleasant metallic taste. There is little or no systemic upset, and mild submandibular lymphadenitis; involvement of the cervical lymph nodes only occurs in severe cases. Generalized fever or malaise is very uncommon.

If the disease is inadequately treated, tissue destruction slows down and the disease may enter a chronic phase with pronounced loss of supporting tissues **(noma)**.

AETIOLOGY

The main predisposing factors of ANUG are:

- poor oral hygiene
- severe malnutrition
- heavy smoking
- emotional stress
- primary herpetic gingivostomatitis
- acquired immunosuppression, such as recent measles infection
- infection with HIV (see Chapter 30).

MICROBIOLOGY

The disease is a specific, anaerobic, polymicrobial infection, mainly due to the combined activity of fusobacteria (*Fusobacterium nucleatum*) and oral spirochaetes (*Treponema* spp.), the so-called **fusospirochaetal complex**. The main evidence for the microbial specificity of ANUG is:

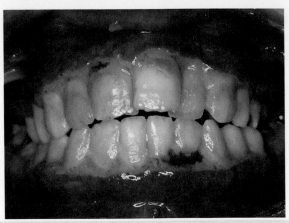

Fig. 33.7 Acute necrotizing ulcerative gingivitis (ANUG). Note the loss of papillae, spontaneous bleeding and gross plaque accumulation.

- microscopical association studies
- the ability of the complex to cause tissue destruction in other body sites, such as the tonsils (Vincent's angina, Chapter 23)
- animal studies
- rapid resolution of the disease and elimination of the fusospirochaetal complex after treatment with metronidazole
- invasion of the gingival soft tissues by both spirochaetes and fusiform bacilli.

Cultural studies indicate that medium-size spirochaetes account for one-third, and fusobacteria less than 5%, of the total flora. The remaining organisms include *Prevotella intermedia*, *Veillonella* spp. and streptococci.

DIAGNOSIS

The clinical appearance together with the offensive smell is pathognomonic. Confirmatory evidence is obtained by microscopy of a Gram-stained, deep gingival smear of the ulcerated lesion. A predominance of **three** components—**fusobacteria**, **spirochaetes** and **leukocytes**—is essential for a confident diagnosis (see Fig. 18.2); some, **but not all three**, of these components may be observed in primary herpetic stomatitis, gonococcal gingivitis, benign mucous membrane pemphigoid, desquamative gingivitis and some forms of leukaemia.

MANAGEMENT

1. Initial local debridement (with ultrasonic scaling, if possible) is essential.
2. Oral hygiene advice should be given, and mouthwashes (e.g., chlorhexidine) should be prescribed.
3. Metronidazole (200 mg three times daily for 4 days) is the drug of choice.

Pericoronitis

Pericoronitis is defined as inflammation of the soft tissues covering or immediately subjacent to the crown of a partially erupted tooth. The condition is frequently seen in the operculum and the soft tissues in erupting lower third molars of young adults.

CLINICAL FEATURES

Pericoronitis could be acute, chronic or recurrent.

- *Acute pericoronitis:* sudden onset and short lived, with significant symptoms such as trismus, extreme pain, especially when opposing tooth causes additional trauma
- *Chronic or recurrent:* repeated episodes of acute pericoronitis; presents with varying degrees of inflammation of the pericoronal flap and adjacent structures, as well as systemic complications.

If the infection is not resolved, a pericoronal abscess may ensue in some cases, especially in the debilitated.

PATHOGENESIS

1. Poor oral hygiene of the space between the tooth and the overlying mucosal tag (the operculum) causes bacterial and food stagnation.
2. If not attended to, spread of infection into the pterygomandibular space (in third lower molar pericoronitis), trismus and swelling of the soft tissues of the posterior mandibular region may result.
3. Further spread of infection into the parapharyngeal space may lead to Vincent's angina and airway obstruction if not immediately treated with high-dose antibiotic therapy (see Chapter 7).

MICROBIOLOGY

Pericoronitis is normally caused by a nonspecific mixture of oral bacteria. Strict anaerobes, such as *Prevotella intermedia*, *Fusobacterium* spp. and anaerobic streptococci are commonly present. Other periodontopathic organisms, such as *Aggregatibacter actinomycetemcomitans* and *Tannerella forsythia*, may also be found.

MANAGEMENT

1. **Mild cases:** local saline irrigation, especially underneath the operculum; trauma relief from the opposing tooth, if any
2. **Moderate to severe cases** (those with trismus, purulence, oedema): antibiotic therapy with penicillin either with or without clindamycin and metronidazole (see also Ludwig's angina, Chapter 34).

NOMA OR CANCRUM ORIS

In some developing countries (e.g., sub-Saharan Africa), an extremely severe form of ANUG—called **noma** or **cancrum oris** or **gangrenous stomatitis**—is seen in children. Typically, the child is less than 10 years old, severely malnourished (especially with regard to protein) and has a recent history of viral infection—for example, measles or another debilitating disease such as tuberculosis. As a result, the specific immune system of the child may be compromised, and the initial necrotic lesion may spread locally

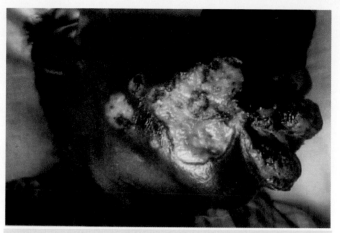

Fig. 33.8 Severe tissue destruction of the orofacial region in an Indian child with cancrum oris or noma.

from the gingivae into the cheek and sometimes to the face, causing extensive tissue loss and severe disfigurement (Fig. 33.8). Noma is extremely rare in developed countries.

Peri-implant Microbiology

Virtually thousands of dental implants are being placed worldwide on a daily basis. In the US alone, more than 3.5 million people currently have dental implants, and the number is increasing by 500,000 annually. This explosive demand for implants is due to the ready availability and accessibility of implant technology, as well as the resultant reduced placement cost of the implants. Hence the dental practitioners will face, in the future, not only an increased demand for dental implants but also a need for dental implant management and rehabilitation subsequent to its placement.

Once an implant is placed, it needs regular maintenance care, and a significant proportion of these prostheses succumb to **peri-implant disease,** which is essentially infectious in nature. However, systemic conditions influence the health of the implants as they do in periodontal diseases.

Although there are wide variations in the reported prevalence of peri-implant disease, which takes the form of either **peri-implant mucositis** or **peri-implantitis** (see below), data indicate that they are a relatively common clinical problem. In one recent report of a large cohort, the prevalence of peri-implant mucositis at the patient and implant levels were 44.4% and 38.2%, respectively. For peri-implantitis, the prevalence at the patient level was 5.6%, while the prevalence at the implant level was 4.0%.

Peri-implant diseases are also characterized by the inflammatory destruction of the implant-supporting, osseo-integrated tissues as a result of plaque biofilm formation on the implant surface.

Under the circumstances, US and European authorities have classified the information on implant complications in four major categories as follows:

- **Peri-implant health:** A lack of visible inflammation and no bleeding upon probing
- **Peri-implant mucositis:** Bleeding on probing and visible signs of inflammation

- **Peri-implantitis:** Inflammation of peri-implant mucosa followed by progressive loss of surrounding bone
- **Hard and soft tissue implant site deficiencies:** Deficiencies of the alveolar ridge caused by natural healing, extraction trauma, infections or a variety of other factors affecting hard and soft tissue.

PERI-IMPLANT DISEASE: PERI-IMPLANTITIS AND PERI-IMPLANT MUCOSITIS

Peri-implant diseases are inflammatory conditions affecting the peri-implant tissues and include **peri-implant mucositis** and **peri-implantitis**. Peri-implant mucositis refers to inflammation of the peri-implant soft tissues without loss of supporting bone. Peri-implantitis is inflammation of the peri-implant soft tissues with loss of supporting bone (Fig. 33.9). Indeed, peri-implant mucositis and peri-implantitis are analogous to gingivitis and periodontitis, both of which affect natural teeth.

Clinical Features

The most common signs and symptoms of peri-implantitis and peri-implant mucositis are:

- colour changes of the gingival tissue around the implant
- bleeding on brushing or probing
- increased pocket depth around the implant
- in severe cases, pus drainage from around the dental implant
- radiological evidence of bone loss around the implant.

Pathogenesis

Biofilm formation on dental implants and the associated supra structures is very similar to biofilm formation around natural teeth, both in its development and role in initiation of disease. As in the case of periodontitis, peri-implantitis can be aggressive with suppuration and bone loss around the infrastructure, and it may lead to loss of the implant.

Microbiology

In Health. Plaque biofilms found in the healthy peri-implant sulci around dental implants are similar in composition to biofilms found in healthy gingival sulci around teeth. There are low levels of bacteria with a predominance of facultative Gram-positive coccoid bacteria.

In Disease. Peri-implant diseases are **mixed microbial infections** and, in most cases, show a similar microflora

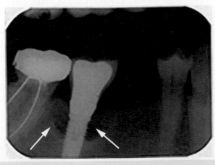

Fig. 33.9 Radiograph showing bone loss owing to peri-implantitis (arrows) around a single tooth implant. (Courtesy Professor Saso Ivanowski.)

to that found in chronic periodontitis, dominated by diverse Gram-negative anaerobic bacteria (*Tannerella forsythia*, *Porphyromonas gingivalis*, *Fusobacterium nucleatum*, *Aggregatibacter actinomycetemcomitans*). However, some studies show high numbers of other organisms such as peptostreptococci, staphylococci (*Staphylococcus aureus*), enteric rods and yeasts in peri-implantitis.

Studies evaluating the dynamics of colonization around dental implants in partially dentate individuals indicate that colonization begins within the first 30 min after exposure of the implant to the oral cavity. With time, a complex microflora gradually develops, which is similar in composition to biofilms found on neighbouring teeth. This underlines the importance of treating already existing periodontitis and establishing a microflora conducive to periodontal health prior to placing dental implants.

Variations in the biofilm composition are observed depending on the implant material, implant design and roughness of the implant surface. The latter in particular impacts biofilm formation with rough-surfaced implants accumulating more biofilms than smooth-surfaced implants.

The peri-implant biofilm microbiota also differs between implants in edentulous patients and those in partially dentate patients. The latter group appears to develop a more 'pathogenic' peri-implant microflora than the edentulous patients. This is not surprising, as partially dentate patients may already harbour a reservoir of subgingival 'periodontopathic' microbiota around their natural teeth that may seed the implant pockets, as opposed to totally edentulous individuals devoid of a microbiome with such pathogenic potential.

The immunopathological events and the composition of the immune cells in peri-implant infections are similar to those of periodontal infections. The lesions are characterized by a predominance of neutrophils and macrophages, as well as T and B cells. Nevertheless, compared to periodontitis, peri-implantitis is marked by a more extensive inflammatory infiltrate and innate immune response, a greater severity of tissue destruction and a faster progression rate, possibly due to the absence of a periodontal ligament and Sharpey's fibres and the rather mechanical nature of osseointegration.

MANAGEMENT

The management principles of peri-implantitis are similar to those of periodontitis. Essentially, plaque biofilm control by the patient, at home, using optimal oral hygiene and mechanical measures, along with professional dental management, are the mainstay of treatment. The rough implant surfaces may pose a challenge in achieving total biofilm control—hence, the critical importance of biofilm control through regular and effective oral hygiene regimens soon after implant placement.

Clinical Implications of Microbiological Tests in Periodontal Disease

Microbiological tests are useful in the management of periodontal disease to **identify** sites of active tissue destruction and to **monitor** the effects of treatment and decide when recall is necessary. The presence of a specific putative pathogen associated with any of the aforementioned periodontal diseases could be detected by:

- **direct microscopy** of one or more smears of samples obtained from the affected site
- **cultural studies** of the predominant cultivable pathogens, using media that select the specific pathogen (e.g., tryptic soy–serum–bacitracin–vancomycin (TSBV) medium to select *Aggregatibacter actinomycetemcomitans*)
- **enzymatic studies** using commercially available test kits that use synthetic substrates (e.g., benzoin arginine naphthylamine (BANA)) to detect arginine-specific proteases liberated by some periodontopathic organisms (e.g., *Porphyromonas gingivalis*, *Tannerella forsythia*, *Treponema denticola*)
- **molecular studies** using principles of PCR to detect specific pathogens. In this context, **NGS technology** and associated rapid diagnostic tests are becoming increasingly fashionable clinical tools as the latter technology could provide **a thumbprint of the patient's oral microbiota**. Looking into the future, it is likely that the oralome and the microbiota of an individual may provide clues on his/her susceptibility for periodontal disease, which may in turn help clinicians to personalize the preventive dental program of the individual.

However, all of the above tests are only useful (a) if the identified organisms are definitively known to cause the disease and (b) if samples can be collected accurately from the site of disease activity (i.e., probably the base of the periodontal pocket in the case of aggressive peridontitis). As this stage has not yet been reached, doubt exists as to the value of these diagnostic tests. Sampling for the presence of *Aggregatibacter actinomycetemcomitans* in aggressive periodontitis and evaluating a Gram-stained smear of the gingival plaque biofilm of suspected ANUG patients for the fuso-spirochaetal complex are perhaps the only microbiological tests that are likely to contribute to the treatment of these diseases at present.

A NOTE ON THE ROLE OF ARCHEA AND VIRUSES IN PERIODONTAL DISEASE

There are a few reports to indicate that viruses and archea may play a role in periodontal disease. Such an association has been suggested for HIV and herpesviruses, especially in view of the aggravation of periodontal diseases in HIV disease (Chapter 30). The demonstration of viral DNA in gingival tissues, crevicular fluid and subgingival plaque in diseased sites has added some credence to this hypothesis. On the other hand, some species of archea such as *Mehtnaosarcina vacuolata* are significantly reduced in periodontal pockets, implying that they may play a role in the homeostasis of this ecosystem. However, conclusive data are warranted to confirm the role of either the archea or viruses in periodontal disease.

Key Facts

- Periodontal disease can be broadly categorized into **gingivitis** and **periodontitis**.
- Clinical features of plaque-related **gingivitis** are **redness**, **oedema** and **bleeding**.
- Periodontitis usually develops from a preexisting gingivitis; however, not every gingivitis develops into periodontitis.
- Periodontitis can be classified into two main groups: **chronic** and **aggressive**. The chronic form is by far the most prevalent disease globally.
- The aggressive form of periodontitis includes those previously categorized as juvenile (localized or generalized), rapidly progressive and prepubertal periodontitis.
- Currently recognized key Gram-negative **periodontopathogens** include *Porphyromonas gingivalis*, *Prevotella intermedia*, *Tannerella forsythia* (formerly *Bacteroides forsythus*) and *Aggregatibacter actinomycetemcomitans*. Some consider *Fusobacterium nucleatum* and *Capnocytophaga* spp. and spirochaetes as equally important (*Note*: *Treponema denticola*, a key periodontopathogen, is Gram neutral).
- The three major, so-called 'red complex' or **'keystone'**, **periodontopathogens** are *Porphyromonas gingivalis*, *Tannerella forsythia* and *Treponema denticola*.
- Disease activity in periodontal disease may range from **slow, chronic progressive destruction** to **brief and acute 'episodic bursts'** with varying intensity and duration (in different sites in the same mouth); hence, microbiological **sampling** for diseased sites or activity is **extremely difficult**.

- In adult periodontitis, the microflora changes from aerobic, nonmotile, Gram-positive cocci to anaerobic, motile, Gram-negative bacilli.
- **Localized or generalized aggressive periodontitis** is strongly associated with *Aggregatibacter actinomycetemcomitans*, either alone or synergistically with *Capnocytophaga* spp. and *Porphyromonas gingivalis*.
- **Necrotizing ulcerative gingivitis** is a specific, anaerobic, polymicrobial infection due to the combined activity of *Fusobacterium nucleatum* and oral spirochaetes (*Treponema* spp.): the **fusospirochaetal complex**.
- In the developing world (e.g., sub-Saharan Africa), an extremely severe, **tissue-destructive sequela** of acute (necrotizing) ulcerative gingivitis (ANUG), called **noma** or **cancrum oris**, is seen mainly in children.
- **Microbiological tests** used in the management of periodontal disease may help **identify** sites of active tissue destruction, **monitor** efficacy of therapy and **decide recall** intervals.
- The presence of putative periodontopathogens could be detected by (1) direct microscopy, (2) microbial cultures, (3) biochemical and immunological methods and (4) molecular methods.
- Periodontal diseases can be treated by plaque control, root surface debridement, periodontal surgery and the prudent use of antimicrobial agents.
- Peri-implant mucositis and peri-implantitis are analogous to gingivitis and periodontitis, respectively, that affect natural teeth.
- Peri-implant diseases are mixed, plaque biofilm–associated infections and in most cases are due to microflora similar to that of chronic periodontitis.

Review Questions (Answers on p. 392)

Please indicate which answers are true and which are false.

33.1. The gingival crevice is a unique ecological niche. Which of the following are true of the gingival crevice?
   a. it is more aerobic than the other locales of the mouth
   b. the presence of gingival crevicular fluid indicates pathology
   c. an increase in the pH promotes the growth of *Porphyromonas gingivalis*
   d. inhabitants of the periodontal pocket are significantly different from those in the gingival crevice
   e. the crevicular flora is polymicrobial, and it comprises both anaerobic and facultative anaerobic organisms

33.2. The pathogenesis of periodontal disease is explained by two contrasting mechanisms: the specific and the nonspecific plaque hypotheses. Indicate which of the following statements supports the specific plaque hypothesis:
   a. necrotizing ulcerative gingivitis responds to treatment with metronidazole
   b. *Aggregatibacter actinomycetemcomitans* is a major agent of aggressive periodontitis
   c. numerous bacterial species are found in advanced periodontal pockets
   d. virulence attributes of a consortium of organisms perpetuate the disease
   e. polymorphs are present in the crevicular fluid

33.3. Which of the following statements on the natural history of periodontal disease are true?
   a. Gram-positive cocci predominate in the healthy gingival crevice
   b. the proportion of Gram-positive rods decreases to nearly 5% in chronic marginal gingivitis
   c. Gram-negative anaerobes predominate in chronic periodontitis
   d. facultative anaerobes predominate in gingivitis
   e. about 75% of the flora in periodontitis is Gram-negative bacilli

33.4. Chronic periodontitis is characterized by:
   a. systemic symptoms such as fever
   b. tooth mobility and migration
   c. gingival recession
   d. bleeding pockets of more than 3 mm depth
   e. absence of pain in general

33.5. Predisposing factors for acute necrotizing ulcerative gingivitis include:
   a. poor oral hygiene
   b. severe malnutrition
   c. heavy smoking
   d. immunodeficiency
   e. diabetes

Further Reading

Armitage, G. C. (1999). Development of a classification system for periodontal disease. *Annals of Periodontology, 4*, 1–6.

Belibasakis, G. N. (2014). Microbiological and immuno-pathological aspects of peri-implant diseases. *Archives of Oral Biology, 59*, 66–72.

Cappuyns, I., Gugerli, P., & Mombelli, A. (2005). Viruses in periodontal disease: A review. *Oral Diseases, 11*, 219–229.

Curtis, M. A., Zenobia, C., & Darveau, R. P. (2011). The relationship of the oral microbiota to periodontal health and disease. *Cell Host & Microbe, 10*, 302–306.

Deng, Z. L., Szafrański, S. P., Jarek, M. et al. (2017). Dysbiosis in chronic periodontitis: Key microbial players and interactions with the human host. *Sci Rep, 7*, 3703. https://doi.org/10.1038/s41598-017-03804-8.

Dietrich, T., Ower, P., Tank, M., West, N. X., Walter, C., Needleman, I., Hughes, F. J., Wadia, R., Milward, M. R., Hodge, P. J., Chapple, I. L. C., & British Society of Periodontology. (2019). Periodontal diagnosis in the context of the 2017 classification system of periodontal diseases and conditions - implementation in clinical practice. *British Dental Journal, 226*(1), 16–22. doi:10.1038/sj.bdj.2019.3. Erratum in *British Dental Journal, 226*(4), 295.

Enwonwu, C. O. (2006). Noma: The ulcer of extreme poverty. *New England Journal of Medicine, 354*, 221–224.

Marsh, P. D., & Marin, M. V. (2009). *Oral microbiology* (5th ed.). Churchill Livingstone.

Mombelli, A., & Samaranayake, L. P. (2004). Topical and systemic antibiotics in the management of periodontal disease. *International Dental Journal, 54*, 3–14.

Socransky, S. S., & Haffajee, A. D. (2003). Microbiology of periodontal disease. In J. Lindhe, T. Karring, & N. P. Lang (Eds.), *Clinical periodontology and implant dentistry* (4th ed., pages: 114–124). Blackwell Munksgaard.

Socransky, S. S., Haffajee, A. D., Cugini, M. A., Smith, C., & Kent, R. L. (1998). Microbial complexes in subgingival plaque. *Journal of Clinical Periodontology, 25*, 134–144.

34 Dentoalveolar and Endodontic Infections

Dentoalveolar infections can be defined as pus-producing (or **pyogenic)** infections associated with the teeth and surrounding supporting structures, such as the periodontium and the alveolar bone. Other terms for these conditions include *periapical abscess, apical abscess, chronic periapical dental infection, dental pyogenic infection, periapical periodontitis* and *dentoalveolar abscess.* The clinical presentation of dentoalveolar infections depends on the **virulence** of the causative microorganisms, the **local** and **systemic defence** mechanisms of the host and the **anatomical features** of the region. Depending on the interactions of these factors, the resulting infection may present as:

- an **abscess** localized to the tooth that initiated the infection
- a diffuse **cellulitis** that spreads along fascial planes
- a **mixture** of both.

Natural History of Dentoalveolar Infections

In health, the dental pulp and the apical periodontium are essentially sterile. The dental pulp can become infected due to dental caries, dental trauma or via extraradicular root canals from deep periodontal pockets. Most frequently, the dental pulp infection is transmitted through dentinal tubules due to a carious lesion. The subsequent inflammation of the pulp tissue is called 'pulpitis'.

If early pulpitis is left untreated, the inflammation develops into an irreversible condition termed **symptomatic irreversible pulpitis**, whence the pulp gradually becomes necrotic. This condition may manifest as occasional sharp pain, usually stimulated by temperature change, and can worsen to spontaneous, constant and dull or severe pain.

Table 34.1 Various Clinical Stages and the Associated Key Clinical Signs and Symptoms During Progression From Pulpitis to Dentoalveolar Infection

Clinical Stage	Characteristic Signs and Symptoms
Symptomatic irreversible pulpitis	Spontaneous pain that may linger with thermal changes due to vital but irreversible pulpitis
Symptomatic apical periodontitis	Pain with mastication and/or percussion or palpation, with or without evidence of radiographic periapical pathology, and without swelling; pulp may still be vital
Pulp necrosis and symptomatic apical periodontitis	Nonvital pulp, and pain with mastication and/or percussion or palpation, with or without evidence of radiographic periapical pathosis, and without swelling
Pulp necrosis and localized acute apical dentoalveolar abscess	Nonvital pulp, with spontaneous pain with or without mastication and/or percussion or palpation, with formation of purulent material, localized swelling, and without evidence of fascial space or local lymph node involvement, fever or malaise
Acute apical dentoalveolar abscess with systemic involvement	Necrotic pulp with spontaneous pain, with or without mastication and/or percussion or palpation, with formation of purulent material, swelling, evidence of fascial space or local lymph node involvement, fever and/or malaise

(Modified from Lockhart, P. B., et al (2019). *Journal of the American Dental Association, 150*(11), 906–921; see further reading section of this Chapter).

Progressive pulp inflammation in the apical region may lead to a necrotic pulp and the infection spreading into the periodontium, a condition termed **symptomatic apical periodontitis**. If untreated, the infection may spread through the alveolar bone to the soft tissues surrounding the jaw to create an **acute apical dentoalveolar abscess**. Depending on the location and the patient's general health, this can further spread into other tissues of the body to cause even **systemic infection** (Table 34.1).

In clinical terms, dental pain and/or intraoral swelling associated with pulpal or subjacent tissue is not only a concern for dental providers but is also the most cited oral health-related reason for a patient contacting an emergency department or physician.

Source of Microorganisms

Most commonly, endogenous oral commensals are the source, usually from the apex of a necrotic tooth or from periodontal pockets as a result of either caries or periodontal disease (Fig. 34.1). Other conditions include accidentally traumatized teeth (e.g., sports injury), pulp exposed teeth due to surgery and so on (see below).

Apical Dentoalveolar Abscess

In a majority of cases, an apical dentoalveolar abscess usually develops by extension of the initial carious lesion into dentine, along with spread of bacteria to the pulp via the dentinal tubules (Figs. 34.1 and 34.2). The pulp responds to infection by rapid **acute inflammation** involving the whole pulp with subsequent sequelae (mentioned above). Bacteria may reach the pulpal compartment through a number of other routes:

- by **traumatic tooth fracture** and pulp exposure
- via **dentinal tubules** due to attrition, abrasion or erosion of dental enamel and exposure of dentine
- by **iatrogenic** traumatic exposure during dental treatment
- through the **periodontal membrane** (periodontitis and pericoronitis) and accessory root canals
- rarely by **anachoresis**—that is, seeding of organisms directly into pulp via the pulpal blood supply during bacteraemia (e.g., tooth extraction at a different site).

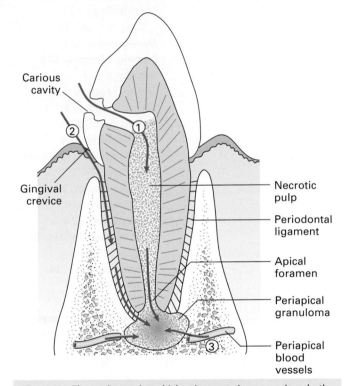

Fig. 34.1 The pathways by which microorganisms may invade the pulp and periapical tissues: (1) from the apical foramen, (2) via the periodontal ligament and (3) via the blood stream (anachoresis).

Labels: Carious cavity; Gingival crevice; Necrotic pulp; Periodontal ligament; Apical foramen; Periapical granuloma; Periapical blood vessels

SEQUELAE

Once pus formation occurs, it may:

1. remain **localized** at the root apex and develop into either an **acute** or a **chronic abscess**
2. lead to low grade alveolar infection and a **focal osteomyelitis**
3. spread into the subjacent subcutaneous tissues leading to **fascial space infection, cellulitis** and eventually **Ludwig's angina,** or **cavernous sinus thrombosis,** if untreated (Figs. 34.2 and 34.3)
4. lead to chronic, low-grade apical infection near the root apex and formation of a **granuloma** and a **periapical cyst**
5. lead to **sinus** formation extraorally onto the skin or intraorally into the maxillary sinus.

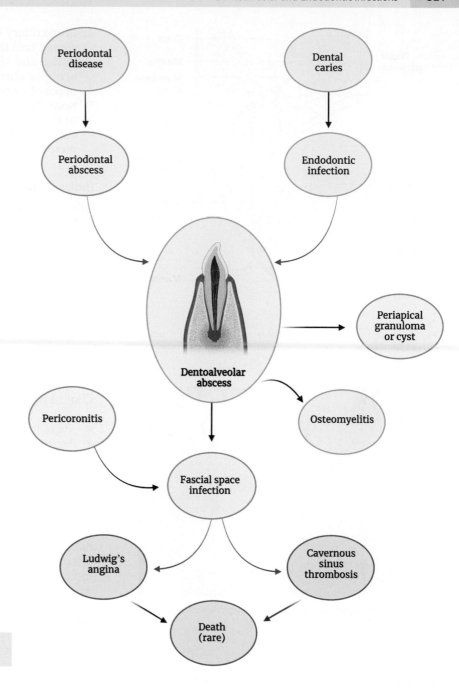

Fig. 34.2 Possible prequelae and sequelae of a dentoalveolar abscess.

6. rarely **death** may ensue due to airway obstruction consequential to Ludwig's angina.

The time required for complete necrosis of the pulp is variable. In some cases, this may happen within days or weeks. However, in others localized, subacute, chronic, insidious infection may be present for many months or even years before the pulp eventually succumbs. The sequelae of this chronic process can be classified further as those due to **direct spread** or indirect spread of infection, as follows.

Direct Spread

1. Spread into the superficial soft tissues may:
   - **localize** as a soft-tissue abscess (Fig. 34.4)
   - extend through the overlying oral mucosa or skin, producing a **sinus** linking the main abscess cavity with the mouth or skin
   - extend through the soft tissue to produce a **cellulitis**.
2. Spread may occur into the adjacent fascial spaces, following the **path of least resistance**; such spread is dependent on the anatomical relation of the original abscess to the adjacent tissues (Table 34.2). Infection via fascial planes often spreads rapidly and for some distance from the original abscess site, and it occasionally may cause severe respiratory distress as a result of occlusion of the airway by oedema (e.g., Ludwig's angina).
3. Infection may extend into the deeper medullary spaces of alveolar bone, producing a spreading **osteomyelitis**; this may occur in compromised patients.

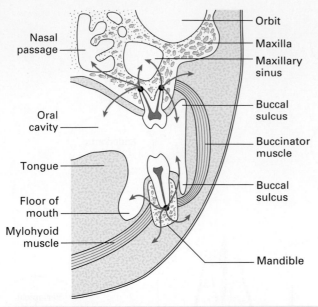

Fig. 34.3 Anatomical pathways (blue arrows) by which pus may spread from an acute dentoalveolar abscess (coronal section, at the first molar tooth level).

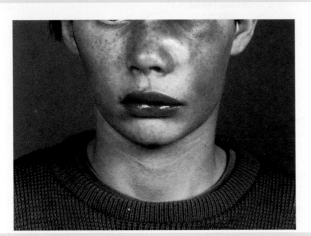

Fig. 34.4 Extension of periapical infection from the left upper canine tooth to the infraorbital region in a teenager.

4. In maxillary teeth, odontogenic infection may directly spread into the maxillary sinus, especially if the sinus lining and the tooth apex are subjacent, leading to acute or chronic **secondary maxillary sinusitis** (as opposed to primary sinusitis due to direct sinus infection). Such infection, if not arrested, may rarely spread to the central nervous system, causing serious complications such as subdural empyema, brain abscesses or meningitis.

Indirect Spread

Other sequelae entail indirect spread via:

- **lymphatic routes**, to regional nodes in the head and neck region (submental, submandibular, deep cervical, parotid and occipital); usually, the involved nodes are tender, swollen and painful, and rarely may suppurate, requiring drainage
- **haematogenous routes**: to other organs such as the brain (rare).

CLINICAL FEATURES

Clinical signs and symptoms depend on the:

- site of infection
- degree and mode of spread
- virulence of the causative organisms
- efficiency of the host defences.

Clinical features may include a nonviable tooth with or without a carious lesion, a large restoration, evidence of trauma, swelling, pain, redness, trismus, local lymph node enlargement, sinus formation, raised temperature and malaise. The latter two symptoms are a direct consequence of increased levels of systemic inflammatory cytokines such as interleukins and tumour necrosis factor in response to bacterial products such as lipopolysaccharides (i.e., endotoxins).

Table 34.2 Sites of Contiguous Spread of Dentoalveolar Infection (see also Fig. 34.3)

Site of Spread	Maxillary Teeth	Mandibular Teeth
Palate	Palatal roots of premolars and molars; also, lateral incisors with a palatally curved root	—
Buccal space	Canines, premolars and molars	Canines, premolars and molars
Infraorbital/periorbital region	Canines mainly	—
Maxillary sinus	Canines, premolars and molars	—
Upper lip	Central and lateral incisors	—
Masseteric space, pterygomandibular space, lateral pharyngeal space	—	Lower third molars
Lower lip	—	Incisors and canines
Submandibular space	—	Root apices below insertion of mylohyoid; usually molars but can also be premolars
Submental space	—	Incisors and canines
Sublingual space	—	Root apices above mylohyoid/geniohyoid; usually incisors, canines and premolars; rarely molars

MICROBIOLOGY

Microbiologically, the dentoalveolar abscess is characterized by the following features:

- infection is usually **polymicrobial** (endogenous), with a mixture of three or four different species
- **monomicrobial** (endogenous) infection (i.e., with a single organism) is unusual
- strict anaerobes are the predominant organisms, and the *viridans* group streptococci are less common than once thought.

The common species isolated from dentoalveolar abscesses are *Prevotella*, *Porphyromonas* and *Fusobacterium* spp., and anaerobic streptococci; facultative anaerobes are the second largest group, for example *Streptococcus milleri* (Table 34.3). There is evidence that some strictly anaerobic bacteria, especially *Porphyromonas gingivalis* and *Fusobacterium* spp., are more likely to cause severe infection than other species, and that synergistic microbial interactions play an important role in the severity of dentoalveolar abscesses.

Apart from the foregoing, culturable bacteria, recent studies have indicated that up to **13%** of the cumulative number of bacteria derived from dentoalveolar lesions are **unculturable**. This suggests that they are likely to play a yet unknown, critical role in the pathogenesis and progression of the disease.

Collection and Transport of Pus Samples

1. Wherever possible, pus should be collected by **needle aspiration** or in a sterile container after external incision. Care must be exercised during recapping the syringe after needle aspiration, and a safety device must be used. In addition, it is important to drain the residual pus once the aspirate has been obtained via an appropriate incision (see Chapter 6).
2. If **swabs** must be used, then a strict **aseptic collection technique** is required. (Because of the indigenous flora on mucosal surfaces, it is difficult, if not impossible, to collect uncontaminated samples when intraoral swabs are used for pus collection.) When the pus sample is contaminated with saliva or dental plaque during collection, this information must be recorded on the request form.

MANAGEMENT

The specific treatment for any given individual will vary. The major management guidelines entail:

Table 34.3 Bacteria Commonly Isolated from Dentoalveolar Abscesses

Facultative anaerobes
   Streptococcus milleri
   Streptococcus sanguinis
   Actinomyces spp.

Obligate anaerobes
   Peptostreptococcus spp.
   Porphyromonas gingivalis
   Prevotella intermedia
   Prevotella melaninogenica
   Fusobacterium nucleatum

1. draining the pus
2. **removing** the source of **infection**
3. prescribing **antibiotics**, probably not required for the majority of localized abscesses, although it may be necessary:
   - when drainage cannot be established immediately
   - if the abscess has spread to the superficial soft tissues
   - when the patient is febrile.

Standard antibiotics include:

- phenoxymethylpenicillin (penicillin V) or short-course, high-dose amoxicillin
- in penicillin-hypersensitive patients: erythromycin or metronidazole (as most infections are due to strict anaerobes).

Ludwig's Angina

Ludwig's angina is defined as a spreading, bilateral infection of the sublingual and submandibular spaces. This is one of the rare situations, in dentistry, when a dental professional can asphyxiate and kill a patient, through slow intervention to relieve immediate airway obstruction.

AETIOLOGY

In the vast majority of cases (about 90%), Ludwig's angina is precipitated by dental or postextraction infection; uncommon sources of infection include submandibular sialadenitis, infected mandibular fracture, oral soft-tissue laceration and puncture wounds of the floor of the mouth. The infection is essentially a **cellulitis** of the **fascial spaces** rather than true abscess formation.

CLINICAL FEATURES

The infection of sublingual and submandibular spaces raises the floor of the mouth and tongue and causes the tissues at the front of the neck to swell. The brawny swelling has a characteristic boardlike consistency, which can barely be indented by the finger. There is severe systemic upset with fever.

Complications include:

- airway obstruction due to either oedema of the glottis or a swollen tongue blocking the nasopharynx
- spread of infection to the masticator and pharyngeal spaces
- death due to asphyxiation, which is a certainty without immediate intervention.

MICROBIOLOGY

Oral commensal bacteria are common agents, especially *Porphyromonas* and *Prevotella* spp., fusobacteria and anaerobic streptococci; it is a **mixed endogenous infection**. Because of the severity of the condition, samples for microbiology assessment should always be obtained, if possible.

MANAGEMENT

1. Ensure that the patient's **airway** remains open (surgically, if necessary).
2. Maintain **fluid balance**.

3. Immediately institute very **high doses of empirical antibiotic therapy** (usually intravenous penicillin, with or without metronidazole).
4. Collect a **sample of pus** before antibiotic therapy, if the patient's condition permits, or immediately afterward.
5. Change the prescribed **antibiotic** if necessary, once the bacteriological results are available.
6. Institute **surgical drainage** in cases of suppurative infection: purulent needle aspirate, crepitus, fluctuance and soft tissue air. The surgical drainage serves two purposes: first, decompressing the fascial compartments of the neck to relieve airway pressure and, second, to evacuate the pus.

Surgical drainage may yield little pus in most cases, particularly in cellulitis.

7. **Eliminate** the primary **source of infection** (e.g., a nonvital tooth).

Pericoronitis (See Chapter 33.)

ALVEOLAR OSTEITIS (DRY SOCKET)

This extremely painful condition called **localized alveolar osteitis,** usually ensues due to a complication of wound healing following a tooth extraction. Alveolar osteitis is seen after approximately 3% of routine extractions and in almost one in five surgical extractions, although these figures may vary in different locales.

AETIOLOGY

Not fully understood; thought to be due to the fibrinolysis of blood clot by anaerobic flora; smoking and oral contraceptives are thought to predispose the condition.

CLINICAL FEATURES

- More common in females
- More common in mandible than maxilla
- Symptoms: severe, throbbing pain, halitosis
- An extraction socket devoid of granulation tissue.

MICROBIOLOGY

Possibly a polymicrobial opportunistic infection with a predominance of anaerobic flora; other causative reasons have been proposed.

MANAGEMENT

- Debridement of socket with chlorhexidine or saline
- Control the pain with analgesics
- Metronidazole may be an option in recalcitrant cases.

Periodontal Abscess

A periodontal abscess is caused by an acute or chronic destructive process in the periodontium, resulting in localized collection of pus communicating with the oral cavity through the gingival sulcus and/or other periodontal sites (and not arising from the tooth pulp).

AETIOLOGY

The abscess probably forms by occlusion or trauma to the orifice of a periodontal pocket, resulting in the extension of infection from the pocket into the supporting tissues. These events might result from **impaction of food** such as a fish bone, or of a detached toothbrush bristle, or from **compression of the pocket wall** by orthodontic tooth movement or by unusual occlusal forces. Normally, the abscess remains localized in the periodontal tissues, and its subsequent development depends on:

- the virulence, type and number of the causative organisms
- the health of the patient's periodontal tissues
- the efficiency of the specific and nonspecific defence mechanisms of the host.

CLINICAL FEATURES

1. Onset is sudden, with swelling, redness and tenderness of the gingiva overlying the abscess.
2. Pain is continuous or related to biting and can be elicited clinically by percussion of the affected tooth.
3. There are no specific radiographic features, although it is commonly associated with a deep periodontal pocket.
4. Pus from the lesion usually drains along the root surface to the orifice of the periodontal pocket; in deep pockets, pus may extend through the alveolar bone to drain through a sinus that opens onto the attached gingiva.
5. Because of intermittent drainage of pus, infection tends to remain localized, and extraoral swelling is uncommon.
6. Untreated abscesses may lead to severe destruction of periodontal tissues and tooth loss.

MICROBIOLOGY

Endogenous, subgingival plaque bacteria are the source of the microorganisms in periodontal abscesses; infection is polymicrobial, with the following bacteria being commonly isolated:

- anaerobic Gram-negative rods, especially black-pigmented *Porphyromonas* and *Prevotella* spp., and fusobacteria
- streptococci, especially haemolytic streptococci and anaerobic streptococci
- others, such as spirochaetes, *Capnocytophaga* spp. and *Actinomyces* spp.

TREATMENT

1. Make a thorough clinical assessment of the patient, including a history of systemic illnesses (e.g., diabetes).
2. If the prognosis is poor, owing to advanced periodontitis or recurrent infection, and it is unlikely that treatment will achieve functional periodontal tissues, then extract the tooth. If the abscess is small and localized, extraction may be carried out immediately; otherwise,

extraction should be postponed until acute infection has subsided.

3. Drainage should be encouraged, and gentle subgingival scaling should be performed to remove calculus and foreign objects.
4. Irrigate the pocket with warm 0.9% sodium chloride solution and prescribe regular hot saline mouthwashes.
5. If pyrexia or cellulitis is present, antibiotics should be prescribed: penicillin, erythromycin and metronidazole are the drugs of choice.

Suppurative Osteomyelitis of the Jaws

Suppurative osteomyelitis is a relatively rare condition that may present as an acute or chronic infection, depending on a variety of factors.

DEFINITION

An **inflammation of the medullary cavity** of the mandible or the maxilla, with possible extension of infection into the cortical bone and the periosteum as a sequela.

AETIOLOGY

Osteomyelitis of the head and neck region is much rarer than dentoalveolar infections, probably because of the good vascular supply to the bone. Accordingly, osteomyelitis of the mandible is more common than of the maxillary region due to the better vascular supply to the latter regions. Conditions that tend to reduce the vascularity of bone predispose to osteomyelitis (e.g., radiation, osteoporosis, Paget's disease, fibrous dysplasia and bone tumours). Drug therapy such as osteoclast inhibitors including denosumab and bisphosphates have resulted in osteonecrosis and related osteomyelitis (Fig. 34.5).

A wide range of organisms have been associated with osteomyelitis of the jaws, including endogenous bacteria (described in the following text) and, rarely, exogenous organisms such as *Treponema pallidum* and *Mycobacterium tuberculosis*.

1. The source of infection is usually a **contiguous focus**, or **haematogenous seeding** of bacteria may occur infrequently.
2. Bacteria multiply in bony medulla and elicit an acute inflammatory reaction.
3. This results in increased intramedullary pressure leading to venous stasis, ischaemia and pus formation.
4. Pus spreads through the Haversian canal system, breaching the periosteum, with resultant **sinus formation** and appearance of **soft-tissue abscesses** on the oral mucosa or skin.
5. If there is no intervention, chronic osteomyelitis results, with new bone (**involucrum**) formation and separation of fragments of necrotic bone (**sequestra**).

CLINICAL FEATURES OF ACUTE OSTEOMYELITIS

Clinical features include pain, mild fever, paraesthesia or anaesthesia of the related skin; loosening of teeth; and

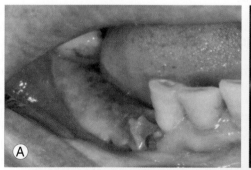
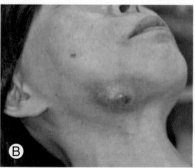
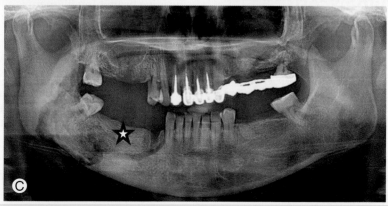

Fig. 34.5 Medication-related osteomyelitis (chronic diffuse type) of the left mandibular region in a female patient taking drugs to prevent bone thinning. (A) Intraoral appearance of the exposed bony mandibular surface, denuded of the mucosa. (B) Associated oral cutaneous fistula. (C) Radiographic image of the radiolucent lesion (asterisk) of the left mandible.
(Courtesy Dr. Yu-Feng Chen and Hong-Po Chang)

exudation of pus from gingival margins or through sinuses or fistulae in the affected skin.

CLINICAL FEATURES OF CHRONIC OSTEOMYELITIS

In chronic osteomyelitis, there is minimal systemic upset, chronic sinuses or fistulae may be present, with little pus, and tender and indurated skin (Fig. 34.5).

MICROBIOLOGY

As the majority of osteomyelitis cases begin as a dentoalveolar infection, the causative organisms of both diseases are similar. **Anaerobes** are the most common isolates— for example, *Tannerella*, *Prevotella* and *Porphyromonas* spp., fusobacteria and anaerobic streptococci; rarely **enterobacteria** may be present. *Staphylococcus aureus*, the most common agent of osteomyelitis in long bones, is infrequently isolated from jaw lesions.

TREATMENT

The management of osteomyelitis is complex. The main principles are:

1. rapid diagnosis of the disease
2. empirical prescription of antibiotics (to prevent further bone destruction and surgical intervention)
3. collection of a pus sample, if feasible, for investigations; collect pus with care when it is exuding from the gingival sulcus, to prevent contamination with commensal bacteria; aspirate pus from contiguous soft-tissue lesions
4. send the sample immediately to the laboratory in anaerobic transport medium for identification and sensitivity testing of causative bacteria
5. drugs of choice are penicillin, penicillinase-resistant penicillins (e.g., flucloxacillin) and, in penicillin-allergic patients, clindamycin and erythromycin
6. other treatment options include tooth extraction, sequestrectomy and resection, and reconstruction of the jaws.

Cervicofacial Actinomycosis

Actinomycosis (see Chapter 13) is an endogenous, granulomatous disease that may occur in the following sites:

- cervicofacial region, most common (60–65%)
- abdomen (10–20%)
- lung
- skin.

AETIOLOGY

In humans, the main infecting organism is *Actinomyces israelii*, which is a common oral commensal present in plaque, carious dentine and calculus. Trauma to the jaws, tooth extraction and teeth with gangrenous pulps may precipitate infection (e.g., calculus or plaque becoming impacted in the depths of a tooth socket at the time of extraction).

CLINICAL FEATURES

Predominantly a disease of younger people, although all ages may be affected, the infection can present in an **acute, subacute** or **chronic form**. There is usually a history of trauma, such as a tooth extraction or a blow to the jaw. Most infections start as an acute swelling indistinguishable on clinical grounds from a dentoalveolar abscess. The chronic form of the disease follows, due to either inadequate or no therapy, or subacute infection related to trauma.

Swelling is common and is either localized or diffuse; if untreated, it may progress into discharging sinuses. Classically, this discharge of pus contains visible granules, which may be gritty to touch, yellow and known as **'sulphur granules'** (a descriptive term, as sulphur is not found in the granules). These granules in pus are almost pathognomonic of the disease.

The submandibular region is most commonly affected; rarely the maxillary antrum, salivary glands and tongue may be involved. Pain is a variable feature. Other features, depending on the site of infection, are multiple discharging sinuses, trismus, pyrexia, fibrosis around the swelling and the presence of infected teeth.

MICROBIOLOGY

The most common agent is *Actinomyces israelii*, although *Actinomyces bovis* and *Actinomyces naeslundii* may occasionally be isolated. In a minority, *Aggregatibacter actinomycetemcomitans* may be isolated in mixed culture with *Actinomyces israelii*.

Laboratory Diagnosis

If a fluctuant abscess is present, collect fluid pus by aspiration using a syringe, or in a sterile container if drainage by external incision is performed. Examine the pus for the presence of 'sulphur granules'; Gram films are made from any part with a lumpy or granular appearance. The granules are washed and crushed in tissue grinders and cultured on blood agar under anaerobic conditions at 37°C for 7 days. **Colonies** often produce a typical **'molar tooth'** morphology (see Fig. 13.1). Pure cultures are then identified using biochemical techniques. A Gram film of a colony will reveal moderate to large clumps of Gram-positive branching filaments.

MANAGEMENT

Acute Lesions

1. Removal of any associated dental focus
2. Incision and drainage of facial abscess
3. A 2- to 3-week course of antibiotics; penicillin is the drug of choice.

Subacute or Chronic Lesions

1. Surgical intervention, as in (1) and (2) above
2. A *longer* antibiotic course, 5–6 weeks on average.

If penicillin cannot be given because of hypersensitivity, erythromycin, tetracycline and clindamycin are good alternatives. The latter drugs penetrate bony tissues well.

Facial Lacerations

On occasion, facial soft-tissue wounds, owing to traumatic or similar injuries, may get infected.

AETIOLOGY

Commensal skin flora such as *Staphylococcus aureus*, *Staphylococcus epidermidis* and *Corynebacterium acnes*.

MANAGEMENT

- Debridement with saline
- Close wound by suturing or adhesive strips, if necessary
- Tetanus vaccine/antibody, if the wound is contaminated, as appropriate
- If infected, swab sample taken for culture and sensitivity
- If infected, antibiotics with known activity against staphylococci (e.g., flucloxacillin)
- Topical application of mupirocin or fucidin cream.

Endodontic Infections

Most common diseases that affect the dental pulp and periapical tissues are bacterial infections originating from the commensal microbiota of the oral microbiome, and hence they are called endogenous infections (*syn.* root canal infections; intraradicular infections), as opposed to exogenous infections caused by bacteria from external sources (e.g., tuberculosis). Root canal or intraradicular or endodontic infections are classic endogenous infections.

Note: Microbiology of endodontic infections is a complex subject and only a thumb sketch is provided here; readers are urged to consult reference texts in this chapter's Further Reading list for fuller accounts of the subject.

For **sources and routes of infection** of pulp and periapical tissue, see above and Fig. 34.1.

PATHOGENESIS OF PULP AND PERIAPICAL INFECTIONS

As described, once bacteria gain access into the sterile pulp chamber, it is extremely difficult for the host defences to completely eliminate them. Resultant acute or chronic inflammation of the pulp, which of course is encased in its mineralized 'tomb', inevitably leads to stasis of the blood supply owing to compressive forces on pulpal blood vessels entering through a narrow apical foramen. Natural pulpal defences on their own cannot cope with this outcome, and in a majority of cases pulpal necrosis is the end result. This, in turn, sets in motion a cascade of events (Fig. 34.6; Table 34.1).

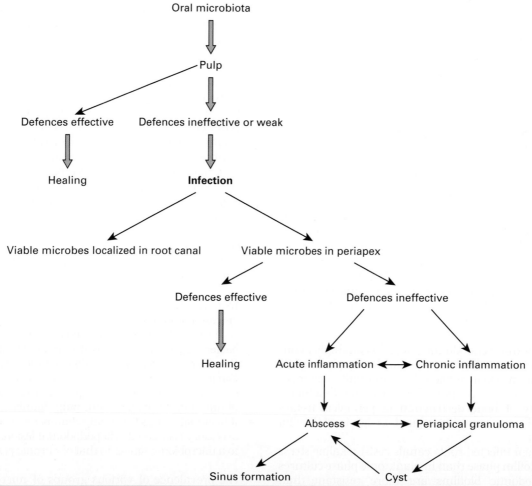

Fig. 34.6 Developmental stages of the infective lesions of the pulp and periapical tissues.

Table 34.4 Microbiota of Primary Endodontic Infections[a,b]

Main Groups	Species
Black pigmented bacteria (60%–70%) saccharolytic species: *Prevotella* asaccharolytic species: *Porphyromonas* *Tannerella forsythia* *Dialister* spp.	*Prevotella intermedia, Prevotella nigrescens, Prevotella tannerae, Prevotella multissacharivorax,* *Prevotella baroniae, Prevotella denticola* *Porphyromonas endodontalis, Porphyromonas gingivalis* *Dialister pneumosintes, Dialister invisus*
Fusobacteria (30%)	***Fusobacterium nucleatum, Fusobacterium periodonticum***
Spirochaetes	Various *Treponema* spp.
Gram-positive anaerobic rods	*Lactobacillus* spp. **(60%)**, *Pseudoramibacter alactolyticus, Filifactor alocis, Actinomyces* spp., *Propionibacterium propionicum, Olsenella* spp., *Slackia exigua, Mogibacterium timidum, Eubacterium* spp.
Streptococci (40%)	*Enterococcus faecalis* **(80%–90% in secondary infections)**, *Parvimonas micra, Streptococcus* *anginosus, Streptococcus mitis, Streptococcus sanguinis*
Campylobacter spp.	*Campylobacter rectus, Campylobacter gracilis*
Miscellaneous cultivable bacteria	*Catonella* spp., *Veillonella parvula, Eikenella corrodens, Granulicatella adiacens, Neisseria mucosa,* *Centipeda periodontii, Gemella morbillorum, Capnocytophaga gingivalis, Corynebacterium matruchotii*
Uncultivable bacterial species	*Dialister pneumosintes, Pseudoramibacter alactolyticus, Filifactor alocis, Catonella morbi, Vagococcus* *fluvialis, Prevotella baroniae, Prevotella multisaccharivorax*
Fungi: *Candida* species	Mainly *Candida albicans*

[a]More common isolates **are in bold** with approximate percentage of isolation rates derived from many studies in parentheses; not an exhaustive list.
[b]Some archaea such as *Methanobrevibacter orali*–like phylotypes and viruses have been isolated on occasion.

HOST DEFENCE MECHANISMS

The host attempts to foil the microbial invasion into pulpal tissue by a variety of mechanisms:

- acute pulpal inflammation with phagocytosis in acute stages and antibody-mediated and cell-mediated immune response at a late stage
- deposition of irregular or sclerotic dentine with minor breaches of defence
- necrosis of the pulp.

MICROBIOLOGY OF ENDODONTIC INFECTIONS

There is a vast literature on this subject and only a summary is given in the following sections.

Endodontic Biofilm: Properties

Endodontic infections are essentially caused by a complex **polymicrobial biofilm** adherent to the root canal surface and formed by microorganisms that have invaded the pulpal space. Conditions under which biofilms develop in root canals are not well understood, and histological data indicate that endodontic biofilm morphology varies between cases, with the following properties:

- biofilm of primary endodontic infections has higher contents of endotoxins (lipopolysaccharides) by virtue of its complex Gram-negative bacterial community (compare with the secondary infections that ensue after treatment)
- the severity of bone destruction in periapical tissues of infected root canals is related to levels of biofilm endotoxins
- bacteria from infected roots canals resist alkaline stress better in biofilm phase than in planktonic phase cultures
- older endodontic biofilms are more resistant than younger biofilms to antimicrobials.

Microbiota of Endodontic Infections

There appears to be a significant difference in the microbiota in primary and secondary endodontic infections, as will be described in the following sections. **Primary endodontic infection** refers to the initial infection of the root canal system, whereas **secondary infection** refers to the infection that ensues after endodontic therapy.

Microbiota of Primary Endodontic Infections. The microbiota of primary endodontic infections is shown in Table 34.4. Primary root canal infections are **complex polymicrobial diseases** with 10–30 bacterial species, and a predominance of obligate anaerobic bacteria. Recent 16S ribosomal RNA (rRNA)–based molecular biological studies have shown uncultivable bacteria such as species of the genera *Dialister* and *Olsenella* and unnamed clones of *Synergistes* in the infected root canals. Clearly, therefore a vast number of organisms can colonize and inhabit the breached pulp chamber, and some organisms are more important than others.

In general, microbial succession from a healthy pulp to a necrotic pulp is as follows:

- In early pulpitis, microflora is simple, dominated by caries-related bacteria.
- As the endodontic biofilm advances, a growth of proteolytic bacteria such as Gram-negative anaerobic species such as *Prevotella, Porphyromonas, Eubacterium, Parvimonas* and *Campylobacter* spp. are seen; this is due to the change in the ecosystem such as its E_h and pH and the ready availability of nutrients within a necrotic pulp chamber.
- If bacterial ingress to the pulp chamber is via extraradicular accessory root canals via periodontal lesions, then it leads to a microbiome similar to that of chronic periodontitis.

The prevalence of various groups of microbiota in primary endodontic infections shown in Table 34.4 is only

Table 34.5 Microbiota of Secondary Endodontic Infections

Main Groups	Species
Gram-negative anaerobic rods	*Fusobacterium nucleatum*, *Prevotella* spp., *Porphyromonas* spp., *Bacteroides* family, *Tannerella*, coliforms
Gram-positive bacteria	*Enterococcus faecalis*, *Lactobacillus* spp., *Streptococcus mitis*, *Streptococcus oralis*, *Parvimonas micra*, *Propionibacterium* spp., *Bifidobacterium* spp., *Actinomyces* spp., *Staphylococcus aureus*
Fungi	Mainly *Candida albicans*

an approximate estimate and differs widely among studies. One reason for this is the quality of microbiological samples delivered for laboratory studies. Aseptic sampling of the infected canal is critical to obviate commensal contaminants, and the generation of spurious data from many studies may be due to contaminated samples. Additionally, the laboratory culture conditions that are not optimal for growth of fastidious bacteria may generate false data.

Some general features of the primary endodontic microbiome are outlined below:

- Distribution of microorganisms in the root canal varies according to which part of the root canal system is being sampled:
  - Apical areas are generally dominated by slow-growing obligate anaerobes.
  - Coronal part of the canal is populated by more rapidly growing facultative anaerobes.
- Gram-negative anaerobic rods (e.g., *Porphyromonas*, *Prevotella* and *Tannerella* spp.) are present in both symptomatic and asymptomatic endodontic infections.
- Eukaryotic yeasts may be seen, and *Candida albicans* is the most common fungus recovered from endodontic infections (approximately 4% of the lesions). Their role in endodontic infections is not clear.
- *Candida* spp. appear to be co-pathogens with bacteria in approximately 1 in 10 patients with endodontic infections. Hence, there is a need to eradicate both bacteria and fungi for successful endodontic therapy.
- Viruses (e.g., Herpes group) have been occasionally isolated from endodontic lesions, but their causal role is questionable.
- Prions causing spongiform encephalopathies are not present in infected pulpal tissue (see Chapter 4).
- Some archaea and uncultivable bacteria have also been detected in infected pulp.

Microbiota of Secondary Endodontic Infections. Secondary endodontic infection may **ensue after unsuccessful treatment** of the affected tooth. This usually occurs due to introduction of microbes into the root canal system during endodontic therapy, especially in cases where the tooth is left open, or leakage from temporary fillings during interappointment periods and/or coronal leakage from defective permanent restorations.

During this phase, certain relatively more potent microbes may enter the root canal system from the oral cavity, or alternatively bacteria that were lying in a dormant state in the canal may assume a more aggressive role due to ecological changes conducive for their survival. For instance, ***Enterococcus faecalis,*** one of the major offenders in secondary endodontic infections, may proliferate within avascular and inaccessible dentinal tubules and evade the

action of all antimicrobial components and medicaments (Table 34.5). The reasons why *Enterococcus faecalis* is common in recalcitrant endodontic infections are:

- its ability to invade dentinal tubules and adhere to collagen
- its ability to grow in high and low pH, high salt concentration and high temperatures (45°C)
- its ability to grow both aerobically and anaerobically
- its resistance to antibiotics as it has plasmids that carry a variety of antibiotic-resistant genes
- expression of virulence factors (e.g., gelatinase, which mediates its adhesion to particulate dentin).

In general, one to five bacterial species have been isolated from root canals after chemomechanical preparation, with the counts ranging from 10^2–10^5 cells per canal. Apart from *Enterococcus faecalis*, anaerobic rods such as *Fusobacterium nucleatum*, *Prevotella* spp., *Campylobacter rectus* and various Gram-positive streptococci can be isolated from such lesions (Table 34.5).

To conclude, it is important to note that the outcome of pulp infection is difficult to predict and depends on the net result of a number of interacting factors such as:

1. the source, route and duration of infection
2. the species, number and toxic end-products of the organisms
3. the specific and nonspecific defence mechanisms of the host
4. the robustness and asepsis of the endodontic interventional procedure, in the case of secondary endodontic infections.

ROLE OF MICROBIOLOGY IN ENDODONTICS

It is generally accepted that the role of endodontic therapy is to render the root canal and periapical tissues 'sterile' and thus ensure the success of the root canal filling. Based on this premise, sterility testing is an attractive proposition as it encourages meticulous clinical technique and assists the clinician in deciding when the canal(s) should be filled. Yet, the rationality of the term 'sterile' in the context of endodontics has been questioned. Sterility is an absolute term (like pregnancy!) and indicates absence of living microbes, and even if a single organism remains in the canal, it cannot be termed sterile. The question then is the magnitude of bacterial numbers that is compatible with clinical success.

There is now clear evidence to show that a few residual bacteria may not cause secondary endodontic infection, and these canals can be restored with good clinical outcomes. Hence, the case for routine culture of endodontic (paper point) samples to elicit the residual microbiological burden after chemomechanical removal of root canal contents is questionable.

There are, however, a number of clinical situations where the microbiological assessment of root canals is justified and helps the clinician. They are:

- patients with a dentoalveolar abscess where endodontic treatment is indicated
- symptomless, nonvital teeth with apical radiolucency
- root canals undergoing treatment with persistent exudate and clinical symptoms.

Some clinicians prefer to keep root canals open without a temporary filling, to encourage pus drainage from a dentoalveolar abscess associated with the tooth. This should be avoided because a complex mixture of oral microbes may then selectively colonize the canal, and eradicating them will often prove difficult.

Microbiological Sampling of Root Canals

If an endodontic sample is required, it should be collected under a rubber dam, using sterile paper points and a strict aseptic technique. Failure to do so may lead to sample contaminations and interpretation of the microbiological findings difficult or almost impossible (see Chapter 6). The following technique will help the clinician to obtain an optimal sample that yields qualitative and quantitative information of an infected root canal and the antibiotic sensitivity of the infecting organisms.

- If the canal is dry, the paper point or the canal should be moistened with sterile saline prior to sampling.
- Place the paper point sample in an anaerobic transport medium and send it directly to the microbiology diagnostic laboratory, for immediate culture if possible. Otherwise, the sample could be refrigerated at 4°C for a few hours.
- In the laboratory, the sample is dispersed by vortex mixing, and a standard inoculum is cultured on blood agar to enable a count of bacteria/mL of medium to be calculated and to ascertain the degree of infestation of the root canal.
- The microbes in the sample are identified after 48–72 h of incubation of the medium. Once a pure culture of the pathogen(s) is obtained, an antibiotic sensitivity profile (antibiogram) of the harvested organisms must be taken to help the clinician decide on the choice antibiotic.

MANAGEMENT OF THE INFECTED CANAL

The most critical part of endodontic therapy is the use of **aseptic technique** to remove mechanically vital, nonvital or infected tissue, and to prepare the canal to insert a root canal filling material and obturate the canal.

Historically, antimicrobial agents were commonly used as an adjunct to endodontic therapy, but their use has declined as the weight of evidence dictates that antibiotics should be used only on the basis of a defined need, such as in cases complicated by severe or recalcitrant infection, as follows.

Systemic Antibiotics in Endodontics: Therapeutic Principles

- The therapeutic use of antibiotics, if at all, must be an adjunct to mechanical treatment.

- Systemic prophylactic antibiotics are only indicated in medically compromised patients. One exception, however is the reimplantation of an avulsed tooth.
- Systemic prophylactic antibiotics, if indicated, must be given preoperatively, preferably as a single high dose.
- There is no case for using antimicrobials as an adjunct to inadequate and careless clinical technique!

If antibiotics are used in endodontics, then they could be administered in three main ways:

1. as **irrigants** to wash out canals during mechanical cleaning procedures
2. as **topical agents** sealed in the root canal for a few days to kill microbes inaccessible to mechanical therapy
3. rarely, as **systemic agents** to destroy microbe within the periapical lesions.

IRRIGANTS IN ENDODONTICS

The irrigants that are currently used in endodontics for cleaning canals can be divided into:

- antibacterials
- decalcifying agents or their combinations
- normal saline sometimes laced with a local anaesthetic.

Salient features of the irrigants, sodium hypochlorite (NaOCl), chlorhexidine, ethylenediaminetetraacetic acid (EDTA), and a mixture of tetracycline, an acid and a detergent (MTAD) are given below:

- **NaOCl:** Commonly called household bleach, NaOCl is the most popular and the most commonly used root canal irrigant. It is an inexpensive, antiseptic lubricant and is used in dilutions ranging from 0.5–5.25%.
  - Advantages of NaOCl include its ability to dissolve organic substances present in the root canal system and its affordability. The major disadvantages of this irrigant are its cytotoxicity when injected into periradicular tissues, foul smell and taste, ability to bleach clothes and ability to cause corrosion of metal objects.
  - Depending on the concentration and the freshness of the solution, it may not kill all the radicular bacteria, nor does it remove all of the smear.
  - Accidental spillover of NaOCl to the periapical region is a not an uncommon complication.
- **Chlorhexidine gluconate (CHX):** CHX has a broad spectrum of antibacterial activity, sustained action and low toxicity. The major advantages of chlorhexidine over NaOCl are its lower cytotoxicity and lack of foul smell and bad taste. However, unlike NaOCl, it cannot dissolve organic debris or necrotic tissues in the root canal system.
- **EDTA:** Chelating agents such as EDTA, citric acid and tetracycline are used for removal of the inorganic portion of the smear. EDTA has little or no antibacterial effect.
- **MTAD (a mixture of a tetracycline isomer, citric acid and a detergent):** MTAD was developed as a final rinse to disinfect the root canal system. It appears to be superior to CHX in antimicrobial activity and has sustained antibacterial activity.

INTRACANAL MEDICAMENTS

These are used to disinfect root canal system between appointments and reduce interappointment pain. They include:

- phenolic compounds (e.g., camphorated monochlorophenol, cresatin)
- aldehydes (e.g., formocresol and glutaraldehyde)
- halides
- calcium hydroxide
- some antibiotics.

These compounds are potent antibacterial agents under laboratory test conditions in vitro, but their efficacy in clinical use is unpredictable. Blood and serum seeping into the canal system are thought to inactivate these agents over time. Some of the aldehyde derivatives have been proposed to neutralize canal tissue remnants and to render them inert.

- **Calcium hydroxide (Ca(OH)$_2$):** Ca(OH)$_2$ is the drug of choice for temporarily sealing the canal; the solution is highly alkaline but not toxic, even affecting robust bacteria such as *Enterococcus faecalis*. It also inactivates bacterial endotoxins and dissolves necrotic tissue remnants, bacteria and their by-products. The antibacterial effect of Ca(OH)$_2$ is owing to its alkaline pH. Extrusion of the material into the periapical tissues can cause tissue necrosis and pain.
- **Corticosteroids:** These anti-inflammatory agents, with no antimicrobial activity, are advocated as intracanal medicaments to reduce postoperative pain.
- **Chlorhexidine gel:** A 2% chlorhexidine gel is used as an intracanal medicament. It can be used alone in gel form or mixed with CaOH$_2$. The gel has sustained antimicrobial activity for up to 21 days. When used in combination with Ca(OH)$_2$, its antimicrobial activity is greater than the combination of Ca(OH)$_2$ and saline.

Key Facts

- Dental caries is the main cause of pulpal and periapical infections; other routes include periodontal pocket and, rarely, **anachoresis** (i.e., haematogenous seeding).
- **Dentoalveolar infections** are usually **polymicrobial** in nature and **endogenous** in origin, with a predominance of strict anaerobes.
- Ideally, **an aspirated sample of pus** should be collected for microbiological examination of a dentoalveolar abscess in the head and neck region.
- **Drainage of pus** is the mainstay of treatment of dentoalveolar and periodontal abscesses; **elimination of the infective focus** and **antibiotic therapy** should be considered on an individual basis.
- **Ludwig's angina** is a spreading, bilateral infection of the sublingual and submandibular spaces; it is a life-threatening infection.
- Prompt intervention and maintenance of the airway are of critical importance in the management of Ludwig's angina; high-dose, empirical, systemic antibiotic therapy is also essential.
- **Periodontal abscess:** an acute or chronic destructive process in the periodontium, resulting in localized collection of pus communicating with the oral cavity through the gingival sulcus and/or other periodontal sites (and not arising from the tooth pulp).
- **Periodontal abscess** is an **endogenous, polymicrobial** infection with a predominantly anaerobic, periodontopathic flora.

- **Alveolar osteitis** (dry socket) is possibly a polymicrobial opportunistic infection with a predominance of anaerobic flora; the exact aetiology is unclear.
- **Suppurative osteomyelitis** of the jaws is **uncommon**; it is mostly seen in immunocompromised patients. Usually a **polymicrobial infection**, it requires both medical and surgical intervention.
- **Cervicofacial actinomycosis** is an **endogenous granulomatous disease**, usually presenting at the angle of the mandible and related to trauma or a history of tooth extraction, mainly caused by *Actinomyces israelii*; 'sulphur granules' may be present in pus.
- Actinomycoses are managed by surgical drainage and long-term antibiotics, preferably penicillin.
- Commensal skin flora such as *Staphylococcus aureus*, *Staphylococcus epidermidis* and *Corynebacterium acnes* may be isolated from infected facial lacerations.
- **Endodontic infections** are **usually endogenous** in nature, caused by infestation of the pulp and the root canals by oral commensal microbiota.
- Most flora of primary endodontic infections are anaerobic in nature.
- *Enterococcus faecalis* is a common pathogen mainly seen in secondary endodontic infections, and its virulence is due to its ability to survive in a high pH and high salt milieu as well as its resistance to antibiotics.
- Infected root canals cannot be 'sterilized'; the mainstay of therapy is to **reduce the bacterial burden** compatible with treatment.

Review Questions (answers on p. 392)

Please indicate which answers are true and which are false.

34.1. Which of the following statements on dentoalveolar abscess are true?
   a. it is often precipitated by bacteria from the systemic route (anachoresis)
   b. it has a polymicrobial aetiology
   c. it is frequently implicated as a cause of brain abscess
   d. it often resolves without antibiotics after adequate drainage
   e. it is a localized collection of pus with an epithelial lining

34.2. Which of the following statements on Ludwig's angina are true?
   a. the majority of cases are due to submandibular sialadenitis
   b. it may warrant an urgent tracheostomy
   c. often the patient is toxic
   d. it needs to be treated with high-dose, parenteral metronidazole and penicillin
   e. a copious amount of pus is yielded on surgical drainage

34.3. Microorganisms that are frequently implicated in the pathogenesis of periodontal abscess include:
   a. *Treponema pallidum*
   b. *haemolytic streptococci*
   c. fusobacteria
   d. staphylococci
   e. *Porphyromonas* spp.

34.4. Which of the following statements on actinomycosis are true?
   a. abdominal lesions are more prevalent than cervicofacial lesions
   b. *Aggregatibacter actinomycetemcomitans* is an associated co-pathogen
   c. lesions contain sulphur
   d. it is caused by a slow-growing, filamentous Gram-positive organism
   e. a 1-week course of penicillin is adequate

Further Reading

Alberti, A., Corbella, S., Taschieri, S., Francetti, L., Fakhruddin, K. S., & Samaranayake, L. P. (2021). Fungal species in endodontic infections: A systematic review and meta-analysis. *PLoS ONE, 16*(7), e0255003. https://doi.org/10.1371/journal.pone.0255003.

Altaie, A. M., Saddik, B., Alsaegh, M. A., Soliman, S. S. M., Hamoudi, R., & Samaranayake, L. P. (2021). Prevalence of unculturable bacteria in the periapical abscess: A systematic review and meta-analysis. *PLoS ONE, 16*(8), e0255485. https://doi.org/10.1371/journal.pone.0255485.

Brook, I. (2005). Microbiology of acute and chronic maxillary sinusitis associated with an odontogenic origin. *The Laryngoscope, 115*, 823–825.

Ingle, J. I., Backland, L. K., & Baumgartner, J. C. (2008). *Endodontics* (6th ed.). BC Decker Inc.

Lewis, M. A. O., MacFarlane, T. W., & McGowan, D. A. (1990). A microbiological and clinical review of the acute dentoalveolar abscess. *British Journal of Oral & Maxillofacial Surgery, 28*, 359–366.

Lockhart, P. B., Tampi, M. P., Abt, E., Aminoshariae, A., Durkin, M. J., Fouad, A. F., Gopal, P., Hatten, B. W., Kennedy, E., Lang, M. S., Patton, L., Paumier, T., Suda, K. J., Pilcher, L., Urquhart, O., O'Brien, K. K., & Carrasco-Labra, A. (2019). Evidence-based clinical practice guideline on antibiotic use for the urgent management of pulpal- and periapical-related dental pain and intraoral swelling: A report from the American Dental Association. *Journal of the American Dental Association, 150*(11), 906–921.e12. https://doi.org/10.1016/j.adaj.2019.08.020.

Marsh, P. D., & Martin, M. V. (2009). *Oral microbiology* (5th ed.). Churchill Livingstone.

Siqueira, J. F., & Rôças, I. N. (2004). Polymerase chain reaction based analysis of microorganisms associated with failed endodontic treatment. *Oral Surgery, Oral Medicine, Oral Pathology, Oral Radiology, and Endodontics, 97*, 85–94.

Siqueira, J. F., & Rôças, I. N. (2009). Diversity of endodontic microbiota revisited. *Journal of Dental Research, 88*, 969–981.

Waltimo, T. M., Sen, B. H., Meurman, J. H., et al. (2003). Yeast in apical periodontitis. *Critical Reviews in Oral Biology and Medicine, 14*, 128–137.

35 · *Oral Mucosal and Salivary Gland Infections*

Oral Mucosal Infections

The oral mucosa, which covers a significant proportion of the oral cavity, is afflicted by a number of infectious diseases. The majority of these are of fungal (candidal) and viral origin and are similar to infections seen in other superficial mucosal surfaces of the body, such as the vagina. In this section, candidal infections are discussed first, followed by viral infections.

It is also noteworthy that some systemic diseases such as syphilis and HIV infection may primarily manifest as oral lesions, as forerunners of subsequent systemic infection.

Hence dentists are well placed to recognise these and alert the patient and his or her phyisician so as to intervene at a very early stage of the infection. Hence a good comprehension of oral manifestations, of systemic diseases, as described in this chapter, is essential for all dental practitioners.

ORAL CANDIDIASIS

Oral candidiasis (*syn:* oral candidosis) is mainly caused by the yeast *Candida albicans*, although other *Candida* species often cause infection. All forms of oral candidiasis are considered to be **opportunistic infections**, and the epithet **'disease of the diseased'** has been applied to these infections, which are seen mainly in the **'very young, the very old and the very sick'**.

Classification

Oral candidiases can be classified as follows (Fig. 35.1):

1. **Primary oral candidiases: localized** candidal infections present **only** in the oral and perioral tissues.
2. **Secondary oral candidiases:** candidal infections that manifest in a **generalized** manner **both in the oral cavity and in other mucous and cutaneous surfaces** (systemic mucocutaneous candidal infections). These are due to rare disorders (except perhaps in candidiasis of human immunodeficiency virus (HIV) infection), such as thymic aplasia and chronic endocrine diseases.

The classic **triad** of (either primary or secondary) oral candidiases are:

I. **pseudomembranous** variant
II. **erythematous** (atrophic) variant
III. **hyperplastic** variant.

In addition, there are a number of other ***Candida-associated lesions*** where the aetiology is multifactorial. These are primary oral candidiases restricted to the oral cavity only. Antifungal therapy alone will not cure these diseases, and underlying cofactors that perpetuate the disease need to be evaluated and eradicated for disease resolution. These diseases are:

- *Candida*-associated denture stomatitis
- angular cheilitis or angular stomatitis
- median rhomboid glossitis
- linear gingival erythema (the microbiological aetiology is not conclusive).

Pseudomembranous Candidiasis

Pseudomembranous candidiasis, classically termed 'thrush' (Fig. 35.2), is an acute infection but may persist intermittently for many months or even years in patients using corticosteroids topically or by aerosol, in HIV-infected individuals and in other immunocompromised patients. It may also be seen in neonates and in the terminally ill, particularly in association with serious underlying conditions such as leukaemia.

Clinical Features. Characterized by white membranes on the surface of the oral mucosa, tongue and elsewhere. The lesions develop to form confluent plaques that resemble

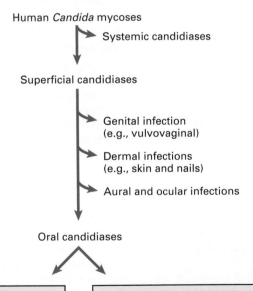

Human *Candida* mycoses
→ Systemic candidiases

Superficial candidiases
→ Genital infection (e.g., vulvovaginal)
→ Dermal infections (e.g., skin and nails)
→ Aural and ocular infections

Oral candidiases

Primary oral candidiases	Secondary oral candidiases
Pseudomembranous Erythematous Hyperplastic *Candida*-associated lesions: 　Denture-induced stomatitis 　Angular stomatitis/cheilitis 　Median rhomboid glossitis 　Linear gingival erythema	Oral manifestations of systemic mucocutaneous candidiasis (due to diseases such as thymic aplasia and candidiasis endocrinopathy syndrome) (Mostly presents as hyperplastic lesions)

Fig. 35.1　Classification of oral candidiasis.

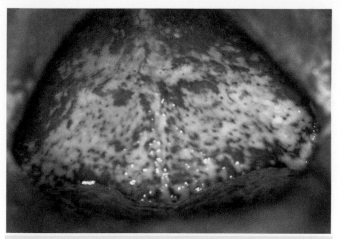

Fig. 35.2 Extensive pseudomembranous candidiasis (thrush) of the palate in a human immunodeficiency virus (HIV)–infected individual.

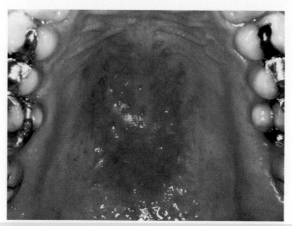

Fig. 35.3 Erythematous candidiasis of the palate in a human immunodeficiency virus (HIV)–infected individual.

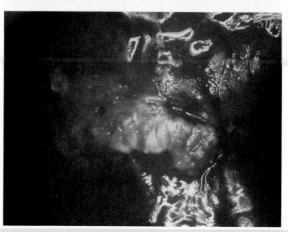

Fig. 35.4 Chronic hyperplastic candidiasis at the commissures of the mouth.

milk curds and can be wiped off to reveal a raw, erythematous and sometimes bleeding base. Hence some consider the pseudomembranous and the erythematous variants a continuum and a single entity (i.e., two stages of the same disease).

Microbiology and Pathology. The white patches consist of necrotic material and desquamated parakeratotic epithelium, penetrated by yeast cells and hyphae, which invade as far as the stratum spinosum. Oropharyngeal thrush may sometimes spread into the adjacent mucosa, particularly that of the upper respiratory tract and the oesophagus. The combination of oral and oesophageal candidiasis is particularly prevalent in HIV disease.

Treatment. Topical antifungal preparations, mainly containing the polyene drugs nystatin and amphotericin, are given as lozenges or pastilles.

Erythematous (Atrophic) Candidiasis

Erythematous candidiasis is a poorly understood condition associated with corticosteroids, topical or systemic broad-spectrum antibiotics, or HIV disease. It may arise as a consequence of persistent acute pseudomembranous candidiasis when the pseudomembranes are shed, or it may develop *de novo*. Erythematous candidiasis of the palate is a common *Candida*-associated lesion frequently observed in elderly people wearing full dentures (*Candida*-associated denture stomatitis; see below).

Clinical Features. The clinical presentation is of one or more asymptomatic erythematous areas, generally on the dorsum of the tongue, palate or buccal mucosa (Fig. 35.3). Lesions on the dorsum of the tongue present as depapillated areas; red areas are often seen on the palate in HIV disease.

There can be associated angular stomatitis, especially in *Candida*-associated denture stomatitis.

Microbiology. Not much is known of the role of yeasts in this condition, although antifungal therapy leads to resolution of the lesions.

Treatment. Topical antifungal treatment, mainly nystatin and amphotericin, is given as lozenges or pastilles. Azole-group agents, such as oral fluconazole tablets, are useful in HIV disease.

Hyperplastic Candidiasis (*Candida* Leukoplakia)

The lesions in hyperplastic candidiasis present as chronic, discrete raised areas that vary from small, palpable, translucent, whitish areas to large, dense, opaque plaques (Fig. 35.4), hard and rough to the touch (plaquelike lesions). Homogeneous areas or speckled areas that do not rub off (nodular lesions) can also be seen. The lesions are often asymptomatic and usually occur on the inside surface of one or both cheeks (retrocommissural area). **Oral cancer supervenes in 9–40%** of cases of hyperplastic candidiasis, as compared with the 2–6% risk of malignant transformation cited for oral white patches in general. Therefore, patients with recalcitrant hyperplastic candidal lesions resistant to therapy should be **kept under regular surveillance**.

Microbiology and Histopathology. Parakeratosis and epithelial hyperplasia occur, with candidal invasion restricted to the upper layers of the epithelium (Fig. 35.5). The condition has been associated in a minority with iron and folate deficiencies and with defective cell-mediated immunity.

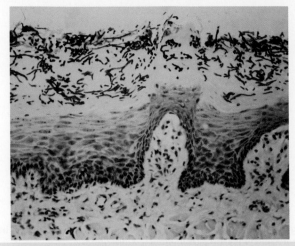

Fig. 35.5   Histopathological section of a chronic hyperplastic candidiasis lesion showing numerous candidal hyphae (pink) infiltrating the superficial layers of the oral epithelium.

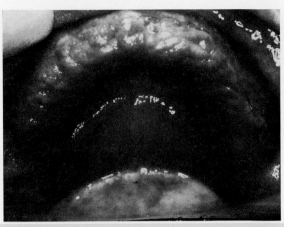

Fig. 35.6   *Candida*-associated denture stomatitis showing the erythematous and oedematous denture-bearing (palatal) mucosa (Newton's type 2 lesion).

Biopsy is important as the condition is premalignant and shows varying degrees of dysplasia.

Treatment. Topical antifungal treatment, mainly nystatin and amphotericin, is given as lozenges or pastilles. Azole group agents, such as oral fluconazole tablets, may help resolve chronic infections. Because of the possibility of malignant transformation, patients should be followed up if the condition is chronic.

CANDIDA-ASSOCIATED LESIONS

Candida-Associated Denture Stomatitis

Candida-associated denture stomatitis (*syn.* chronic atrophic candidiasis, denture sore mouth) is one of the most common ailments in wearers of full dentures; in some areas, such as Scandinavia, 60% of wearers over 60 years old were reported to suffer from the condition. It is also associated with patients wearing orthodontic appliances or obturators for cleft palate. The characteristic presenting signs are erythema and oedema of the mucosa that is in contact with the fitting surface of the upper denture. The mucosa underneath the lower dentures is hardly ever involved, possibly due to the good salivary flow relative to the upper denture bearing mucosa.

Clinical Features. The patient may occasionally experience slight soreness but is usually **asymptomatic**; the only presenting complaint is sometimes an associated angular stomatitis. Depending on the severity of inflammation, the lesions may appear as:

- **pinpoint erythema** of the denture-bearing mucosa (Newton's type 1)
- diffuse and **confluent erythema** and oedema of the denture-bearing mucosa (Newton's type 2; Fig. 35.6)
- **papillary hyperplasia** and inflammation, commonly involving the central part of the hard palate and the alveolar ridge (Newton's type 3; Fig. 35.7).

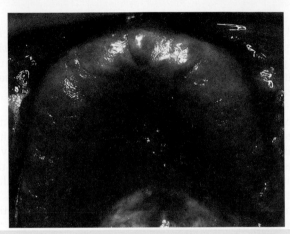

Fig. 35.7   *Candida*-associated denture stomatitis showing palatal papillary hyperplasia (Newton's type 3 lesion).

Aetiology

1. **Local factors:** poor denture hygiene, ill-fitting dentures, traumatic dentures, carbohydrate-rich diets, xerostomia (e.g., Sjögren's syndrome)
2. **Systemic factors:** iron and folate deficiency, diabetes mellitus, immune defects.

Microbiology and Histopathology. It is generally considered to be due to accumulation of plaque biofilms with **yeasts and bacteria** on the fitting surface of the denture and the underlying mucosa. In the papillary hyperplastic variety, *Candida* species do not invade the epithelium. Other aetiological factors, such as mechanical irritation or an allergic reaction to the denture base material, may be involved.

Treatment. The condition is treated by:

- scrupulous denture hygiene and removal of dentures at night (these measures alone, without antifungals, are adequate in the majority of cases)
- regular disinfection of dentures by steeping them in sodium hypochlorite or chlorhexidine to eradicate the reservoir of candidal cells in the prosthesis
- review of the fit of the denture to relieve trauma, if any

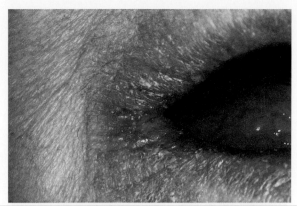

Fig. 35.8   Angular cheilitis in a denture wearer. Note the yellow crusting due to staphylococcal infection.

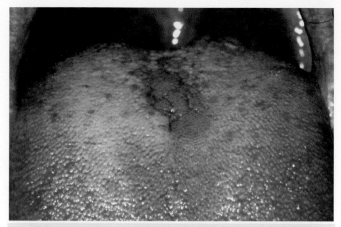

Fig. 35.10   Median rhomboid glossitis showing the characteristic diamond-shaped lesion on the mid-dorsal region of the tongue. Note the depapillated, relatively smooth lesion.

- a diet with a low content of fermentable carbohydrates
- polyene antifungals—nystatin, amphotericin (lozenges, pastilles, etc.).

Angular Stomatitis

The lesions of angular stomatitis (*syn.* perleche, angular cheilitis) are seen in one or both angles of the mouth (Fig. 35.8), especially as a complication of *Candida*-associated denture stomatitis.

Clinical Features. Characterized by soreness, erythema and fissuring, this condition is commonly associated with denture-induced stomatitis. Both **yeasts and bacteria** (especially *Staphylococcus aureus*) are involved as interacting predisposing factors. However, angular stomatitis is very occasionally an isolated initial sign of anaemia or vitamin deficiency, such as vitamin B$_{12}$ deficiency, and resolves when the underlying disease has been treated. The condition is also seen in HIV-associated disease (Fig. 35.9).

Microbiology. *Candida* spp. are present with or without coinfection with *Staphylococcus aureus*. The presence of yellow crusting may indicate staphylococcal infection.

Treatment

1. Elimination of the intraoral reservoir of infection in concurrent denture stomatitis.
2. Adjustment of vertical dimension of the dentures to prevent saliva retention and moisture at the angles of the mouth. (*Note:* Moist body surfaces encourage the growth of *Candida*.)

3. Topical antifungal therapy with nystatin, amphotericin B or miconazole (miconazole has both antifungal and antistaphylococcal activity and is useful for mixed infections); antistaphylococcal preparations (dictated by microbiological investigation) include fusidic acid and neomycin/chlorhexidine.
4. Investigate for possible underlying disease: iron or vitamin B$_{12}$ deficiency; HIV infection, etc.

Median Rhomboid Glossitis

Midline glossitis, or **glossal central papillary atrophy**, is characterized by an area of papillary atrophy that is elliptical or rhomboid in shape and symmetrically placed centrally at the midline of the tongue, anterior to the circumvallate papillae (Fig. 35.10). Occasionally, median rhomboid glossitis presents with a hyperplastic exophytic or even lobulated appearance. In addition to fungal infection, a number of predisposing cofactors, including smoking, steroid inhalation and remnants of the tuberculum impar, have been proposed.

Microbiology and Management. The condition frequently shows a mixed bacterial–fungal microflora and responds to antifungals and/or improvement in oral hygiene. The lesion may also spontaneously remit. Patients are often worried about the appearance and are cancerphobic. In this event, reassurance is essential.

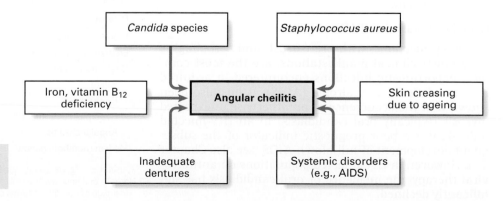

Fig. 35.9   The aetiological factors implicated in angular cheilitis. AIDS, acquired immune deficiency syndrome.

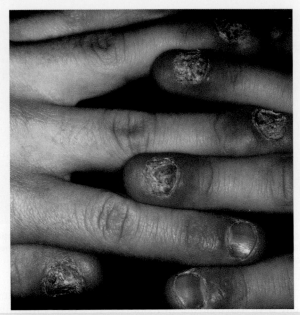

Fig. 35.11   Candidal paronychia in a patient with chronic mucocutaneous candidiasis. (*Note*: This patient also had scalp and oral involvement.)

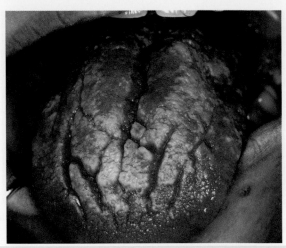

Fig. 35.12   Chronic mucocutaneous candidiasis: hyperplastic lesions of the tongue in the same patient shown in Fig. 35.11.

Linear Gingival Erythema

This condition, defined as a localized or generalized erythematous band extending along the gingival margins (between adjacent gingival papillae), was first described in HIV-infected individuals; it is, however, not confined to this group. Although *Candida* is implicated in the pathogenesis, and lesions resolve after antifungal therapy in some cases, it is likely that other cofactors such as oral hygiene play an equally important role.

CANDIDIASIS AND IMMUNOCOMPROMISED HOSTS

A few patients have chronic candidiasis from an early age, sometimes with a definable immune defect (e.g., chronic mucocutaneous candidiasis) (Figs. 35.11 and 35.12). Candidal infections in these patients are seen in the oral mucosa, skin and other body parts. These secondary oral candidal infections have increased recently because of the high prevalence of attenuated immune response, consequent to diseases such as HIV infection, haematological malignancy and treatment protocols, including aggressive cytotoxic therapy.

Oral Candidiasis in HIV Disease

Candidal infections, with oral thrush and oesophagitis as frequent clinical manifestations, are the most common opportunistic infections encountered in acquired immune deficiency syndrome (AIDS). It has also been shown that the occurrence of an otherwise unexpected mycosis (typically oral candidiasis) in an HIV-infected individual is a poor prognostic indicator of the subsequent development of full-blown AIDS (see also Chapter 30). However, in HIV-infected populations on antiretroviral therapy, the incidence of oral candidiasis has significantly declined.

Systemic Candidiasis

Candidiasis is usually restricted to the skin and mucous membranes but may occasionally spread and manifest systemically (multisystem involvement). Systemic forms of candidiasis may affect only one organ or be disseminated (candidal septicaemia, candidaemia). This occurs mainly in compromised patients (e.g., up to 30% of all patients with acute leukaemia die with systemic candidal infections).

Laboratory Diagnosis

A summary of the specimens required for the laboratory diagnosis of oral candidal infections is given in Table 35.1.

Oral Manifestations of Systemic Mycoses

A number of systemic fungal infections may manifest as oral **ulcerations or granulomas**. Many of these are caused by dimorphic fungi and are uncommon in the West, but are seen in developing countries. These oral lesions are usually **secondary diseases**, the primary lesions being confined to the lungs and/or the skin. Because the primary lesion is internal, it may go unnoticed until the secondary oral lesion presents as the apparently initial manifestation

Table 35.1   Specimens Required for the Laboratory Diagnosis of Oral Candidal Infections

Disease	Smear	Swab	Biopsy
Pseudomembranous candidiasis	+	+	−
Erythematous candidiasis	±	+	−
Denture stomatitis			
Palate	+	+	−
Denture	+	+	−
Hyperplastic candidiasis	+	±	+
Angular cheilitis	+	+	−
Median rhomboid glossitis	+	+	−

+, useful; ±, may be useful; −, inappropriate.
Note: An oral rinse (with 10 ml saline) for 1 min is required to evaluate the oral carriage of Candida in terms of colony-forming units per millilitre (CFU/ml).

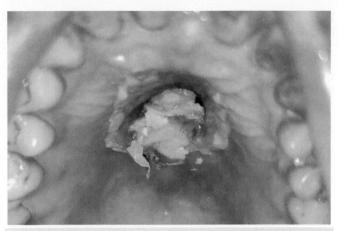

Fig 35.13 Palatal perforation due to maxillary sinus infection with *Mucor* spp., in an immunocompromised patient. Note the grey-black necrotic palatal tissue.

of the infection (e.g., histoplasmosis). Usually, the lesions heal without causing illness, but in progressive disease, sometimes related to lung cavitation, infection can disseminate to the skin, mucosae and internal organs. In a majority of patients, the initial lesion heals, often asymptomatically, and delayed hypersensitivity develops, with a positive skin test reaction to the appropriate antigen. A majority all of these infections present in the oral cavity as ulcerations.

Diagnosis. Direct demonstration of yeast-like forms of the fungi in exudate, sputum or biopsy specimens; isolation in appropriate culture media and/or serology.

Treatment. Almost all dimorphic fungi are sensitive to amphotericin; fluconazole may be an alternative.
Some examples of these infections follow.

EXAMPLES OF ORAL MANIFESTATIONS OF SYSTEMIC FUNGAL INFECTIONS

Mucormycosis

Agent. *Mucorales* spp.

Main Oral Sites Affected. Nasal or sinus congestion when the maxillary sinus is affected. If untreated, palatal perforation may occur with oroantral fistula formation. (Fig. 35.13) In extreme cases the lesions on nasal bridge or palatal surface may perforate into the orbital area, leading to blindness.

Clinical Features. One-sided facial swelling; sinus congestion; headache.

Frequency of Oral Infection. There has been a recrudescence of mucormycoses during the COVID-19 pandemic. Particularly, oral and maxillofacial mycoses have frequently been reported either concurrently with COVID-19 symptoms or during the immediate postrecovery period. Numerous cases were reported from the Indian subcontinent during the COVID-19 panedmic.

Histoplasmosis

Agent. *Histoplasma capsulatum*, a dimorphic fungus.

Main Oral Sites Affected. Oral mucosa, tongue, palate, gingiva, periapical region.

Clinical Features. Nodular indurated or granular masses and ulceration; tissue destruction with bone erosion.

Frequency of Oral Infection. In 40–50% of cases.

Paracoccidioidomycosis

Agent. *Paracoccidioides brasiliensis*, a dimorphic fungus (more common in western countries than in Asia).

Main Oral Sites Affected. Tongue, hard and soft palate, gingiva.

Clinical Features. Papules or vesicles leading to ulceration.

Frequency of Oral Infection. Common.

Penicilliosis

Agent. *Penicillium marneffei*, a dimorphic fungus, common in Southeast Asia.

Main Oral Sites Affected. Palate, gingiva, labial mucosa, tongue, oropharynx.

Clinical Features. Erosions or shallow ulcers covered with a white slough.

Frequency of Oral Infection. Very common.

Oral Viral Infections

The majority of virus infections of the oral mucosa are due to the **herpes group of viruses**. Occasionally, other viruses, such as coxsackieviruses, papillomaviruses and paramyxoviruses (which cause measles and mumps), may manifest with oral symptoms (see Chapter 21).

PRIMARY HERPES SIMPLEX INFECTION: HERPETIC STOMATITIS

Herpetic stomatitis is the most common viral infection to affect the mouth; it is caused by human herpesviruses 1 and 2 (HHV-1 and HHV-2). The incubation period is about 5 days, and the virus is transmitted by contact with skin lesions or infected saliva. Children may carry the virus asymptomatically, or as convalescent carriers, in saliva for several months, but the virus is rarely isolated from adults once the primary lesion heals. The early-childhood infection is usually subclinical, frequently dismissed as 'teething', but if the infection occurs in adults, the symptoms are obvious and severe. In countries with high standards of hygiene, there is an increasing frequency of adults presenting with primary herpes.

Clinical Features

In the initial stages, there is mild to severe fever and enlarged lymph nodes, with pain in the mouth and throat; then, a variable number of vesicles develop haphazardly on the oral mucosa, the tongue and gingivae. These vesicles rupture quickly to form small round or irregular superficial ulcers with erythematous haloes and greyish-yellow bases. The gingivae are inflamed, and the infection may be confused with acute necrotizing ulcerative gingivitis (ANUG) of bacterial origin. In some, ANUG may develop secondary to primary herpetic stomatitis. The mouth is very painful and eating and swallowing may be difficult. The lesions resolve without scarring within 5–10 days.

POST-PRIMARY HERPES SIMPLEX INFECTION: HERPES LABIALIS (HHV-1 AND HHV-2)

About one-third of the patients who have had primary infection develop herpes labialis (cold sore) in later life as a result of **reactivation of the latent virus**, which usually resides in the trigeminal ganglion. Other synonyms used for the disease entity are secondary or recrudescent herpes. The stimulus for post-primary infection and the reactivation of the virus could be:

- stress
- trauma
- exposure to sunlight
- menstruation
- debilitating disease.

The lesion commonly develops at the **mucocutaneous junction of the lip** or on the skin adjacent to the nostrils. Characteristically, the lesions are preceded, some 24 hours before, by a premonitory sign of itching, prickling or a burning sensation. Blisters then develop, enlarge, coalesce, rupture, become encrusted and heal within 10–14 days (see Fig. 21.3).

Intraoral recurrent herpetic infections are infrequent; they involve the hard palate, alveolar ridges and gingiva. These lesions develop in a similar manner to those of the lips and appear as a cluster of small, shallow ulcers with red, irregular margins. Pain is not a common feature, and the intraoral lesions may or may not recur intermittently for years.

HERPETIC DERMATITIS AND HERPETIC WHITLOW (HHV-1 AND HHV-2)

Primary herpetic dermatitis is localized and characterized by pruritus, burning and pain. Multiple vesicles appear, persist for 4–5 days and burst, with resultant crusting scabs that heal within 2–3 weeks. Dentists who escaped exposure in childhood may contract herpetic dermatitis from patients who have either primary or secondary herpes. Infection may take the form of a **herpetic whitlow on the finger**, resulting in an intensely painful lesion (see Fig. 21.2). Herpetic whitlow may recur, but less frequently than the perioral infection.

Laboratory Diagnosis of Herpetic Infection

See also Chapter 6.

Direct Examination. Smears should be stained with monoclonal fluorescent antisera to herpes simplex virus type 1 or 2 (HHV-1 or HHV-2). This technique is specific and rapid.

Culture. Herpes simplex virus is readily isolated from samples of oral lesions in a variety of tissue culture systems, but this is now supplanted by molecular biological analyses

Serology. In primary infection, a fourfold or greater increase in antibody titre between the acute and convalescent sera is indicative of recent infection with herpes simplex virus. The demonstration of immunoglobulin M (IgM) antibodies by immunofluorescence techniques in a single sample can also be used in diagnosis.

Management

Moderate to severe primary herpetic stomatitis is treated with oral and topical aciclovir, together with symptomatic measures. However, the use of aciclovir in recurrent herpetic infections should be limited to immunocompromised patients and those who have a past history of severe, extensive or frequently recurring lesions. The patients should apply the drug *before* vesicles form to obtain the best results.

VARICELLA AND ZOSTER (HHV-3)

Primary infection with the varicella-zoster virus causes chickenpox. Zoster or shingles is the **secondary** (*syn.* postprimary, reactivation) **infection** due to the reactivation of the virus hiding in the latent form in sensory ganglia (e.g., the trigeminal ganglion for the facial region; see Fig. 21.3).

Chickenpox

Chickenpox is a common infectious disease and is usually contracted in childhood.

Oral Manifestations. Before the typical skin rash develops, lesions may be found in the mouth, especially on the hard palate, pillars of the fauces and uvula, although any area of the oral mucosa may be involved. The characteristic skin rash—which is centripetal and progresses from macular to papular, vesicular and pustular, and forms before scabbing—helps to differentiate chickenpox from other causes of oral ulceration. The oral lesions consist of small ulcers surrounded by an area of erythema. The vesicles are quickly ruptured in the mouth and therefore are rarely noticed. The lesions may be painful in adults, but children rarely complain of discomfort.

Shingles (Zoster)

Shingles is a localized eruption due to the reactivation of the herpes zoster virus. It involves an area of **skin supplied by one or more sensory ganglia** in which the virus is residing. In some 10% of cases, zoster reflects an underlying immune-deficiency state, possibly a neoplasm such as lymphoma or HIV disease.

Oral Manifestations. The trigeminal nerve is affected in about 15% of cases, with the ophthalmic, maxillary and mandibular divisions involved in that order of precedence. The lesions of shingles may be found on the skin, on the oral mucosa or both. Severe localized oral pain often precedes the rash and mimics the pain of toothache. The most common intraoral sites affected are the anterior half of the tongue, the soft palate and the cheek. The vesicles break down intraorally within a few hours to give very painful ulcerated areas with a yellowish-grey surface and erythematous borders. The oral lesions heal more quickly than the skin lesions and rarely scar.

Laboratory Diagnosis of Chickenpox and Shingles

The clinical presentation is characteristic, but in unusual circumstances the disease can be confirmed in the laboratory by submitting:

- vesicle fluid for electron microscopy and virus isolation
- smears from an ulcer for immunofluorescence
- acute or convalescent sera to test for the presence of specific IgM antibodies by immunofluorescence.

Management

Chickenpox is self-limiting, but an effective vaccine is available to prevent infection. For zoster, high-dose aciclovir (800 mg five times daily) should be prescribed as soon as possible, especially in immunocompromised patients.

EPSTEIN–BARR VIRUS INFECTIONS (HHV-4)

Epstein–Barr virus is the agent of a number of infections, including infectious mononucleosis, nasopharyngeal carcinoma, Burkitt's lymphoma, oral hairy leukoplakia and posttransplant lymphoproliferative diseases.

Infectious Mononucleosis

Infectious mononucleosis is an acute infectious disease, mainly of children and young adults. The agent, the Epstein–Barr virus, is present in the oropharyngeal secretions of patients suffering or convalescing from infectious mononucleosis; the disease is transmitted by kissing. The virus has also been demonstrated in the oropharynx of healthy carriers.

Oral Manifestations. At the onset, the throat is painful and congested but exudate is absent. An enanthem consisting of clusters of fine petechial haemorrhages may be seen at the junction of the hard and soft palates (these lesions are also found in other virus infections of the respiratory tract). Subsequently, a white pseudomembrane may develop on the tonsil and on other parts of the oral mucosa, and oral ulceration may occur. Other presenting signs may be submandibular lymphadenitis and mild fever.

Laboratory Diagnosis. The diagnosis of infectious mononucleosis may be possible on the typical clinical presentation. Laboratory tests required to confirm the diagnosis include:

- **haematology:** differential white blood cell count to demonstrate the lymphocytosis and atypical mononuclear cells (20%)
- **serology:**
  - testing an acute serum sample for the presence of IgM antibodies to the Epstein–Barr virus capsid antigen (using an immunofluorescence technique)
  - the monospot or Paul–Bunnell tests.

HAIRY LEUKOPLAKIA

See Chapter 30.

ORAL MANIFESTATIONS OF OTHER HERPESVIRUSES (HHV-5 TO HHV-8)

Other herpesvirus infections are generally of minor consequence, except for Kaposi's sarcoma caused by HHV-8 (see Chapter 21).

COXSACKIEVIRUS INFECTIONS

Two diseases caused by group A coxsackieviruses produce oral signs and symptoms:

- **hand, foot and mouth disease**, caused mainly by coxsackievirus A16 and, less commonly, by types A4, A5, A9 or A10
- **herpangina**, caused by coxsackieviruses A2, A4, A5, A6 and A8.

Oral Manifestations of Herpangina

This febrile disease is characterized by sore throat, dysphagia, anorexia and occasionally a stiff neck. Accompanying oral signs and symptoms are small, papulovesicular lesions about 1–2 mm in diameter, with a greyish-white surface surrounded by red areolae, especially in the palate. The disease lasts for about 3–4 days, the fever abates and the oral lesions heal promptly.

PARAMYXOVIRUS INFECTIONS

Measles, mumps, parainfluenza and respiratory syncytial viruses are categorized as paramyxoviruses. Of these, measles and mumps are of concern in dentistry as they commonly manifest with oral signs or symptoms. Measles is discussed in Chapter 21; mumps is described later in this chapter (see Viral Infections of Salivary Glands).

Oral Manifestations of Bacterial Infections

SYPHILIS

Syphilis is reemerging as a relatively common disease due to the HIV pandemic and the increasing promiscuity associated with affluence worldwide. As oral manifestations are the early signs of the disease, dental practitioners should pay particular attention to these.

Primary Syphilis

Chancre is the characteristic sign of primary syphilis and normally appears in the genitalia, but extragenital lesions, mostly in the oral cavity, occur in some 10% of cases. The common sites affected are the lips and tongue, and, to a lesser extent, the gingival and tonsillar areas. The lesions heal spontaneously about 5 weeks after appearing. The regional lymph nodes are usually enlarged.

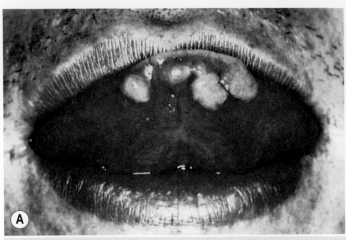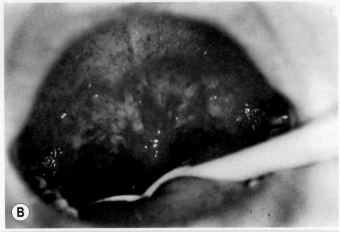

Fig. 35.14   Mucous patches of secondary syphilis on the tongue (A) and soft palate (B). Note the greyish-white, glistening lesions.

Table 35.2	Oral Manifestations and Infectivity of Syphilis	
Stage	**Orofacial Manifestations**	**Infectivity**
Primary	Chancre of lip, tongue, gingiva	Extremely high
Secondary	Mucous patches on tonsil, tongue, soft palate, cheek; 'snail-track' ulcers; rubbery, enlarged cervical lymph nodes	High
Tertiary	'Gumma' of palate; rarely osteomyelitis; syphilitic leukoplakia leading to carcinoma	Nil
Congenital	Hutchinson's incisors; 'mulberry' molars; facial deformities with open bite or dish face	Nil

Secondary Syphilis

Oral manifestations are slightly raised, greyish-white glistening patches on the mucosa—the so-called **'mucous patches'** of the tonsils, soft palate, tongue and cheek (Fig. 35.14); gingivae are rarely involved. The surface membrane covering the lesions is grey and easily removed, and contains many spirochaetes. The mucous patches may later coalesce to produce a serpiginous lesion (**'snail-track' ulcer**). The cervical lymph nodes are enlarged and rubbery in consistency. The lesions heal spontaneously 2–6 weeks after appearing. However, typical lesions may not always be present because of unrelated antibiotic therapy.

Tertiary Syphilis

The characteristic sign of this stage is the syphilitic **gumma**. The most common oral site of gumma formation is the hard palate, but the soft palate, lips and tongue may be involved (Table 35.2). The lesion starts as a small, pale, raised, painless area that ulcerates and rapidly progresses to a large, necrotic zone with exposure of bone and, in the case of the palate, may eventually perforate into the nasal cavity. The palatal lesions are usually midline; in rare cases, the soft palate may be involved. No spirochaetes are found in gummata.

Atrophic or **interstitial glossitis** is another oral manifestation of tertiary syphilis. Clinically, there is atrophy of the filiform and fungiform papillae, which results in a smooth, sometimes wrinkled, lingual surface. Subsequent leukoplakia may develop.

Late and Quaternary Syphilis

The quaternary stage of syphilis, which may develop 10–20 years after primary syphilis, is characterized by two main clinical forms: cardiovascular syphilis and neurosyphilis. No specific oral manifestations are seen at this stage.

Congenital Syphilis

The dental lesions are a result of infection of the developing tooth germ by *Treponema pallidum*. The deciduous teeth are minimally affected; the permanent teeth may be malformed or fail to develop. The most common dental manifestations of congenital syphilis are **Hutchinson's incisors** and **'mulberry' molar** teeth. In the former, upper central incisors are mostly involved; the teeth are barrel shaped and have a crescentic notch at the incisal edge. In the latter, the first permanent molar teeth have a roughened dirty, yellow, hypoplastic occlusal surface, with poorly developed cusps resembling the surface of a mulberry. Other manifestations of congenital syphilis include frontal bossing and saddle nose.

TUBERCULOSIS

Oral lesions of tuberculosis are usually **secondary to primary infection** elsewhere, commonly the lungs. Primary infections of the oral mucosa by *Mycobacterium tuberculosis* are rare. In the case of secondary infection, the sources of infection are contaminated sputum or blood-borne bacilli. Lesions are found more commonly in the posterior area of the mouth, and it has been suggested that this may be due to the relative propensity of lymphoid tissue in this region. The major oral lesions are:

- oral ulceration
- tuberculous lymphadenitis
- periapical granulomas and bone infections.

Oral Ulceration

There is a wide spectrum of tuberculous lesions of the oral mucosa, including indolent **ulcers**, diffuse inflammatory lesions, **granulomas** and **fissures**; pain may be mild or absent. The tongue is most commonly affected, but lesions have been noted on the buccal mucosa, gingivae, floor of the mouth, lips, and the hard and soft palates. Primary tuberculosis of the oral mucosa is more common in children and adolescents than in adults and usually presents as a single, painless indolent ulcer, commonly on the gingiva, with enlarged cervical lymph nodes, or as a white patch.

Tuberculous Lymphadenitis

The cervical glands are most commonly affected, and in patients with pulmonary tuberculosis, the route of infection is probably by lymphatic or haematogenous spread, or via an abrasion of the mouth. In patients with no evidence of systemic infection, the route is probably via the tonsils or oral mucosa. The typical presentation is a lump in the neck, which may be painful. The size may vary, and in the early stages the swelling is firm but mobile. Later, the mass becomes fixed, with the formation of an abscess and sinus—a **cold abscess**. The lesions may be unilateral, bilateral, single or multiple.

Periapical Granuloma and Bone Infections

In patients with active tuberculosis, tubercle bacilli are seen in periapical granulomas. Tooth extraction may lead to delayed healing of the socket, which fills with '**tuberculous granulations**'.

Bone infections are not uncommon in tuberculosis: secondary tuberculous osteomyelitis may involve the maxilla or mandible. Here, the bacilli may gain access to the bone by:

- haematogenous spread
- direct spread from an oral lesion
- infected saliva entering an extraction socket or fracture.

Tuberculous osteomyelitis of the jaws is chronic in nature, usually with severe pain and the production of bony sequestra.

Tuberculosis of the Salivary Glands

See below.

LEPROSY

Leprosy, a granulomatous disease caused by *Mycobacterium leprae*, is of two main types: the tuberculoid and the lepromatous variants (see Chapter 19).

Tuberculoid Leprosy

Tuberculoid leprosy does not directly affect the oral mucosa, but the associated neurological features may affect the mouth and face. Such manifestations vary from loss of eyebrows to nodular involvement of all facial cutaneous and subcutaneous structures. If the trigeminal nerve is involved, **hyperaesthesia** or **paraesthesia** of the face, lips, tongue, palate, cheeks or gingiva may be present; secondary **ocular changes** may occur, with subsequent corneal and conjunctival sensory loss. The facial lesions of tuberculoid leprosy comprise dry, hairless, anaesthetic plaques, with a well-defined and raised border, that are red on white skin and hypopigmented on dark skin.

Lepromatous Leprosy

In lepromatous leprosy, *Mycobacterium leprae* is present in many tissues of the body, and multiple, erythematous, bilateral and symmetrical lesions are found on the skin of the face, arms and legs. The lesions are anaesthetic. The **nasomaxillary complex is the primary area of destruction** in the facial region. Facial skeletal changes, such as saddle nose, atrophy of the anterior nasal spine and premaxillary bone recession, are common, with or without tooth loss (see Fig. 19.3). Dental deformities are limited to a pink discoloration of the upper incisors due to invasion of the pulp by infected granulomatous tissue, which can produce pulpitis and pulp death.

The incidence of oral lesions in lepromatous leprosy varies from 10% to 60%. Intraoral nodules have been described as yellowish-red, soft to hard, sessile, single or confluent lesions, which tend to ulcerate. Healing is by secondary intention with fibrous scars. The sites most commonly involved are the premaxillary gingivae, the hard and soft palates, uvula and tongue. Tongue lesions, particularly on the anterior two-thirds, consist of single or multiple nodules, giving a 'cobblestone' appearance, or in some instances they may resemble a geographic tongue with erythematous areas denuded of papillae. As the saliva of patients with oral lesions commonly contains *Mycobacterium leprae*, this could be a possible source of infection.

Salivary Gland Infections

Inflammation of the salivary glands – **sialadenitis** – due to infective causes is not an uncommon phenomenon. Sialadenitis can be:

- viral (in the majority)
- bacterial (in the minority).

The parotid glands are more commonly infected than the submandibular glands, and infections of the accessory salivary glands are very rare (Table 35.3). Apart from mumps, the majority of salivary gland infections are seen in adults.

Table 35.3 Classification of Salivary Gland Infections

Type of Infection	Gland Usually Affected	Predisposing Factor(s)
Mumps (endemic parotitis)	Parotid	No prior exposure to virus
Acute suppurative parotitis	Parotid	Severe xerostomia (e.g., Sjögren's syndrome), localized and diffuse abnormalities of the salivary glands
Obstructive sialadenitis	Submandibular	Sialoliths, foreign bodies, ductal strictures, mucus plugs
Suppurative and chronic recurrent parotitis of childhood	Parotid	Congenital or acquired abnormality of ductal system
Rare miscellaneous disorders (e.g., tuberculosis, actinomycosis and fungal infections)	Parotid or submandibular	Systemic infection by specific agents (e.g., *Mycobacterium tuberculosis*)

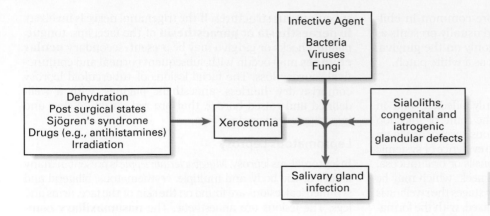

Fig. 35.15   **Factors important in the pathogenesis of salivary gland infections.**

PATHOGENESIS

Initiation and progression of salivary gland infections depend on the **decrease in host resistance** to infection:

- **general:** debility, dehydration
- **local:** obstruction of ducts due to sialoliths (salivary stones), strictures or other pathology and the **virulence** of the causative organism; factors important in salivary gland infections are shown in Fig. 35.15.

VIRAL INFECTIONS OF SALIVARY GLANDS

Mumps (Endemic Parotitis)

Mumps is caused by an **RNA paramyxovirus**, which infects circulating lymphocytes, especially activated T cells. These spread in the blood, 'targeting' **salivary duct epithelial cells** and replicating in them, leading to acinar disintegration, periductal oedema and a mononuclear infiltrate (Fig. 35.16). Subsequently, the virus is shed in saliva and spreads into the blood stream, causing a viraemia.

Epidemiology. The disease is frequently seen in winter and spring. Clinical or subclinical infection may occur at all ages but is most common in childhood.

Incubation Period and Infectivity. Approximately 14–28 days; the saliva of patients incubating mumps (during the prodromal period) is infectious for a few days before parotitis develops and up to 2 weeks after the onset of clinical symptoms. Mumps is transmitted by direct contact with saliva and by droplet spread, and hence the disease may be contracted in the dental clinic environment.

Clinical Features. These include:

- pyrexia, sore throat, furred tongue, trismus and earache, commonly
- pain on chewing and/or pain and tenderness on upward pressure beneath the angle of the lower jaw (pain may be acute during salivation)
- reddening of the opening of the parotid duct
- increase in glandular size, and varying consistency of the gland from normal to very hard
- low salivary flow rate leading to nonspecific stomatitis and halitosis

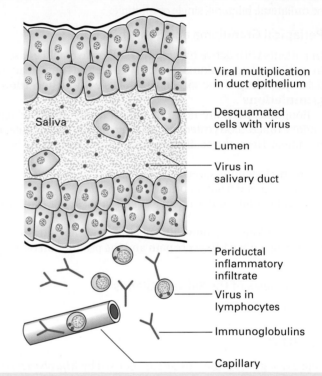

Fig. 35.16   **Mumps virus multiplication in salivary duct and shedding into saliva.**

- trismus and earache due to parotid involvement
- either one or both parotid glands may be involved, with a delay of up to 5 days in between; salivary glands other than the parotid may be enlarged in some 10% of cases
- the clinical course of mumps varies widely, from a mild upset lasting a day or two to a severe illness with high fever lasting up to 2 weeks; complete recovery is usual.

Complications. Complications are due to involvement of other glands or tissues, leading to meningoencephalitis (30%) and orchitis (25% of adult males); rarely, thyroiditis, neuritis, myocarditis and nephritis.

Diagnosis. Diagnosis is normally made on clinical grounds. On unusual clinical presentation, laboratory investigations may be required and include:

- **serology:** to demonstrate antibodies to mumps virus antigens using serological tests (e.g., the detection of IgM antibodies using immunofluorescence)
- **electron microscopy:** saliva (pure parotid saliva collected by cannulation) may be examined for typical virus particles.

Salivary Gland Disease in HIV Infection

Salivary gland disease may occur in a minority of HIV-infected individuals. **Xerostomia** and/or **enlargement** of the major salivary glands are the two main presentations: xerostomia is present in some 10% of cases, while major gland enlargement may be accompanied by illness resembling Sjögren's syndrome.

The histological picture is variable, with lymphocytic sialadenitis, hyperplasia of salivary lymph nodes, Kaposi's sarcoma or lymphoma. The aetiology of HIV-induced salivary gland disease is not clear.

Other Viral Infections of Salivary Glands

Mumps is the most common viral cause of sialadenitis, but a member of the herpesvirus group, cytomegalovirus, can also cause a clinical disease, **cytomegalic inclusion disease** (salivary gland inclusion disease), which affects newborns, children and adults and has multiple systemic manifestations, including salivary gland enlargement. The disease is so called because of the large, doubly contoured **'owl-eye' inclusion bodies** seen within the nucleus or cytoplasm of duct cells of the parotid gland.

Rarely, other viruses such as parainfluenza virus types 2 and 3, echoviruses and coxsackieviruses have been implicated in nonsuppurative sialadenitis.

BACTERIAL INFECTIONS OF SALIVARY GLANDS

Acute Suppurative Parotitis (Bacterial Sialadenitis)

Acute suppurative parotitis is seen mostly in adults with salivary gland abnormalities. In the past, it was primarily a disease of dehydrated or postoperative patients, but with the introduction of proper fluid balance and antibiotic prophylaxis, suppurative parotitis in these groups is now rare.

Aetiology and Pathogenesis. In health, potential oral pathogens cannot ascend the salivary ducts and invade the glandular tissue because of the flushing action of saliva. However, if the flow of saliva is greatly reduced or stopped, a retrograde infection via the salivary duct may ensue. Predisposing factors include:

- drugs that reduce salivary flow (e.g., diuretics, certain antihistamines, tranquillizers and anticholinergics)
- localized salivary gland abnormalities (e.g., calculus, mucus plug or benign strictures)
- generalized sialectasis (e.g., in patients who become dehydrated after gastrointestinal surgery or patients with Sjögren's syndrome); a progressive degenerative disease affecting salivary gland tissue.

Clinical Features

1. Unilateral or bilateral swelling of the parotid glands may be present for days or weeks. Swelling may be limited to the gland or, in more severe infections, extend locally, involving the pre- and postauricular areas. The earlobes may be displaced laterally.
2. Purulent salivary secretions occur at the duct orifice.
3. Trismus results from pain and swelling.
4. Usually, there are no systemic symptoms, but occasionally fever, chills and leukocytosis may be seen.
5. In chronic infection, recurrent bouts of acute exacerbation of infection followed by periods of remission may lead to replacement fibrosis.

Investigations

- If possible, pus should be aspirated through a fine, small-bore, polythene catheter attached to a syringe, or collected aseptically on a cotton-wool swab by 'milking' the duct, and sent immediately to the laboratory. The ductal orifice and the subjacent mucosa should be decontaminated with an antiseptic such as chlorhexidine prior to swab collection of pus.
- Catheter collection of pus should not be performed during the acute stage.
- Pus should be collected before antibiotics are prescribed.

Microbiology. Both monomicrobial and polymicrobial infections may occur. The organisms most commonly isolated are α-haemolytic streptococci; the frequency of isolation of *Staphylococcus aureus* is gradually diminishing (Table 35.4).

Treatment. The treatment of choice is parenteral antibiotic therapy, guided by culture of pus and sensitivity tests. Amoxicillin is the agent of choice, or erythromycin in patients hypersensitive to penicillins. A Gram-stained smear of the pus is useful in deciding initial antibiotic therapy.

Thorough oral hygiene is extremely important. Salivation should be encouraged by increased fluid intake (rehydration) and the use of **sialagogues** (e.g., lemon juice). In severe cases, consider surgical drainage of pus.

Once the acute condition has resolved, the patient should be referred for **sialographic investigation** of the affected gland or glands to identify correctable salivary gland abnormalities (e.g., mucus plugs, benign strictures and calculi), which lead to recurrence of infection. *Note:*

Table 35.4 Bacteria Commonly Isolated From Bacterial Parotitis

Common isolates[a]
α-haemolytic streptococci
Staphylococcus aureus
Less common isolates
Haemophilus spp.
Eikenella corrodens
Bacteroides spp.
Anaerobic streptococci
Rare isolates
Neisseria gonorrhoeae
Mycobacterium tuberculosis
Actinomyces spp.
Treponema pallidum

[a]Polymicrobial infections are common.

Sialography should never be attempted during the acute phase of the illness.

Subsequent treatment options include duct dilation, removal of ductal obstructions or surgical revision of ducts.

Sequelae. If acute bacterial parotitis is untreated, severe complications may ensue, especially in debilitated patients. These are:

- extension of inflammation and oedema into the neck and resultant respiratory obstruction
- cellulitis of the face and neck
- osteomyelitis of adjacent facial bones
- rarely, septicaemia and death.

Submandibular Sialadenitis

Submandibular sialadenitis is less common than acute suppurative bacterial parotitis. Most bacterial infections of the submandibular glands are associated with obstructive ductal disease (e.g., sialoliths and ductal strictures). The aetiology, microbiology and management of submandibular (submaxillary) sialadenitis are similar to those of bacterial parotitis.

Neonatal Suppurative Parotitis and Recurrent Parotitis of Childhood

These rare diseases, with unknown aetiology, are confined to the first decade of life. In recurrent parotitis, the child experiences repeated acute episodes of painful parotid gland enlargement. The suggested predisposing factors include congenital abnormalities of the ductal system, preceding mumps and foreign bodies in the parotid duct. Management includes removal of the aetiological agent, symptomatic therapy and antibiotics, if necessary.

Rare Bacterial Infections of Salivary Glands

Salivary gland infections by organisms such as *Treponema pallidum*, *Neisseria gonorrhoeae*, *Actinomyces israelii* and *Mycobacterium tuberculosis* have been rarely described. These may be due to:

- endogenous, ascending infection via salivary ducts (e.g., *Actinomyces israelii*)
- infection via an adjacent, contiguous focus (e.g., *Treponema pallidum*)
- reactivation of an old lesion (e.g., *Mycobacterium tuberculosis*).

Key Facts

- **Oral candidiasis**, an opportunistic infection, is the most common oral fungal infection in humans, and it is usually seen in the **very young**, the **very old** and the **very sick**.
- **Oral candidiasis**, classified as a superficial (as opposed to systemic) mycosis, can be broadly subdivided into primary and secondary disease: **primary disease** is strictly confined to the oral cavity, whereas **secondary disease** is present in both the oral and other superficial body sites.
- The classic disease triad of oral candidiasis comprises **pseudomembranous** (thrush), **erythematous** and **hyperplastic** variants.
- Other common ***Candida*-associated lesions** are denture stomatitis, angular cheilitis and median rhomboid glossitis.
- **Herpesviruses** (eight are now recognized) cause the majority of oral viral infections.
- In general, **herpes simplex viruses** types 1 and 2 (human herpesviruses 1 and 2 (HHV-1 and HHV-2)) cause infections above and below the belt, respectively (i.e., oral and genital infections).
- Herpetic gingivostomatitis is the primary infection, and herpes labialis is the reactivation (*syn.* post- primary, secondary) infection caused by HHV-1.
- Varicella-zoster virus (HHV-3) causes chickenpox (primary infection) and zoster/shingles (reactivation infection) affecting well-defined dermatomes ('belt of roses from hell').
- **Epstein–Barr virus** (HHV-4) causes **infectious mononucleosis** or glandular fever, common in young adults, and a number of other diseases.
- Group A **coxsackieviruses** cause **hand, foot and mouth disease** of children and **herpangina**; oral lesions are papulovesicular, small and greyish-white.

- Oral manifestations of syphilis include **chancre** (primary syphilis), **mucous patches** and **snail-track ulcers** (secondary), and **gumma** and **interstitial glossitis** (tertiary).
- **Mulberry (moon) molars** and **Hutchinson's incisors** can be seen in congenital syphilis, due to infection of the tooth germ by *Treponema pallidum*; other manifestations are frontal bossing and saddle nose.
- Oral ulceration, lymphadenitis, periapical granulomas and bone infection are the common oral manifestations of tuberculosis; these are secondary to primary infection of the lungs.
- **Leprosy**, a chronic granulomatous disease, manifests as tuberculous and lepromatous variants; intraoral nodules, which ulcerate and heal with fibromatous scars, and gross facial disfiguration are seen in the lepromatous variant.
- The most common salivary gland infection is caused by the mumps virus; bacterial infections of salivary glands are relatively uncommon.
- **Mumps** is characterized by the enlargement and inflammation of one or both parotid glands, reddening of the parotid duct orifice, pyrexia and (sometimes) earache.
- Xerostomia and enlargement of major salivary glands are seen in HIV infection.
- **Acute suppurative parotitis**, caused mainly by α-haemolytic streptococci and *Staphylococcus aureus*, is exquisitely painful.
- **Management** of bacterial parotitis entails **antibiotic** therapy, good **oral hygiene**, **rehydration**, **sialagogues** and, if necessary, surgical drainage.
- Less commonly, salivary gland infections are caused by *Mycobacterium tuberculosis*, *Actinomyces* spp., *Neisseria gonorrhoeae* and *Treponema pallidum*.

Review Questions (Answers on p. 392)

Please indicate which answers are true and which are false.

35.1. A 70-year-old asthmatic who is on inhaled budesonide (a steroid) for the last 15 years presents with a white patch on the buccal mucosa that could be easily removed, revealing a red patch underneath. Which of the following statements are true?
   a. it is likely that this patient is having an opportunistic infection
   b. culturing a swab from the white patch on blood agar will aid in the diagnosis
   c. the drug treatment to the patient's medical condition is likely to have caused the white/red patch
   d. administration of amoxicillin might worsen the condition
   e. nystatin lozenges are the treatment of choice

35.2. Seeing a patient with mucocutaneous candidiasis with oral lesions should prompt you to:
   a. look for a cause for immunodeficiency
   b. start antiretroviral therapy
   c. isolate the patient as he/she may spread the infection to others
   d. enquire about the family history of the disease
   e. start topical antifungal treatment for the oral lesions

35.3. *Candida*-associated denture stomatitis (*syn:* chronic atrophic candidiasis):
   a. is usually symptomatic
   b. frequently presents with angular stomatitis
   c. can be treated by improving denture hygiene and not wearing dentures at night
   d. is common on both the upper and the lower denture-bearing mucosa
   e. palatal papillary hyperplasia may be seen in advanced cases

35.4. Which statements about infections of the oral cavity due to human herpesviruses are true?
   a. infection with human herpesvirus 2 (HHV-2) is common in children
   b. reactivation leads to herpes stomatitis in one-third of patients
   c. infection with HHV-8 may cause Kaposi's sarcoma
   d. severe toothache may follow oral herpes zoster infections
   e. palatal petechiae are pathognomonic of Epstein–Barr virus (EBV) infections

35.5. Match the stage of syphilis that will demonstrate the appropriate clinical feature:
   a. chancre
      primary/secondary/tertiary/congenital
   b. gumma of hard palate
      primary/secondary/tertiary/congenital
   c. snail-track ulcer
      primary/secondary/tertiary/congenital
   d. mulberry molar teeth
      primary/secondary/tertiary/congenital
   e. mucous patches
      primary/secondary/tertiary/congenital
   f. saddle nose
      primary/secondary/tertiary/congenital

35.6. Which of the following statements related to infections of the salivary glands are true?
   a. mumps is common among children
   b. acute suppurative parotitis is common among postoperative patients
   c. in mumps, parotid glands are primarily involved
   d. mumps might lead to orchitis and pancreatitis
   e. β-haemolytic streptococci are the major aetiological agent for acute bacterial parotitis

Further Reading

Lamey, P. J., Boyle, M. A., MacFarlane, T. W., et al. (1987). Acute suppurative parotitis in out-patients: Microbiological and post-treatment sialographic findings. *Oral Surgery, Oral Medicine, and Oral Pathology, 63,* 37–41.

Reichart, P., Samaranayake, L. P., & Philipsen, H. P. (2000). Pathology and clinical correlates in oral candidiasis and its variants: A review. *Oral Diseases, 6,* 85–91.

Samaranayake, L. P., Cheung, L. K., & Samaranayake, Y. H. (2002). Candidiasis and other fungal diseases of the mouth. *Dermatologic Therapy, 15,* 252–270.

Samaranayake, L. P., Fakhruddin, K. S., Ngo, H. C., Bandara, H. M. N. M., & Leung, Y. Y. (2022). Orofacial mycoses in Coronavirus Disease-2019 (COVID-19): A systematic review. *International Dental Journal, 72,* 607–620.

Samaranayake, L. P., & MacFarlane, T. W. (Eds.). (1990). *Oral candidosis.* Wright.

Sitheeque, M., & Samaranayake, L. P. (2003). Chronic hyperplastic candidiasis (candidal leukoplakia). *Critical Reviews in Oral Biology and Medicine, 14,* 253–267.

Soysa, N. S., Samaranayake, L. P., & Ellepola, A. N. B. (2008). Antimicrobials as a contributory factor in oral candidosis: A brief overview. *Oral Diseases, 14,* 138–143.

PART 6

CROSS-INFECTION AND CONTROL

The theoretical and practical aspects of infection control described in this part will undoubtedly regulate the daily clinical regime of any dental practice. Thus, the students are strongly advised to be thoroughly conversant with this subject matter, and to supplement this section with further reading from the lists of recommended books and articles.

Further, the infection control regimentation in dentistry came under intense scrutiny during the COVID-19 pandemic, as SARS-CoV-2, swiftly spreads though aerosols causing respiratory infections. Thus, the profession was subjected to additional, further stringent infection control measures that are currently in force throughout the world. These measures are likely to be modified and downgraded in the future due to the waning of the pandemic.

Every effort has been made here to outline the extant international infection control guidelines. However, as new infections are constantly emerging, the protocol described may be necessarily modified or indeed totally revised. Therefore, students are urged to pay heed to the changing scenarios in infection control and stay current by visiting appropriate sources of information such as the Centers of Disease Control and Prevention and the British Dental Association websites in USA and UK, respectively, and local and regional advisory guidelines such as National Infection Prevention and Control Manual (NIPCM) of Scotland.

- General principles of infection control, standard precautions and transmission-based precautions
- Standard infection control procedures in dentistry Part I: personal protection, sharps injuries protocol and immunization
- Standard infection control procedures in dentistry Part II: sterilization, disinfection and antisepsis, with a summary of transmission-based infection control procedures

36 *General Principles of Infection Control, Standard Precautions and Transmission-Based Precautions*

This chapter outlines the basics of how infections spread in a clinic environment, the infection control recommendations now termed Standard Precautions, and the further add-on stringent precautions known as Transmission-Based Precautions when patients have diseases that are spread through contact, droplet or airborne routes (e.g., skin contact, sneezing, coughing), such as COVID-19.

The Centers for Disease Control and Prevention (CDC) in the US has been the prime mover in formulating and promulgating these recommendations as well as introducing subsequent modifications as various infections have emerged over time. In general, these recommendations are directly adapted in many jurisdictions of the world, some with minor variations. Hence, the details in this and other chapters are essentially adapted from the CDC recommendations of 2018.

General Principles of Infection Control

CROSS-INFECTION

Cross-infection may be defined as the transmission of infectious agents between patient and patient, and patient and staff, *within a clinical environment*. Transmission may result from person-to-person contact or via contaminated objects, termed **fomites**, as well as through the airborne route via splatter, aerosols or a common source such as dental unit waterlines (Fig. 36.1). Organisms capable of causing cross-infection in humans are derived from:

■ other human sources (the most important)
■ animal sources, i.e., **vectors** (less important)
■ inanimate sources, i.e., **fomites** (of least importance).

(Note: animal vectors of infection are not dicussed here).

GENERAL PRINCIPLES OF INFECTION TRANSMISSION

Transmission of infection from one person to another requires:

1. a **source** of infection: the person with the infection is called the index case
2. a **mode** or **vehicle** by which the infective agent is transmitted—for example, blood, droplets of saliva, instruments contaminated with blood, saliva and tissue debris. (Though not relevant to dentistry, animals, birds or insects are the largest vectors of infection transmission (e.g., mosquitoes in malaria, dengue, and Zika).)
3. a **route** of transmission, for example inhalation, ingestion.

It can be helpful to think of these steps in the transmission of infection as a *'chain of infection'* that can lead to disease unless it is interrupted by infection prevention and control measures. Links in the chain need to be broken to halt further transmission and to prevent disease spread. Vaccinations are used to protect health care workers from the infected 'source patient,' and once infected, drug therapy with antimicrobials is used to treat the disease.

Infection control and prevention measures such as personal protective equipment (PPE) can block the vehicles of transmission and prevent access of microbes to the mucosa of the respiratory tract, mouth or gut.

The source, mode and route of infection are discussed next.

SOURCES OF INFECTION

The sources of infection in clinical dentistry are mainly human; they include:

1. **People with overt asymptomatic infections.** Such individuals liberate large numbers of organisms into the environment (e.g., droplets and discharges from the mouth or other portals; wounds, ulcers and sores on the skin). Fortunately, in routine clinical dentistry, few patients with acute life-threatening diseases are seen. Common infections circulating in the community can be transmitted in the dental environment from patients or staff with *overt infections*, such as SARS-CoV-2 and seasonal influenza.

2. **People in the prodromal stage of certain infections.** During the *prodrome or the incubating period,* the organisms multiply without evidence of infection; although patients are healthy at this stage, they could be highly infectious. Viral infections, such as measles, mumps and chickenpox (varicella), are easily spread in this manner. Persons incubating mumps or measles are infectious for 5–6 days before symptoms appear and they are aware of their illness. A significant proportion of patients with prodromal illness may attend for dental treatment, as neither they nor the healthcare provider is unaware of the insidious disease they harbour. Hence, for instance, the requirement for occupational vaccination of all dental health care workers and students, with the mumps, measles and rubella (MMR) vaccine and varicella vaccine.

3. **People who are healthy carriers of pathogens.** Such persons can be classified as:
   ■ convalescent carriers
   ■ asymptomatic carriers.

Convalescent carriers are those who suffer an illness and apparently recover, although blood and secretions of the individual act as persistent reservoirs of infective organisms. For example, following diphtheria or streptococcal sore throat, the organisms may persist in the throat for some time and infect others or, in the case of hepatitis B, patients may recover fully, although they may carry the infectious agent in the blood for a considerable period. The latter are called **chronic carriers**.

Asymptomatic carriers give no history of infection as they may have unknowingly had a nonapparent or subclinical infection (recognized merely because of the presence of specific antibodies in the person's blood). Nevertheless, these individuals may carry infective microbes in the saliva, blood and other body secretions.

Hepatitis B and hepatitis C are classic examples of diseases that may manifest with or without symptoms, and thus, for example, the clinician may be faced with either a convalescent or an asymptomatic carrier of hepatitis B or C virus. *Note:* A convalescent carrier can be identified from the history of infection, as opposed to an asymptomatic carrier who cannot be diagnosed in this way. In the case of hepatitis C, a carrier may not be identified for decades before they present to their doctor with liver disease or liver cancer, but during that period they may have unwittingly transmitted their infection to many others.

MODES OF INFECTION

Transmission of infection may occur in one of two modes:

■ **Directly through inhalation of aerosols or droplets** containing infectious agents is the most common mode of infection in general either in the clinic or the community. An alternative, less common mode of infection transmission in the clinic is through **contaminated saliva, secretions and blood**, as in the case of an ungloved practitioner with a cut on the finger performing an extraction, or during an exposure-prone procedure during which the gloved hand of the clinician is pierced by a sharp instrument or tooth.

■ **Indirectly via contaminated sharps and instruments** occurs when materials have been improperly decontaminated (Fig. 36.1).

Some of the infectious agents of concern in dentistry and their possible routes of transmission are given in Table 36.1.

AIRBORNE INFECTION

Airborne infective organisms in the form of infectious aerosols may be inhaled, causing diseases such as COVID-19, influenza, the common cold and tuberculosis. When aerosols are created, for example by high-speed instruments, different sizes of droplets are produced. Their fate depends on their size.

Droplets greater than 100 μm in diameter are called **splatter** (or spatter) and settle very quickly on surfaces as a result of gravitational pull; they contaminate whatever is immediately in front of and below the patient within a 1–2-m radius. **Droplets** or particles between **20 μm and 100 μm** in size fall from airborne suspension within seconds. Usually generated during coughing or sneezing, the latter contain numerous microbes. True **aerosols**, by contrast, comprise very small particles **less than 5 μm** or droplet nuclei (fluid droplets that evaporate rapidly and shrink to less than 5 μm) that remain suspended or **entrained** in the air for many hours and travel long distances on air currents. Small droplets of less than 100 μm in diameter account for the majority of droplets created in the dental surgery (Table 36.2).

Droplet nuclei, which consist of dried salivary, sputum or serum secretions and any organisms they may contain, eventually fall to the ground or are inhaled into the alveoli of the lungs with the potential to cause respiratory infections. In practical terms, this underscores the importance of adequate ventilation of the clinical environment and wearing face masks, particularly during the use of aerosol-creating instruments and the routine disinfection of surgery surfaces.

INFECTION VIA SHARPS AND NEEDLE-STICK INJURIES OR SURFACE CONTACT

The major route of cross-infection in the dental surgery is through the skin or mucosa due to accidents involving sharps or needle-stick injuries (Fig. 36.1). There is evidence that hepatitis B, hepatitis C and HIV transmission from patient to dentist, and *vice versa*, has occurred by this means. Improperly disinfected clinical surfaces may also act as reservoirs of infection, as in the case of COVID-19.

Routes of Infection

Transmission of the pathogen to the new host is sometimes by **direct contact** but is more often an **indirect process**

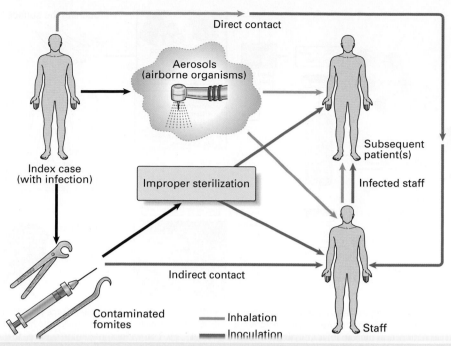

Fig. 36.1   Routes and modes by which infection may spread in the dental clinic.

Table 36.1   Some Infectious Agents of Concern in Dentistry and Their Routes of Transmission

Microorganism	Major Transmission Route
Viruses	
Cytomegalovirus	Inhalation
Hepatitis viruses	Inoculation
Hepatitis B	Inoculation
Hepatitis C	Inoculation
Delta hepatitis (hepatitis D)	Inoculation
Herpes simplex virus types 1 and 2	Direct contact
Human immunodeficiency virus (HIV)	Inoculation
Measles and mumps viruses	Inhalation
Respiratory Viruses	
Influenza virus	Inhalation
Rhinovirus	Inhalation
Adenovirus	Inhalation
Rubella virus	Inhalation
Bacteria	
Neisseria gonorrhoeae	Inoculation
Treponema pallidum (syphilis)	Inoculation
Mycobacterium tuberculosis	Inoculation/inhalation
Streptococcus pyogenes	Inhalation

Table 36.2   Characteristics of Aerosols Produced by High-Speed Instrumentation

	Particles	Droplet Nuclei
Diameter	>100 μm	<100 μm
Time spent airborne	Minutes	Hours
Penetration into respiratory tract	Unlikely	Possible
Possible mode of transmission	Direct contact or from dust	Inhalation

Inhalation, inoculation and, rarely, direct contact are the modes by which the pathogens gain access to the host tissues in the dental clinic environment.

SARS-CoV-2 infection typifies the many routes by which infections could spread either in the clinic or the community, as exemplified in Fig. 36.2.

Standard Infection Control Precautions

From the foregoing, it is clear that it is impossible to ascertain whether the patient who attends for dental treatment is a carrier of infectious agents. Therefore, *all patients should be treated as if they are reservoirs of pathogens.* The infection control procedures involved in such treatment are termed **standard precautions** (previously termed 'universal precautions'), and all clinical procedures performed on **any patient** should be conducted using **standard precautions**.

The corollary of this is that no additional infection control precautions should be necessary when a patient who is a carrier of infection such as hepatitis C or human immunodeficiency virus (HIV) attends the clinic. *The importance of*

involving various vehicles of infection (see above). Once the organism has approached the new host, it may gain ingress via a number of routes:

- **inhalation**
- inoculation or **injection**
- **ingestion** (e.g., diarrhoeal diseases; see Chapter 26)
- **transplacental** (e.g., congenital syphilis, congenital Zika syndrome or HIV acquired in utero).

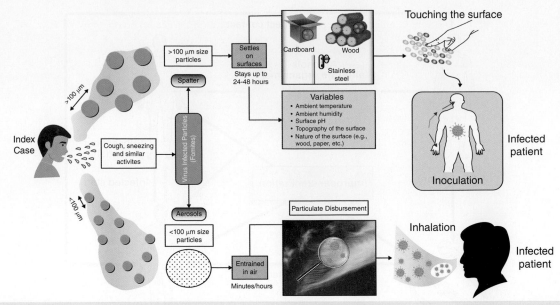

Fig. 36.2 A schematic diagram depicting the aerosol and droplet spread of SARS-CoV-2 from an index case (source patient or asymptomatic individual) to two different patients through the droplet route (sequence above) and the aerosol route (sequence below). Note how the particle size determines the route of infection dissemination, and the variables affecting the survival of SARS-CoV-2 on various inanimate surfaces that eventually act as vectors of viral spread (fomites).

this concept cannot be overemphasized and should be noted by all who practice dentistry.

EVOLUTION OF UNIVERSAL PRECAUTIONS, STANDARD PRECAUTIONS AND TRANSMISSION-BASED PRECAUTIONS

The first set of recommendations on infection control in dentistry, issued in the late 1980s, focused primarily on the transmission of blood-borne pathogen transmission in dental care and other clinical settings and was termed **universal precautions**. These recommendations, which were formulated during the AIDS pandemic, emphasized the need to treat *blood and other bodily fluids contaminated with blood* from all patients as potentially infectious.

However, the realization that moist body substances—that is, secretions and excretions such as semen, saliva, tears and breast milk (but not sweat)—*irrespective of whether they are contaminated with blood or not,* are equally important in disease transmission led to the development of **standard precautions** in the mid-1990s. Thus, standard precautions are similar to universal precautions, as they are designed to reduce the risk of infection transmission from both recognized and unrecognized sources of infection to patients and clinicians.

The standard precautions apply to contact with:

- blood
- all body fluids, secretions and excretions (except sweat), *regardless of whether they are blood contaminated*
- nonintact skin
- mucous membranes.

For the overwhelming majority of infectious diseases, including those possibly encountered routinely in dental settings, the application of standard precautions will arrest disease transmission.

However, in special situations in which a patient with a known infection or an asymptomatic carrier of such an infection, which has a high transmission potential, is suspected or encountered, **transmission-based precautions** or **additional precautions** have to be implemented. These include situations dealing with patients either having or suspected to be infected with virulent pathogens that are transmitted through:

- air or droplets (e.g., COVID-19 or other coronaviruses such as SARS, MERS, tuberculosis, influenza, chickenpox, mumps)
- indirect or direct contact with contaminated sources (e.g., methicillin-resistant *Staphylococcus aureus* (MRSA) or multidrug-resistant *Mycobacterium tuberculosis*).

These so-called transmission-based precautions include patient isolation, adequate room ventilation, respiratory protection of workers and postponement of nonemergency dental care procedures. It should, however, be realized that in routine dentistry, application of standard precautions would be the norm.

However, with the advent of COVID-19, which is highly transmissible, this situation changed considerably, and the latter additional layer of transmission-based infection controls had to be applied, particularly during the pandemic period. Usually, though, additional transmission-based precautions need to be implemented only in special situations, such as during outbreaks of highly contagious viral infections or virulent bacterial infections. Some examples of infections that require this additional layer of infection control—such as coronavirus infections, tuberculosis, measles, chickenpox and multidrug-resistant *Staphylococcus aureus* infections—are shown in Table 36.3.

Table 36.3 Some Infections for Which Transmission-Based Precautions Are Required (not an exhaustive list)

Airborne Transmission

- COVID-19 and other coronavirus infections (SARS, MERS)
- Active/open pulmonary tuberculosis
- Measles
- *Varicella* (chickenpox)
- *Streptococcus pyogenes* (scarlet fever)
- Influenza
- Pertussis (whooping cough)
- Rubella
- Meningococcal infection

Droplet Transmission

- *Streptococcus pyogenes* (scarlet fever)
- Influenza
- Pertussis (whooping cough)
- Rubella
- Meningococcal infection

Note: Patients with these infections should not undergo elective dental treatment unless in emergency situations.

Although applied during the pandemic period, for reasons of absolute necessity, the persistent, long-term application of transmission-based precautions (e.g., airborne precautions for patients with suspected tuberculosis) in dental settings is clearly not feasible due to the added financial burden both for the patient and the clinician and engineering controls required for clean air, as well as spatial facilities for separation of index patients from routine attendees. A saving grace here for routine dentistry is that patients do not usually seek routine dental outpatient care when acutely ill with diseases requiring transmission-based precautions.

Nonetheless, all dental surgeries should have systems for early detection and management of potentially infectious patients at initial points of entry to the dental clinic at all times (e.g., thermal body temperature scanners and alerting devices). This also includes rescheduling nonemergency dental care until the patient is no longer infectious and/or referral to a local or regional dental setting such as a hospital dental clinic, with appropriate infection prevention precautions.

Note on COVID-19 pandemic and infection control: With the waning of the pandemic worldwide, at the time of this writing, a return to standard infection control measures in routine dentistry is likely to be reintroduced by various authorities. This again depends on the regional prevalence of the disease and sporadic flare-up of COVID-19 that is predicted to occur from time to time in the future. Hence, DCWs, should keep abreast of all the current regional data on highly transmissible diseases such as COVID-19 and/or any other new infectious diseases that may pose a threat of infection transmission in the clinic, as these impact the level of infection control that should be implemented (i.e., either standard precautions or transmission-based precautions).

A detailed discussion of the standard precautions and transmission-based precautions are provided in the next two chapters. The outlines of these are given below and in Fig. 36.3.

STANDARD PRECAUTIONS: BASICS

Standard precautions are the minimum infection prevention practices that apply **to all patient care**, regardless of suspected or confirmed infection status of the patient. These are designed to both protect DCWs and prevent dental personnel from spreading infections among patients. The main features of standard precautions are:

- hand hygiene
- use of personal protective equipment (e.g., gloves, masks, eyewear)
- respiratory hygiene/cough etiquette
- sharps safety (engineering and work practice controls)
- safe injection practices (i.e., aseptic technique for parenteral medications)

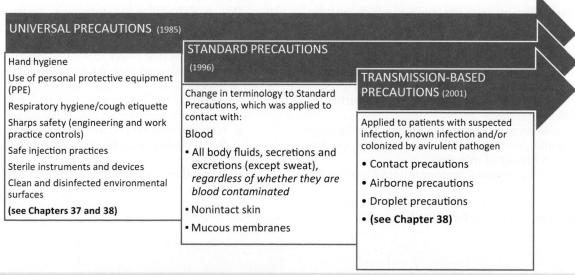

Fig. 36.3 • **Evolution of infection control recommendations over the last few decades.**

- sterile instruments and devices
- clean and disinfected environmental surfaces
- education, lifelong learning and training.

- contact precautions
- airborne precautions
- droplet precautions.

TRANSMISSION-BASED PRECAUTIONS: BASICS

The basic features of transmission-based precautions (Fig. 36.3) are:

These key features of the foregoing are described in detail in the next two chapters with a summary box of key recommendations for each item.

Key Facts

- Cross-infection may be defined as the transmission of infectious agents between patients and staff **within a clinical environment**.
- The **animate** (e.g., insects, humans) and **inanimate** sources (e.g., blood, saliva) that carry and transmit infection are called **vectors** and **fomites**, respectively.
- **Transmission of infection** from one person to another requires a **source** of infection (the index case), a **mode** or **vehicle** of transmission (e.g., vectors and fomites) and a **route** of transmission (e.g., inhalation, percutaneous).
- Transmission of infection in dentistry could occur by direct contact, airborne spread or via contaminated sharps.
- The **sources** of infection in clinical dentistry are mainly humans and constitute those (1) with **overt infections**, (2) in the **prodromal** stage of infections and (3) who are healthy **carriers** of pathogens.
- The infective agents may gain entry into the body by **inhalation**, **inoculation** (or injection) or **ingestion**.
- Healthy carriers of pathogens are of two types: **convalescent** carriers and **asymptomatic** carriers.
- **Standard infection** control precautions uphold the concept of **treating every patient as a potential carrier of infectious disease** and that all body fluids except sweat are potentially infectious.
- All patients in dentistry, irrespective of whether they carry apparent infections or not, should be treated under a standard infection control protocol.
- In special situations where a patient with a known virulent infection or an asymptomatic carrier of such an infection with a high transmission potential is suspected or encountered, **transmission-based precautions** or **additional precautions** have to be implemented.
- Transmission-based precautions incorporate the triad of **contact precautions, airborne precautions** and **droplet precautions.**
- With the waning of the COVID-19 pandemic, practitioners using transmission-based infection control recommendations currently applied in routine dentistry are likely to revert to the standard infection control measures. However transmission-based controls must be reintroduced if a flare-up of COVID-19 occurs or if and when another new, highly transmissible infection emerges in the future.

Review Questions (Answers on p. 392)

Please indicate which answers are true and which are false.

36.1. Which of the following statements related to cross-infection are true?
  a. blood and saliva are regarded as fomites with respect to infection transmission
  b. viral infections are unlikely to spread during the prodromal stage
  c. convalescent carriers are different from asymptomatic carriers in that asymptomatic carriers have a history of infection
  d. prions are resistant to conventional sterilization methods
  e. droplet nuclei less than 100 μm in diameter are entrained in the air for many hours

36.2. Which of the following statements are true?
  a. the first person that is traced to have begun an infection is called the index case
  b. overt infection refers to a situation in which the carrier is unaware that he/she is having a specific infection
  c. convalescent carriers of infection harbour the infectious agent for an extremely long period
  d. standard infection control precautions are applied when dealing with blood, body fluids, sweat and saliva
  e. inhalation is a major route through which infections are transmitted in dentistry

Further Reading

Centers for Disease Control and Prevention (CDC). (2016). *Summary of infection prevention practices in dental settings: Basic expectations for safe care*. CDC, US Department of Health and Human Services. https://www.cdc.gov/oralhealth/infectioncontrol/pdf/safe-care2.pdf.

Goering, R., Dockrell, H., Zuckerman, M., et al. (2012). Hospital infection, sterilization and disinfection. In Goering, R., Dockrell, H., Zuckerman, M., Roitt, I. M., & Chiodini, P. L. (Eds.), *Mims' medical microbiology*, (5th ed., Chap. 36). Saunders/Elsevier.

National Health Service. (2021). *(HTM 01–05) Decontamination in primary care dental practices* (2nd ed.). https://www.england.nhs.uk/publication/decontamination-in-primary-care-dental-practices-htm-01-05.

Pankhurst, C. L., & Coulter, W. A. (2017). *Basic guide to infection prevention and control* (2nd ed.). Wiley-Blackwell.

Samaranayake, L., & Fakhruddin, K. (2021). Pandemics, past present and future: Their impact on oral health care. *Journal of the American Dentistry Association, 152*(12), 972–980. https://doi.org/10.1016/j.adaj.2021.09.008.

Samaranayake, L., & Fakhruddin, K. (2023, May). Epidemics, pandemics and dentistry: A commentary. https://doi.org/10.12968/denu.2023.50.5.454.

Samaranayake, L., & Peiris, M. (2004). Severe acute respiratory syndrome and dentistry: A retrospective view. *Journal of the American Dentistry Association, 135*(9), 1292–1302.

Samaranayake, L. P., Scheutz, F., & Cottone, J. (1991). *Infection control for the dental team*. Munksgaard.

37 Standard Infection Control Procedures in Dentistry Part I: Personal Protection, Sharps Injuries Protocol and Immunization

Implementation of **standard infection control** precautions in dentistry (previously termed 'universal precautions') entails prevention of infection transmission within the dental clinic environment and **assumes that ALL patients are carriers of infectious diseases**. Such a policy protects both patients and staff, reduces staff concerns and prevents discrimination against patients. In this chapter, the major features reflecting the best current practice of standard infection control are outlined, but the reader is strongly advised to keep abreast with the literature because of the constant flux and changes that are bound to happen in this space, due to the emergence of new infectious diseases, as well as the advances in applied technology. Apart from the general features related to practice management vis-à-vis infection control recommendations, this chapter provides key guidance for the standard infection control recommendations. The next chapter is a continuum of infection control and outlines sterilization, disinfection and antisepsis as applied in dentistry.

Practice Management and Staff Development

All staff who join a practice should undergo a **formal education programme** that includes the theory and practice of infection control in dentistry. In addition, a written **infection control protocol** specific for the practice **should be available for inspection** by patients and other interested parties. Practitioners may be subjected to litigation in some jurisdictions if such documentation is not available and readily accessible.

An **in-service training** programme, updating techniques and material, should be provided for the staff. This may take the form of regular attendance at local scientific meetings, continuing education programs and access to current information such as journals and the Internet.

Infection Control: Specific Practical Features

A comprehensive infection control protocol includes a number of elements:

- patient evaluation
- personal protection
- hand and respiratory hygiene
- instrument decontamination: cleaning, disinfection, sterilization and storage
- use of disposables (single-use devices and personal protective equipment (PPE))
- disinfection of the environment
- clinical and laboratory asepsis

- disposal of waste
- staff training, including continuing education.

PATIENT EVALUATION

A thorough **medical history** should be taken from each patient and updated at each recall visit. It is not only good clinical practice but may also reveal disease that is important in relation to cross-infection and relevant to the dental procedure to be undertaken. If a questionnaire is used for this purpose, it should always be supported by direct discussions with the patient. The medical history should not be used to categorize patients as high risk or low risk, as was the procedure prior to the introduction of standard infection control precautions. In taking a history, the practitioner should identify the infectious disease of concern, and relevant questions should be asked in an environment conducive to the disclosure of sensitive personal information. It is also important that:

- all staff are trained in the **proper management of records**, including keeping them away from the public view in the front office, safe storage and maintenance with due regard to appropriate data protection legislation
- a written **policy on confidentiality** should be signed by all staff members
- personal **medical or dental details are not disclosed** to other health care workers without the consent of the patient.

PERSONAL PROTECTION AND PERSONAL PROTECTIVE EQUIPMENT

Personal protection and PPE are discussed under the following headings:

- Personal Hygiene
- Clinic Clothing
- Barrier Protection (gloves, eye shield, face masks, rubber dam isolation)
- Immunization Procedures.

Personal Hygiene

The personal hygiene of all members of staff who are either directly or indirectly in contact with patients should be scrupulous. A rigidly followed **code of hygiene** will greatly reduce cross-infection in the dental clinic. In general, when working with patients, dental personnel should observe the following precautions:

- Refrain from touching anything not required for the particular procedure. Specifically, staff should keep their hands away from their eyes, nose, mouth and hair, and they should avoid touching sores or abrasions.
- Cover cuts and bruises on fingers with dressings (because they serve as easy portals for pathogens).
- Hair should be kept short or tied up; otherwise, a hair net should be worn.

Hand Hygiene. Fingers are the most common vehicles of infection transmission. This fact is poorly recognized by all. The World Health Organization (WHO) promotes the '**5 Moments for Hand Hygiene**', which recommends that health care workers clean their hands (Fig. 37.1):

1. before touching a patient
2. before clean/aseptic procedures
3. after body fluid exposure/risk (e.g., saliva, blood or other bodily fluid)
4. after touching a patient
5. after touching patient surroundings.

The whole dental team should pay attention to meticulous hand care:

- A dedicated clean and **clutter-free sink** should be provided in the clinic for hand-washing, and the taps should be operated by elbow or foot controls or sensors (no-touch technique). The sink should have no overflows or plugs to prevent contamination of the faucets with *Pseudomonas* spp. and other environmental microbes resident in sink traps and U-bends. Wall-mounted hand hygiene solutions should be dispensed in disposable rather than refillable cartridges/bottles.
- Keep **fingernails** short and clean. Dental personnel should work '**bare below the elbow**' in order to facilitate good hand hygiene. **Jewellery** such as rings and watches should be removed as rings tend to entrap organisms and damage gloves. Do not wear nail polish, artificial fingernails or extenders when having direct contact with patients. If long-sleeved clothing is worn, it should be rolled up above the elbow.
- For routine dental examinations and nonsurgical procedures, use water and plain soap (hand-washing) or antimicrobial soap (hand antisepsis) specific for health care settings or use an alcohol-based hand rub. Thoroughly clean the hands before putting on and removing gloves and before and after treating each patient.
- **Alcohol-based hand rubs** are effective for hand hygiene in health care settings. Alcohol-based hand rubs have the advantage of causing less skin dehydration than soaps, are faster to use and do not require running water. However, hand rubs are only effective as hand disinfectants on visibly clean hands—that is, in the absence of blood or dirt. Plain soap and water are used to wash dirty hands. Hands should also be cleaned before leaving the surgery for any purpose and upon return.
- A **good hand-hygiene technique**, as shown in Fig. 37.1, which can be used with hand rubs or soaps, should be developed by all staff so that all areas of the hands and wrists are cleaned consistently Finger tips, finger and thumb webs, backs of hands and the wrists are often missed when cleaning hands (Fig. 37.2).
- Any obvious cuts or abrasions must be covered with adhesive waterproof dressings.
- Liquid (not bar) soap should be used for routine hand-washing, and antimicrobial liquids should be used for hand-washing prior to surgical procedures. A surgical scrub, also referred to as antisepsis scrub, is a more extensive disinfection of the hands and arms that reduces the numbers of resident bacteria to a minimum; however, it is **not possible to achieve sterilization of the skin**.

Duration of the entire procedure: 40–60 sec.

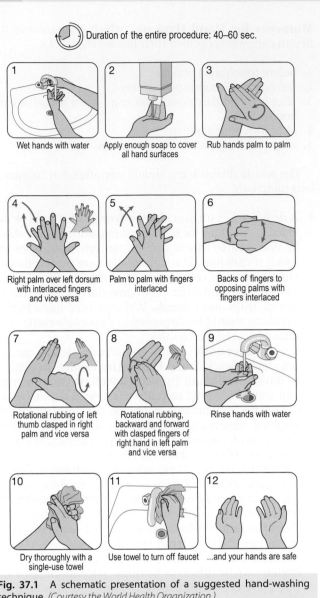

Fig. 37.1 A schematic presentation of a suggested hand-washing technique. *(Courtesy the World Health Organization.)*

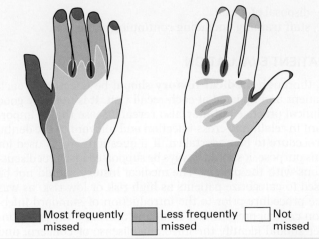

| ■ Most frequently missed | ■ Less frequently missed | □ Not missed |

Fig. 37.2 Areas of the hand that are not thoroughly washed owing to poor hand-washing technique.

at least daily, and more frequently if they become visibly contaminated. Renewable overgarments should be washed at an appropriate temperature (e.g., 60°C) in a well-maintained washing machine. Grossly contaminated clothing should be dealt with separately.

Wear overgarments ***only* in the clinic premises**, not in corridors, canteens or lifts. An additional waterproof vinyl apron could be worn to protect the overgarment if there is a risk of exposure to body fluids during dental treatment, when working in the instrument-cleaning area or working in the laboratory (e.g., denture trimming).

Barrier Protection

Personal hygiene measures reduce the level of possible pathogens on our bodies and clothes, although they do not completely eliminate them. In order to minimize further the spread of organisms from staff to patients (and vice versa), the following **personal protective equipment (PPE)**, which form a protective barrier, should be used. Dental staff should be trained to select and don and remove the appropriate PPE so that the risk of clothing or skin contamination is reduced:

- gloves
- eye shields (goggles or visors)
- face masks
- rubber dam isolation.

Hand hygiene is always the final step after removing and disposing of PPE. Always remove PPE before leaving the work area.

Gloves. All dentists and close support personnel should routinely wear disposable **nitrile, latex or vinyl gloves**. In many countries, nitrile gloves have replaced the use of latex gloves in dentistry to prevent latex allergy being triggered in the dental team and susceptible patients. The main aim of wearing gloves in routine dentistry is not to achieve consistent surgical sterility but to establish reasonable standards of hygiene in order to safeguard both the dental personnel and the patient.

The efficacy of gloves greatly diminishes if they are **perforated**. As gloves may perforate during surgical procedures,

- Hands washed with soaps and antimicrobial solutions should be dried thoroughly using disposable paper towels, and gloves should be donned as the last step before treatment commences.
- **Moisturizing cream** should be used as a routine at the end of each treatment session to maintain a healthy skin. Take care not to contaminate the cream during use by not sharing moisturizers and by using elbow-operated dispensers.
- Consider the compatibility of lotions and antiseptic products and the effect of petroleum or other oil emollients on the **integrity of gloves** during product selection and glove usage.
- A **ready reckoner** for hand hygiene and antisepsis is provided in Table 37.1, and key CDC recommendations for hand hygiene in dental settings are in Box 37.1.

Clinic Clothing

A freshly laundered **uniform or overgarment** should be worn by all clinical personnel. Garments should be changed

Table 37.1   A Ready Reckoner for Hand Hygiene and Antisepsis

Methods	Agent	Purpose	Area	Duration (minimum)	Indications
Routine hand-wash	Water and nonantimicrobial detergent (e.g., plain soap)	Remove soil and transient microorganisms	Fingertips to the wrist	30–40 s	■ Before and after treating each patient (e.g., before wearing gloves and after glove removal)
Routine hand antisepsis Antiseptic hand-wash	Water and antimicrobial agent/detergent (e.g., chlorhexidine, iodine and iodophors, chloroxylenol, triclosan)	Remove or destroy transient microorganisms and reduce resident flora	Fingertips to the wrist at a minimum	30–40 s	■ After bare-handed touching of inanimate objects likely to be contaminated by blood or saliva
or Antiseptic hand rub	Alcohol-based hand rub			Rub hands until the agent is dry (15–20 s)	■ Before leaving the dental operatory ■ When visibly soiled ■ Before regloving, after removing gloves that are torn, cut or punctured
Surgical hand antisepsis	Water and antimicrobial agent/detergent (e.g., chlorhexidine, iodine and iodophors, chloroxylenol, triclosan)	Remove or destroy transient microorganisms and reduce resident flora (persistent effect)	Hands and forearms up to the elbows	2 min	■ Before donning sterile surgical gloves for surgical procedures
	Water and nonantimicrobial detergent (e.g., plain soap) followed by an alcohol-based hand rub with persistent activity			Follow manufacturer's instructions for alcohol-based hand rub	

Box 37.1   Key CDC Recommendations for Hand Hygiene in Dental Settings

1. Perform hand hygiene—
   a. When hands are visibly soiled.
   b. After barehanded touching of instruments, equipment, materials, and other objects likely to be contaminated by blood, saliva or respiratory secretions.
   c. Before and after treating each patient.
   d. Before putting on gloves and again immediately after removing gloves.
2. Use soap and water when hands are visibly soiled (e.g., blood, body fluids); otherwise, an alcohol-based hand rub may be used.
3. For surgical procedures, perform a surgical hand scrub before putting on sterile surgeon's gloves.
   (Oral surgical procedures involve the incision, excision, or reflection of tissue that exposes the normally sterile areas of the oral cavity (e.g., biopsy, periodontal surgery, apical surgery, implant surgery and surgical extractions of teeth; removal of erupted or nonerupted tooth requiring elevation of mucoperiosteal flap, removal of bone or section of tooth, and suturing, if needed).

(From Centers for Disease Control and Prevention. (2018). *Summary of infection prevention practices in dental settings.* https://www.cdc.gov/oralhealth/infectioncontrol/summary-infection-prevention-practices/standard-precautions.html)

it is advisable to change gloves at least **hourly** during long operative procedures on the same patient. Gloves should be **checked for visible defects** immediately after wearing them, and immediately changed when breaches occur; never wash and reuse gloves. Irritant and contact dermatitis and allergies to chemicals and gloves used in dentistry are relatively commonly seen in dental team or can develop in sensitized patients. Skin creams, a spray-on microfilm on the skin or a cotton glove liner may help these individuals.

There are three main types of gloves used in dentistry; their different uses should be clear:

1. Clean, high-quality, **protective nitrile or latex gloves** should be used whenever examining a patient's mouth or providing routine dental treatment when no blood-letting procedures are undertaken.
2. **Sterile gloves** should be used for surgical procedures or procedures that may lead to blood-letting. The wearing of two pairs of gloves during oral surgical procedures leads to a lower frequency of inner glove perforation and visible blood on the surgeon's hands; however, the effectiveness of the latter procedure in preventing disease transmission has not been demonstrated.
3. **Heavy-duty utility gloves** should be used for cleaning instruments or surfaces or handling chemicals.

Care should be taken to prevent contact between gloves and incompatible material (e.g., some impression materials) or naked flames.

Gloves should be removed as soon as patient contact is over. The hands should then be cleaned, and **hand cream** should be applied to prevent excessive drying of the skin. In addition, dental personnel should wash their hands with an alcohol-based hand rub or soap and water before leaving the clinic. Dental personnel with **exudative lesions** or **weeping dermatitis** should refrain from all direct patient care and from handling equipment until the condition resolves.

A new pair of gloves should be worn for each patient. Gloves should **never be reused**, as this will result in defects that will diminish their value as an effective barrier, and adequate removal of previous patients' pathogens cannot be guaranteed. Treat gloves as surgical waste and dispose of them accordingly (Box 37.2).

Box 37.2 Key CDC Recommendations for Personal Protective Equipment in Dental Settings

1. Provide sufficient and appropriate personal protective equipment (PPE) and ensure that it is accessible to DCWs.
2. Educate all DCWs on proper selection and use of PPE.
3. Wear gloves whenever there is potential for contact with blood, body fluids, mucous membranes, nonintact skin or contaminated equipment.
   - Do not wear the same pair of gloves for the care of more than one patient.
   - Do not wash gloves. Gloves cannot be reused.
   - Perform hand hygiene immediately after removing gloves.
4. Wear protective clothing that covers skin and personal clothing during procedures or activities where contact with blood, saliva, or other potentially infectious material (OPIM) is anticipated.
5. Wear mouth, nose, and eye protection during all dental operative procedures.
6. Remove PPE before leaving the work area.

(From Centers for Disease Control and Prevention. (2018). *Summary of infection prevention practices in dental settings.* https://www.cdc.gov/oralhealth/infectioncontrol/summary-infection-prevention-practices/standard-precautions.html)

Contact Dermatitis and Latex Hypersensitivity. All health care workers should be educated on the signs, symptoms and diagnoses of **skin reactions** associated with frequent hand hygiene and glove use. Patients should be screened for **latex allergy** through a health history questionnaire and referred for medical consultation when latex allergy is suspected. Emergency treatment kits with **latex-free products** should be available at all times.

Eye Shields. Eye shields (goggles or visors) should be worn by dentists and close support personnel during all procedures to protect the conjunctivae from spatter and debris generated by high-speed handpieces, scaling (manual or ultrasonic) and polishing and cleaning of instruments:

- Eyewear and face shields should be cleaned regularly and when visibly soiled.
- It is preferable to use eyewear with side protection.
- A patient's eyes should always be protected during examination and treatment.

Face Masks. Wearing a face mask, such as a surgical mask, is a necessary hygienic measure, particularly during high-speed instrumentation, as it acts as a barrier to reduce the inhalation of contaminated splatter and aerosols that might lead to both upper and lower respiratory tract infections. The filtration efficacy of such aerosols depends upon:

- the **material** used for mask manufacture (paper masks are inferior to respirator masks)
- the **length of time** the mask is worn: the useful life of a mask is thought to be about 30–60 min, particularly if the mask is wet. Thus masks are considered single-use items and a clean mask should be worn for each patient.

Always ensure that masks are **well adapted** so that the nose and mouth are completely covered. Masks with metal inserts are preferable as they can be tailored to fit the individual's profile.

Masks should not be touched with gloves during treatment or worn outside the treatment zone; they should be worn beneath face shields as the latter provide only minimal protection from aerosols.

Although surgical masks have partial particulate filtration properties, only respirator masks have the filtering efficiencies required for adequate respiratory protection against contaminated aerosols generated when treating a patient with an infection transmitted by the airborne route—for example, *Mycobacterium tuberculosis.*

Respirator masks are manufactured with a range of filtering efficiencies. Masks with the highest filtering efficiency FFP3 (equivalent to N99 in USA) with 98% filtering efficiency are recommended for protection against infectious aerosols in health care. Respirator masks must be **fit tested** before use and checked by the wearer for facial seal according to the manufacturer's instructions. Finally, provide sufficient and appropriate PPE and ensure that it is accessible to all direct care workers (DCWs).

Respiratory Hygiene/Cough Etiquette

Respiratory hygiene/cough etiquette infection prevention measures are designed to limit the transmission of respiratory pathogens spread by droplet or airborne routes discussed above. These strategies target primarily patients and individuals accompanying patients to the dental clinic who might have undiagnosed transmissible respiratory infections, but they equally **apply to any dental care worker** with signs of illness, including cough, congestion, runny nose or increased production of respiratory secretions. All DCWs, including administrative staff, should be educated on preventing the spread of respiratory pathogens when in contact with symptomatic persons. The key CDC recommendations for respiratory hygiene/cough etiquette in dental settings is given in Box 37.3.

Rubber Dam Isolation. As far as possible, a rubber dam should be used in operative procedures to minimize saliva and blood-contaminated aerosol production. Use of a rubber dam during operative procedures:

- provides a **clear visual field** as the tissues are retracted
- minimizes instrument **contact with the mucosa** (thus minimizing tissue injury and subsequent bleeding)
- reduces **aerosol formation**, as saliva pooling does not occur on the rubber dam surface
- minimizes the **retraction of contaminated oral fluids** into the dental unit water systems as the rubber dam prevents pooling of oral fluids and the possibility of suck-back into the water lines.

A Note on Preprocedural Mouthrinses. Chlorhexidine gluconate (0.1–0.2%), essential oils or povidone–iodine mouthwash prior to a surgical procedure is recommended, by some, to reduce the intraoral microbial load leading to systemic bacteraemias as well as the number of airborne pathogens. There is **no firm scientific evidence** to indicate

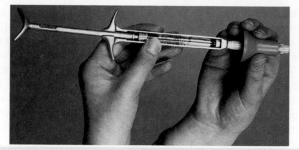

Fig. 37.3   A needle-resheathing device.

that preprocedural mouth rinsing prevents or reduces clinical infections due to oral microbes, either among care providers or patients. However, studies have demonstrated that a preprocedural rinse with an antimicrobial product can reduce the level of oral microorganisms in aerosols and spatter generated during routine dental procedures with rotary instruments (e.g., dental handpieces or ultrasonic scalers).

Aspiration and Ventilation. Routine use of efficient **high-speed aspirators** with external vents and good ventilation will minimize cross-infection from aerosols. Aspirator tips should be single use and the lines regularly cleaned according to the manufacturer's instructions.

Handling Sharps and Related Injuries

Numerous objects with sharp edges are used in dentistry (e.g., needles, blades, burs, endodontic files, orthodontic wires and matrix bands). Most sharps exposures in dentistry are preventable or avoidable either when (i) using the item/s, (ii) during cleanup and decontamination and (iii) during disposal. Hence, every dental practice should have policies and procedures in place that address the safety of sharps.

A **list of all the types of sharps** used in the practice should be kept, identifying those that are disposable and those that may be reused and hence need to be processed. Further, each dental practice should have policies and procedures available that address sharps safety. DCWs should be aware of the risk of injury whenever sharps are exposed.

Items of equipment designated as single use carry the international symbol of a '2' crossed through with a line (2) and are not designed to withstand decontamination and are likely to fail if reused. **Sharps containers** of the approved type should be used in each working area and kept as close as possible to the point of use. They should not be overfilled, and the lid must be kept in the closed position when not in use, then locked prior to disposal to prevent tampering. Containers must be disposed of as clinical waste, ideally by incineration.

Two main approaches are used to reduce sharps injuries: **engineering controls and administrative or work-practice controls**.

Engineering controls should be used as much as possible as the primary method to reduce sharps exposures to blood-borne pathogens. Engineering controls remove or isolate a hazard in the workplace and are frequently **technology based** (e.g., self-sheathing anaesthetic needles, safety scalpels and needleless IV ports; robust sharps containers and needle recapping devices; Fig. 37.3). Employers should involve those DCWs who are directly responsible for patient care (e.g., dentists, hygienists, dental assistants) in identifying, evaluating and selecting devices with engineered safety features at least annually and as they become available.

Administrative or work-practice controls are behaviour based and intended to reduce the risk of blood exposure by changing the way DCWs perform tasks, such as using a one-handed scoop technique for recapping needles between uses and before disposal. Similar work practice controls include:

- not bending or breaking needles before disposal
- not passing a syringe with an unsheathed needle by hand
- removing burs before disassembling the handpiece from the dental unit
- using instruments in place of fingers for tissue retraction
- palpation during suturing and administration of anaesthesia.

All used disposable syringes and needles, scalpel blades and other sharp items should be placed in appropriate **puncture-resistant containers** located close to the area where they are used. Sharps containers should be disposed of according to state and local regulated medical waste rules.

The dental team should be conversant with all sharps handling procedures, which should be an integral part of ongoing staff education.

Sharps Injury Protocol. It is normally recommended for the practice to **nominate a person** to coordinate the

administration of staff health and the reporting and recording of accidents and near misses within the practice. All sharps injuries should be recorded in a **designated register** (accident book) and followed up. A standard protocol for sharps injury should be displayed clearly. However, in the event of an accident, a detailed risk assessment of the incident and counselling should be provided by a specialist in occupational health or a microbiologist to allay any concerns, undertake serological testing and recommend a suitable prophylaxis regimen, if indicated. Guidelines for the management of sharps injuries are shown in Table 37.2; a ready reckoner and an action plan for postexposure prophylaxis is given in Fig. 37.4, showing the relative risk of contracting blood-borne virus infections through a sharps injury. Finally, key CDC recommendations for sharps safety in dental settings is given in Box 37.4.

Safe Injection Practices

DCWs inject virtually millions of doses of local anaesthesia on a daily basis worldwide. Safe injection practices are intended to prevent transmission of infections between one patient and another, or between a patient and DCW during preparation and administration of these injections via routes such as subcutaneous, submucosal, intravenous or intramuscular. Hence, it is paramount that all DCWs not only adopt safe injection protocols but also are aware of these (Box 37.5).

Table 37.2   Principles Guiding the Management of Sharps Injuries

First Aid

- Wash puncture site thoroughly with soap and warm water; antiseptics may be used in addition
- Encourage bleeding by squeezing the injured area
- Dry aseptically and report to supervisor according to the local regulations

Further Action

- Review hepatitis B, C and human immunodeficiency virus (HIV) risk of source patient
- Inform source patient of the incident and counsel patient regarding HIV test, if indicated
- Arrange for venesection of the patient
- Contact occupational health authority, as per local regulations

Action by Occupational Health Authority

- Record in detail circumstances of the sharps injury (i.e., demographic information of the exposed worker, details of the exposure)
- Check hepatitis B vaccination status of staff; if unvaccinated or hepatitis B vaccine non-responder, immediately commence hepatitis B vaccination procedure together with intramuscular hepatitis B immunoglobulin
- Offer counselling to the recipient with regard to HIV risk; if there is significant exposure, commence HIV prophylaxis drugs and continue for 28 days; serological monitoring at 4 weeks (and in some instances additional testing at 8 weeks)
  There is no prophylaxis available for hepatitis C; antiviral therapy is available following seroconversion to hepatitis C virus (HCV)
- Arrange venesection of the recipient for baseline serum antibody levels
- Arrange follow-up antibody testing at 6 months for hepatitis B virus (HBV) and 6, 12 and 24 weeks for HCV
- Return details to the occupational health authority and the infection control team as appropriate

---

DCWs routinely use needles and cartridges containing local anaesthetics for a single patient only, and thereafter the dental cartridge syringe is cleaned and heat sterilized between patients. Other such practices used in dentistry may include use of parenteral medications combined with fluid infusion systems, such as for patients undergoing conscious sedation.

Immunization Procedures

Practitioners should have a **written policy** on the vaccination (including administration of boosters) of all staff and maintain an **up-to-date immunization record** of themselves and their staff, which should be kept confidential. In the US, recommended immunizations for dental health care personnel include hepatitis B, MMR (measles, mumps, and rubella), varicella (chickenpox) and Tdap (tetanus, diphtheria, pertussis).

In the UK, dental staff must comply with national regulations for preemployment standard health clearance checks and vaccinations. For those staff performing exposure-prone procedures as part of their role, then compliance with additional health clearance checks is mandatory. A list of vaccines that are available to dental health care workers is shown in Chapter 10 (Table 10.2). In the UK, vaccination against hepatitis B virus, tuberculosis (TB), MMR and varicella has been recommended for clinical dental staff, in addition to routine immunization against tetanus, poliomyelitis and diphtheria. An annotated outline of vaccines available to dental personnel is given in the following sections.

Bacille Calmette–Guérin Vaccine

Organism. Active against *Mycobacterium tuberculosis*. The vaccine contains live *Mycobacterium bovis* (termed 'bacille Calmette–Guérin' (BCG)) **attenuated by propagation** in a bile-potato medium. Killed vaccines do not produce the cell-mediated immune response essential for protection against TB.

Indications. In the UK, the BCG vaccination is used as an occupational vaccine for those working in health care whose tuberculin test indicates no reaction. Until 2005, UK schoolchildren were vaccinated against TB at the age of 12–14 years. This vaccination schedule was replaced with a targeted, risk-based immunization protocol for susceptible neonates and infants who may be exposed to TB from family members or in locations where there are high rates of TB. The most effective use of BCG vaccination is to give it as soon as possible after birth to prevent infants at increased risk of exposure to TB. These infants include those who are at increased risk of developing severe disease, such as miliary TB and TB meningitis. BCG is less effective at protecting against adult-type disease in older age groups.

Administration. Single dose intradermally in the deltoid muscle.

Poliomyelitis Vaccine

Organism. Poliomyelitis is an acute illness that follows invasion through the gastrointestinal tract by one of the three serotypes of polio virus (serotypes 1, 2 and 3). The virus replicates in the gut and has a high affinity for nervous

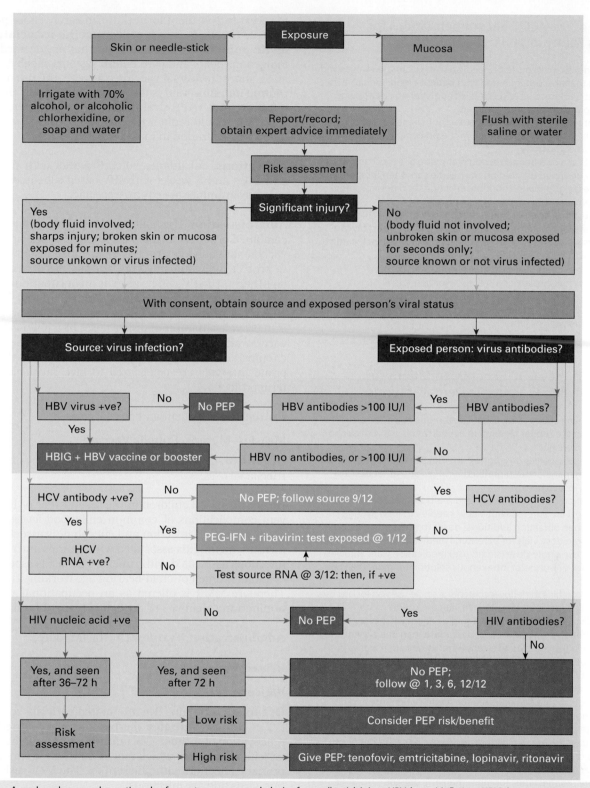

Fig. 37.4 A ready reckoner and an action plan for postexposure prophylaxis of a needle-stick injury. HBV, hepatitis B virus; HBIG, hepatitis B immunoglobulin; HCV, hepatitis C virus; HIV, human immunodeficiency virus; PEP, postexposure prophylaxis PEG-IFN, Pegylated interferon.

tissue. Transmission is through contact with the **faeces or pharyngeal secretions** of an infected person. Polio virus replicates for longer periods and it can be excreted for 3–6 weeks in faeces and 2 weeks in saliva. There are two types of vaccine. **The Salk vaccine**, an **inactivated (killed) poliovirus** (IPV), is a trivalent vaccine (with all three serotypes), which is delivered by intramuscular (IM) injection. The alternative vaccine is the **Sabin vaccine** (oral poliovirus vaccine (OPV)), which is an **oral live attenuated vaccine** that has been utilized for the Global Polio Eradication Initiative because of the ease of delivery. The OPV live attenuated vaccine virus retains the potential

Box 37.4   Key CDC Recommendations for Sharps Safety in Dental Settings

1. Consider sharp items (e.g., needles, scalers, burs, lab knives and wires) that are contaminated with patient blood and saliva as potentially infective, and establish engineering controls and work practices to prevent injuries.
2. Do not recap used needles by using both hands or any other technique that involves directing the point of a needle toward any part of the body.
3. Use either a one-handed scoop technique or a mechanical device designed for holding the needle cap when recapping needles (e.g., between multiple injections and before removing from a nondisposable aspirating syringe).
4. Place used disposable syringes and needles, scalpel blades, and other sharp items in appropriate puncture-resistant containers located as close as possible to the area where the items are used.

(From Centers for Disease Control and Prevention. (2018). *Summary of infection prevention practices in dental settings.* https://www.cdc.gov/oralhealth/infectioncontrol/summary-infection-prevention-practices/standard-precautions.html)

Box 37.5   Key CDC Recommendations for Safe Injection Practices in Dental Settings

1. Prepare injections using aseptic technique in a clean area.
2. Disinfect the rubber septum on a medication vial with alcohol before piercing.
3. Do not use needles or syringes* for more than one patient (this includes manufactured prefilled syringes and other devices such as insulin pens).
4. Medication containers (single and multidose vials, ampules and bags) are entered with a new needle and new syringe, even when obtaining additional doses for the same patient.
5. Use single-dose vials for parenteral medications when possible.
6. Do not use single-dose (single-use) medication vials, ampules, and bags or bottles of intravenous solution for more than one patient.
7. Do not combine the leftover contents of single-use vials for later use.
8. The following apply if multidose vials are used:
   ■ Dedicate multidose vials to a single patient whenever possible.
   ■ If multidose vials will be used for more than one patient, they should be restricted to a centralized medication area and should not enter the immediate patient treatment area (e.g., dental operatory) to prevent inadvertent contamination.
   ■ If a multidose vial enters the immediate patient treatment area, it should be dedicated for single-patient use and discarded immediately after use.
   ■ Date multidose vials when first opened and discard within 28 days, unless the manufacturer specifies a shorter or longer date for that opened vial.
9. Do not use fluid infusion or administration sets (e.g., IV bags, tubings, connections) for more than one patient.

Note on Administering Local Dental Anaesthesia: When using a dental cartridge syringe to administer local anaesthesia, do not use the needle or aesthetic cartridge for more than one patient. Ensure that the dental cartridge syringe is appropriately cleaned and heat sterilized before use on another patient.

(From Centers for Disease Control and Prevention. (2018). *Summary of infection prevention practices in dental settings.* https://www.cdc.gov/oralhealth/infectioncontrol/summary-infection-prevention-practices/standard-precautions.html)

to revert to a virulent form that can rarely cause paralytic disease. This rare event is called **vaccine-associated paralytic polio** (VAPP). In countries that are deemed free of indigenous polio, and with health systems capable of delivering almost universal vaccine coverage, the use of IPV for routine immunization is favoured as this avoids the risk of infection from VAPP strains. However, WHO recommends that OPV should remain the vaccine of choice for routine infant immunization in most countries.

Indications. All infants, after 6 weeks with OPV-based schedules and 8 weeks with IPV-based schedules, but the exact programmes are country specific.

Administration. The polio vaccine is only given as part of combined products injected IM in the UK. The appropriate vaccine for each age group is determined also by the need to protect individuals against tetanus, pertussis, Hib and diphtheria. Td/IPV can be used as an occupational vaccine or as a booster to protect against polio in adults.

The objective of the primary immunization programme is to provide a minimum of five doses of a polio-containing vaccine at appropriate intervals for all individuals. In most circumstances, a total of five doses of vaccine at the appropriate intervals are considered to give satisfactory long-term protection.

Protection. Excellent for both vaccines.

Measles–Mumps–Rubella Vaccine

Organism. Live-attenuated strains of measles, mumps and rubella viruses.

Indications. All children in the second year of life, to prevent complications of common childhood fevers, such as respiratory tract infection and encephalitis associated with measles, meningitis associated with mumps and congenital infections associated with rubella. The last is especially relevant for women of child-bearing age working in dentistry. Therefore MMR is offered as an occupational vaccine to nonimmune members of the dental team of both sexes.

Administration. Two doses by the IM route.

Protection. Good.

Varicella

Organism. Contains live attenuated varicella zoster virus (VZV) strains. **Shingles** (herpes zoster) is caused by the reactivation of a latent VZV infection, resulting in a painful, vesicular skin rash, which may occur many years after the primary infection with chickenpox. The VZV vesicles contain virus and are infectious.

Following primary VZV infection, the virus enters the sensory nerves and travels along the nerve to the sensory dorsal root ganglia and establishes a permanent latent infection (Chapters 4 and 21). The risk and severity of shingles increase markedly with age and are associated with very painful **post-herpetic neuralgia,** which can be difficult to manage successfully. Furthermore, **chickenpox** can cause severe maternal disease, and 10–20% of pregnant women infected later in pregnancy may develop **varicella**

pneumonia, which can be fatal. For these reasons varicella vaccine is universally recommended.

Indications. Vaccine is used as a childhood vaccine, occupational vaccine to prevent the primary disease chickenpox and prophylactically to prevent recurrence of shingles in the elderly greater than 70 years of age. When used as an occupational vaccine in health care professionals, evidence of natural immunity should be tested serologically and vaccination provided only to the nonimmune health care workers.

Administration. Immunization comprises two doses of the live attenuated vaccine 4–8 weeks apart. Varicella vaccine is contraindicated in pregnancy and, as a precaution, pregnancy should be avoided for 1 month following the last dose of varicella vaccine. Different strength vaccines are used for primary immunization and vaccination of the elderly due to waning immunity and vaccine response in older people.

Protection. Good.

Triple Vaccine: Diphtheria–Tetanus–Pertussis

Organism. Three-in-one vaccine for prevention against diphtheria caused by *Corynebacterium diphtheriae*, whooping cough caused by *Bordetella pertussis* and tetanus caused by *Clostridium tetani*. Contains killed *Bordetella pertussis* and diphtheria and tetanus toxoid.

Indications. All infants and as an occupational vaccine in the US.

Administration. Three spaced doses by injection; subsequent booster doses of diphtheria and tetanus toxoids only.

Protection. Effective, but booster doses of tetanus and diphtheria are required to maintain immunity.

Tetanus Toxoid

Organism. Contains the toxin of *Clostridium tetani* that has been formol treated.

Indications. Active immunization of the entire population. Although the disease is rare, tetanus can develop after very trivial wounds.

Administration. Three spaced injections in infancy, as a component of the triple vaccine. Booster doses at 5 years and in the event of injury.

Protection. Excellent.

Hepatitis B Vaccine

Organism. Contains the hepatitis B surface antigen (HBsAg; see Chapter 29), manufactured in yeasts by genetic recombination and absorbed on to aluminium salt. Successful vaccination also offers protection against delta hepatitis (hepatitis D).

Indications

All health care workers who are at special risk, including dentists, dental hygienists, dental surgery assistants, medical laboratory workers and those handling blood products. Currently, to prevent early childhood hepatitis B (HBV) infection and to eventually protect adolescents and adults from infection, the WHO recommends universal administration at birth to newborns with hepatitis B. This approach has been adopted in the US, many countries in Europe and in Southeast Asian countries where the disease is endemic, with the aim of eradicating the disease worldwide. Chronically infected persons are at increased lifetime risk for cirrhosis and hepatocellular carcinoma (HCC) and also serve as the main reservoir for continued HBV transmission.

Administration. Three doses (two doses at an interval of 1 month, followed by a third 6 months later) IM in the deltoid.

Protection. Approximately 10–15% of adults fail to respond to three doses of vaccine or respond poorly. Poor responses are mostly associated with individuals over age 40, obesity, smoking and advanced liver disease. If antibody levels are suboptimal, then a fourth (booster) dose may be given. Nonresponders to the vaccine are tested for markers of current or past infection with HBV in order to exclude asymptomatic carriers.

Individuals having the initial course of vaccination should undergo pre- and postimmunization tests, and those who fail to seroconvert should be followed up as appropriate.

Vaccine protection is very good, offering approximately 95% protection. There is controversy over the necessity of reinforcing booster doses. Some authorities in the UK advocate boosters after 5 years, whereas others, especially in the US, contend that booster doses are unnecessary because of the anamnestic response of the immune system.

Passive Immunization with Hepatitis B Immunoglobulin. Passive immunization with hepatitis B immunoglobulin (HBIG) should be instituted within 48 h if an unprotected health care worker sustains an accident with blood or saliva containing hepatitis B antigens. This should be followed by a complete course of the hepatitis B vaccine, the first dose of which may be administered immediately or within 7 days of the accident. If the person declines the vaccine, then a second dose of HBIG should be administered 1 month after the first dose.

Influenza Vaccine

Organism. Three types are currently available: live attenuated, inactivated or recombinant influenza vaccines. These are derived from different influenza viruses that are prevalent in the specific geographic region (e.g., northern or southern hemisphere). The quadrivalent flu vaccines are currently the most common in the West. They are so named because they protect against four different flu viruses, two influenza A viruses and two influenza B viruses. It is important to recognize, because of the phenomenon of antigenic 'drift' and 'shift' seen in influenza viruses, that the vaccine composition needs to be reviewed and altered each year, which is a formidable task.

Indications

In recent years the indications for influenza vaccination have widened from elderly individuals, those people living in residential facilities or long-stay hospitals, to include pregnant women, infants and people with underlying health conditions such as respiratory or cardiac disease, chronic neurological conditions or immunosuppression. All these groups are prone to develop a range of more serious respiratory infections with influenza. Influenza during pregnancy may also be associated with perinatal mortality, prematurity, smaller neonatal size and lower birth weight. In many countries, seasonal influenza vaccination is recommended for frontline health care workers, including dental health care workers (DHCWs).

Administration

One dose by injection, repeated each winter, which is the usual period of outbreak.

Protection

Relatively short (approximately a year).

COVID-19 Vaccine

Organism. SARS-CoV-2 and variants such as the currently prevalent Omicron variant or its derivatives are the active ingredients of COVID-19 vaccine (see Chapter 10; Fig. 10.11).

The **bivalent COVID-19 vaccine** has two genetic (mRNA) components: (1) the original strain of the virus that broadly confers protection against the disease and (2) the other corresponding to Omicron variants BA.4 and BA.5 that are descendants (lineages) from the parental Omicron variant.

Other vaccine delivery modes that are likely to be available in the immediate future are **nasal spray vaccines** and **oral vaccines** currently undergoing trials. They should prove popular as injections are not required.

Indications

In the US the COVID-19 Treatment Guidelines Panel recommends COVID-19 vaccination as soon as possible for everyone who is eligible, such as those with chronic diseases and elderly, as well as front-line health care workers, including dentists. A primary series of COVID-19 vaccinations is recommended for everyone aged ≥6 months in the US.

Administration

The primary vaccine series of COVID-19 comprises three doses (two doses at an interval of 1 month, followed by a third 6 months later) depending on the vaccine type. Vaccination is IM in the deltoid. Booster doses are indicated for vulnerable populations and DHCWs.

The boosters are indicated 4 or more months after the primary series of COVID-19 vaccines. The latter guidance was current at the time of this writing but is highly likely to change in the future, depending on the disease prevalence and endemicity of the virus in different regions of the world. The type and dose of vaccine and the timing of such additional booster doses depend on the recipient's age and underlying medical conditions. DCWs are urged to keep abreast of these vaccine requirements by referral to local guidelines as and when necessary.

OCCUPATIONALLY ACQUIRED INFECTIONS

Health care workers routinely run the risk of acquiring infections by virtue of their profession: so-called 'occupationally acquired infections'. Particular concerns for health care workers are blood-borne viral infections, including hepatitis B and C, and human immunodeficiency virus (HIV) infection. Hepatitis B infection used to be about 10 times more common among DCWs than among the public, but with the advent of the extremely effective hepatitis B vaccine, this danger is now minimal. The average risks of transmission of these diseases after exposure to blood are:

- 0.3% for percutaneous exposure to HIV-infected blood
- 0.1% for mucocutaneous exposure to HIV-infected blood
- 0.5–1.8% for percutaneous exposure to hepatitis C virus (HCV)–infected blood with detectable RNA
- 6.0% for hepatitis B of a nonimmune individual to an HBsAg-positive source
- 30% for percutaneous exposure of a nonimmune individual to a hepatitis B 'e' antigen (HBeAg)-positive source.

(*Note:* Hepatitis B is most infectious, and the least infectious in this context is HIV.)

Other than viral infections, rarely bacterial infections such as tuberculosis and legionella infections may be acquired by exposed DCWs.

Additionally, it should be noted that certain features of a percutaneous injury carry a particularly high risk of infection transmission, as follows:

- a deep injury
- terminal HIV-related illness in the source patient
- visible blood on the device that caused the injury
- injury with a needle that had been placed in a source patient's artery or vein.

When considering the source patient, the risk is higher than average in people who are:

- from countries where the condition is endemic
- have had multiple blood transfusions
- dialysis patients
- intravenous drug users.

Key Facts

- The policy of **standard infection control** or standard precautions, which assumes that **ALL** patients are potential carriers of infectious diseases and all body fluids except for sweat are potentially infectious, should be the norm in dental practice.
- The main features in a **comprehensive infection control protocol** are patient evaluation, personal protection, instrument cleaning, sterilization and storage, use of disposables, cleaning and disinfection of surfaces, laboratory asepsis, and disposal of waste and staff training, including continuing education.
- **Personal protection** should incorporate appropriate clinic clothing, personal hygiene, barrier protection (gloves, eye shield, face masks, rubber dam isolation) and immunization procedures.
- As far as possible, a **rubber dam** should be used in operative procedures to minimize saliva/blood-contaminated aerosol production.

- Use of efficient high-speed **aspirators** will minimize cross-infection from aerosols.
- To avoid sharps injuries, be conversant with all **sharps handling procedures**, which should be an integral part of staff education.
- Have a **written policy on the vaccination** of all staff, and maintain a confidential, up-to-date immunization record for all staff members.
- The threat of COVID-19 appears to be receding worldwide. Nevertheless DCWs have a duty of care to keep abreast of the current disease prevalence data in the jurisdictions where they practice and to take all necessary measures to mitigate SARS-CoV-2 transmission, such as implementing transmission-based precautions and booster vaccinations as dictated by their local professional organizations.

Review Questions (Answers on p. 392)

Please indicate which answers are true and which are false.

37.1. Which of the following procedures can be regarded as optimal for controlling cross-infection in a dental clinic?
   a. wearing a single face mask for 3 h
   b. wearing headgear for all operational procedures
   c. washing gloves and reusing them after visual examination of a patient
   d. wearing gloves after removal of all hand jewellery
   e. changing clinic attire once in 3 days

37.2. Which of the following vaccines would you recommend to a dental surgery assistant who is starting to work with you?
   a. hepatitis A
   b. measles–mumps–rubella (MMR)
   c. hepatitis B immunoglobulin
   d. tetanus toxoid
   e. flu vaccine

37.3. You treat a human immunodeficiency virus (HIV)–infected patient in your surgery. Your dental surgery assistant sustains a needle-stick injury while attempting to resheath the needle used for local anaesthetic of this patient. You will:
   a. blame the dental surgery assistant for resheathing the needle
   b. wash the puncture site thoroughly with soap, warm water and a disinfectant
   c. review the infection control procedures that led to this situation
   d. review the patient's medical history to check their hepatitis B status
   e. record in detail the circumstances of the injury

37.4. The following infectious agents are likely to be transmitted in dental care settings:
   a. hepatitis G
   b. *Streptococcus pyogenes*
   c. *Candida albicans*
   d. hepatitis C
   e. influenza

Further Reading

Beltrami, E. M., Williams, I. T., Shapiro, C. N., et al. (2000). Risk and management of blood-borne infections in health care workers. *Clinical Microbiology Reviews, 13,* 385–407.

Centers for Disease Control and Prevention (CDC). (2023). *Infection prevention & control in dental settings.* CDC, US Department of Health and Human Services. https://www.cdc.gov/oralhealth/infectioncontrol/index.html.

Coia, J. E., Ritchie, L., Adisesh, A., et al. (2013). Guidance on the use of respiratory and facial protection equipment. *Journal of Hospital Infection, 85,* 170–182.

Loveday, H. P., Wilson, J. A., Pratta, R. J., et al. (2014). Epic3: National evidence-based guidelines for preventing healthcare-associated infections in NHS hospitals in England. *Journal of Hospital Infection, 86S1,* S1–S70.

Pankhurst, C. L., & Coulter, W. A. (2017). *Basic guide to infection prevention and control* (2nd ed.). Wiley-Blackwell.

Public Health England. (2021). *Immunisation against infectious disease – The green book* (3rd ed.). https://www.gov.uk/government/collections/immunisation-against-infectious-disease-the-green-book.

Samaranayake, L. P., Scheutz, F., & Cottone, J. (1991). *Infection control for the dental team.* Munksgaard.

Samaranayake, L., & Scully, C. (2013). Needlestick and occupational exposure to infections: A compendium of current guidelines. *British Dental Journal, 215,* 163–166.

Sax, H., Allegranzi, B., Larson, E., et al. (2007). My five moments for hand hygiene: A user-centered design approach to understand, train, monitor and report hand hygiene. *Journal of Hospital Infection, 67,* 9–21.

38 Standard Infection Control Procedures in Dentistry Part II: Sterilization, Disinfection and Antisepsis, with a Summary of Transmission-Based Infection Control Procedures

Chapter 37 outlined the key principles involved in personal protection of the dental health care worker (DHCW) such as personal protective equipment (PPE), how to avoid sharps injuries in the clinic, the protocol and strategic planning related to injuries so sustained and the vaccines that are important for DHCWs. This chapter, a continuum of standard infection controls, outlines sterilization, disinfection and antisepsis as applied in dentistry. In addition, the final subsection of the chapter outlines the transmission based precautions in dentistry that should be implemented in special circumstances. These are all equally important aspects of infection control for all involved in the practice of clinical dentistry.

Sterilization, Disinfection and Antisepsis

The reader should clearly bear in mind the following basic definitions of sterilization, disinfection and antisepsis as these terms are frequently used in clinical dentistry.

- **Sterilization** is a process that kills or removes all organisms (and their spores) in a material or an object.
- **Disinfection** is a process that kills or removes pathogenic organisms in a material or an object, **excluding bacterial spores**, so that they pose no threat of infection.
- **Antisepsis** is the application of a chemical agent externally on a live surface (skin or mucosa) to destroy organisms or to inhibit their growth. Thus all antiseptics could be used as disinfectants, but all disinfectants cannot be used as antiseptics because of toxicity.

In general, sterilization involves extensive treatment of equipment and materials, and it is costly and labor intensive. It is dependent on:

- knowledge of the death curves of bacteria or spores when they are exposed to the inactivation process; spores vary in their resistance to sterilizing agents: spores of *Bacillus stearothermophilus* are used to test the efficacy of steam autoclaves and unsaturated chemical vapour, and *Bacillus subtilis* spores are used to test the efficacy of dry heat and ethylene oxide sterilization
- the penetrating ability of the inactivating agent: steam penetrates more effectively than dry heat
- the ability of the article to withstand the sterilizing process, with no appreciable damage to instruments and other materials (e.g., corrosion of sharp, cutting edges of instruments)
- a procedure that is simple but efficient and relatively quick (so that there is a readily available supply of sterile instruments and materials); thus, the temperature of sterilization is of crucial importance, as is the period for which the instrument or material is held at a given temperature—both of these factors dictate the efficacy of the chosen sterilization method
- the effects of organic matter, such as saliva and blood, which enhance the survival of bacteria and interfere with the sterilization process; all articles must be clean before sterilization.

All instruments and appliances used in dentistry should ideally be **sterilized**, although some items of equipment and certain surfaces (e.g., bracket tables attached to the dental chair) do pose problems. In such circumstances, the best alternative is to **disinfect** the items or surfaces concerned. In some instances, hard to decontaminate dental equipment can be replaced with equivalent single-use devices. Single-use devices are labelled by the manufacturer for only a single use and therefore do not have reprocessing instructions. Use single-use devices for one patient only and dispose of appropriately.

Decontamination

Decontamination (*syn.* reprocessing) is the process by which **reusable items are rendered safe** for further use and for staff to handle. Decontamination is required to minimize the risk of cross-infection between patients and between patients and staff. The term 'decontamination' (as opposed to 'sterilization' and 'disinfection') has gained popularity particularly in European regions and is less widely used in North America. Decontamination is a complex and an exacting process and entails:

- cleaning
- disinfection
- sterilization (Fig. 38.1A).

Decontamination of Instruments

RECEIVING, CLEANING AND DECONTAMINATION

The removal of contaminated instruments and equipment from the treatment area should follow a set routine, avoiding cross-contamination between the soiled and sterilized instruments. Once an effective method of instrument or equipment flow has been worked out, one should adhere strictly to this method.

Reusable instruments, supplies and equipment should be **received, sorted, cleaned** and **decontaminated**, in that particular order, in a dedicated section of the **processing area**. Cleaning should precede all disinfection and sterilization processes and should involve removal of debris as well as organic and inorganic contamination.

Removal of debris and contamination is achieved either by:

- cleaning using a thermal **washer disinfector** (most preferred method)
- manual cleaning combined with ultrasonic cleaning
- manual cleaning (the least preferred)

If visible debris, whether inorganic or organic matter, is not removed, it will interfere with microbial inactivation and can compromise the disinfection or sterilization process. After cleaning, instruments should be rinsed with water to remove chemical or detergent residue.

Considerations in selecting cleaning methods and equipment include:

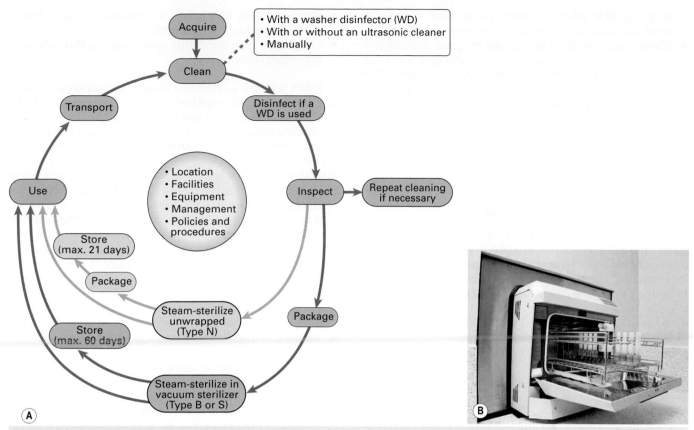

Fig. 38.1 (A) A diagram showing the instrument decontamination cycle. (B) A thermal washer disinfector. ((A) From National Health Service. (2021). (HTM 01–05) *Decontamination in primary care dental practices.* https://www.england.nhs.uk/publication/decontamination-in-primary-care-dental-practices-htm-01-05, with permission; Crown Copyright.)

- **efficacy** of the method, process and equipment
- **compatibility** with items to be cleaned
- **occupational health** and exposure risks.

Note that the use of automated cleaning equipment such as an **ultrasonic cleaner** or thermal **washer disinfector** does not require presoaking or scrubbing of instruments. These instruments therefore:

- increase cleaning efficacy and productivity
- reduce danger of aerosolization of infectious particles
- reduce incidence of sharps injuries and are hence safer
- reduce manual labour.

PRESTERILIZATION CLEANING

Whenever possible, cleaning should be performed using an automated and validated process in preference to manual cleaning. Manual cleaning should only be considered where manufacturer's instructions specify that the device is not compatible with automated processing. Heavy-duty household utility gloves must be used when cleaning instruments; plastic aprons, eye protection and face masks are also desirable. Instruments should be cleaned as soon as possible after use. If immediate cleaning is not feasible, placing instruments in a puncture-resistant container and soaking them with detergent, a disinfectant/detergent or an enzymatic cleaner will prevent drying of patient material

and make cleaning easier and less time consuming. Use of a liquid chemical sterilant/high-level disinfectant (e.g., glutaraldehyde) as a holding solution is not recommended.

Reusable dental hand instruments with a sharp or cutting edge should be handled with extreme care during scrubbing to prevent hand injury. Dental cements on instruments should be removed in the surgery before setting solid. Uncapped needles should never be left on the instrument tray, and after use these and other single-use disposable sharps should be placed directly in puncture-resistant containers.

AUTOMATED CLEANING USING WASHER DISINFECTORS

A thermal washer disinfector (Fig. 38.1B) is the preferred method for cleaning dental instruments as it offers the best option for the control and reproducibility of cleaning; a typical thermal washer disinfector cycle for instruments includes the following five stages:

- **Flush**—removes gross contamination, including blood, tissue and solid debris, bone fragments and other fluids. A water temperature of less than 45°C is used to prevent protein coagulation and fixing of soil to the instrument.
- **Wash**—removes any remaining soil. Mechanical and chemical processes loosen and break up contamination adhering to the instrument surface. Detergents should

be compatible with the instruments used in order to avoid discolouration, staining, corrosion and pitting.

- **Rinse**—removes detergent used during the cleaning process. This stage can contain several substages. The quality of water used is important as otherwise it may lead to long-term problems such as spotting of instruments.
- **Thermal disinfection**—the temperature of the load is raised and held at the preset disinfection temperature for the required disinfection holding time: for example 80°C for 10 min or 90°C for 1 min.
- **Drying**—purges the load and chamber with heated air to remove residual moisture.

PREPARATION AND PACKAGING

In a separate section of the processing area, cleaned instruments and other supplies should be **inspected**; **assembled** into sets or trays; and **wrapped**, **packaged** or placed into container systems as appropriate for sterilization. Instruments used in dentistry may be packaged for sterilization using:

- an open-tray system sealed with a see-through sterilization bag
- perforated trays with fitted covers wrapped with sterilization paper
- individual packaging in commercially available sterilization bags.

Prior to packaging, all hinged instruments should be opened and unlocked. An **internal chemical indicator** should be placed in every package. In addition, an external **chemical indicator** (e.g., chemical indicator tape) should be used when the internal indicator cannot be seen from outside the package. For unwrapped loads, at a minimum, an internal chemical indicator should be placed in the tray or cassette with items to be sterilized. Dental practices should refer to the manufacturer's instructions regarding use and correct placement of chemical indicators. Critical and semicritical instruments that will be stored should be wrapped or placed in containers (e.g., cassettes or organizing trays) designed to maintain sterility during storage.

Sterilization

THE STERILIZATION PROCESS

In dentistry, sterilization is usually achieved by moist heat using steam under pressure in an autoclave.

Other sterilization methods, not used in dentistry, are ethylene oxide gas and gamma-irradiation (employed by commercial suppliers of plastic goods) and filtration (used for sterilization of injectable drugs). Hot air ovens and chemiclaves were once popular in dentistry, but they are no longer used or recommended due to quality control and environmental issues.

MOIST HEAT STERILIZATION (STEAM UNDER PRESSURE)

Steam under pressure is a very effective sterilizing agent as it:

- liberates latent heat when it condenses to form water, potentiating microbicidal activity
- contracts in volume during condensation, thus reinforcing penetration.

When water is heated in a closed environment, its boiling point is raised, together with the temperature of the generated steam—for example, at 104 kPa (15 psi), the steam temperature is 121°C. This phenomenon is utilized in steam sterilization by the **autoclave** (Fig. 38.2). Put simply, an autoclave is a glorified domestic pressure cooker with a double-walled or jacketed chamber; steam circulates under high pressure inside the chamber, in which the objects for sterilization (the **load**) have been placed. Once the sterilization cycle is complete, drying the load is accomplished by evacuating the steam. Drying can be accelerated by the suction of warm, filtered air into and through the chamber. It is important to expel the air in the chamber at the beginning of a sterilization cycle because:

- the temperature of an air–steam mixture at a given pressure is lower than that of pure steam
- air pockets interfere with steam penetration.

There are two types of autoclaves:

1. **Vacuum autoclaves** in which air is evacuated from a metal chamber by vacuum pump are now becoming popular in dentistry due to wide availability of small, bench-top units. In central sterile supply units in hospitals, they are sometimes referred to as 'porous load autoclaves'. These vacuum autoclaves are more desirable for routine dentistry than the gravity displacement type for the sterilization of hollow devices such as dental handpieces.
2. **Gravity displacement autoclaves** are small, automatic benchtop autoclaves. They work on the principle of downward displacement of air as a consequence of steam entering at the top of the chamber.

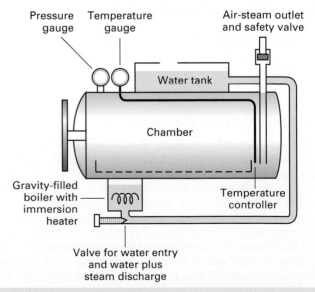

Fig. 38.2 Principal features of a small autoclave used in dentistry.

In general, a sterilization cycle with a holding period of 134°C for 3–4 min at 207 kPa is recommended for both **wrapped and unwrapped dental instruments**. The temperature and heating/holding/cooling periods are set as default settings, especially the benchtop steam autoclaves manufactured for dental use.

AUTOCLAVES USED IN DENTISTRY

Three different types of autoclaves are used in dentistry; these are categorized into three classes (or types): classes B, S and N.

- **Class B** —These are the most advanced type of autoclave, and most commonly used in dentistry. They incorporate a **vacuum stage** and are designed to reprocess load types such as hollow, air-retentive and packaged loads. A number of different cycles may be provided. Each cycle should be fully validated and used in accordance with instructions provided by both the sterilizer manufacturer and the instrument manufacturer(s).
- **Class S** —These sterilizers are specially designed to reprocess specific load types and are an intermediate type, between Class B and N autoclaves (see below). The manufacturer of the sterilizer will define exactly which load, or instrument, types are compatible, and the equipment should be used strictly in accordance with these instructions. Autoclaves of this class have a vacuum pump, enabling total air removal from the chamber before starting the sterilization process. However, only a single-stage prevacuum is used here; it is less effective than the vacuum used in class B autoclaves.
- **Class N** —This is the lowest-class device and can be used only as an auxiliary unit or a stand-by device. The sterilization process here is different as it does not have a vacuum pump (which is present in class B and class S autoclaves), and hence can only sterilise instruments with a solid structure (not bore type, hollow instruments). Class N sterilisers also do not have an effective drying option, unlike more advanced autoclaves.

THE STERILIZATION CYCLE

The sterilization cycle can be divided into three periods (Fig. 38.3): the **heating-up period**, the **holding period** and the **cooling period**. For the N-type nonvacuum benchtop autoclave (routinely used in dentistry), this entails:

1. removal of air by a vacuum pump or downward displacement of air by incoming steam while the chamber is heated to the selected temperature
2. 'holding' the load, which is sterilized, for the appropriate period at the selected temperature and pressure
3. drying the load to its original condition by a partial vacuum (this is assisted by the heat from the jacket)
4. restoration of the chamber to atmospheric pressure by rapid exhaustion of steam.

NOTES ON THE PROPER USE OF BENCHTOP AUTOCLAVES

- Autoclaves should not be overloaded with instruments.

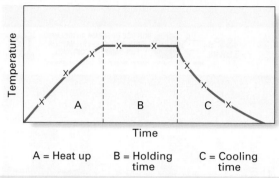

Fig. 38.3 The stages of a full sterilization cycle. (A) Heat up. (B) Holding time. (C) Cooling time.

- The water reservoir should be filled at the start of the day with water that is fresh distilled or put through reverse osmosis to prevent buildup of residues or lubricant. Do not use tap water, which can lead to biofilm formation in the reservoir and accumulation of lime scale. Sterilizers are designed either with an automated single-use water cycle and drainage or with a water reservoir that should be drained manually at the end of the day with the reservoir cleaned with fresh purified water and left to dry overnight.
- Autoclaves should be validated and serviced annually, and a logbook of daily process monitoring, validation, autoclave maintenance and defects should be kept (in the UK, these records must be maintained for a minimum of 2 years).
- The mechanical indicators of the autoclave (temperature, pressure and holding time) should be monitored routinely at the start of the day and the results recorded in the machine log book as part of the practice's quality control procedures.
- When using a vacuum autoclave, a drying cycle should be used for bagged instruments.

MONITORING STERILIZATION

Achievement of the requisite temperature and pressure, as indicated by the gauges of the autoclave (or any other sterilizer), does not guarantee that the entire load has been sterilized. All sterilization procedures must therefore be carefully and regularly monitored so that failures are detected and sterility is ensured. The indicators used for checking sterility are (Fig. 38.4):

- **Process monitoring:** using mechanical indicators (i.e., the temperature, holding time and pressure gauges of the autoclave)
- **Chemical indicators:** colour-changing solutions or paper cards, paper strips, adhesive tape
- **Biological indicators/monitors.**

Chemical indicators: These are materials (either liquid or paper) that irreversibly change colour on exposure to the appropriate sterilization cycle, indicating that the load has been processed. They are manufactured as colour-changing solutions or paper cards/strips, or adhesive tape (Fig. 38.4).

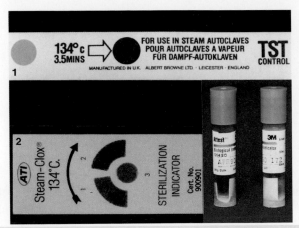

Fig. 38.4 Chemical indicators (1, 2) and a biological indicator (3) used for autoclave monitoring.

The colour change of the solution/paper occurs after exposure to normal autoclave operating temperatures of 121°C at 15 psi. Note that **there is no time factor** that causes this colour change. Chemical indicators provide a **quick visual reference** for heat penetration inside the load. They are usually positioned near the centre of each load, and toward the bottom front of the autoclave.

Chemical tape indicators: As opposed to chemical indicators that could be placed inside a load, these are adhesive-backed paper tape or sterilization pouches on which the chemically treated areas darken upon reaching a specified temperature to form dark diagonal lines and may display words, such as 'sterile' or 'autoclaved'. These markings only appear when the tape indicator has been exposed to even a few minutes (i.e., even before the specified holding period is reached) to standard autoclave temperatures.

Tape indicators should be used on all material decontaminated by autoclaving to show that the material has been processed. A 3- to 4-inch strip of autoclave tape placed on the outside of the autoclave pan, bag or individual container is sufficient. If the temperature-sensitive tape undergoes no colour change (i.e., does not indicate that the desired temperature was reached during the sterilization process), the load is not considered decontaminated and needs to be reprocessed.

Note that process indicators **do not prove** sterilization but merely verify that the items have been subjected to the processing conditions; thus, the main function of a process indicator is to ensure the operator that the material has gone through a sterilization cycle. At least one process indicator should be cycled with every sterilization load, and the results should be documented in a sterility control file.

Biological indicators/monitors: In contrast to process indicators, these are designed to **prove** that sterilization conditions have been reached (i.e., both the time and temperature requirement). The indicators used for this purpose are bacterial spores (e.g., *Bacillus stearothermophilius*), which require high temperatures for extended periods to lose their viability (the corollary is that if the spores are killed, then less-resistant microbes are killed more readily, and sterility is achieved).

Biological monitoring or **spore tests** (Fig. 38.4): These tests are usually contained in a vacuum-sealed

vial and should be used on a **weekly basis** in dentistry. The monitor should be placed in the sterilizer at a point where sterilization is most difficult to achieve (e.g., commonly on the bottom shelf of the autoclave near the drain). After cycling, each vial with the indicator organism should be sent for culture or cultured in the clinic according to the manufacturer's instructions. The results of biological monitoring should be routinely recorded and kept in a **sterility control file**. Spore tests should also be done (a) when commissioning a new autoclave, (b) after servicing or repairs and (c) as part of the training of new staff.

QUALITY CONTROL OF SMALL BENCHTOP AUTOCLAVES

Small autoclaves should be operated to ensure that they are:

- compliant with the local safety requirements, as well as the manufacturer's instructions
- installed, commissioned, validated, maintained and operated appropriately in compliance with the manufacturer's instructions.

DAILY TESTS OF SMALL AUTOCLAVES

The daily tests should be performed by the user and will normally consist of:

- a warmup cycle before instruments can be processed (for some autoclaves)
- a steam penetration test—Helix or Bowie–Dick (vacuum sterilizers only)
- an automatic control test according to manufacturers' instructions
- the above outcomes should be recorded in the logbook together with the date and signature of the operator.

The Bowie–Dick or Helix test is used in vacuum autoclaves to check the steam penetration into the centre of the autoclave load and to signal the presence of any air pockets.

STORAGE AND CARE OF STERILE INSTRUMENTS/ DEVICES

Once sterilized, the instruments or devices should be maintained in a sterile state until they are used again. The proper storage of sterile instruments is therefore as important as the sterilization process itself; improper storage would break the **'chain of sterility'** and introduce the possibility of **pathogenic recolonization risk**. A barrier(s) should be maintained between the instruments and the general practice environment. The following guidelines should be followed in storing sterile instruments/devices:

- Maintain rigorous records to identify all instruments, packs and their contents, and their storage times.
- Use a 'first-in first-out principle' when removing instruments from storage areas.
- Store sterilized instruments in purpose-built storage cabinets that can be easily cleaned.

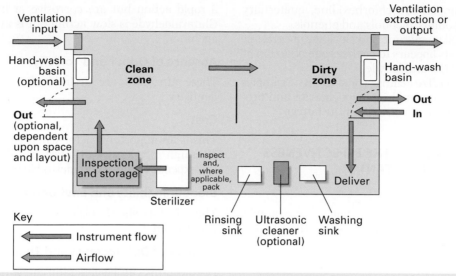

Fig. 38.5   Example layout for a single decontamination room. (*Principle:* No clean material in dirty zones and no dirty material in clean zones.) ((A) From National Health Service. (2021). (HTM 01–05) *Decontamination in primary care dental practices.* https://www.england.nhs.uk/publication/decontamination-in-primary-care-dental-practices-htm-01-05, with permission; Crown Copyright.)

- The instrument storage area should be dedicated for that purpose and situated ideally in the clean area of the decontamination room (Fig. 38.5).
- Instruments should be stored above floor level away from direct sunlight and water in a secure, dry and cool environment.
- Appropriately coded labels should be used to indicate the contents, cycle number and expiration dates on packs that are nontransparent.
- Before using the stored instruments, check them to ensure that the packaging is intact and dry.
- Do not reuse wrapped instruments stored for more than 1 year from the date of sterilization. These have to be cleaned and resterilized (Fig. 38.1).

Disinfection

Methods of disinfection consist of:

- heat (pasteurization; boiling in water)
- physical methods (ultrasonics)
- chemical methods.

DISINFECTION BY HEAT

Pasteurization

Pasteurization is named after Louis Pasteur's discovery that mild heating prevents the spoilage of wine by selective killing of unwanted microbes. A similar treatment is now applied to milk to delay souring due to microbial activity. Milk is raised to a temperature of either 63°C –66°C for 30 min or (in the flash method) to 72°C for 15 s. This procedure renders the milk safe from contamination with *Mycobacterium tuberculosis*, *Campylobacter* spp. and other pathogens. It should be noted that pasteurization is not a sterilization process.

Boiling Water

If the boiling period is short, bacterial spores can survive; boiling water is therefore inadequate for sterilization of dental instruments.

DISINFECTION BY PHYSICAL METHODS: ULTRASONICS

Ultrasound is an effective way of disrupting microbial cell membranes and is used for removing debris before autoclaving. The ultrasonic bath generates high-frequency sound waves that create alternating regions of high and low pressure within the bath. The bath is filled with a detergent or enzymic solution, and the sound waves produce bubbles in the detergent under low pressure that implode when the pressure changes from low to high, thereby dislodging debris adhering to the instrument. Ultrasonic baths are particularly useful when cleaning complex, hinged or serrated devices.

DISINFECTION BY CHEMICAL METHODS

Choosing a chemical disinfectant should be done carefully because a disinfectant used for one purpose may not be equally effective for another. Further, the antimicrobial activity of a chemical disinfectant falls drastically in the presence of organic debris. Products that usually disinfect items or surfaces may not do so when there is heavy contamination, particularly with resistant microbes in large numbers. The residual levels of organisms following disinfection may still represent an infection risk to unusually susceptible patients.

Mode of Action of Chemical Disinfectants

The chemicals used as disinfectants generally behave as 'protoplasmic poisons' in three different ways:

1. Membrane-active disinfectants **damage the bacterial cell membrane** with resultant egress of the cell

constituents; examples are chlorhexidine, quaternary ammonium compounds, alcohols and phenols.

2. **Fixation** of the cell membrane and blockage of egress of cellular components appears to be the mode of action of formaldehyde and glutaraldehyde.

3. Oxidizing agents **oxidize** cellular constituents; examples are halide disinfectants such as hypochlorite and bromides (the former is more active than the latter).

CONDITIONS DETERMINING THE EFFECTIVENESS AND CHOICE OF A DISINFECTANT

Spectrum of Activity

Disinfectants vary widely in their activity—for example, some are more active against Gram-positive than Gram-negative bacteria (Table 38.1).

Satisfactory Contact

All contaminated surfaces should come into contact with the disinfectant for the specified period. Organic debris, air and greasy material may prevent this, hence the importance of thorough cleaning of the material or instrument before disinfection.

Concentration

Adequate concentration of disinfectants is essential, and they should always be accurately dispensed. It is important to use the manufacturer's stated dilution of the disinfectant.

pH

The activity of a disinfectant is often dependent on pH (e.g., glutaraldehydes act only at alkaline pH, whereas phenols work best at acid pH).

Neutralization

A wide range of substances, including blood and saliva, hard water, soaps and detergent, may neutralize the disinfectant.

Stability

Not all disinfectants are stable, especially when diluted, and may deteriorate with age or storage. Solutions should be freshly prepared for use and marked with an expiration date.

Speed of Action

In general, disinfectants act slowly, and their activity depends on the concentration used. Hypochlorites have a rapid action but are corrosive at high concentrations. Glutaraldehyde is slow acting but is an effective sporicidal agent.

Absence of Odour and Toxicity

These attributes are desirable for disinfectants used in dentistry.

Cost

This is an important factor when choosing a disinfectant, although inexpensive disinfectants should not be used at the expense of those with desirable properties.

Biodegradability and Environmental Impact

These factors should also be considered when choosing a disinfectant.

Potency of Disinfectants and Their Uses

Disinfectants can be generally categorized as having **high**, **intermediate** or **low potency**, depending on their ability to kill various groups of organisms:

- **High-level disinfectants** are active against Gram-positive and Gram-negative bacteria, spores and *Mycobacterium tuberculosis* (Table 38.1).
- **Intermediate-level disinfectants** destroy *Mycobacterium tuberculosis*, vegetative bacteria, most viruses and fungi, but few, if any, spores.
- **Low-level disinfectants** kill most bacteria and most fungi, but not *Mycobacterium tuberculosis* or spores.

A rough guide to the use of these three categories of disinfectants is given below.

Step 1

Categorize the items that require disinfection or sterilization into three groups (Table 38.2):

- **critical items**—those that penetrate the skin or mucosa and/or touch exposed tissues, including bone (e.g., surgical instruments and periodontal scalers and burs)
- **semicritical items**—those that come in contact with mucous membranes or nonintact skin, such as exposed skin that is abraded or has dermatitis (e.g., mouth mirrors, amalgam condensers)
- **noncritical items**—those that only come into contact with skin (e.g., radiograph head/cone, blood pressure cuff, facebow)

Table 38.1   Properties of Disinfectants Used in Dentistry

| Disinfectant | ACTIVITY AGAINST | | | | INACTIVATED BY | | |
	GPC	GNB	Spores	TB	Protein	Soap	Corrosive action
Glutaraldehyde	++	++	++	++	±	−	+
Chlorine compounds	++	++	++	+	++	−	++ or ±Θ
Iodophors	++	++	± or −	+	+	−	−
Phenolics	++	++	−	+	±	−	+ or ±
Alcohol (70%)	++	++	−	+	++	−	−
Chlorhexidine	++	+	−	−	+	++	−

GPC, Gram-positive cocci; GNB, Gram-negative bacilli; TB, tubercle bacilli; ++, high; +, moderate; ±, low; −, nil; Θ, buffered solutions.

Table 38.2   Categories of Patient-Care Items and How They Should Be Processed After Usage

Category	Definition	Process by	Examples
Critical	Penetrate soft tissue, contact bone, enter into or contact the blood stream, or other normally sterile tissue of the mouth	Sterilization	Surgical instruments, sealers, dental handpieces
Semicritical	Contact mucous membranes, but will not penetrate soft tissue, contact bone, enter into or contact the blood stream, or other normally sterile tissue of the mouth	Sterilization or use single-use items, or high-level disinfection	Dental mouth mirror, amalgam condenser, reusable dental impression trays
Noncritical	Contact with intact skin	Low- to intermediate-level disinfection	Blood pressure cuff, cuff stethoscope, pulse oximeter

Step 2

Use the appropriate technique (Table 38.2):

- steam sterilization for all critical items as they have the greatest risk of transmitting infection
- steam sterilization for heat tolerant semicritical items (e.g., dental handpieces); for heat-sensitive items replace with a heat-tolerant or disposable alternative. If there is no alternative, use a high-potency disinfectant
- intermediate (intermediate-level (i.e., tuberculocidal claim) or low-potency hospital disinfectants for noncritical items.

DISINFECTANT AND ANTISEPTIC AGENTS COMMONLY USED IN DENTISTRY

Alcohols

Ethyl alcohol or propyl alcohol (70%) in water is useful for skin antisepsis prior to cannulation, injection and surgical hand-scrubbing. Alcohol combined with disinfectants is used in dentistry for surface disinfection, but authorities in the US do not recommend alcohol for this purpose as it evaporates relatively quickly and leaves no residual effect. Other disadvantages are its flammability, limited sporicidal activity and ready inactivation by organic material. Yet, alcohols are still popular because they are cheap, fast acting, readily available and water soluble.

Aldehydes

Glutaraldehyde is perhaps the most popular disinfectant used in dentistry in some regions, whereas it is banned in others. It is both a skin irritant and a sensitization agent, which results in both long-term and short-term health effects. It is mainly used for so-called 'cold sterilization' or the high-level disinfection of equipment (such as fibre-optic instruments) that does not withstand autoclaving procedures. All aldehydes are high-potency disinfectants.

The free aldehyde groups of glutaraldehyde react strongly with the free amino groups of proteins in a pH-dependent manner. This leads to the effective microbicidal activity, sensitization of skin and, incidentally, cross-linking with proteins such as collagen when used as a component of dentine-bonding systems. Hence, as the pH decreases, the activity of glutaraldehyde declines while its stability increases. Conversely, when the pH is alkaline, the activity is higher and it becomes less stable. Hence, in practice, glutaraldehyde is commercially available as a 2% acidic solution, to which an 'activator' has to be added to bring the solution to the 'in-use' alkaline pH of 8.0. Although the activated solution has a shelf-life of up to 14 days, this should be interpreted with caution as the solution may become prematurely ineffective due to other factors. In regions where glutaraldehyde is banned, then alternative, nongluteraldehyde-containing products are used for high-level disinfection (e.g., ortho-phthalaldehydes, peracetic acid and hydrogen peroxide).

Bisguanides

Chlorhexidine is an example of a bisguanide disinfectant; it is widely used in dentistry as an antiseptic and a plaque-controlling agent. For example a 0.4% solution in detergent is used as a surgical scrub (Hibiscrub); 0.2% chlorhexidine gluconate in aqueous solution is used as an antiplaque agent (Corsodyl); and at a higher concentration (2%), it is used as a denture disinfectant. It is a cationic bisguanide molecule, usually prepared as salts of acetate, digluconate, hydrochloride and nitrate.

As chlorhexidine has two positive charges at its polar ends, it is highly active against both Gram-positive and Gram-negative organisms. (*Note:* All bacteria possess negatively charged cell walls in nature.) It also kills *Candida* (but not *Mycobacterium tuberculosis*). Due to ingress of the disinfectant, the cell membrane permeability is altered with resultant leakage of cell contents and precipitation of the cytoplasm leading to cell death. Its **substantivity** (i.e., prolonged persistence) in the oral cavity is mainly due to absorption onto hydroxyapatite and salivary mucus.

Halogen Compounds

Hypochlorites are oxidizing agents and act by releasing halide ions. Although cheap and effective, hypochlorites readily corrode metal and are quickly inactivated by organic matter (e.g., proprietary preparations include Chloros and Domestos). *Note:* Available chlorine is a measure commonly used to indicate the oxidizing capacity of hypochlorite agents and is expressed as the equivalent amount of elemental chlorine. Thus, the equivalence of 1% available chlorine corresponds to 10,000 ppm available chlorine. Chlorine releasing granules (e.g., sodium hypochlorite/sodium dichloroisocyanurate) or a liquid solution of hypochlorite at a concentration of 10,000 ppm (1%) is used to disinfect surfaces contaminated by blood and body fluid spills. Disposable chlorine-releasing wipes (equivalent to 1000 ppm or 0.1% free chlorine) are employed to clean blood spots from dental chairs.

Phenolics

Phenolic disinfectants are clear, soluble or black/white fluids (black/white fluids are not used in dentistry). They do not irritate the skin and are used for gross decontamination because they are not easily degraded by organic material. They are poorly virucidal and sporicidal. As most bacteria are killed by these agents, they are used widely in hospitals and laboratories (e.g., Clearsol and Stericol.)

Chloroxylenol is also a nonirritant phenolic used universally as an antiseptic; it has poor activity against many bacteria, and its use is limited to domestic disinfection (e.g., Dettol).

A sterilization and disinfection guide for items commonly used in dentistry is given in Table 38.2.

Environmental Disinfection

The dental clinic setting should always be kept free of potential pathogens by appropriate environmental infection control measures. In general, when using environmental disinfectants:

- The manufacturers' instructions for correct use of cleaning and disinfecting products must be strictly adhered to.
- High-level disinfectants for disinfection of environmental (clinical contact or housekeeping) surfaces should not be used as they pose a health hazard to workers.
- Always use appropriate PPE when cleaning and disinfecting environmental surfaces (e.g., puncture- and chemical-resistant gloves, disposable plastic apron, protective eyewear/face shield and mask).

CLINICAL CONTACT SURFACES

Clinical contact surfaces can be directly contaminated from patient materials either by direct spray or spatter generated during dental procedures or by contact with contaminated gloved hands of the dental personnel. These surfaces can subsequently contaminate other instruments, devices, hands or gloves. Examples of such surfaces include:

- light handles
- switches
- dental radiograph equipment
- dental chairside computers
- reusable containers of dental materials
- drawer handles
- faucet handles
- countertops
- doorknobs.

Barrier protection of surfaces and equipment can prevent contamination of clinical contact surfaces, but it is particularly effective for those that are difficult to clean. Barriers include clear plastic wrap, bags, sheets, tubing and plastic-backed paper or other materials impervious to moisture. Because such coverings can become contaminated, they should be removed and discarded between each patient, with gloved hands. After removing the barrier, the surface must be cleaned and disinfected. The barrier makes cleaning easier and faster. After removing gloves and performing hand hygiene, barriers on these surfaces should be replaced with clean ones before the next patient.

If barriers are not used, surfaces should be cleaned and disinfected between patients by using either low-level or intermediate-level disinfectant wipes. Disinfectant sprays are to be avoided where possible as repeated use of sprays can lead to hypersensitivity reactions in staff or trigger allergic reactions in susceptible patients.

HOUSEKEEPING SURFACES

- The dental practice should train staff to undertake daily cleaning of exposed housekeeping surfaces (e.g., floors, walls, cupboard doors and sinks) with detergent and warm water or with registered hospital disinfectant/detergent. An alternative cleaning method widely used in hospitals is cleaning with a microfibre cloth and water. Microfibre cloths are formed of very fine fibres at a high density, which produces a vast surface area that acts to remove and trap dirt and microbes. The cloths, which are reusable, are then laundered in a washing machine at 60°C–90°C to remove and destroy the pathogens.
- Clean mops and cloths after use and allow to dry before reuse, or use single-use, disposable materials. Cloths and mops used to clean housekeeping surfaces in heavily contaminated patient treatment areas should be separated from those used to clean nonclinical areas in order to prevent cross-contamination. This can be achieved by colour coding of cleaning materials (e.g., mops, cloths and buckets) according to the room where they are to be used.
- It is critical that fresh cleaning or disinfecting solutions are made daily or according to manufacturer's instructions.
- Walls, blinds and curtains in patient-care areas should be cleaned weekly to avoid buildup of dust or soil.
- A nominated person in the dental practice should train staff to inspect and audit the cleaning undertaken throughout the dental premises.

Dental Unit Water Lines: Disinfection and Management

The question of the quality of water in dental unit water lines (DUWLs) attached to handpieces, ultrasonic sealers and air/water syringes has been debated widely. The source of water to the dental unit is either directly from municipal supply or from water reservoir bottles usually filled with distilled or reverse osmosis water attached to the dental chair. After entering the unit, it passes through a multichannel control box that distributes the water to hoses (DUWLs) feeding various attachments, such as the high-speed handpiece, the air/water syringe and the ultrasonic scaler.

Unfortunately, certain properties of the DUWLs promote bacterial growth. The lines have a very small bore but a high surface area, and this, accompanied by the intermittent, slow flow rate, may result in the whole column of water in the DUWL becoming stagnant for long periods of time. In addition, suck-back of oral fluids may occur during use. Hence, bacteria tend to form **biofilms** within a few hours on the internal surfaces of DUWLs unless they are regularly cleaned and disinfected (Chapter 31). In general, these organisms are mostly nonpathogenic and saprophytic and may not cause disease in healthy individuals.

However, there is some risk to the health of dental staff and patients from opportunistic and respiratory pathogens such as *Legionella* spp., nontuberculous mycobacteria (NTM) and pseudomonads. These organisms can mutiply in the biofilm to reach infective concentrations, with the potential for inhalation-associated respiratory infections or direct contamination of surgical wounds. As mentioned, the majority of microbes isolated from DUWLs are innocuous environmental saprophytic bacteria. Legislation has provided guidelines for the upper limits of bacteria and, hence, the quality of the water resources that service the DUWLs. Generally, the water entering the DUWL contains very few organisms: 0–100 colony-forming units (CFUs)/mL. However, water exiting the handpiece may contain 100,000–1,000,000 CFU/mL, mainly because of the organisms that are picked up from the bacterial biofilms growing within the lines.

The guidelines from the Centers for Disease Control and Prevention (CDC) in the US recommend that water delivered to patients from a DUWL during **nonsurgical dental procedures** should meet drinking water standards, i.e., ≤500 CFU/mL of aerobic, mesophilic heterotrophic bacteria. In the UK, the current recommendation for dental unit water quality is more stringent and is set at 100–200 cfu/mL of aerobic heterotrophs at 22°C.

To allow dentists to have better control over the quality of the water used in patient care, integrated water reservoirs—or water-bottle systems that are independent of the public water supply—are recommended. As these systems on their own may not be adequate commercial products, devices are available that can improve and maintain water quality (discussed in the next section). Furthermore, independent engineering control systems such as a type A air-gap—a physical gap that prevents back siphonage of contaminated water into the municipal main supply—should be considered if the latter is the source of the water.

RECOMMENDATIONS ON CARE OF WATER LINES

- The quality of water used for routine dental treatments should match that of the national standards for drinking water **(range: ≤100–200 CFU/mL (UK) or ≤500 CFU/mL (US) of heterotrophic water bacteria)**.
- Independent reservoir and water bottle systems are recommended to be filled with freshly produced (i.e., less than 12 hours old) reverse osmosis or distilled water. These purified waters are not sterile but are less likely

to contain the *Legionella* spp., nontuberculous mycobacteria and pseudomonads found in ordinary potable tap water.

- In the UK, national guidelines recommend that dental surgeries/offices should drain down, clean, flush and disinfect all system components, pipework and bottles twice daily. Independent water storage bottles should be cleaned, rinsed with reverse osmosis-derived or distilled water, dried and stored dry and inverted overnight.
- All DUWLs should be **flushed for 2 min at the beginning of each day**, prior to commencing treatment and at the end of the day.
- The DUWL should be **flushed for 20–30 s between patients** to reduce temporarily the microbial count, as well as to clean the water line of materials that may have entered from the patient's mouth. This includes handpieces, ultrasonic scalers and air/water syringes.
- All DUWLs should be **fitted with nonretractable devices,** to prevent suck-back (backflow/back-siphonage) of material into the municipal water supply.
- Water from DUWLs should **never** be used as an irrigant in procedures involving breaches of the **mucosa and bone exposure**. During **surgical procedures use sterile solutions** of coolant/irrigant administered by an appropriate delivery device (e.g., sterile bulb syringe, sterile tubing that bypasses dental unit waterlines or sterile single-use devices).
- The dental unit manufacturer should be consulted for appropriate methods and equipment to maintain the recommended quality of dental unit water and its recommendations followed for monitoring and sustaining water quality; the need for periodic maintenance of anti-retraction mechanisms should also be verified with the manufacturer.

MAINTAINING QUALITY OF DENTAL UNIT WATER

This could be achieved currently using antiretraction valves, filters, flushing, chemicals or water purifiers.

Antiretraction Valves

Antiretraction valves (check valves) are now the norm in all modern dental units and dental handpieces and prevent the reaspiration (or suck-back or back-siphonage) of fluid contaminated with oral flora of patients into the water line. However, it is now known that the antiretraction valves are very inefficient unless they are regularly maintained and replaced periodically. Check valves on the dental unit help prevent back-siphonage into the potable water system.

Filters

Filters may be installed—for instance, between the water line and the dental instrument. These have no effect on the biofilm in the water lines but will remove microorganisms as the water is delivered to the patient. Filters are inefficient as they must be replaced periodically, and the frequency depends on the amount of biofilm in the water lines.

Flushing

This is a simple and efficient means of temporarily reducing the bacterial load in the water line. It is recognized that regular flushing prior to patient treatment will discharge the stagnant water, reduce the impact of oral suck-back and draw up fresh biocide into the DUWL, facilitating disinfection of the waterline. Staff should be alert to signs of change in water quality such as malodor, cloudiness and bad taste imparted to the water by microbial contamination, all of which are particularly noticeable after periods of stagnation. These signal that conditions may be appropriate to support the growth of legionella. The dental practice should seek further advice on microbial sampling for legionella detection.

Although flushing can reduce the numbers of bacteria in expelled water, the effect is transient and has no impact on the water-line biofilm. Care should be taken to avoid splatter and aerosol exposure during DUWL flushing, and masks and eyewear should be donned. Irregularly used dental units should be flushed on a routine basis (at least weekly) to prevent stagnation.

Biocides and Chemicals

These remove, inactivate or prevent the formation of biofilm. Chemicals can either be continuously infused into or be intermittently added to the dental unit water by varying technologies. Disinfectants deployed in DUWLs must be active against the range of microorganisms found in the DUWL, including *Legionella* spp., be nontoxic to patients and not damage the water lines or handpieces (e.g., alkaline or hydrogen peroxide, hydrogen peroxide/silver ions, peracetic acid formulations, tetrasodium EDTA, chlorhexidine formulations, iodine, quarternary ammoniums and chlorine dioxide). Hypochlorite, once popular for disinfecting DUWLs, leads to corrosion of handpieces and is now used for "shock treatment" eradication of microbiologically proven legionella contamination. Concerns here are the possible development of bacteria resistant to chemicals and environmental pollution.

Water Purifiers

Water purifiers treat the water coming into the dental unit (source water). They kill or remove microorganisms by methods such as filtration, electrolyzed water or ultraviolet light. One advantage of these technologies is that they may delay biofilm formation on water lines or synergize other treatment methods.

Miscellaneous

Other, rather expensive methods for delivery of quality water include the use of sterile water and autoclavable systems.

Boil-Water Advisories

A boil-water advisory is issued by authorities when the public water supply is likely to be contaminated with pathogenic organisms or the number of microbes in the system is above that which is compatible with health. During such periods, the following apply:

- Do not deliver water from the public water system to the patient through the dental unit, ultrasonic scaler or other dental equipment connected to that system.
- Do not use water from the public water system for dental treatment, patient-rinsing or hand-washing. For the latter purpose, antimicrobial-containing products that do not require water can be used (e.g., alcohol-based

hand rubs). If hands are visibly contaminated, use bottled water and soap for hand-washing or an antiseptic hand towel.
- Once the advisory is cancelled, follow guidance given by the local water utility on adequate flushing of water lines. If no guidance is provided, flush dental water lines and faucets for 1–5 min before resuming patient care. Disinfect DUWLs as recommended by the dental unit manufacturer.

Recommendations on Care of Handpieces and Other Devices Attached to Air and Water Lines

- Clean and steam-sterilize handpieces and other intraoral instruments that can be removed from the air and water lines of dental units after each patient treatment session. Their surfaces should be cleaned, and the internal elements cleaned and lubricated according to the manufacturer's instructions before sterilization.
- Do not surface-disinfect or use liquid chemical sterilants or ethylene oxide on handpieces and other intraoral instruments that can be detached from the air and water lines of dental units.
- The handpiece should be stored as appropriate according to national guidelines and run to remove excess lubricant immediately before use on patients.

Dental Radiology

- Always wear gloves when exposing radiographs and handling contaminated film packets. If spattering of blood or other body fluids is likely, use appropriate protective wear such as eyewear and mask.
- Use heat-tolerant or disposable intraoral devices whenever possible (e.g., film-holding and positioning devices). Clean and heat-sterilize heat-tolerant devices between patients. If heat-sensitive material is used, then high-level disinfection for semicritical items must be employed.
- Transport and handle exposed radiographs in an aseptic manner to prevent contamination of developing equipment.
- **Digital radiography sensors**: depending on the manufacturer's recommendations, either clean and heat-sterilize or high-level disinfect the sensor between patients. The sensor is usually a barrier-protected, semicritical item. If the item cannot tolerate these procedures, then a recommended barrier system has to be employed or cleaned and disinfected with an intermediate-level (i.e., tuberculocidal) activity. Manufacturer's recommendations must be adhered to for disinfection and sterilization of digital radiology sensors and for the protection of related computer hardware.

Laboratory Asepsis

Dental practitioners regularly send clinical material to the laboratory—for example, impression material, dentures sent to the technology laboratory or pathological samples such as pus or biopsy specimens referred to pathology laboratories. The dentist is obliged to deliver all such items in a manner that obviates infectious hazards, whether during transport or within the laboratory. Blood and saliva must be carefully cleaned from the impressions and denture work by washing under running water and disinfection, and, if appropriate, placed in plastic bags before transport to the laboratory. Proprietary disinfectant soaking solutions are preferred to sprays for decontaminating the microbes retained on impression surfaces.

The dental laboratory itself should be regarded as a clean (not contaminated) area, and appropriate protocols for disinfection of surfaces and material, as well as regular and timely renewal of disinfectant solutions, should be established. Smoking and eating should be prohibited.

Microbiological specimens sent to the laboratory should be securely bagged to avoid contamination of personnel who handle the items. The request form should be separately enclosed to prevent contamination. Biopsy specimens should be put in a sturdy container with a secure lid to prevent leakage during transport. Care should be taken when collecting specimens to avoid contamination of the external surface of the container. If specimens are to be transported by post or courier, then they should be placed in an outer padded leakproof postal packet clearly marked with the words 'PATHOLOGICAL SPECIMEN – FRAGILE – HANDLE WITH CARE', along with the name and address of the sender (and person to be contacted in case of leakage or queries) and that of the recipient.

Office/Surgery Design and Maintenance

Proper office or surgery design is the cornerstone of an effective infection control programme (Fig. 38.6). Major features of such a design are:

1. There is a clear demarcation between the **contaminated or dirty** and **clean zones** (i.e., the surgery and the sterilizing and storage areas, respectively).
2. Treatment areas and the laboratory should have few, if any, wood surfaces, porous or heavy draperies, or textured wall coverings, in order to facilitate cleaning and disinfection.
3. No eating or smoking is allowed in contaminated zones.
4. Carpets should not be used in the treatment areas, where flooring should be covered with seamless, disinfectant-resistant vinyl in order to minimize dust and microbial burden and to withstand frequent cleaning.
5. Ideally, ventilation in the surgical and peripheral areas should be centrally controlled (air renewal 12–15 air changes per hour) and planned to minimize cross-currents of air from one area to another. The air filter, if any, should be periodically changed, and special venting should be installed to scavenge noxious chemical vapour.

Infection control requirements should always be borne in mind when selecting new equipment.

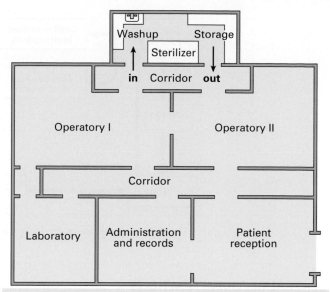
Fig. 38.6 Floor plan of a dental clinic designed to minimize cross-infection.

Instrument Recirculation and Office Design

In order to conduct an efficient and routine sterility programme, it is important to organize the various arms of the infection control programme outlined above in the most effective manner. Therefore, it is essential to design the dental office and instrument decontamination areas (washing up, sterilizing and storage) to achieve this aim. The instrument decontamination area should be organized in order to:

- separate contaminated objects from sterile or clean objects
- store sterile items until required
- facilitate easy cleaning and disinfection
- facilitate a smooth flow of items between contaminated and clean zones
- design the ventilation of the air so that it flows from the clean to the dirty area.

A suitable instrument recirculation profile is shown in Fig. 38.7. Other noteworthy points are:

- If possible, the instrument decontamination centre should be close to the clinic for ease of use.
- The work surfaces of the area should be smooth, nonporous and seamless.
- An air evacuation system (low-volume) with continuous movement of air upward from the working surface should be operational to reduce airborne microbes and noxious chemical vapours (these should be regularly serviced, and filters should be replaced as appropriate).

Disposal of Clinical Waste

Any waste material that has been in contact with human sources is contaminated with potentially pathogenic microbes or will possibly support their growth.

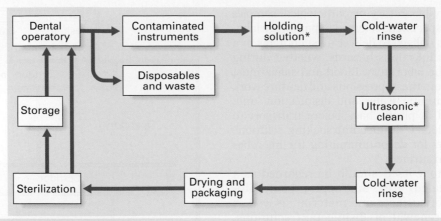

Fig. 38.7 A suggested scheme for instrument recirculation. (* See text for other options.)

GENERAL RECOMMENDATIONS

Develop a good clinical waste management programme, per local guidelines. Disposal of regulated clinical waste, both hazardous and nonhazardous, must follow these local and federal regulations. Ensure that DHCWs who handle and dispose of potentially infective wastes are trained in appropriate handling and disposal methods and informed of the possible health and safety hazards. In the UK, all dental workers who handle waste, including cleaners, must be vaccinated against hepatitis B.

CLINICAL WASTE IN DENTAL HEALTH CARE FACILITIES

Before disposal and making safe, use a colour-coded and/or labelled container that prevents leakage (e.g., biohazard bag) to contain nonsharp, regulated clinical and medicine waste according to national guidelines on waste classification—either by incineration or alternative temperature technologies. Incineration is required for the safe disposal of medicine waste.

All sharp items (especially needles), tissues or blood should be considered as particularly dangerous and should be handled and disposed of with special precautions. **Disposable needles, scalpels or other sharp items must be placed intact into puncture-resistant containers** before disposal and incineration.

If permitted by local regulations, carefully discard blood, suctioned fluids or other liquid waste into a drain connected to a sanitary sewer system. Wear appropriate protective attire while performing this task. Clinical waste should never be mixed with domestic waste, as this is a dangerous practice; it may also lead to litigation, therefore national clinical waste disposal guidelines should be strictly adhered to.

Transmission-Based Precautions

When patients have either a documented infection or are suspected of having an infection with *specified* **highly transmissible pathogens** for which standard infection control precautions are inadequate to prevent infection

transmission (Table 38.3), an additional tier of **transmission-based precautions *on top of standard infection control protocol*** must be implemented.

Usually, such patients are managed in hospital settings and infrequently in community ambulatory care clinic settings. However, this situation changed dramatically with the advent of the COVID-19 pandemic, as asymptomatic patients harbouring SARS-CoV-2 may attend the clinic seeking routine dental care. Apart from COVID-19, several other infections and conditions that may not be treated in a community/ambulatory clinic but in hospitalized patients that require transmission-based precautions are shown in Table 38.3.

These categories of patients should always be **treated on an *elective basis*** until their disease or the condition is resolved. If emergency surgical intervention is required, then transmission-based precautions must be applied on top of standard infection control protocols.

In addition, as some dental professionals are hospital based, they may have to attend to patients infected with highly transmissible agents and, hence, a good understanding of transmission-based precautions is essential.

Furthermore, transmission-based precautions are sometimes recommended for use on an empiric, transient basis until a diagnosis of a new, emerging infection can be made. Finally, it should be borne in mind that transmission-based precautions are an additional layer of protection for the DHCW and ***always should be used in conjunction with standard precautions***.

CLASSIFICATION

There are essentially three categories of transmission-based precautions:

- **Airborne precautions**—prevent transmission of infectious agents that are very small (<100 µm) and remain viable and suspended in the air over long periods and distances (e.g., measles, tuberculosis, COVID-19, chicken pox)
- **Droplet precautions**—prevent transmission of diseases spread by large respiratory droplets (>100 µm) through coughing, sneezing, or talking (e.g., seasonal influenza, whooping cough)

Table 38.3   Some Examples of Conditions and Diseases Requiring Transmission-Based Precautions (in addition to standard precautions)

Disease/Condition	Contact Precautions	Droplet Precautions	Airborne Precautions	Duration of Precautions
COVID-19 SARS MERS	Yes	Yes	Yes	Variable but usually 10 days after fever resolution provided respiratory symptoms are absent or improving
Herpes simplex (mucocutaneous, disseminated or primary, severe)*	Yes	NA	NA	Until lesions are dry and crusted
Herpes (varicella) Zoster (Chicken Pox)*	Yes	NA	Yes	Until lesions are dry and crusted
Seasonal Influenza	NA	Yes	NA	5 days, except in immunocompromised
Measles (Rubeola)	NA	NA	Yes	4 days after onset of rash, except DI in people who are immunocompromised
Mumps	NA	Yes	NA	9 days after symptom resolution
Pertussis	NA	Yes	NA	5 days after symptom resolution
Rubella	NA	Yes	NA	Day 7 after onset of rash
Methicillin (MRSA) and vancomycin Resistant *Staphylococcus aureus* (VRSA)	Yes	NA	NA	Unresolved
Tuberculosis (open) Pulmonary or laryngeal	NA	Yes	Yes	Usually three consecutive sputum smears negative for acid-fast bacilli

NA: Not applicable; * Recurrent oral herpetic lesions only require standard precautions.
Note: Transmission-based precautions typically remain in effect only while there is risk of the infectious agent being transmitted or for the duration of the illness.

■ **Contact precautions**—prevent diseases that are spread by either direct contact with the patient or indirect contact with the patient's environment such as bedding, cabinet tops, and so on.

More than a single transmission-based precaution category may apply at the same time because some diseases are transmitted via multiple routes.

It is noteworthy, that some items of standard infection control and transmission-based precautions are overlapping and do not differ much from the routine infection control practices of dentists. This is because dentists have to wear PPE as they are frequently exposed to blood and blood-contaminated saliva during dental procedures. On the other hand, nurses or physicians may not always wear a complete ensemble of PPE for all patient interactions and, hence, transmission-based precautions are applied as blanket recommendations for all DHCWs.

Contact Precautions: For Ambulatory Clinic Settings

Contact with patients with known or suspected infections represents an increased risk for contact transmission.

Examples of conditions requiring contact precautions include, but are not limited to, herpes simplex and mutidrug-resistant organisms (MDROs)—for example,

methicillin-resistant *Staphylococcus aureus* (MRSA) or vancomycin-resistant *Staphylococcus aureus* (VRSA)—and for patients in ambulatory care settings who have uncontrolled wound drainage or other syndromes representing increased risk of contact transmission.

■ **Ensure appropriate patient placement**. Place patients requiring contact precautions in a room separate from the general clinic or a dedicated examination room or cubicle as soon as possible.

■ **Use PPE appropriately** (Chapter 37). This includes masks, gloves and gowns. Don PPE upon room entry and properly discard before exiting the patient room to contain pathogens; use hand hygiene as appropriate,

■ **Limit transport and movement of patients** outside of the room to medically necessary purposes. When transport or movement is necessary, cover or contain the infected or colonized areas of the patient's body. Remove and dispose of contaminated PPE and perform hand hygiene prior to transporting patients on contact precautions.

■ **Use disposable or dedicated patient-care equipment.** If common use of equipment for multiple patients (e.g., blood pressure cuffs) is unavoidable, clean and disinfect such equipment before use on another patient.

■ **Prioritize cleaning and disinfection of the rooms** of patients on contact precautions, ensuring rooms are frequently cleaned and disinfected (e.g., daily or prior to use by another patient) and focusing on frequently touched surfaces and equipment in the immediate vicinity of the patient. Remove all unnecessary items, such as furniture, magazines, magazine racks and decorative material.

Droplet Precautions: For Ambulatory Clinic Settings

Technically, droplet transmission is considered a form of contact transmission because some infectious agents transmitted via this route also may be transmitted by direct or indirect contact (see Fig. 36.2).

For patients known or suspected to be infected with pathogens transmitted by respiratory droplets that are generated by a patient who is coughing, sneezing, or talking:

- **Source control:** Put a mask on the patient.
- **Ensure appropriate patient placement:** Place patient in an exam room or cubicle as soon as possible and instruct patient to follow respiratory hygiene/cough etiquette recommendations.
- **Use PPE appropriately:** Don mask and eye protection before entry into the patient room or patient space.
- **Limit transport and movement of patients:** If transport or movement outside of the room is necessary, limit it to medically necessary purposes and instruct the patient to wear a mask and follow respiratory hygiene/cough etiquette.

Airborne Precautions: For Ambulatory Clinic Settings

For patients known or suspected to be infected with pathogens transmitted by the airborne route (e.g., COVID-19, tuberculosis, measles, chickenpox, disseminated herpes zoster):

- **Source control**: Put a mask on the patient.
- **Ensure appropriate patient placement in an airborne infection isolation room (AIIR)** with proper air filtration controls. If this is not feasible, masking the patient and placing the patient in a private room with the door closed will reduce the likelihood of airborne transmission until the patient is either transferred to a facility with an AIIR or returned home.
- **Restrict susceptible healthcare personnel from entering the room** of patients known or suspected to have measles, chickenpox, or disseminated zoster if other immune health care personnel are available.
- **Use PPE appropriately**, including a *fit-tested* National Institute for Occupational Safety and Health (NIOSH)–approved N95 or higher-level respirator for healthcare personnel.
- **Limit transport and movement of patients** outside of the room to medically necessary purposes. If transport or movement outside an AIIR is necessary, instruct patients to wear a surgical mask, if possible, and observe respiratory hygiene/cough etiquette.
- Immunize susceptible persons as soon as possible following unprotected contact with vaccine-preventable infections (e.g., COVID-19, measles, varicella).

Key Facts

- **Decontamination** is the process by which reusable items are rendered safe for further use and for staff to handle. Decontamination is required to minimize the risk of cross-infection between patients and between patients and staff. Decontamination includes cleaning, disinfection and sterilization steps.
- **Sterilization** is a process that kills or **removes all** organisms (and their spores) in a material or an object.
- **Disinfection** is a process that kills or removes **pathogenic organisms** in a material or an object, **excluding bacterial spores**, so that they pose no threat of infection.
- **Antisepsis** is the application of a chemical agent externally on a **live surface** (skin or mucosa) to destroy organisms or to inhibit their growth (all antiseptics are disinfectants but not all disinfectants are antiseptics).
- Sterilization can be divided into four stages: **presterilization cleaning, packaging**, the **sterilization process** and **aseptic storage**.
- In dentistry, sterilization is usually achieved by **moist heat** (steam under pressure in an autoclave). The sterilization cycle (either in an autoclave or in a hot-air oven) can be divided into the **heating-up period**, the **holding period** and the **cooling period**.
- The three classes of sterilizers Class B, S and N, and the Class B and S are vacuum autoclaves commonly used in dentistry.
- The indicators that must be routinely used for checking sterility are **mechanical** process indicators (i.e., the temperature and pressure gauges of the autoclave), **chemical** indicators and **biological** indicators/monitors.

- Regular decontamination audits should be conducted of all areas of the dental premises where instrument and device reprocessing occurs.
- The key mode of disinfection are **physical** (ultrasonics) and **chemical** (disinfectants) methods (most used in dentistry).
- Disinfectants can be generally categorized as having **high, intermediate** or **low potency**, depending on their ability to kill various groups of organisms.
- Water in dental unit water lines for nonsurgical procedures should not contain more than **100–200 CFU/mL** (UK) and **>500 CFU/mL** (US) of aerobic, heterotrophic bacteria.
- When sending clinical **material to the laboratory, obviate infectious hazards** during transport and within the laboratory.
- Dispose of **clinical waste**, including sharps, medicines and personal protective equipment in a safe manner.
- **Proper office/surgery design** is the cornerstone of an effective infection control programme.
- **Transmission-based precautions** must be instituted when patients have either a documented infection or are suspected of having an infection with *specified* **highly transmissible pathogens** for which standard infection control precautions are inadequate to prevent infection transmission.
- There are three categories of transmission-based precautions: contact, airborne and droplet.
- Transmission-based precautions are an **additional layer of protection for the health care worker (HCW)** and must be applied on top of the routine universal precautions.

Review Questions (Answers on p. 392)

Please indicate which answers are true and which are false.

38.1. Which of the following modes of sterilization are permitted by legislation for use in a small dental clinic?
   a. steam (autoclave)
   b. dry heat
   c. unsaturated chemical vapour
   d. radiation
   e. glutaraldehyde exposure for 30 min

38.2. Which of the following statements on disinfectants is true?
   a. alcohol is active against bacterial spores
   b. glutaraldehyde is active against both gram positive and gram negative organisms
   c. chlorhexidine is not inactivated by either soap or proteins
   d. glutaraldehyde is a medium level disinfectant
   e. hypochlorites kill organisms by their reducing action

38.3. Which of the following statements related to disinfection/sterilization is/are true?
   a. a dental mirror could be classified as a critical item
   b. all critical items must be sterilized
   c. semi critical items may be used in dentistry after high level disinfection
   d. the head rest of a dental chair could be classified as a semi-critical item
   e. A high level disinfectant must be used for disinfecting house keeping surfaces

38.4. Which of the following statements with regards to dental unit water lines (DUWL)is/are true/false
   a. The quality of water used for dental treatment must match that of the standards of drinking water
   b. Water from DUWL may be used for cleansing the wound during a surgical removal of a third molar tooth
   c. The water of DUWL may contain upto 500 CFU/mL of heterotrophic bacteria
   d. Legionella infection can be transmitted to patients from DUWL
   e. The biofilms in DUWL can be removed by flushing the water line regularly

Further Reading

Centers for Disease Control and Prevention. (2016). *Summary of infection prevention practices in dental settings: Basic expectations for safe care*. https://www.cdc.gov/oralhealth/infectioncontrol/summary-infection-prevention-practices.

Franco, F. F. S., Spratt, D., Leao, J. C., & Porter, S. R. (2005). Biofilm formation and control in dental unit water lines. *Biofilms, 2*, 9–17.

Health & Safety Executive. (2013). *Legionnaires' disease: The control of legionella bacteria in water systems: Approved code of practice and guidance* (4th ed.). https://www.hse.gov.uk/pubns/books/l8.htm.

National Health Service. (2021). (HTM 01–05) *Decontamination in primary care dental practices*. https://www.england.nhs.uk/publication/decontamination-in-primary-care-dental-practices-htm-01-05.

Pankhurst, C. L., & Coulter, W. A. (2017). *Basic guide to infection prevention and control* (2nd ed.). Wiley-Blackwell.

Pankhurst, C. L., Scully, C., & Samaranayake, L. (2017). Dental unit water lines and their disinfection and management. *Dental Update, 44*, 284–292.

Samaranayake, L. P., Scheutz, F., & Cottone, J. (1991). *Infection control for the dental team*. Munksgaard.

Answers to Review Questions

2.1

A. F
B. F
C. T
D. T
E. T

2.2

A. T
B. T
C. T
D. T
E. F

2.3

A. 1 and 7
B. 4
C. 3
D. 5
E. 8
F. 6
G. 2

3.1

A. T
B. F
C. F
D. F
E. T

3.2

A. T
B. T
C. T
D. T
E. F

3.3

A. T
B. F
C. T
D. T
E. F

4.1

A. F
B. T
C. F
D. T
E. F

4.2

A. T
B. T
C. F
D. T
E. T

4.3

A. T
B. T
C. T
D. F
E. T

4.4

A. T
B. T
C. F
D. T
E. F

4.5

A. F
B. T
C. T
D. T
E. T

5.1

A. T
B. T
C. F
D. T
E. T

5.2

A. T
B. T
C. T
D. T
E. T

5.3

A. T
B. F
C. T
D. T
E. T

5.4

A. F
B. F
C. T
D. T
E. T

6.1

A. T
B. F
C. T
D. F
E. T

6.2

A. T
B. T
C. T
D. T
E. F

6.3

A. 5
B. 2
C. 1
D. 3
E. 4

6.4

A. 2
B. 1
C. 5
D. 3
E. 4

6.5

A. F
B. F
C. F
D. F
E. T

7.1

A. T
B. T
C. T
D. F
E. T

7.2

A. T
B. F
C. F
D. T
E. T

7.3

A. T
B. F
C. T
D. F
E. T

7.4

A. T
B. T
C. F
D. T
E. T

7.5

A. T
B. F
C. F
D. T
E. T

7.6

A. T
B. T
C. T
D. F
E. T

7.7

A. T
B. F
C. T
D. T
E. F

8.1

A. F
B. T
C. F
D. F
E. T

8.2

A. F
B. F
C. F
D. T
E. F

8.3

A. F
B. T
C. F
D. T
E. F

8.4

A. F
B. F
C. F
D. T
E. F

8.5

A. F
B. F
C. F
D. F
E. T

8.6

A. T
B. F
C. T
D. T
E. T

8.7

A. T
B. T
C. F
D. T
E. T

8.8

A. T
B. F
C. T
D. F
E. T

8.9

A. T
B. T
C. F
D. T
E. F

8.10

A. F
B. F
C. F
D. T
E. T

8.11

A. T
B. F
C. T
D. F
E. T

8.12

A. F
B. F
C. T
D. T
E. T

8.13

A. F
B. F
C. F
D. F
E. T

8.14

A. F
B. T
C. F
D. F
E. F

8.15

A. F
B. T
C. T
D. T
E. T

8.16

A. F
B. T
C. T
D. F
E. T

9.1

A. F
B. T
C. F
D. F
E. F

9.2

A. T
B. T
C. T
D. F
E. T

9.3

A. F
B. T
C. F
D. F
E. F

9.4

A. F
B. F
C. T
D. F
E. F

10.1

A. T
B. T
C. T
D. F
E. T

10.2

A. T
B. T
C. T
D. F
E. T

10.3

A. T
B. F
C. T
D. T
E. T

11.1

A. T
B. T
C. F
D. T
E. F

11.2

A. T
B. T
C. T
D. F
E. F

11.3

A. T
B. T
C. F
D. T
E. F

11.4

A. T
B. T
C. T
D. T
E. F

12.1

A. T
B. T
C. T
D. F
E. F

12.2

A. F
B. T
C. F
D. T
E. T

12.3

A. T
B. F
C. T
D. T
E. T

12.4

A. F
B. T
C. F
D. F
E. F

13.1

A. F
B. T
C. F
D. F
E. T

13.2

A. T
B. T
C. F
D. F
E. T

13.3

A. T
B. F
C. T
D. T
E. F

13.4

A. F
B. T
C. T
D. T
E. T

13.5

A. F
B. F
C. T
D. T
E. T

14.1

A. T
B. T
C. F
D. F
E. T

14.2

A. F
B. F
C. T
D. T
E. F

14.3

A. T
B. T
C. F
D. T
E. F

14.4

A. T
B. T
C. T
D. T
E. T

14.5

A. F
B. T
C. T
D. T
E. F

14.6

A. T
B. T
C. F
D. T
E. T

15.1

A. F
B. F
C. T
D. F
E. T

15.2

A. T
B. T
C. T
D. T
E. T

15.3

A. F
B. T
C. T
D. T
E. F

15.4

A. T
B. T
C. F
D. F
E. T

16.1

A. T
B. T
C. F
D. F
E. F

16.2

A. T
B. F
C. F
D. T
E. T

16.3

A. T
B. T
C. F
D. T
E. T

17.1

A. F
B. F
C. F
D. T
E. F

17.2

A. T
B. F
C. T
D. T
E. F

17.3

A. T
B. F
C. F
D. T
E. F

18.1

A. T
B. F
C. T
D. T
E. T

18.2

A. F
B. T
C. T
D. T
E. T

18.3

A. T
B. T
C. T
D. T
E. F

19.1

A. F
B. T
C. T
D. F
E. T

19.2

A. T
B. F
C. T
D. T
E. F

19.3

A. T
B. F
C. F
D. T
E. T

19.4

A. F
B. T
C. T
D. F
E. T

20.1

A. T
B. T
C. T
D. F
E. T

20.2

A. T
B. T
C. T
D. T
E. F

20.3

A. T
B. T
C. T
D. F
E. T

21.1

A. T
B. T
C. F
D. T
E. F

21.2

A. F
B. T
C. T
D. T
E. F

21.3

A. T
B. F
C. T
D. T
E. F

21.4

A. T
B. T
C. T
D. F
E. T

21.5

A. T
B. F
C. T
D. T
E. T

21.6

A. T
B. F
C. T
D. F
E. T

21.7

A. T
B. T
C. F
D. T
E. T

21.8

A. F
B. T
C. T
D. T
E. T

21.9

A. T
B. T
C. T
D. F
E. F

22.1

A. T
B. T
C. F
D. T
E. F

22.2

A. T
B. T
C. F
D. T
E. F

22.3

A. T
B. T
C. T
D. F
E. F

23.1

A. F
B. F
C. T
D. F
E. T

23.2

A. T
B. F
C. T
D. T
E. T

23.3

A. T
B. T
C. F
D. F
E. T

23.4

A. T
B. T
C. T
D. T
E. T

23.5

A. T
B. T
C. F
D. T
E. T

23.6

A. T
B. T
C. T
D. F
E. T

23.7

A. F
B. T
C. F
D. F
E. T

23.8

A. F
B. T
C. T
D. T
E. F

24.1

A. T
B. T
C. T
D. T
E. T

24.2

A. T
B. T
C. T
D. F
E. T

24.3

A. F
B. T
C. T
D. T
E. F

24.4

A. F
B. F
C. T
D. T
E. T

24.5

A. T
B. T
C. T
D. F
E. F

25.1

A. T
B. F
C. T
D. F
E. F

25.2

A. T
B. T
C. T
D. T
E. T

25.3

A. T
B. F
C. T
D. F
E. T

25.4

A. T
B. T
C. T
D. F
E. T

25.5

A. F
B. T
C. T
D. F
E. T

25.6

A. F
B. T
C. T
D. F
E. F

25.7

A. T
B. F
C. T
D. T
E. T

26.1

A. T
B. F
C. T
D. F
E. F

26.2

A. F
B. F
C. T
D. F
E. T

26.3

A. T
B. T
C. F
D. T
E. T

26.4

A. A T
B. T
C. F
D. T
E. F

26.5

A. 3
B. 1
C. 2
D. 4
E. 5

27.1

A. T
B. T
C. T
D. T
E. T

27.2

A. T
B. F
C. F
D. T
E. T

27.3

A. F
B. T
C. T
D. F
E. T

27.4

A. F
B. T
C. F
D. T
E. F

27.5

A. T
B. F
C. F
D. F
E. T

28.1

A. T
B. F
C. T
D. T
E. F

28.2

A. T
B. F
C. T
D. T
E. T

28.3

A. T
B. T
C. T
D. F
E. T

28.4

A. F
B. T
C. T
D. T
E. T

28.5

A. 1
B. 2
C. 3
D. 2
E. 5

29.1

A. F
B. T
C. T
D. F
E. T

29.2

A. T
B. T
C. T
D. F
E. T

29.3

A. T
B. T
C. T
D. F
E. T

29.4

A. F
B. F
C. T
D. F
E. T

29.5

A. T
B. T
C. F
D. T
E. T

30.1

A. T
B. T
C. F
D. T
E. F

30.2

A. F
B. T
C. F
D. T
E. F

30.3

A. T
B. T
C. T
D. T
E. T

30.4

A. F
B. T
C. T
D. F
E. T

30.5

A. F
B. T
C. T
D. F
E. T

31.1

A. F
B. T
C. T
D. F
E. T

31.2

A. T
B. T
C. T
D. T
E. F

31.3

A. F
B. T
C. T
D. T
E. F

31.4

A. F
B. F
C. T
D. F
E. T

32.1

A. F
B. F
C. F
D. T
E. T

32.2

A. T
B. F
C. T
D. T
E. F

32.3

A. T
B. T
C. F
D. T
E. F

32.4

A. F
B. T
C. T
D. F
E. T

32.5

A. F
B. T
C. T
D. F
E. T

33.1

A. F
B. F
C. T
D. T
E. T

33.2

A. T
B. T
C. F
D. F
E. F

33.3

A. T
B. F
C. T
D. T
E. T

33.4

A. F
B. T
C. T
D. T
E. T

33.5

A. T
B. T
C. T
D. T
E. F

34.1

A. F
B. T
C. F
D. T
E. F

34.2

A. F
B. T
C. T
D. T
E. F

34.3

A. F
B. T
C. T
D. F
E. T

34.4

A. F
B. T
C. F
D. T
E. F

35.1

A. T
B. F
C. T
D. T
E. T

35.2

A. T
B. F
C. F
D. F
E. F

35.3

A. F
B. T
C. T
D. F
E. T

35.4

A. F
B. T
C. T
D. F
E. F

35.5

A. primary
B. tertiary
C. secondary
D. congenital
E. secondary
F. congenital

35.6

A. T
B. T
C. T
D. T
E. F

36.1

A. T
B. F
C. F
D. T
E. T

36.2

A. T
B. T
C. F
D. F
E. F

37.1

A. F
B. F
C. F
D. T
E. F

37.2

A. F
B. T
C. F
D. F
E. F

37.3

A. F
B. T
C. T
D. T
E. T

37.4

A. F
B. F
C. F
D. T
E. T

38.1

A. T
B. F
C. F
D. F
E. F

38.2

A. F
B. T
C. F
D. F
E. F

38.3

A. F
B. T
C. T
D. F
E. F

38.4

A. T
B. F
C. T
D. T
E. F

Glossary of Terms and Abbreviations

16SRNA gene The small subunit of the bacterial and archaeal ribosome: The DNA sequence of this gene is the most commonly used taxonomic marker for microbial communities

abscess A localized collection of pus; *see* pus

acidophile An organism that prefers acidic environments; such an organism is said to be acidophilic

acquired immune deficiency syndrome (AIDS) The final stage of infection with the human immunodeficiency virus in which the patient has a low count of CD4⁺ T cells and suffers from opportunistic infections, opportunistic malignancies and/or encephalitis/dementia

acquired immunity Immunity or resistance acquired at some point in an individual's lifetime

active acquired immunity Immunity or resistance acquired as a result of the active production of antibodies and activated T cells

active immunization Stimulation of the immune system by intentional vaccination with foreign antigens

acute disease A disease having a sudden onset and short duration

acute-phase proteins Proteins whose concentration rises rapidly in body fluids following tissue injury or infection and which reduce inflammatory tissue damage

adaptive immunity The development of specifically activated B and/or T cells following exposure to antigen

adhesion molecule Cell surface molecule that enhances intercellular interactions

adjuvant A substance that enhances the immune response to an antigen

aerotolerant anaerobe An organism that can live in the presence of oxygen but grows best in an anaerobic environment (one that contains no oxygen)

affinity maturation Introduction of point mutations into immunoglobulin V genes that increases the strength of binding of antibody to antigen

agammaglobulinaemia Absence of, or extremely low levels of, the gamma fraction of serum globulin; sometimes used to denote the absence of immunoglobulins

ageusia Total absence of taste

agglutination The clumping of particles (including cells and latex beads) in solution

agglutination test Laboratory procedure that results in agglutination, usually following reaction with antibodies and antigenic determinants on particles

AIDS *See* acquired immunodeficiency syndrome

allergen An antigen to which one may become allergic

allergy Immediate hypersensitivity reaction in susceptible persons caused by release of pharmacological mediators from mast cells and basophils following interaction of surface-bound immunoglobulin E with allergen

α₁-antitrypsin An acute-phase protein that neutralizes proteases released by bacteria or damaged tissue

αβ T cells T lymphocytes bearing T cell receptors consisting of α and β chains

alternative pathway Complement activation independent of antibody, often induced by bacterial products such as endotoxin and lipopolysaccharide

amino acids The basic units or building blocks of proteins

anaerobe An organism that does not require oxygen for survival; can exist in the absence of oxygen

Analytical Profile Index (API) a commercially available system to speciate and identify different bacteria

anamnestic response An immune response following exposure to an antigen to which the individual is already sensitized; also known as a secondary response or memory response

anaphylactic shock Severe immune reaction mediated by immunoglobulin E, which may be fatal owing to constriction of bronchial smooth muscles

anaphylatoxin Complement split products C3a, C4a and C5a that directly cause smooth-muscle contraction and mast cell degranulation

anaphylaxis An immediate, severe, sometimes fatal, systemic allergic reaction

anergy Nonresponsiveness to antigen; T cells may become specifically anergic when exposed to antigen in the absence of activation signal 2

angioedema Collections of fluid (oedema) in the skin, mucous membrane, or viscera due to overproduction of anaphylatoxins

ångström A unit of length, equivalent to 0.1 nm; roughly the diameter of an atom

anosmia Absence or total loss of smell

antagonism The killing, injury or inhibition of one microorganism by products of another

antibiotic A substance produced by a microorganism that inhibits or destroys other microorganisms

antibody Immunoglobulin (a glycoprotein) molecule produced by B lymphocytes in response to an antigen; binds specifically to the antigen that induced its secretion; often protective

antibody-dependent cell-mediated cytotoxicity Killing of antibody-coated target cells by polymorphs, monocyte/macrophages or natural killer cells that have surface receptors for the Fc portion of immunoglobulin G

anticodon The trinucleotide sequence that is complementary to a codon; found on a transfer RNA molecule

antigen Any molecule that can induce an immune response; sometimes called an immunogen

antigen presentation Display of short peptides bound to major histocompatibility complex molecules on antigen-presenting cells for recognition by T cells

antigen-presenting cells (APCs) Cells that are able to present peptides on major histocompatibility complex molecules to T cells and activate them

antigen processing Digestion of complex antigen molecules into short peptides, assembly of peptide–major histocompatibility complexes and transport of complexes to the cell surface of antigen-presenting cells

antigenic determinant   The smallest part of an antigen capable of stimulating the production of antibodies or activating T cells; *see also* epitope

antigenic disguise   Binding of normal, nonimmunogenic, self molecules to the surface of a parasite so that its foreignness is masked

antigenic drift   Minor structural changes of viral antigens due to point mutations

antigenic modulation   Loss of antigen from cell surfaces following binding of antibody

antigenic shift   Exchange of large segments of genetic material between viruses resulting in major changes in antigenicity

antigenic variation   Modification of the structure of pathogen antigens

anti-idiotype vaccine   Anti-antipathogen antibody with immunostimulating properties similar to those of the pathogen

anti-idiotypic antibody   Antibody against V regions of antibodies, B cell or T cell receptors

antimicrobial agent   A drug, disinfectant or other substance that kills microorganisms or suppresses their growth

antisepsis   Prevention of infection by inhibiting the growth of pathogens

antiseptic   An agent or substance capable of effecting antisepsis; usually refers to a chemical disinfectant that is safe to use on living tissues

antiserum   Serum containing a particular antibody or antibodies; also called immune serum

antisialagogue   Substance that prevents salivation

antitoxin   An antibody produced in response to a toxin; often capable of neutralizing the toxin that stimulated its production

APC   *See* antigen-presenting cell

API   *See* Analytical Profile Index

apicectomy   An operation in which the apex of a tooth is removed

apoptosis   A form of programmed cell death in which products of cell disintegration are packaged as membrane-bound particles that are readily phagocytosed

approximal   Surface between adjacent teeth

archaeome   Constituent archaeal component of the (oral) microbiome mostly of methane-producing archaea

aseptic technique   Measures taken to ensure that living pathogens are absent

asymptomatic disease   A disease having no symptoms

asymptomatic infection   The presence of a pathogen in or on the body, without any symptoms of disease

atrophy   Shrinkage in size of an organ or tissue by reduction in size of its cells

attenuated live vaccine   Live vaccine containing organism of reduced virulence due to culturing under unfavourable conditions

autochthonous population   A characteristic member of the microbial community of a habitat

autoclave   An apparatus used for sterilization by steam under pressure

autogenic succession   Bacterial succession influenced by microbial factors; for example, the metabolism of pioneer species lowers the redox potential during plaque development; this allows obligate anaerobes to colonize

autoimmune disease   A disease in which the body produces antibodies directed against its own tissues

autoimmunity   Diseases caused by pathogenic immune reactions against self antigens

autoradiography   Exposure of a gel or blot to radiographic film to identify the position of a radioactive probe

autotroph   An organism that uses carbon dioxide as its sole carbon source

avirulent   Not virulent

axial filament   An organelle of motility possessed by spirochaetes

B7   Molecules (B7.1 and B7.2) present on 'professional' antigen-presenting cells that bind to CD28 (to signal for activation) or CTLA-4 (to signal for inactivation) on T cells

bacillus (*pl.* bacilli)   A rod-shaped bacterium; also a member of the genus *Bacillus* (aerobic, Gram-positive, spore-forming rods)

bacteraemia   The presence of bacteria in the blood stream

bacteria (*sing.* bacterium)   Primitive, unicellular, prokaryotic microorganisms

bacterial succession   Pattern of development of a microbial community

bactericidal agent   A chemical agent or drug that kills bacteria; a bactericide

bacteriocins   Proteins produced by certain bacteria (those possessing bacteriocinogenic plasmids) that can kill other bacteria

bacteriome   Constituent bacterial component of the microbiome

bacteriophage   A virus that infects a bacterium; also known simply as a *phage*

bacteriostatic agent   A chemical agent or drug that inhibits the growth of bacteria

bacteriuria   Multiplication of bacteria in urine within the renal tract (more than 10^5 organisms per millilitre of urine is considered to be significant bacteriuria, i.e., evidence of urinary tract infection)

basophil   Type of polymorphonuclear leukocyte with granules that stain with basic dyes

B cell   *See* B lymphocyte

B cell receptor (BCR)   Surface Ig molecules on B cells that recognize and bind antigens

bcl-2   An inhibitor of programmed cell death

β₂-microglobulin   A polypeptide associated with major histocompatibility complex I molecules

binary fission   A method of reproduction whereby one cell divides to become two cells

B lymphocyte   Bone marrow–derived lymphocyte responsible for production of antibodies

blotting   Transfer of proteins onto nitrocellulose following electrophoresis

bone marrow   Primary lymphoid organ; the site of production and development of blood cells

botulinum toxin   The neurotoxin produced by *Clostridium botulinum*; causes botulism

candidiasis   Infection with, or disease caused by, a yeast in the genus *Candida* (usually *C. albicans*); formerly called *moniliasis*; also called *candidosis*

candidosis (*pl.* candidoses or candidiases)   *See* candidiasis

capnophile   An organism that grows best in the presence of increased concentrations of carbon dioxide

capsid   The external protein coat or covering of a virion

capsomeres   The protein units that make up the capsid of some virions

capsule   An organized layer of glycocalyx, firmly attached to the outer surface of the bacterial cell wall

cariogenic   Dental caries inducing (e.g., bacteria, carbohydrate-rich diets, etc.)

carrier   An individual with an asymptomatic infection that can be transmitted to other susceptible individuals

CD28   Surface molecule on T cells that binds to B7 on 'professional' antigen-presenting cells to transmit T cell activation signal 2

CD3   A group of proteins associated with the T cell receptor that help transmit activation signals following engagement of T cell receptors by major histocompatibility complex (MHC) peptide

CD4   Surface molecule on a subset of T cells that binds to major histocompatibility complex II molecules during antigen recognition; the receptor for human immunodeficiency virus

CD40   Surface molecule on 'professional' antigen-presenting cells that binds to CD40L on T-helper cells to transmit B cell activation signal 2

CD40 ligand (CD40L)   Molecule present on T-helper cells that binds to CD40 on 'professional' antigen-presenting cells and can transmit signal 2 for activation

CD45RA   A molecule found on naive T-helper cells

CD45RO   A molecule found on memory T-helper cells

CD8   Surface molecule on a subset of T cells that binds to major histocompatibility complex I molecules during antigen recognition

cell membrane   The protoplasmic boundary of all cells; controls permeability and serves other important functions

cell wall   The outermost rigid layer of the cell (bacterial, fungal and plant cells)

cellulitis   Spreading infection of subcutaneous tissues

centriole   Tubular structure thought to play a role in nuclear division (mitosis) in animal cells and the cells of lower plants

cervicitis   Inflammation of the neck of the uterus, the cervix uteri

chemokine   One of a family of low-molecular-weight cytokines involved in lymphocyte trafficking

chemotaxis   Migration of cells, especially phagocytes, towards a high concentration of a chemotactic factor

chitin   A polysaccharide found in fungal cell walls but not found in the cell walls of other microorganisms

chromatin   The genetic material of the nucleus; consisting of DNA and associated proteins; during mitotic division, the chromatin condenses and is seen as chromosomes

chromosome   A condensed form of chromatin; the location of genes; bacterial cells usually contain only one chromosome, which divides to become two just prior to binary fission

chronic disease   A disease of slow progress and long duration

cilia (*sing.* **cilium**)   Thin, hairlike organelles of motility

cistron   The smallest functional unit of heredity; a length of chromosomal DNA associated with a single biochemical function; a gene may consist of one or more cistrons; sometimes used synonymously with the term *gene*

clade   A group of organisms descended from a common ancestor, corresponding to a single branch on the tree of life

classical pathway   Activation of complement by antigen–antibody complexes

climax community   Stable complex microbial community that develops by, and is the final product of, the process of bacterial succession

clonal selection   The process whereby an antigen induces proliferation of a single antigen-specific lymphocyte to produce large numbers of identical antigen-reactive daughter cells

coaggregation   The attachment of a cell to a preattached organism by specific molecular interactions

coagulase   A bacterial enzyme that causes plasma to clot or coagulate

coccus (*pl.* **cocci**)   A spherical bacterium

codon   A sequence of three nucleotides in a strand of messenger RNA that provides the genetic information (code) for a certain amino acid to be incorporated into a growing protein chain

coenzyme   A substance that enhances or is necessary for the action of an enzyme; several vitamins are coenzymes; a type of cofactor

collagenase   A bacterial enzyme that causes the breakdown of collagen

colonization resistance   The ability of the resident microflora to prevent colonization by exogenous species

colony-stimulating factor   Cytokines that stimulate haematopoiesis

commensalism   An interbacterial interaction beneficial to one population but with a neutral effect on the other

communicable disease   A disease capable of being transmitted

community-acquired infection   Any infection acquired outside of a hospital setting

competition   Rivalry among bacteria for growth-limiting nutrients

complement   An enzyme cascade consisting of over 25 components (including C1–C9); involved in inflammation, chemotaxis, phagocytosis and lysis of microorganisms

conjugation   As used in this book, the union of two bacterial cells, for the purpose of genetic transfer; not a reproductive process

convalescent carrier   A person who no longer shows the signs of a particular infectious disease but continues to harbour and transmit the pathogen during the convalescence period (e.g., hepatitis B)

co-stimulator molecule   Molecule that stimulates second signals for activation

COVID-19   Coronavirus disease-2019

C-reactive protein   An acute-phase protein that promotes phagocytosis of bacteria

C region   Constant region of an antibody, B cell receptor or T cell receptor polypeptide

cross-reactivity   Binding of antibody, B cell receptor or T cell receptor with antigen other than the one that induced activation

CTLA-4   Like CD28, binds to B7, but unlike the former induces T cell inactivation

cyst   A fluid-filled pathological cavity lined by epithelium

cystitis infection of the bladder

cytokine Soluble hormonelike messenger of the immune system (e.g., lymphokines, monokines)

cytoplasm The portion of a cell's protoplasm that lies outside the nucleus of the cell

cytotoxic Detrimental or destructive to cells

cytotoxin Toxic substance that inhibits or destroys cells (e.g., verocytotoxin of *Escherichia coli*)

demineralization Dissolution of enamel or cementum by acid

dendritic cell A type of 'professional' antigen-presenting cell present in secondary lymphoid tissues that expresses high levels of major histocompatibility complex I and II molecules

dental caries Localized dissolution of the enamel or root surface by acid derived from the microbial degradation of dietary carbohydrates

dental plaque Tenacious deposit on the tooth surface comprising bacteria, their extracellular products and polymers of salivary origin

deoxyribonucleic acid (DNA) A macromolecule containing the genetic code in the form of genes

dermatophyte Fungal organism causing superficial mycosis of the skin, hair or nails

diplococci Cocci arranged in pairs

disinfect To destroy pathogens in or on any substance or to inhibit their growth and vital activity

disinfectant A chemical agent used to destroy pathogens or inhibit their growth; usually refers to a chemical agent used on inanimate material

disinfection A process that kills or removes pathogenic organisms in a material or an object, excluding bacterial spores, so that they pose no threat of infection

diversity (D) gene Selectable V-region genes of B cell receptor H chains, T cell receptor β chains and T cell receptor δ chains, which contribute to the diversity of B and T cell repertoires

DNA *See* deoxyribonucleic acid

dysgeusia A condition in which a foul, salty, rancid or metallic taste sensation persists in the mouth

ecology The branch of biology concerned with interrelationships among living organisms; encompassing the relationships of organisms to each other, to the environment and to the entire energy balance within a given ecosystem

ecosystem An ecological system that includes all the organisms and the environment within which they occur naturally

empirical therapy Therapy (usually antibiotics) prescribed without the benefit of laboratory tests

encephalitis Inflammation or infection of the brain

encephalomyelitis Inflammation or infection of the brain and spinal cord

endemic disease A disease that is always present in a particular community or region

endogenous processing The processing of intracellular proteins, including those of intracellular pathogens, onto major histocompatibility complex I molecules for recognition by cytotoxic T cells

endoplasmic reticulum The network of cytoplasmic tubules and flattened sacs in a eukaryotic cell

endospore A resistant body formed within a bacterial cell

endotoxin The lipid portion of the lipopolysaccharide found in the cell walls of Gram-negative bacteria; intracellular toxin

enriched medium Culture medium that enables isolation of fastidious organisms from samples or specimens and growth in the laboratory

enterotoxin A bacterial toxin specific for cells of the intestinal mucosa

eosinophil Type of polymorphonuclear leukocyte with granules that stain with acidic dyes, such as eosin

epidemic disease A disease occurring in a higher-than-usual number of cases in a population during a given time interval

epidemiology The study of relationships among the various factors that determine the frequency and distribution of diseases

episome An extrachromosomal element (plasmid) that may either integrate into the host bacterium's chromosome or replicate and function stably when physically separated from the chromosome

epitope The portion of an antigen that binds to the V region of an antibody, B cell receptor or T cell receptor

erythrogenic toxin A bacterial toxin that produces redness, usually in the form of a rash

eukaryotic cell A cell containing a true nucleus; organisms having such cells are referred to as *eukaryotes*

exogenous processing Processing of endocytosed extracellular proteins onto major histocompatibility complex II molecules for recognition by T-helper cells

exotoxin A toxin that is released from the cell; an extracellular toxin (opposite of endotoxin)

exudate Any fluid (e.g., pus) that exudes (oozes) from tissue, often as a result of injury, infection or inflammation

fastidious bacterium A bacterium that is difficult to isolate or grow in the laboratory owing to its complex nutritional requirements

Fc receptors Cell surface molecules on phagocytes and natural killer cells that bind to antibody-coated target cells

fermentation An anaerobic biochemical pathway in which substances are broken down and energy and reduced compounds are produced; oxygen does not participate in the process

fimbria (*pl.* fimbriae) Fine, short, hairlike filaments that extend from the bacterial cell surface; synonymous with pili; *see* pili

flagellum (*pl.* flagella) A whiplike organelle of motility

fomite An inanimate object or substance capable of absorbing and transmitting a pathogen (e.g., bed linen, towels)

fungicidal agent A chemical agent or drug that kills fungi; a fungicide

fungus (*pl.* fungi) Eukaryotic, nonphotosynthetic microorganism that is saprophytic or parasitic

GALT *See* gut-associated lymphoid tissue

γδ T cells T cells using γ and δ instead of α and β T cell receptor genes; probably important in defence against bacteria

gene A functional unit of heredity that occupies a specific space (locus) on a chromosome; capable of directing the formation of an enzyme or other protein

generalized infection An infection that has spread throughout the body; also known as a systemic infection

generation time   The time required for a cell to split into two cells; also called *doubling time*

genetic vaccines   Pathogen-specific RNA or DNA segments capable of inducing pathogen protein expression and both humoural and cell-mediated immunity

genomics   The study of genes and their functions

genotype   The complete genetic constitution of an individual; all of that individual's genes

genus (*pl.* genera)   The first name in binomial nomenclature; contains closely related species

germinal centre   The site of B cell activation and differentiation in secondary lymphoid tissue

gingival crevice   Protected habitat formed where the teeth rise out of the gum

gingival crevicular fluid   Serum-like exudate bathing and flushing the gingival crevice. It has a considerable influence on the ecology of this region by introducing (1) nutrients for the microbial community and (2) components of the immune system and other host defences

gingivitis   Inflammation or infection of the gingiva (gums)

glycocalyx   Extracellular material that may or may not be firmly attached to the outer surface of the cell wall (e.g., capsule, slime layers)

gnotobiotic animal   Germ-free animal deliberately infected with a known bacterial population or microflora

gp120   A component of the envelope of human immunodeficiency virus, responsible for binding to CD4

gp41   A component of the envelope of human immunodeficiency virus, responsible for fusion with target cell membranes

Gram stain   A differential staining procedure named for its developer, Hans Christian Gram, a Danish bacteriologist; differentiates bacteria into those that stain purple (Gram-positive) and those that stain pink/red (Gram-negative)

granulocyte   A granular leukocyte; neutrophils, eosinophils and basophils are examples

granuloma   Collection of macrophages, epithelioid cells, giant cells and fibroblasts formed in response to chronic immune stimulation—for example, following persistent infection of macrophages

granzymes   Granular proteases found in cytotoxic T cells and natural killer cells

growth curve   A graphic representation of the change in size of a bacterial population over a period of time; includes a lag phase, a log phase, a stationary phase and a death phase

gut-associated lymphoid tissue (GALT)   Accumulations of secondary lymphoid tissue associated with the gastrointestinal tract

haematopoietic stem cell   Multipotent progenitor of all types of blood cells

haemolysin   A bacterial enzyme capable of lysing erythrocytes and releasing their haemoglobin

haemolysis   Destruction of red blood cells (erythrocytes) in such a manner that haemoglobin is liberated into the surrounding environment

hapten   A small, nonantigenic molecule that becomes antigenic when combined with a large molecule

HBV   Hepatitis B virus; the aetiological agent of serum hepatitis

HCV   Hepatitis C virus; the aetiological agent of hepatitis C

HDV   Hepatitis D virus; the aetiological agent of hepatitis D or delta hepatitis

hepatitis   Inflammation of the liver

heterotroph   An organism that uses organic chemicals as a source of carbon; sometimes called an *organotroph*

HGV   Hepatitis G virus; the aetiological agent of hepatitis G

HIV   Human immunodeficiency virus; the aetiological agent of acquired immunodeficiency syndrome

HLA   *See* human leukocyte antigen

hopanoids   Sterol-like molecules present in bacterial plasma membranes

host   The organism on or in which a parasite lives

human immunodeficiency virus (HIV)   The virus that causes acquired immunodeficiency syndrome

human leukocyte antigen (HLA)   Product of the major histocompatibility complex in humans

hyaluronic acid   A gelatinous mucopolysaccharide that acts as an intracellular cement in body tissue

hyaluronidase   A bacterial enzyme that breaks down hyaluronic acid; sometimes called diffusing or spreading factor, because it enables bacteria to invade deeper into the tissue

hybridoma   Hybrid cell produced by fusing an antibody-producing cell with a myeloma cell; hybridomas are immortal and produce monoclonal antibody

hyperimmune globulin   Preparation containing specific antibodies used to prevent disease after exposure to a pathogen

hyperplasia   Increase in the size of an organ by increase in the number of cells

hypersensitivity   A condition in which there is an exaggerated or inappropriate immune reaction that causes tissue destruction or inflammation

hypha (*pl.* hyphae)   Long, branching, threadlike tubes containing the fungal cytoplasm and its organelles; intertwining structural units of moulds

hypogeusia   Partial loss of taste

hyposmia   Decreased sense of smell

hypogammaglobulinaemia   Decreased quantity of the gamma fraction of serum globulin, including a decreased quantity of immunoglobulins

ICAM   *See* intercellular adhesion molecule

idiotype   Antibody, B cell receptor and T cell receptor V regions

IFN   *See* interferon

IgA   Immunoglobulin class with the major function of protecting mucosal surfaces against pathogens

Igα, Igβ   Proteins associated with the B cell receptor that help transmit B cell activation signals

IgD   Immunoglobulin class found on mature B cell surfaces

IgE   Immunoglobulin class that protects against helminths and is responsible for symptoms of allergy

IgG   Major antibody class of the secondary immune response

IgM   Major antibody class of the primary immune response

IL   *See* interleukin

immune complex   Complex of antigen with antibody

immune deviation   Suppression of an ongoing immune response by a switch from type 1 to type 2 or type 2 to type 1 cytokine production

immunocompetent Able to produce a normal immune response

immunocompromised The state of being susceptible to infection by virtue of impairment or malfunction of the immune system

immunodeficiency A state in which the immune system is deficient in a particular type of immune response

immunodiagnostic procedures Diagnostic test procedures that utilize the principles of immunology; used to detect either antigen or antibody in clinical specimens

immunoglobulin Proteins, consisting of two light polypeptide chains and two heavy chains that function as antibodies

immunological synapse The signalling complex formed between an antigen-presenting cell and a T cell

immunostimulating complex (ISCOM) Preparation of antigen combined with saponin, cholesterol and phosphatidylcholine that induces strong T and B cell immune responses

immunosuppression A condition in which individuals are unable to mount a normal immune response owing to suppression or depression of their immune system

inactivated vaccine Killed whole organisms, products of organisms or subunits of organisms that induce protective immune responses

inclusion body Distinctive structure frequently formed in the nucleus and/or cytoplasm of cells infected with certain viruses

indigenous microflora Microorganisms that live on and in the healthy body; also called *indigenous microbiota, normal flora*

infective endocarditis Infection of the lining of the heart (endocardium)

inflammation A pathological process comprising a dynamic complex of cytological and histological reactions induced by injury or abnormal stimulation by physical, chemical or biological agents

innate immunity The natural protective mechanisms present before contact with antigen

intercellular adhesion molecule (ICAM) Molecule that interacts at cell surfaces to promote cell–cell contact

interferon (IFN) A class of small, antiviral glycoproteins, produced by cells infected with an animal virus; cell specific and species specific—but not virus specific; interferons are mediators that increase resistance to viral infection: IFN-α is produced by leukocytes, IFN-β by fibroblasts and IFN-γ by activated T cells and natural killer cells; IFN-γ has numerous effects in modulating immune responses

interleukin (IL) A mediator involved in signalling between cells of the immune system

intravenous immunoglobulin Pooled antibodies from normal donors used to provide passive protection against infection in patients with antibody deficiencies

invariant chain A molecule that stabilizes 'empty' major histocompatibility complex II molecules, which can be replaced by antigenic peptides

in vitro In an artificial environment, such as a laboratory setting

in vivo In a living organism; used in reference to what occurs within a living organism

ISCOM *See* immunostimulating complex

isotype Immunoglobulin class, dependent on the type of heavy-chain C gene used

isotype switching The change from expression of a 5′ immunoglobulin C_H gene by a B cell to expression of a downstream C_H gene

joining (J) gene Selectable V-region genes of B cell receptors and T cell receptors that contribute to the diversity of B and T cell repertoires

κ (kappa) light chain One of two types of immunoglobulin light chain

keystone pathogens Organisms that cause a disproportionately large effect on their natural environment relative to their abundance (e.g., *P. gingivalis* in periodontal disease)

lag phase That part of a bacterial growth curve during which multiplication of the organisms is very slow or scarcely appreciable; the first phase in a bacterial growth curve

λ (lambda) light chain One of two types of immunoglobulin light chain

latency Incorporation of viral genes into those of the host cell without overt production of virions

latent infection An asymptomatic infection capable of manifesting symptoms under particular circumstances or if activated

lecithin A name given to several types of phospholipids that are essential constituents of animal and plant cells

lecithinase A bacterial enzyme capable of breaking down lecithin

leukocidin A bacterial enzyme capable of destroying leukocytes

leukocyte function-associated antigen (LFA) Molecule that interacts at cell surfaces to promote cell–cell contact

lipopolysaccharide A macromolecule of combined lipid and polysaccharide, found in the cell walls of Gram-negative bacteria

log phase Logarithmic phase; a bacterial growth phase during which maximal multiplication is occurring by geometrical progression; plotting the logarithm (log) of the number of organisms against time produces a straight upward-pointing line; the second phase in a bacterial growth curve; also known as the exponential growth phase

lophotrichous bacteria Bacteria possessing two or more flagella at one or both ends (poles) of the cell

lymphadenitis Inflammation of a lymph node or lymph nodes

lymphadenopathy A disease process affecting a lymph node or lymph nodes

lymph node Secondary lymphoid tissue that drains fluids from the tissues and concentrates foreign antigens onto antigen-presenting cells

lymphocyte Cell that expresses immunological specificity and is responsible for adaptive immune responses

lymphocytosis An increased number of lymphocytes in the blood

lymphokines Soluble protein mediators released by sensitized lymphocytes; examples include chemotactic factors and interleukins; lymphokines represent one category of cytokines

lymphotoxin Proinflammatory cytokine, also known as tumour necrosis factor-β

lyophilization Freeze-drying; a method of preserving microorganisms and foods

lysogenic conversion Alteration of the genetic constitution of a bacterial cell due to the integration of viral genetic material into the host cell genome

lysosome Membrane-bound vesicle found in the cytoplasm of eukaryotic cells, containing a variety of digestive enzymes, including lysozyme

lysozyme A digestive enzyme found in lysosomes, tears and other body fluids; especially destructive to bacterial cell walls

lytic cycle Process occurring when a virus takes over the metabolic machinery of the host cell, reproduces itself and ruptures (lyses) the host cell to allow the newly assembled virions to escape

MAC *See* membrane attack complex

macrophage A large phagocytic cell that arises from a monocyte

major histocompatibility complex (MHC) A complex genetic system coding for cell surface molecules that bind peptides for presentation to T cells

malaise A generalized feeling of discomfort or unease

MALT *See* mucosa-associated lymphoid tissue

mast cell Cells that bind immunoglobulin E and release mediators of inflammation and allergy

membrane attack complex (MAC) The final stage of complement activation that can result in target cell lysis

memory The survival of certain T and B cells after initial encounter with antigen, which are able to produce an accelerated and enhanced immune response on subsequently encountering the same antigen

meningitis Inflammation or infection of the meninges

MERS **M**iddle **E**ast **R**espiratory **S**yndrome

mesophile A microorganism having an optimum growth temperature between 25°C and 40°C; such an organism is said to be mesophilic

mesosome A prokaryotic cell organelle (an infolding of the cytoplasmic membrane) possibly involved in cellular respiration

messenger RNA (mRNA) The type of RNA that contains the exact same genetic information as a single gene on a DNA molecule

metabolomics The global analysis of metabolites, small molecules generated in the process of metabolism

metagenome/metatranscriptome The total genomic DNA or RNA transcripts of all organisms within a specific microbial community

MHC *See* major histocompatibility complex

MHC I The class of major histocompatibility complex antigens (-A, -B and -C) that present peptides to CD8$^+$ T cells

MHC II The class of major histocompatibility complex antigens (-DP, -DQ and -DR) that present peptides to CD4$^+$ T cells

microbial antagonism The killing, injury or inhibition of one microbe by the substances produced by another

microbial homoeostasis The natural stability of the resident microflora of a site

microbicidal agent A chemical or drug that kills microorganisms; a microbicide

microbiome The total microbial community, including biomolecules, within a defined ecosystem, such as the human body or individual body site or habitat

micrometre A unit of length, equal to one-millionth of a metre (µm)

minimum infective dose The minimum number of microorganisms required to cause an infection

mitosis A process of cell reproduction consisting of a sequence of modifications of the nucleus that result in the formation of two daughter cells with exactly the same chromosome and DNA content as that of the original cell

monoclonal antibodies Antibodies produced by hybridomas; such antibodies are of exceptional purity and specificity

monocyte A relatively large mononuclear leukocyte; monocytes present in the blood differentiate into tissue-resident macrophages

monokine Soluble protein mediator released by activated monocytes and macrophages; monokines represent one category of cytokines

monotrichous Possessing only one flagellum

motile Possessing the ability to move

mRNA *See* messenger RNA

mucocutaneous Affects both skin and mucous membranes

mucosa-associated lymphoid tissue (MALT) Nonencapsulated dispersed aggregates of lymphoid cells positioned to protect the main passages by which microorganisms gain entry to the body (alimentary, respiratory and urogenital tracts)

muramyl dipeptide A constituent of mycobacteria that is a potentially useful adjuvant for human vaccines

mutant A phenotype in which a mutation is manifested

mutation An inheritable change in the character of a gene; a change in the sequence of base pairs in a DNA molecule

mutualism A symbiotic relationship in which both parties derive benefit

mycelium (*pl.* mycelia) A fungal colony; composed of a mass of intertwined hyphae

mycobiome Constituent fungal component of the microbiome

mycology The branch of science concerned with the study of fungi

mycosis (*pl.* mycoses) A fungal disease

myelitis Inflammation or infection of the spinal cord

myocarditis Inflammation of the myocardium (the muscular walls of the heart)

nanometre A unit of length, equal to one-billionth of a metre (nm)

natural killer (NK) cell A type of cytotoxic human blood lymphocyte that kills cells (e.g., virus-infected cells, tumour cells) expressing low levels of major histocompatibility complex molecules

necrosis Death of tissues or cells

negative selection Depletion of thymocytes bearing T cell receptors that bind strongly to major histocompatibility complex + self peptides

neoplasia Literally 'new growth' of cells, but usually applied to benign or malignant cancers

nephritis Inflammation of the kidneys

neurotoxin A bacterial toxin that attacks the nervous system

neutrophil A type of granulocyte found in blood; its granules contain neutral substances that attract neither acidic nor basic dyes; also called a *polymorphonuclear cell* (*PMN*)

niche   The function or role of an organism in a habitat; species with identical niches will, therefore, be in competition

nitric oxide   A major cytotoxic product of phagocytic cells, responsible for killing microorganisms

NK   *See* natural killer; a type of lymphocyte

nosocomial infection   Infection acquired while hospitalized

N-region addition   The insertion of small numbers of nontemplated nucleotides at junctions between B cell receptor and T cell receptor V(D)J segments

nuclear membrane   The membrane that surrounds the chromosomes and nucleoplasm of a eukaryotic cell

nucleic acid   Macromolecule consisting of linear chains of nucleotides (e.g., DNA, mRNA, tRNA, rRNA)

nucleolus   A dense portion of the nucleus, where ribosomal RNA (rRNA) is produced

nucleoplasm   That portion of a cell protoplasm that lies within the nucleus

nucleotide   The basic unit or building block of nucleic acids; each nucleotide consists of a purine or pyrimidine combined with a pentose (ribose or deoxyribose) and a phosphate group

nucleus (*pl.* nuclei)   That portion of a eukaryotic cell that contains the nucleoplasm, chromosomes and nucleoli

obligate aerobe   An organism that requires 20% oxygen (the amount found in atmospheric air) to survive

obligate anaerobe   An organism that cannot survive in oxygen

occlusal   Surface on the top of the tooth

oedema   Swelling due to an accumulation of watery fluid in cells, tissues or body cavities

oligonucleotide   A compound made up of a small number of nucleotides, used to probe for complementary sequences within a gene

oncogene   Gene expressed in malignant cells, the product of which may cause abnormal growth regulation

oncogenic   Capable of causing cancer

oophoritis   Inflammation or infection on an ovary

operational taxonomic unit (OTU)   A cluster of organisms similar at a defined sequence identity threshold within some region such as the whole 16S gene, used in the absence of a named species, genus, etc.

opportunist   A microbe with the potential to cause disease when an opportunity arises (e.g., in human immunodeficiency virus infection when resistance is low) but which does not do so under ordinary circumstances; also called an *opportunistic pathogen*

opportunistic infection   Infection that only occurs in immunosuppressed or immunodeficient patients

opsonin   A substance (such as an antibody or complement component) that enhances phagocytosis

opsonization   Coating of particles with antibody or complement products to permit binding to Fc or C-receptors on phagocytes

oral microbiome   The totality of the oral microbes, their genetic information, and the oral environment in which they interact

oral mycobiome   (Greek: *mykes,* fungus) The totality of the oral fungi, their genetic information, and the oral environment in which they interact

oral microbiota   All living microbes residing within the oral microbiome

oral virome (*syn.* oral virobiome)   The totality of the oral viruses, their genetic information, and the oral environment in which they interact

osteomyelitis   Inflammation of bone caused usually by infection

passive immunization   Transfer of preformed antibodies to a nonimmune individual—for example, placental transfer of immunoglobulin G antibodies to the foetus

PCR   *See* polymerase chain reaction

perform   Molecule released by cytotoxic T cells and natural killer cells that polymerizes on target cell membranes, forming transmembrane channels

pericoronitis   Infection around the crown of an erupting tooth

peri-implantitis   A destructive inflammatory process affecting both the soft and hard tissues surrounding dental implants (comparable to periodontitis)

peri-implant mucositis   An inflammatory lesion of the soft tissues surrounding an endosseous implant in the absence of loss of supporting bone or continuing marginal bone loss (comparable to gingivitis)

periodontopathogen   An organism implicated in the aetiology of periodontal disease

peripheral tolerance   Induction of specific nonresponsiveness in anti-self T cells that have survived negative selection in the thymus

Peyer's patches   Aggregations of lymphoid tissue in the lower ileum

phageome   A community of bacteriophages and their metagenomes localized in a particular environment

phagocyte   A cell that can engulf particles and digest them in cytoplasmic vacuoles

phenotype   The properties shown by a body or cell that are due to expression of its genotype

pili (*syn.* fimbriae)   a specialized pilus called the sex pilus can form a link between recipient and donor cells during bacterial conjugation (mainly in Gram-negative bacteria)

pleiotropy   Having several different activities; used especially in describing cytokines

polyclonal activation   Induction of a state of activation in a high proportion of lymphocytes (as opposed to the very low proportion activated by a given antigen)

polymerase chain reaction (PCR)   A method of producing multiple copies of DNA using polymerase enzymes; this amplification process can be used to detect a microbe present in low cell numbers

polymorphonuclear leukocyte   A phagocytic cell whose nucleus is composed of two or more lobes

positive selection   The process of allowing those thymocytes whose T cell receptors bind with low affinity to major histocompatibility complex molecules + self peptides to survive

postbiotics   A mixture of dead microorganisms and/or their components that confers a health benefit on the host

pre-B cells   Cells that are committed to the B cell lineage but have not yet expressed mature B cell receptors

prebiotics   A substrate that is selectively utilized by host microorganisms conferring a health benefit on the host

probiotics   Live microorganisms that confer health benefits when consumed or applied to the body

primary lymphoid organs   The sites of lymphocyte development: bone marrow and thymus

primary response   The immune response that occurs on first exposure to a given antigen

prion   Proteinaceous infectious particle that is the agent of slowly progressive chronic diseases such as variant Creutzfeldt–Jakob disease (vCJD); smallest known infectious agent

prodromal phase   The period between infection and the appearance of the symptoms

programmed cell death   Self-destruction of cells that do not receive special signals for survival

prophylaxis   Prevention of a disease or a process that can lead to a disease

proteomics   The large-scale study of proteins, particularly their structures and functions

proteosome   Organelle responsible for processing of cytoplasmic proteins into peptides for antigen presentation

protoplasm   The semifluid matter within living cells; cytoplasm and nucleoplasm are examples

protozoa (*sing.* protozoan)   Unicellular eukaryotes found in water and soil; some are pathogens (e.g., *Entamoeba oralis*, found in the mouth)

purine   A molecule found in certain nucleotides and, therefore, in nucleic acids; adenine and guanine are purines found in both DNA and RNA

pus   A fluid product of inflammation, containing leukocytes, tissue debris, and dead and dying bacteria

pyelonephritis   infection of the pelvis and parenchyma of the kidney, most often the result of bacterial infection

pyogenic   Pus producing; causing the production of pus

pyrimidine   A molecule found in certain nucleotides and, therefore, in nucleic acids; thymine and cytosine are pyrimidines found in DNA; cytosine and uracil are pyrimidines found in RNA

pyrogen   An agent that causes a rise in body temperature; such an agent is said to be pyrogenic

pyuria   presence of pus cells (polymorphs) in urine

reactive oxygen intermediaries   Cytotoxic products of phagocytes responsible for killing microorganisms

recombinant DNA technology   The artificial manipulation of segments of DNA from one organism into the DNA of another organism, to allow cloning of the gene and synthesis of the specific gene product

recombinant vaccine   A vaccine produced by recombinant DNA technology

red complex bacteria   Three bacterial species that appear later during biofilm development and are considered keystone periodontal pathogens (i.e., *Porphyromonas gingivalis*, *Treponema denticola* and *Tannerella forsythia*)

redundancy   Having the same activity as several other molecules. Used especially in describing cytokines

reservoir of infection   Living or nonliving material in or on which a pathogen multiplies and/or develops

resident microflora   Members of the indigenous microflora that are more or less permanent

restriction enzyme   Enzyme that breaks DNA at a specific nucleotide sequence

retrovirus   A virus that transcribes its RNA into DNA and back again; this is accomplished by the presence of the enzyme reverse transcriptase

reverse transcriptase   An enzyme that converts RNA into DNA

ribonucleic acid (RNA)   A macromolecule of which there are three main types: messenger RNA (mRNA), ribosomal RNA (rRNA) and transfer RNA (tRNA); found in all cells, but only in certain viruses (RNA viruses)

ribosomal RNA (rRNA)   The type of RNA molecule found in ribosomes

ribosome   Organelle that is the site of protein synthesis in both prokaryotic and eukaryotic cells

RNA polymerase   The enzyme necessary for transcription; *see* transcription)

rRNA   Ribosomal RNA

salivary leukocyte protease inhibitor (SLPI)   A proline-rich protein found in the saliva that inhibits viruses such as human immunodeficiency virus

saprophyte   An organism that lives on dead or decaying organic matter; such an organism is said to be saprophytic

SARS-CoV-2   **s**evere **a**cute **r**espiratory **s**yndrome 2

secondary disease   A disease that follows the initial disease

secondary lymphoid organs   Lymph nodes, spleen and mucosa-associated lymphoid tissue, the sites where lymphocytes encounter and respond to antigen

secondary response   The immune response that occurs when memory T or B cells encounter antigen for a second or subsequent time

selective medium   Culture medium that allows a certain organism or group of organisms to grow while inhibiting growth of all other organisms

septicaemia   A disease consisting of chills, fever, prostration; the presence of large quantities of bacteria and/or their toxins in the blood

sequestered antigen   Self antigen that is normally hidden from the immune system and does not induce neonatal tolerance. Following tissue damage, these antigens may be released and stimulate an autoimmune response

sequestrum   A necrotic piece of bone

serological procedure   Immunodiagnostic test procedure performed using serum

serology   Branch of science concerned with serum and serological procedures

sex pilus   A specialized pilus through which one bacterial cell (the donor cell) transfers genetic material to another bacterial cell (the recipient cell) during conjugation

sialadenitis   Infection of the salivary glands

sialagogue   Substance that encourages saliva production

sialolith   Stone in the salivary gland

signal 1   An activation signal delivered through the B cell receptor or T cell receptor, which alone is not sufficient for B cell or T cell activation

signal 2   A second activation signal required for lymphoid cell activation; for T cells, this is mediated by binding of CD28 to B7 on an antigen-presenting cell, for B cells CD40 must bind to CD40L on T-helper cells

sinus   A tissue tract or space lined with epithelium from which pus or fluids drain

Sjögren's syndrome   A syndrome with dry mouth (xerostomia), dry eyes and rheumatoid arthritis

slime layer   A nonorganized, nonattached layer of glycocalyx surrounding a bacterial cell

SLPI   *See* salivary leukocyte protease inhibitor

species   A specific member of a given genus (e.g., *Porphyromonas gingivalis* is a species of the genus *Porphyromonas*); the name of a particular species consists of two parts: the generic name (the first name) and the specific epithet (the second name); a singular species is abbreviated 'sp.', and plural species is abbreviated 'spp.'

specific epithet   The second part (second name) in the name of a species

spirochaete   Spiral-shaped bacterium (e.g., *Treponema denticola*)

spleen   Secondary lymphoid organ important in the induction of immune responses to antigens present in the blood

sporadic disease   A disease that occurs occasionally, usually affecting one person; neither endemic nor epidemic

sporicidal agent   A chemical agent that kills spores; a sporicide

sporulation   Production of one or more spores

stationary phase   Bacterial growth phase during which organisms are dying at the same rate at which new organisms are being produced; the third phase in a bacterial growth curve

sterile   Free of all living microorganisms, including spores

sterilization   The destruction of all microorganisms, including spores

streptokinase   A kinase produced by streptococci

subgingival   Below the gingival (gum) margin—for example, pertaining to a sample taken from the gingival crevice or periodontal pocket

substrate   The substance that is acted upon or changed by an enzyme

subunit vaccine   Vaccine that employs only immunogenic subunits of a pathogen, rather than the whole organism

superantigen   Molecule that stimulates a subset of T cells by binding to T cell receptor Vβ and major histocompatibility complex II

superinfection   An overgrowth of one or more particular organisms—often organisms that are resistant to an antimicrobial agent that the patient is receiving

surrogate light chains   Polypeptides that, together with the constant region of immunoglobulin M, produce a primitive receptor on the surface of pre-B cells

symbiosis   The living together or close association of two dissimilar organisms

syncytium   Multinucleate giant cell formed by fusion of several cells

synbiotics   Combination prebiotic and probiotic mixtures comprising live microorganisms and substrate(s) selectively utilized by host microorganisms that confer a health benefit on the host

synergism   As used in this book, the correlated action of two or more microorganisms so that the combined action is greater than that of each acting separately (e.g., when two microbes accomplish more than either could do alone)

synthetic peptide vaccine   Vaccine that employs only peptide epitopes of a pathogen

systemic infection   *See* generalized infection

taxon   The microbes belonging to a taxonomic category, typically of low level, such as genus or species

taxonomy   The systematic classification of living things

T cell   *See* T lymphocyte

T cell receptor (TCR)   Heterodimers (αβ or γδ) on the surface of T cells that recognize and bind antigenic peptides presented by major histocompatibility complex molecules on antigen-presenting cells

T-cytotoxic cells   A subset of T cells that recognize antigenic peptides presented by major histocompatibility complex I molecules and can kill the peptide-bearing cell

teichoic acid   Polymer found in the cell walls of Gram-positive bacteria

terminal deoxynucleotidyl transferase   An enzyme that causes the addition of nucleotides to the junctions between B cell receptor and T cell receptor V(D)J segments

tetanolysin   Neurotoxin produced by tetanus bacillus

tetanospasmin   Neurotoxin produced by *Clostridium tetani*; causes tetanus

TGF   *See* transforming growth factor

T$_H$0   A newly activated T-helper cell that secretes a wide range of lymphokines

T$_H$1   A T-helper cell that produces interleukin-2, interferon γ and lymphotoxin and induces macrophage activation

T$_H$2   A T-helper cell that produces interleukin-4 (IL-4), IL-5 and IL-10 and induces B cell activation

T-helper cell   T cell subset required for activating the effector functions of macrophages, B cells, natural killer cells and other T cells

thermophile   An organism that thrives at a temperature of 50°C or higher; such an organism is said to be thermophilic

thrombus   A blood clot within a vessel

thymic selection   Deletion of potentially self-reactive thymocytes and retention of thymocytes able to recognize foreign peptides presented by major histocompatibility complex molecules

thymocyte   Precursor of mature T cells

thymus   Organ in the mediastinal cavity anterior to and above the heart; primary lymphoid organ for T-lymphocyte development

T lymphocyte   Subset of lymphocytes that recognizes antigenic peptides in the context of major histocompatibility complex I or II molecules; *see* T-cytotoxic cell, T-helper cell, T-suppressor cell

TNF   *See* tumour necrosis factor

tolerance   Specific nonreactivity to an antigen

tonsils   Secondary lymphoid tissue in the pharynx

toxaemia   The presence of toxins in the blood, especially during septicaemia

toxigenicity   The capacity to produce toxin—a measure of virulence; a microorganism capable of producing a toxin is said to be toxigenic

toxin   As used in this book, a poisonous substance produced by a microorganism

toxoid   A toxin that has been modified artificially to destroy its toxicity but retain its antigenicity; toxoids are used as vaccines (e.g., tetanus toxoid)

transcription   Transfer of the genetic code from one type of nucleic acid to another; usually, the synthesis of an mRNA molecule from a DNA template

transcriptomics   The study of the transcriptome, the complete set of RNA transcripts produced by the genome at any one time

transduction   Transfer of genetic material (and its phenotypic expression) from one bacterial cell to another via bacteriophages

transfection   Introduction of a segment of DNA into the genes of another organism

transfer RNA (tRNA)   The type of RNA molecule that is capable of combining with (and thus activating) a specific amino acid; involved in protein synthesis (translation); the anticodon on a tRNA molecule recognizes the codon on an mRNA molecule

transformation   In microbial genetics, transfer of genetic information between bacteria via uptake of naked DNA; bacteria capable of taking up naked DNA are said to be 'competent'

transforming growth factor beta (TGF-β)   Cytokine with generally suppressive activity against cytokine-secreting cells

transient microflora   Temporary members of the indigenous microflora that are 'in transit' (e.g., *Escherichia coli* in the oral cavity)

translation   The process by which mRNA, tRNA and ribosomes affect the production of proteins from amino acids; protein synthesis

transporter associated with antigen processing (TAP)   Molecule responsible for transporting peptides from proteosome to endoplasmic reticulum for association with major histocompatibility complex I

T-regulator cell   T cell subset that suppresses immune reactions by producing mainly transforming growth factor-β and/or interleukin-10

T-suppressor cell   T cell subset that negatively regulates immune responses, usually by interfering with T-helper cell function

tuberculocidal agent   A chemical or drug that kills *Mycobacterium tuberculosis*, the agent of tuberculosis

tumour necrosis factor (TNF)   Cytokine that can damage tumour cells; TNF-α and TNF-β (also known as lymphotoxin) are important mediators of inflammation and have other immune regulatory functions

universal precautions   Safety precautions taken by health care workers to protect themselves from cross-infection, whereby all patients are treated as if they are carrying an infection

urethritis   Inflammation or infection of the urethra

urticaria   A vascular reaction of the skin often caused by an allergic reaction

vaccination   Stimulation of a specific immune response against a pathogen in order to provide protection against natural exposure to that pathogen

vacuole   Membrane-bound storage space in the cell

vector   An invertebrate animal (e.g., mite, mosquito) capable of transmitting pathogens among vertebrates

vegetation   Blood clot on the heart lining or endocardium

V genes   Genes encoding the variable region of antibodies, B cell receptors and T cell receptors

virion   A complete, infectious viral particle

virome (virobiome)   Constituent viral component of the microbiome

virucidal agent   A chemical or drug that kills viruses; a virucide

virulence   A measure of pathogenicity; invasiveness and toxigenicity contribute to virulence

virus   Acellular microorganism that is smaller than a bacterium; an intracellular parasite

V region   The part of an antibody, B cell receptor or T cell receptor responsible for binding to a specific epitope

xerostomia   Dryness of the mouth, usually due to impairment of the salivary gland function

zoonosis (*pl.* zoonoses)   An infectious disease or infestation transmissible from animals to humans

Index

Note: Page numbers followed by '*f*' indicate figures and '*t*' indicate tables.